SKILLS FOR MIDWIFERY PRACTICE

AUSTRALIA AND NEW ZEALAND

SKILLS FOR MIDWIFERY PRACTICE

AUSTRALIA AND NEW ZEALAND

2nd edition

Ruth Johnson, BA(Hons) RGN RM
Clinical Midwife,
Formerly Senior Lecturer Midwifery,
University of Hertfordshire, UK
Supervisor of Midwives

Wendy Taylor, BSc (Hons) MSc RN RM
Clinical Midwifery Educator,
Whangarei, New Zealand
Formerly Senior Lecturer Midwifery,
University of Hertfordshire, UK

Australian and New Zealand authors:

Sally de-Vitry Smith PhD RN RM
Assistant Professor (Clinical) Midwifery
School of Nursing Midwifery and Public Health
Faculty of Health
University of Canberra
Canberra, ACT

Sara Bayes PhD RN RM
Professor in Midwifery and Head of Midwifery
School of Nursing, Midwifery and Paramedicine
Faculty of Health Sciences
Australian Catholic University
Melbourne, VIC

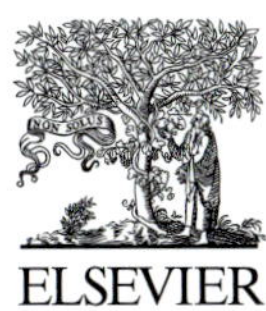

ELSEVIER

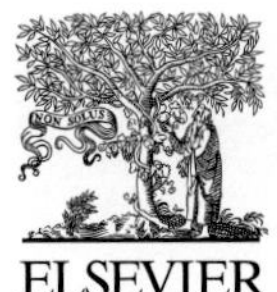

Elsevier Australia, ACN 001 002 357
(a division of Reed International Books Australia Pty Ltd)
Tower 1, 475 Victoria Avenue, Chatswood, NSW 2067

Skills for Midwifery Practice

ISBN: 978-0-7020-6187-5

This adaptation of *Skills for Midwifery Practice*, 4e by Ruth Johnson and Wendy Taylor, was undertaken by Elsevier Australia and is published by arrangement with Elsevier Ltd.

Skills for Midwifery Practice, Australian and New Zealand 2nd edition

ISBN: 978-0-7295-4379-8

Notice

The adaptation has been undertaken by Elsevier Australia at its sole responsibility. Practitioners and researchers must always rely on their own experience and knowledge in evaluating and using any information, methods, compounds or experiments described herein. Because of rapid advances in the medical sciences, in particular, independent verification of diagnoses and drug dosages should be made. To the fullest extent of the law, no responsibility is assumed by Elsevier, authors, editors or contributors in relation to the adaptation or for any injury and/or damage to persons or property as a matter of products liability, negligence or otherwise, or from any use or operation of any methods, products, instructions, or ideas contained in the material herein.

National Library of Australia Cataloguing-in-Publication Data

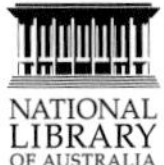

A catalogue record for this book is available from the National Library of Australia

Senior Content Strategist: Libby Houston
Content Project Manager: Shruti Raj
Edited by Leanne Peters
Proofread by Melissa Faulkner
Cover by Georgette Hall
Index by SPi Global
Typeset by GW Tech India
Printed in China by 1010 Printing International Ltd

CONTENTS

PREFACE

Welcome to the second Australia and New Zealand edition of *Skills for Midwifery Practice*. We hope this text proves a useful resource for your practice. Each chapter is underpinned by evidence related to midwifery care and updated to reflect best practice at the time of writing.

We have attempted to capture a comprehensive range of woman-centred midwifery skills, but recognise further advances in midwifery practice will continue as midwives strive to improve outcomes for women and babies. We understand knowledge is rapidly superseded as new research emerges.

As midwives we are inspired by and privileged to accompany women, babies and families on their journey through the birth process. We also recognise the demands of our work and the importance of midwives caring for their health and emotional wellbeing in a safe work environment.

Theory and evidence sections precede each skill. Australian and New Zealand guidelines, policies, standards, statistics, terminology, models of care and cultural considerations are reflected. Each chapter addresses woman, baby and midwife as relevant. We also recognise individuals have gender diverse identities. Terms such as *pregnant person, childbearing people* and *parent* can be used to avoid gendering birth and those who give birth as feminine. However, because women continue to be marginalised and oppressed around the world, we have continued to use the terms *woman, mother* and *maternity* in this edition. By using these terms, we do not mean to exclude those who give birth and do not identify as a woman.

Sally de-Vitry Smith and Sara Bayes

AUTHORS – AUSTRALIA AND NEW ZEALAND EDITION

Sally de-Vitry Smith RN, RM, PhD
Assistant Professor (Clinical) Midwifery
School of Nursing Midwifery and Public Health
Faculty of Health
University of Canberra
ACT, Australia

Sara Bayes PhD RN RM
Head of Midwifery
School of Nursing, Midwifery and Paramedicine
Faculty of Health Sciences
Australian Catholic University
VIC, Australia

ACKNOWLEDGEMENT

Contributors to Australia and New Zealand Edition

Janene Antney RN, RM
Lecturer in Nursing and Midwifery, College of Healthcare Sciences, Division of Tropical Health and Medicine, James Cook University, Townsville, Qld, Australia

Dianne Bloxsome RN, RM, BNurs, PGDipMidwifery, MResarchPractice
Midwifery Lecturer, School of Nursing and Midwifery, Edith Cowan University, Joondalup, WA, Australia

Natalie Cusens RN, RM, BSc(Nurs), GradDipMidwifery, MNurs(Leadership and Management)
Lecturer in Nursing and Midwifery, School of Nursing and Midwifery, College of Healthcare Sciences, Division of Tropical Health and Medicine, James Cook University, Townsville, Qld, Australia

Clare Davison RN, RM, GradDipMidwifery, MPhil(Nursing and Midwifery)
Privately Practising Endorsed Midwife and Lecturer in Midwifery, School of Nursing and Midwifery, Edith Cowan University, Joondalup, WA, Australia

Elizabeth Emmanuel RM, MHN, BNurs, MNurs(Midwifery), PhD
Senior Lecturer, School of Health and Human Sciences. Southern Cross University, Bilinga, Qld, Australia

Susan Lennox RN, RM, BA(Phil), MMidwifery(Applied), PhD
Professional Supervisor/Mentor Adjunct Research Associate, Graduate School of Nursing, Midwifery and Health, Victoria University of Wellington, Wellington, New Zealand

Robyn Maude RN, RM, BNurs, MA(Applied), PhD
Midwifery Senior Lecturer, Graduate School of Nursing, Midwifery and Health, Faculty of Health, Victoria University of Wellington, Wellington, New Zealand

Sarah Nicholls RM, MPhil(Research), BSc(Hons) Midwifery, Clinical Community Midwife, WA, Australia

PART 1

GENERAL SKILLS

Section 1: Principles of infection control

Section 2: Vital signs

Section 3: Screening and testing

Section 4: Principles of elimination management

Section 5: Principles of drug administration

Section 6: Skills for supporting antenatal wellbeing

Section 7: Skills for preparing women for labour, birth and early parenting

SECTION 1

PRINCIPLES OF INFECTION CONTROL

CHAPTER 1

STANDARD PRECAUTIONS AND HAND HYGIENE

Learning outcomes

Having read this chapter, the reader should be able to:

- discuss standard precautions and the midwife's role and responsibilities
- minimise risk of transmission of infectious agents
- discuss the principles of general hand care
- discuss the benefits and usage of alcohol-based hand rub
- discuss the role and responsibilities of the midwife in relation to hand hygiene
- identify specific situations when personal protective equipment (PPE) should be used
- describe transmission precautions.

HEALTHCARE-ASSOCIATED INFECTIONS

Healthcare-associated infections (HAIs) are preventable, yet every year in Australia over 165,000 patients develop HAIs (National Health and Medical Research Council [NHMRC] 2019). HAIs are infections acquired as a direct or indirect consequence of care from healthcare services. Healthcare-associated bloodstream infections (**bacteraemia**) cause significant morbidity, leading to increases in hospital stay, long-term disability, antibiotic-resistant microorganisms and social and economic costs for families (World Health Organization [WHO] 2011) and a mortality rate of 12–32% (Goto & Al-Hansan 2013). In the maternity setting, invasive procedures such as epidural anaesthesia, urinary catheterisation and caesarean section expose women to an increased risk of infection. HAIs are a serious threat to women, infants and families; therefore, strict adherence to infection control is essential.

In Australia and New Zealand serious infections caused by multiple antibiotic-resistant organisms (multidrug resistant organisms [MROs]), such as **methicillin-resistant *Staphylococcus aureus* (MRSA)** and **vancomycin-resistant enterococci (VRE)** are increasing. *S. aureus* can infect intravenous cannulas and surgical wounds leading to serious bloodstream infections (bacteraemia) such as sepsis and endocarditis (Kwiecinski & Horswill 2020). *Staphylococcus aureus* bloodstream infections are also known as staphylococcus aureus bacteraemia (SAB), *S. aureus* or 'golden staph'. The term *Staphylococcus aureus* bloodstream infections is now preferred to *Staphylococcus aureus* bacteraemia (Australian Institute of Health and Welfare [AIHW] 2021).

Australia has agreed on a national benchmark of no more than two cases per 10,000 days of patient care (AIHW 2021). *S. aureus* bloodstream infections have a high mortality rate and are more common in the Australian Indigenous population (Hewagama et al 2016). High *S. aureus* colonisation rates have been found in New Zealand school children, with almost 52% colonised (Hewagama et al 2016). The incidence of community-acquired MRSA has been increasing and is no longer an infection occurring primarily in the hospital setting. Approximately 33% of people carry *S. aureus* on their skin or in their nose with no ill effects; however, 2–3% carry MRSA, which is difficult to treat because of its antibiotic resistance (Centers for Disease Control and Prevention 2015). In 2019–20, Australian public hospitals reported 1428 *S. aureus* bloodstream infections; 83% of these infections were methicillin-sensitive *Staphylococcus aureus* (MSSA) and able to be treated with antimicrobials (AIHW 2021).

MRSA is spread by direct contact with a contaminated surface (e.g. mobile phone, pen), clothing or skin-to-skin (Turner et al 2019). MRSA spread is reduced by handwashing and the use of alcohol-based hand rub. *Clostridioides difficile* (previously called *Clostridium difficile*) is another bacterial source of HAIs and is found in the intestine of approximately 3% of the population. When the normal gut bacteria which usually prevent *C. difficile* from multiplying are destroyed by antibiotics, *C. difficile* numbers increase, releasing toxins that damage the intestinal wall and cause diarrhoea. *C. difficile* can be found on surfaces such as bedside tables and the hands of healthcare workers.

New pathogens are emerging and spreading, causing global health emergencies (Storr et al 2017). Middle East respiratory syndrome coronavirus (MERS-CoV) and severe acute respiratory syndrome associated coronavirus (SARS-CoV) have occurred. In 2020 a novel coronavirus outbreak occurred due to the spread of a respiratory virus called SARS-CoV-2. The WHO declared the outbreak a public health emergency of international concern (PHEIC) in January 2020 and in March Coronavirus COVID-19 was declared a global pandemic (WHO 2020). As of 26 August 2021 the number of confirmed COVID-19 cases globally has exceeded 213 million and the death rate is approaching 4.5 million (WHO 2021).

Outbreaks of the mosquito-borne **Zika virus** have caused great concern for pregnant women. The Zika virus can be transmitted from mother to fetus and may result in congenital Zika syndrome which can cause significant morbidity, including microcephaly, intellectual disability and impaired vision and hearing (Turienzo & Brown 2016). Zika virus may cause minimal symptoms and can be transmitted through sexual contact when people are unaware they have been infected (Oster et al 2016). The Zika virus has been identified in the Pacific with both Australians (Australian Nursing & Midwifery Federation [ANMF] 2016) and New Zealanders infected, generally while travelling (Public Health Surveillance NZ 2017).

The WHO has developed recommendations on the core components of infection prevention and control measures, and the containment of antimicrobial resistance (Storr et al 2017). These measures include infection prevention and control (IPC) education for all healthcare workers using team-based and task-based strategies. All healthcare workers have a responsibility for IPC, and to understand the chain of infection.

The National Health and Medical Research Council (NHMRC) developed the *Australian Guidelines for the Prevention and Control of Infection in Healthcare* (2019) to provide an evidence-based approach to infection control. In 2011, New Zealand established the Hand Hygiene New Zealand (HHNZ) steering group to deliver a national hand hygiene program (Freeman et al 2016). Both programs are based on the WHO approach and outline the work practices used to minimise transmission of infectious agents. The New Zealand hand hygiene program has led to significant increases in compliance, with the five moments for hand hygiene becoming the social norm (Freeman et al 2016). In the clinical setting, a two-tiered approach encompasses standard precautions and transmission-based precautions.

STANDARD PRECAUTIONS

Standard precautions are the first line of defence for protecting everyone from the transmission of infectious agents and are applied universally, in all environments, whether infection is evident or not (Fig 1.1). It is the midwife's responsibility to understand modes of HAI transmission, apply standard precautions and practice in a manner that minimises transmission of infection and is compliant with relevant standards (NHMRC 2019). Standard precautions are always used because the possibility of pathogen transmission or contact with bodily fluids such as blood, vaginal and seminal secretions, urine or faeces, amniotic fluid, cerebrospinal fluid, saliva, breast milk or other infectious agents exists. Sweat is considered an exception. Midwives have frequent and close physical contact with women and babies and commonly work in clinical situations where there is potential for infection transmission (e.g. birth, vaginal examination, rupture of membranes, caesarean section, injections, perineal repair, venepuncture and cannulation). The NHMRC (2019) states that standard precautions consist of:

- hand hygiene
- personal protective equipment
- safe handling and disposal of sharps
- environmental controls including routine environmental cleaning
- reprocessing of reusable medical equipment and instruments
- respiratory hygiene and cough etiquette
- aseptic non-touch technique
- waste management
- appropriate handling of linen (pp. 26–7).

HAND HYGIENE

Hand hygiene is critical and is recognised as the single-most important strategy to preventing HAIs (Kingston et al 2017). Hand hygiene includes washing hands with soap and water (non-antimicrobial or antimicrobial) or applying an alcohol-based hand rub (ABHR) (Hand Hygiene Australia [HHA] 2021).

Correctly performed hand hygiene reduces the number of microorganisms present on hands and helps decrease transmission of infectious organisms (Australian Commission on Safety and Quality in Health Care [ACSQHC] 2021). Midwives must remain vigilant and ensure hand hygiene is a habitual part of

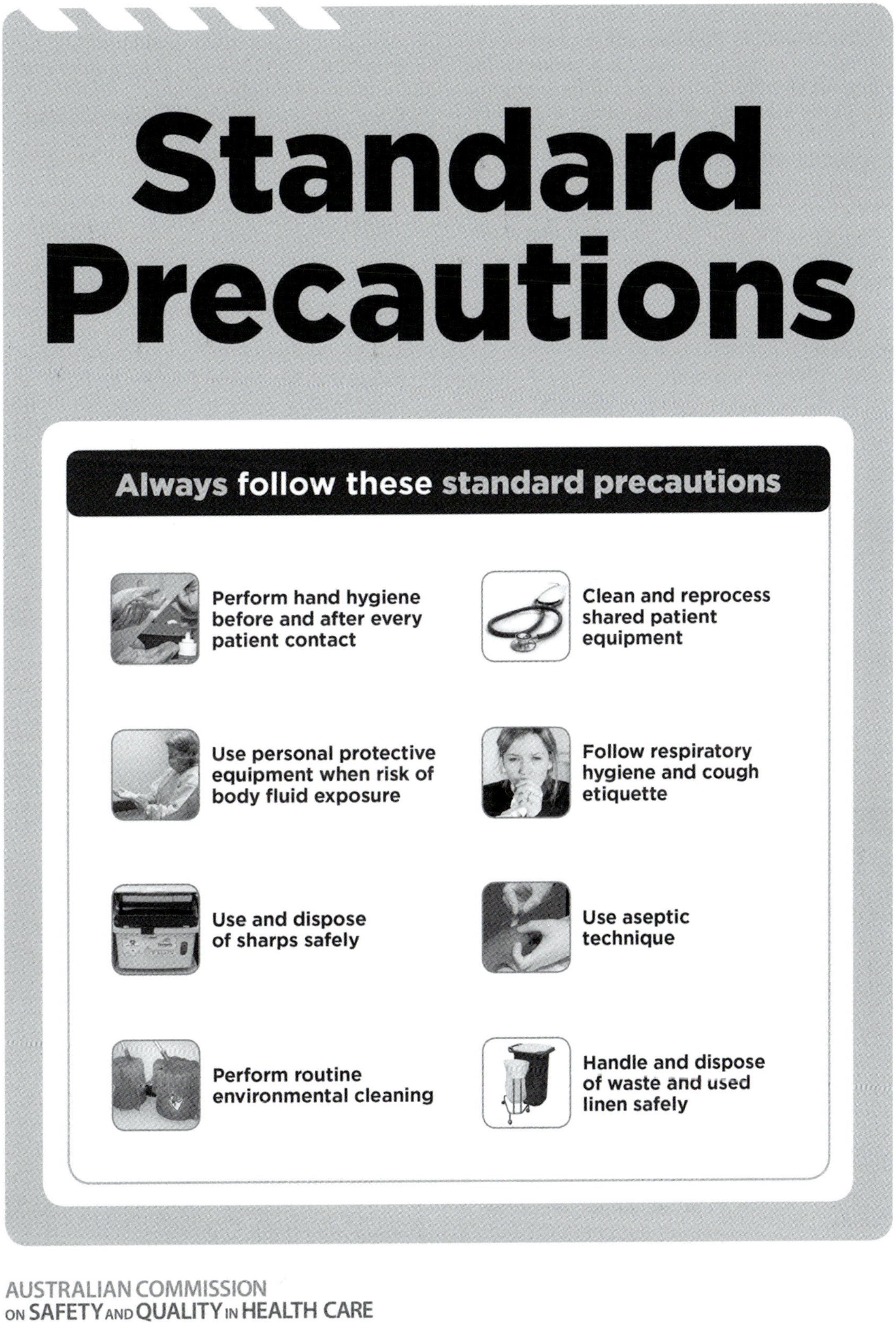

Standard Precautions

Always follow these standard precautions

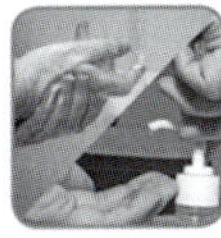
Perform hand hygiene before and after every patient contact

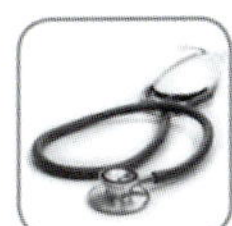
Clean and reprocess shared patient equipment

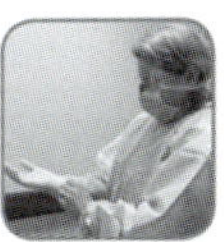
Use personal protective equipment when risk of body fluid exposure

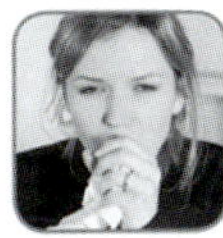
Follow respiratory hygiene and cough etiquette

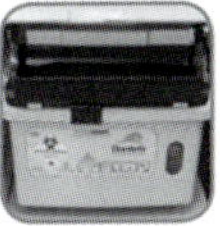
Use and dispose of sharps safely

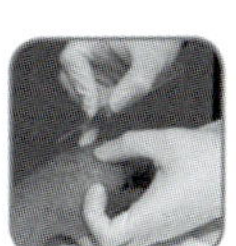
Use aseptic technique

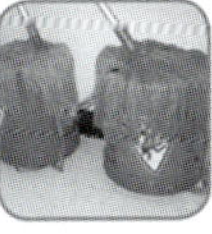
Perform routine environmental cleaning

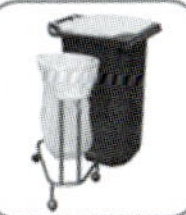
Handle and dispose of waste and used linen safely

AUSTRALIAN COMMISSION ON SAFETY AND QUALITY IN HEALTH CARE

FIGURE 1.1 Standard precautions.
Source: Reproduced with the permission of the Australian Commission on Safety and Quality in Health Care.

work practice. A strong correlation exists between hand hygiene compliance and incidence of hospital-acquired MRSA (Jian et al 2016). Midwives and nurses have the highest rates of compliance with the **5 moments for hand hygiene** (HHA 2021). Barriers to hand hygiene compliance include lack of time and forgetfulness (White et al 2015).

Continuity of care in midwifery has known benefits for women, and midwives are increasingly seeing women in their homes for antenatal care, birth and postnatal care. In recognition of the shift from hospital to home care, the WHO has released guidelines for hand hygiene in outpatient and home settings. Midwives must continue to follow standard precautions in the home and community setting. Hand hygiene is the most effective, least expensive way to prevent HAIs (Wilson et al 2015).

The five critical moments when routine hand hygiene needs to be performed, as identified by the WHO and the *Australian Guidelines for the Prevention and Control of Infection in Healthcare* (NHMRC 2019), are (Fig 1.2):

1. before touching a patient
2. before a procedure
3. after a procedure or body substance exposure risk
4. after touching a patient
5. after touching patient surroundings.

In addition, hand hygiene should also be performed in the following situations.

- Before starting work and before leaving work.
- Prior to and after eating or handling food or drinks.
- Before and after using a computer keyboard in a clinical area.
- When hands are visibly soiled.
- After visiting the toilet.
- Before putting on or removing gloves.
- After handling laundry/equipment/waste.
- After blowing, wiping or touching nose and mouth.
- Postnatal women should be advised to wash their hands before and after changing sanitary pads to reduce the risk of sepsis (Harper 2011).

Hand hygiene needs to be performed correctly to reduce the number of microorganisms on hands.

- Cuts or abrasions on the skin should be covered with a waterproof dressing to provide a barrier to viruses and bacteria.
- Arms should be bare below the elbows.

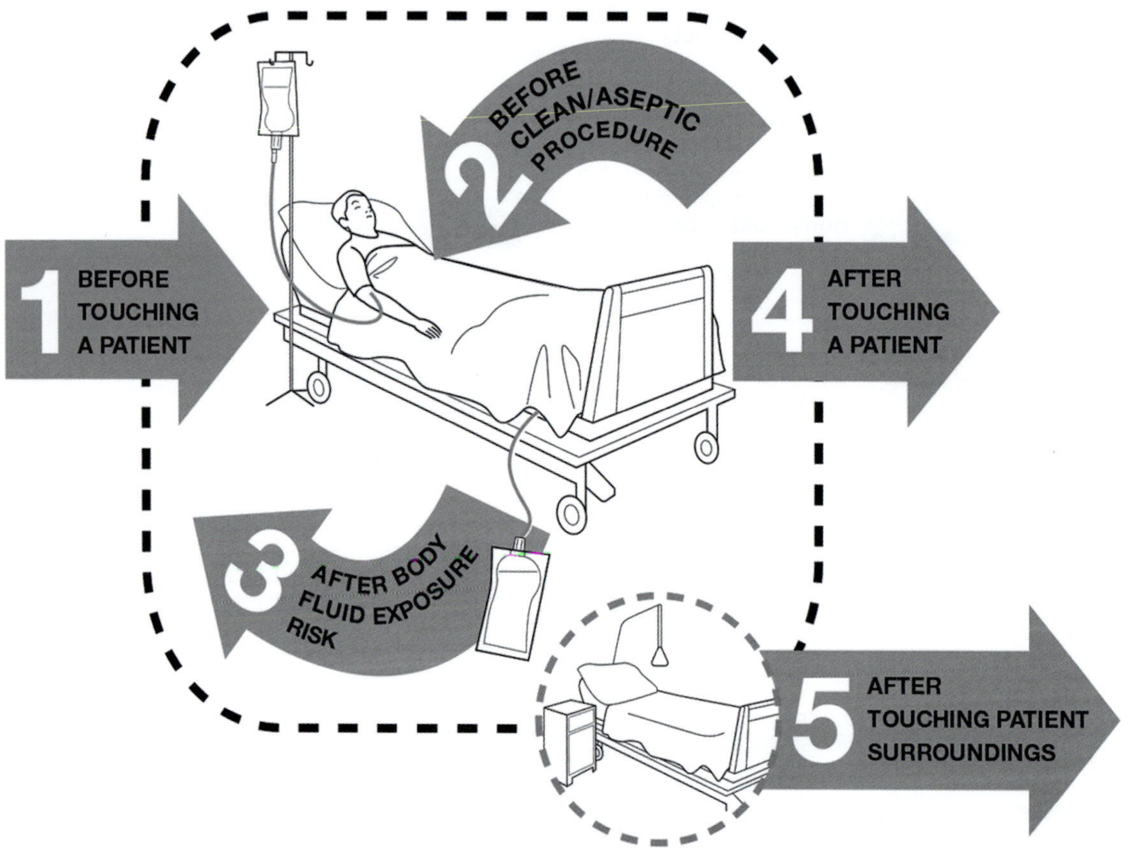

FIGURE 1.2 **Five moments of hand hygiene.**
Source: Reprinted from World Health Organization (WHO): Guidelines on hand hygiene in health care, 2009b. WHO, Geneva.

Alcohol-based hand rub

Alcohol-based hand rub (ABHR) is recommended for clinical situations when hands are visibly clean. It is preferable for ABHR to contain 60–80% ethanol and meet the European Standard EN 1500 (ACSQHC 2019, NHMRC 2019). If hands are contaminated, visibly soiled or exposed to any potentially spore-forming organisms, or after using the toilet, hands should be washed with soap and water (HHA 2021).

ABHR has multiple advantages, including a greater reduction in bacteria than soap and water. It is quick to use, less irritating to the skin, readily accessible and cost-effective (Fig 1.3). The amount of ABHR required for effective hand hygiene is 2–3 mL, which takes 15–20 seconds to dry. Hands should be dry prior to using ABHR as wet hands dilute the solution and decrease effectiveness. ABHR can be used multiple times as there is no limit to its usage before handwashing with soap and water is required. Cutaneous alcohol absorption is minimal; however, if for religious reasons ABHR use is a concern, isopropanol can be used in preference to

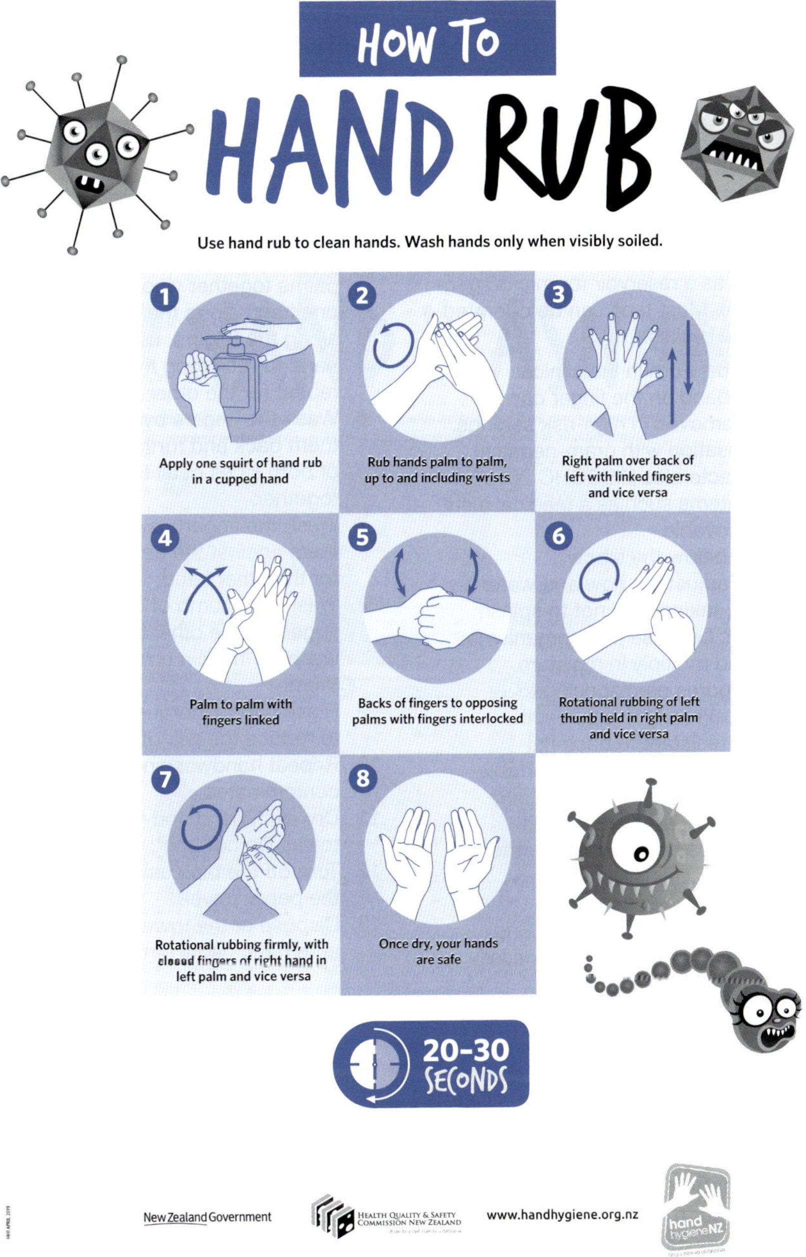

FIGURE 1.3 How to use alcohol-based hand rub.
Source: New Zealand Government, Health Quality & Safety Commission New Zealand (HQSC), Hand Hygiene NZ.

SKILL 1.2 General hand care

- Hands should be examined daily for cuts, grazes, dermatitis and torn cuticles as these increase the risk of infection to the midwife. Any skin breaches should be covered with a waterproof dressing (ACSQHC 2019). Damaged skin increases the midwife's risk of infection and can increase the number of microorganisms present, thereby increasing the risk of infection being transmitted to others.
- Nails should be kept short (≤ 0.5 cm, or no longer than the end of the finger) and filed smoothly as long or ragged nails can scratch women and babies or tear gloves. Dirt and secretions, which can harbour microorganisms, may be found under fingernails.
- Nail polish, artificial nails, nail art or nail extensions should not be worn by any midwife who has direct contact with women and infants (Clinical Excellence Commission 2020).
- Artificial nails increase the number of gram-negative pathogens. Most bacteria are found along the 1 mm of nail next to the subungual skin. Microorganisms can flourish in the ridge that appears as the nail grows. Nail polish does not increase bacterial numbers but chipped nail polish has the potential to harbour pathogens (ACSQHC 2019).
- Nail polish is not recommended due to the potential for harbouring bacteria.
- Apply an emollient hand cream or moisturiser that is compatible with the antiseptics and barrier products used to clean the hands on a regular basis to prevent them from drying out and cracking. The product should list water as its first ingredient and contain no anionic-based chemicals or petroleum.

Hand hygiene increases the risk of health workers developing occupation-related skin problems. A retrospective analysis at a metropolitan dermatology clinic in Victoria found the most common diagnoses were irritant and allergic-contact dermatitis from rubber glove chemicals, preservatives, heat and sweating, with a lower incidence occurring in health workers using ABHR (Higgins et al 2016).

Irritated skin can become chafed and cracked, which causes pain and damage to the protective barrier of the skin and encourages bacterial colonisation. This risk can be reduced if the ABHR contains an emollient to reduce skin damage, dryness and irritation (ACSQHC 2019). Many skin issues are due to irritant contact dermatitis (ICD) from handwashing, soaps, paper towels and hot water which may cause dry skin. Other causes include sweating from long periods of glove use and the powder used in gloves. A lotion containing oil or a barrier cream used at least three times per day can help protect the hands against dryness and irritation (ACSQHC 2019).

Bare below the elbow

Long sleeves can become contaminated with pathogens and make handwashing less effective; therefore, most healthcare facilities recommend their staff are 'bare below the elbow' when providing direct patient care. If exposure of the forearms is unacceptable for religious reasons, the sleeve should not be loose or dangling and must be rolled or pulled back securely during handwashing and direct patient care (National Institute for Health and Care Excellence [NICE] 2014).

Rings, bracelets and watches should not be worn (Goldberg 2017). The skin under rings has increased microorganisms compared to bare skin. A plain flat band can be worn during routine care, but should be removed in a high-risk setting. Although compliance with hand hygiene is high, there appears to be a knowledge gap related to wearing jewellery on the hands and wrists (Accardi et al 2017).

PERSONAL PROTECTIVE EQUIPMENT

Personal protective equipment (PPE) refers to the barriers used to help protect healthcare practitioners from being infected and prevent the potential transfer of infection from one person to another via staff members. PPE includes gloves, gowns, aprons, masks, goggles, visors, caps and theatre footwear. Barriers to PPE use have been described as discomfort, compromised dexterity, fogging of eyewear, emergency situations and the belief that prescription glasses provide adequate eye protection (Olson et al 2016). Although wearing protective clothing can feel disruptive to the relationship between midwives and women, this can be overcome by education about the important role of preventing transmission of infection. The choice of PPE is based on an assessment of the risk of transmission of infection. The following factors need to be considered:

- likelihood of exposure to blood and bodily fluids
- type of substance involved
- probable route of transmission of an infectious agent.

SKILL 1.3 Sequence for putting on and removing PPE (donning and doffing)

PPE should be readily available at the point of use and should be donned and removed correctly. After PPE is put on, work from clean to dirty and limit touching surfaces; keep hands away from the face and hair. PPE should be changed if it becomes torn or contaminated. Always perform hand hygiene before and after putting on PPE. Contamination of skin and clothing occurs frequently, particularly if PPE is removed incorrectly (Tomas et al 2015). The *Australian Guidelines for the Prevention and Control of Infection in Healthcare* (NHMRC 2019) recommend the following order for donning PPE (Fig 1.6):

1. hand hygiene
2. gown
3. face mask or respirator mask
4. eye protection, goggles, face shield
5. gloves pulled over the sleeves of the gown (double gloving recommended for Ebola).

For removing PPE, the following sequence is recommended (NHMRC 2019):

1. gloves
2. eye protection, goggles or face shield
3. gown
4. face mask or respirator
5. perform hand hygiene.

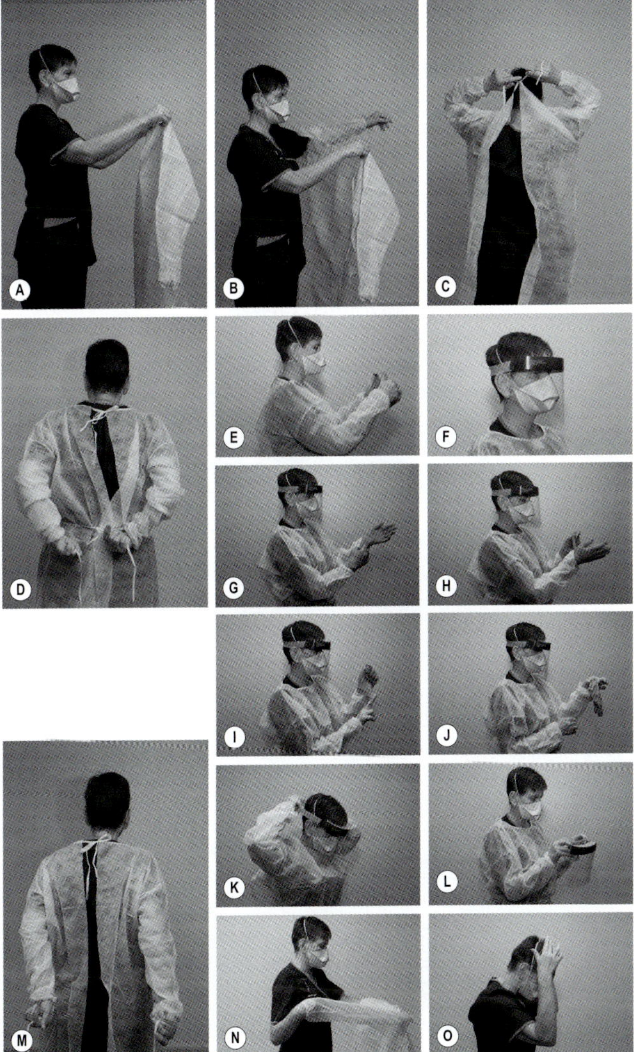

FIGURE 1.6 Correct sequence for donning and doffing PPE. **A–F**, Put on mask followed by gown, face shield then gloves. **G–O**, Remove equipment in reverse order, gloves, face shield, gown and lastly mask.

PPE is considered contaminated once the midwife has entered the patient room, and should be removed before leaving the patient care area. An exception is if the use of a respirator is required; this is removed after leaving the patient care room and closing the door (Mata et al 2015).

Gloves

Gloves should be selected according to the task to be undertaken and be the correct size (Fig 1.7). Incorrect glove size can have a detrimental effect on dexterity and lead to increased muscle fatigue. Gloves should be stored correctly, used before the expiry date and meet Australian and New Zealand standards (Standards Australia 2014). Non-sterile, single-use medical gloves are available in synthetic materials such as nitrile and natural rubber latex (NRL). Non-powdered gloves are preferable as they decrease exposure to latex proteins through respiratory and contact routes and reduce the risk of latex allergy. For many routine tasks, gloves are not required (e.g. vital sign observations, subcutaneous [SC] injections). Non-sterile examination gloves should be worn when handling body fluids (e.g. emptying catheter bags, removing vomit and testing urine), while sterile gloves are worn for childbirth, surgery and any procedures in which an aseptic non-touch technique (ANTT) causes the hands to be in close proximity to key sites or key parts.

Gloves are also worn to protect the hands from repeated exposure to chemicals or situations, such as using surface wipes to clean trays and trolleys. Hand hygiene is performed before putting gloves on and when gloves are removed. Gloves should be worn once only, removed as soon after use as possible, removed correctly and disposed of in the clinical waste. Inappropriate use of gloves can increase the risk of cross infection and includes not removing gloves after a procedure is completed and touching other surfaces such as curtains (Wilson & Loveday 2015) or light switches.

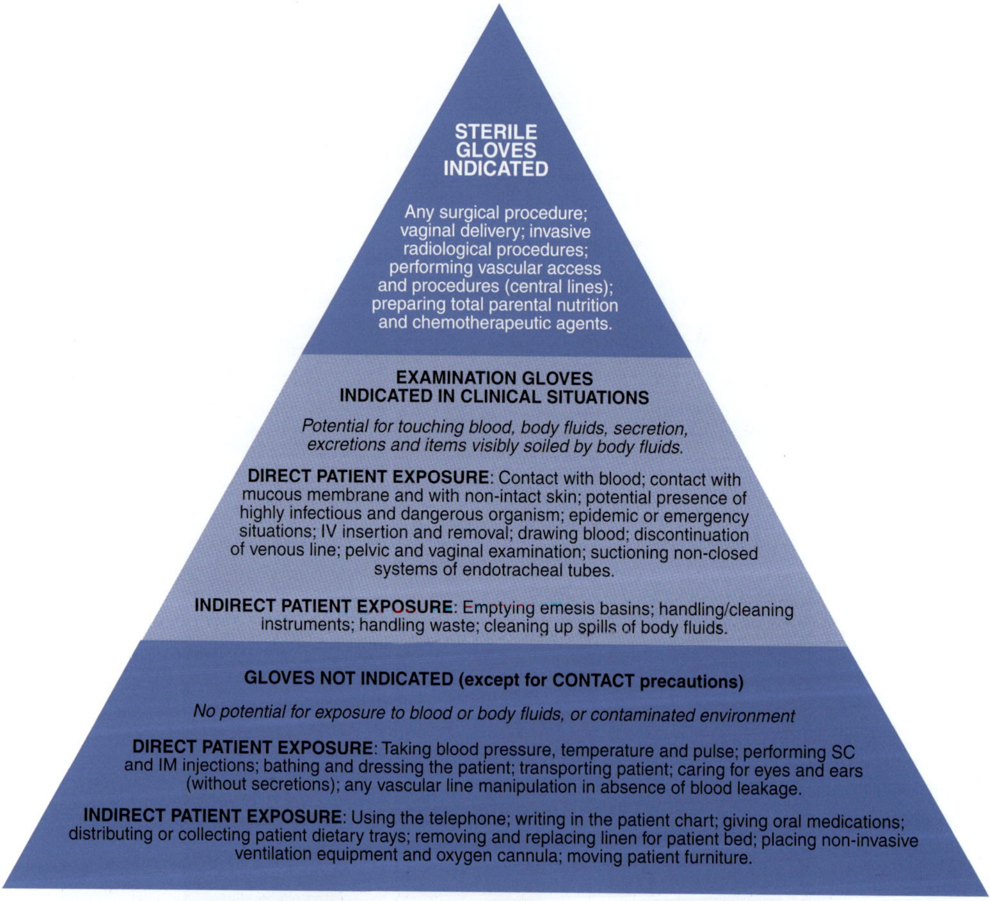

STERILE GLOVES INDICATED

Any surgical procedure; vaginal delivery; invasive radiological procedures; performing vascular access and procedures (central lines); preparing total parental nutrition and chemotherapeutic agents.

EXAMINATION GLOVES INDICATED IN CLINICAL SITUATIONS

Potential for touching blood, body fluids, secretion, excretions and items visibly soiled by body fluids.

DIRECT PATIENT EXPOSURE: Contact with blood; contact with mucous membrane and with non-intact skin; potential presence of highly infectious and dangerous organism; epidemic or emergency situations; IV insertion and removal; drawing blood; discontinuation of venous line; pelvic and vaginal examination; suctioning non-closed systems of endotracheal tubes.

INDIRECT PATIENT EXPOSURE: Emptying emesis basins; handling/cleaning instruments; handling waste; cleaning up spills of body fluids.

GLOVES NOT INDICATED (except for CONTACT precautions)

No potential for exposure to blood or body fluids, or contaminated environment

DIRECT PATIENT EXPOSURE: Taking blood pressure, temperature and pulse; performing SC and IM injections; bathing and dressing the patient; transporting patient; caring for eyes and ears (without secretions); any vascular line manipulation in absence of blood leakage.

INDIRECT PATIENT EXPOSURE: Using the telephone; writing in the patient chart; giving oral medications; distributing or collecting patient dietary trays; removing and replacing linen for patient bed; placing non-invasive ventilation equipment and oxygen cannula; moving patient furniture.

FIGURE 1.7 **Glove use.**
Source: Reprinted from World Health Organization (WHO): Glove use information leaflet, 2009a. Online 29 Dec 2017. Available: www.who.int/gpsc/5may/Glove_Use_Information_Leaflet.pdf.

SKILL 1.4 Donning non-sterile gloves

1. Wash hands or use ABHR.
2. Take glove from its original box.
3. Touch only the top edge of the glove.
4. Don first glove.
5. Take second glove from box with the bare hand and touch only the area near the cuff.
6. Avoid touching the skin of the forearm with the gloved hand, turn the external surface of the glove to be donned on the folded fingers of the gloved hand and pull the glove up without touching any skin.
7. Once the gloves are donned do not touch anything that is not defined by indications and conditions for glove use (Fig 1.8).

SKILL 1.5 Removing gloves (doffing)

1. Using the dominant hand to grasp the outside wrist of the other glove, pull it off so that it becomes inside out (Fig 1.9).
2. Keep hold of it with the gloved hand, then slide the ungloved thumb inside the cuff of the other glove.
3. Remove the glove, turning it inside out. This contains the glove, inside out, within the second glove.
4. Perform hand hygiene.

Removing gloves correctly (whether sterile or non-sterile) prevents the hands from being contaminated from the gloves and contains contamination within the gloves. Gloves that are just 'ripped off' spread contamination into the air and onto nearby surfaces. Wilson and Loveday (2014) suggest that gloves put on too early or removed too late add to the transmission of microorganisms.

Gloves do not provide 100% protection as hand contamination may occur due to small perforations in gloves or contamination during glove removal. When wearing gloves, they should not be washed or have ABHR applied as these actions reduce glove integrity and can create pinholes or cause gloves to rupture (Clinical Excellence Commission 2021). Double gloving is not recommended as it can increase dermatological side effects including overhydration of hands, latex allergies, eczema and irritant dermatitis (Victoria State Government 2020). Double gloving can be used to transition from a dirty to a clean procedure quickly or in theatre settings (Clinical Excellence Commission 2021).

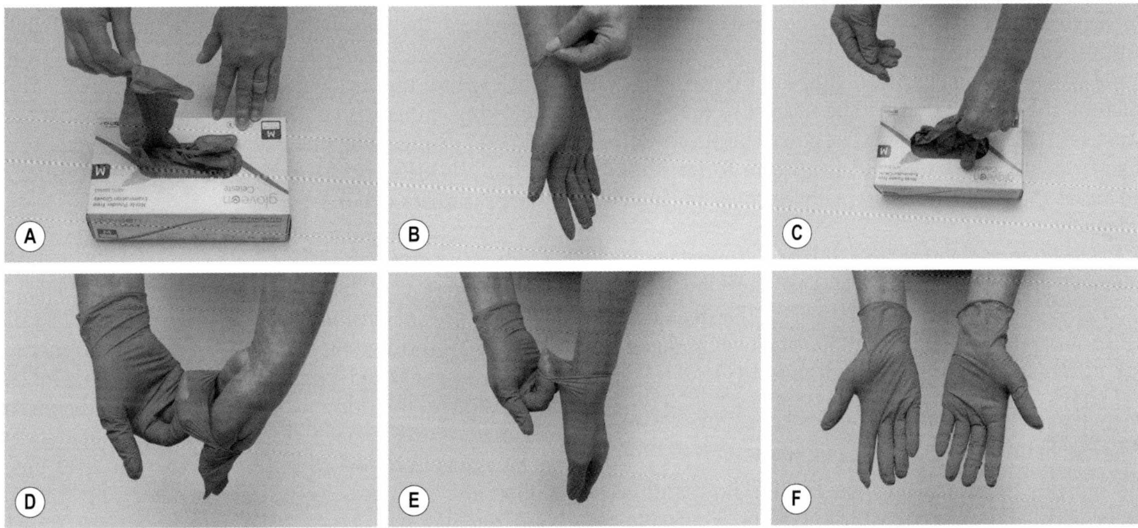

FIGURE 1.8 **A–F, Donning (putting on) gloves.**

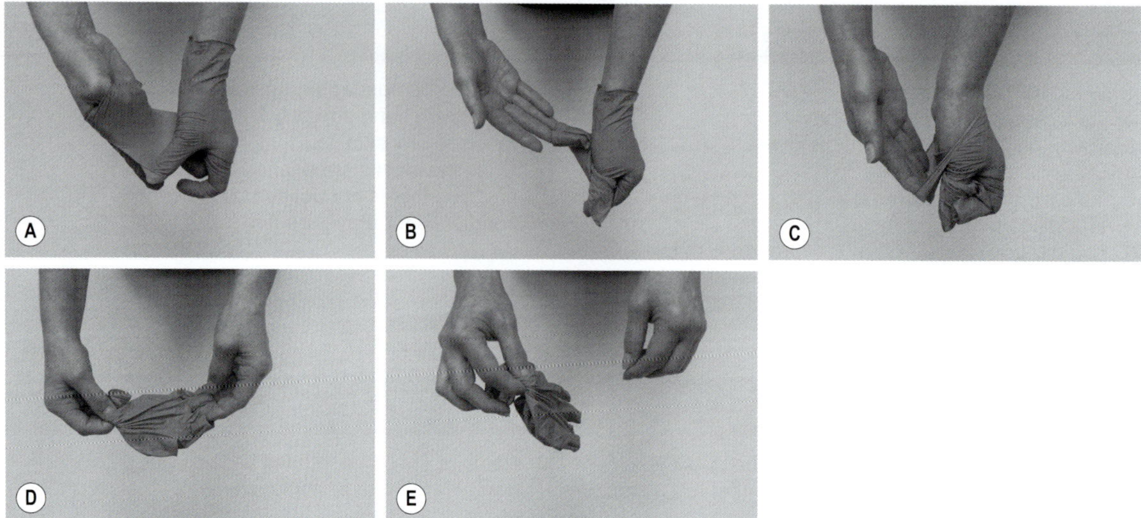

FIGURE 1.9 **A–E, Doffing (removing) gloves.**

Plastic aprons

Disposable, single-use plastic aprons should be worn when there is a possibility of sprays or spills that risks contaminating the midwife's clothing (Loveday et al 2014). An apron should not touch the hair when being put on and should be worn loosely (Criscitelli 2014). At the end of the procedure it should be removed after the gloves by breaking the cleaner parts (e.g. neck ties and sides), then folded 'in' so that the potentially contaminated area does not touch the clothing. Hand decontamination should then be undertaken.

Full-body gowns

Gowns protect the healthcare worker from contamination with potentially infectious substances such as blood and bodily fluids. Sterile gowns are worn for surgical procedures and procedures requiring an aseptic field, including perineal repair and epidurals. Sterile gowns are folded in so they are put on without touching the outside that will be nearest to the woman (Martirani & Weaving 2011). The gown should cover the torso from neck to knees and from arm to wristband, and tie at the neck and waist. Gloves cover both wrist and gown.

A study investigating the relative importance of universal glove and gown use and hand hygiene in the intensive care unit found 44% of the decrease in MRSA was related to universal use of gloves and gowns and 38.1% was due to improved hand hygiene (Harris et al 2017).

Masks, face and eye protection

The mucous membranes of the mouth, nose and eyes can provide a point of entry for infectious agents. Fluid-repellent protective eyewear, face shields and masks decrease exposure to splashes of blood and body fluids. To put on a mask, secure the ties or elastic bands of the mask at the back of the head and at the neck (Fig 1.10). The flexible noseband should fit over the bridge of the nose and be pinched to fit correctly. The mask fits the face snugly and extends below the chin. The eyewear or face shield is put on after the mask and adjusted to fit the face correctly. Eye covering and masks are removed after gloves and aprons and are always removed by handling the ties/frame at the sides and back of the head, rather than touching the front, which is likely to be contaminated.

SHARPS

Sharps injuries carry a serious risk of harm and are a common but preventable cause of injury to midwives (Griffith 2015). A sharps injury is one that occurs as a result of the skin being broken by a medical sharp such as needles, scalpels and stitch cutters. The injury can expose the midwife to blood-borne infections including hepatitis B virus, hepatitis C virus and human immunodeficiency virus (HIV). According to the NHMRC (2019, p. 53) the highest number of sharps injuries occur:

- during use of a sharp device on a patient (41%)
- after use and before disposal (40%)
- during or after disposal of sharp devices (15%).

The use of hollow-bore sharps is of particular concern as residual blood is associated with an increase in the risk for blood-borne virus transmission. Hollow-bore sharps includes needles attached to disposable syringes, butterfly needles, intravenous catheter stylets, multi-sample blood collection needles, arterial blood collection syringes, aspiration needles and injector pen needles (NHMRC 2019, p. 53). Sharps injuries commonly involve a contaminated needle which has been used for injection or phlebotomy (NSW Health

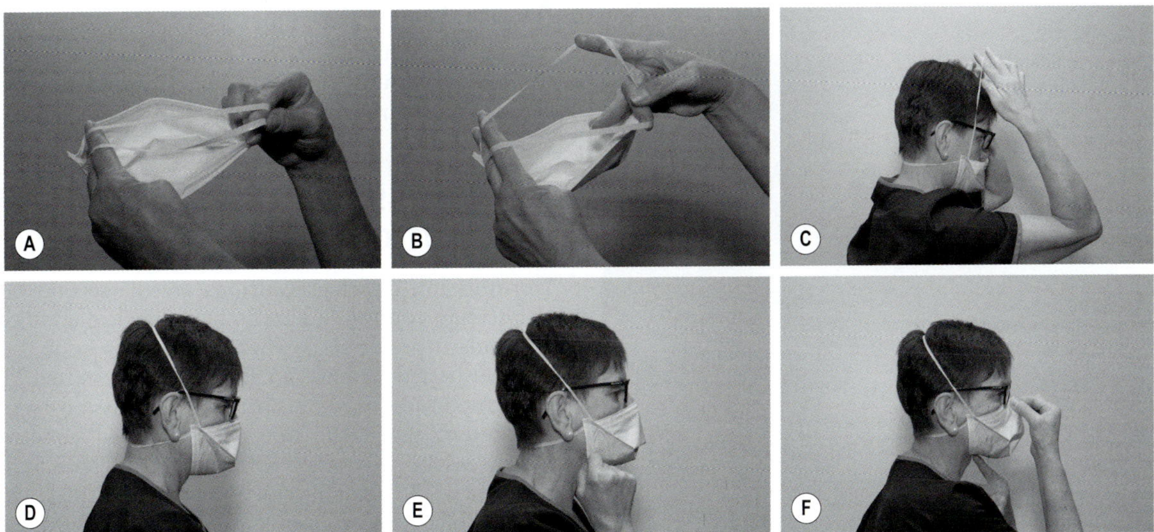

FIGURE 1.10 **A–F, Sequence for donning and doffing a P2 respirator mask. (Note: Sequence is reversed for doffing.)**

2018). It is estimated that approximately 18,700 needlestick injuries occur in Australian hospitals every year, or around 2.86 incidents per 100 full-time equivalent staff (Murphy 2014). Employers have a responsibility to reduce the risk and incidence of sharps injuries by educating employees, providing safety-engineered sharps wherever practical and having a protocol for prophylactic exposure treatment in place.

The handling of sharps must be kept to a minimum. The use of needles and other sharps should be eliminated or reduced by use of needleless devices and safety-engineered components such as retractable devices.

Exposure-prone procedures (EPPs)

If the potential exists for contact between the skin of the midwife and a sharp, the midwife should know their HIV and hepatitis C virus (HCV) status. Midwives who are positive for HIV or HCV must not perform EPPs (Clinical Excellence Commission 2020).

Midwives who have direct contact with women or neonates require immunological protection against diphtheria, tetanus, pertussis, hepatitis B virus, measles, mumps, rubella and chickenpox, and an annual influenza vaccine is usually recommended (Clinical Excellence Commission 2020).

SKILL 1.6 Disposing of sharps

- Avoid using needles when possible.
- Never re-sheath (recap) used needles.
- Fit safety engineered devices (needle-free vial adapters, retracting lancets, etc.).
- Use instruments to grasp needles, retract tissue and load or unload needles or scalpels.
- Place all sharps directly into an approved sharps box at the point of care (Fig 1.11).
- Fill sharps box to the level that indicates it is full, then secure and dispose of contents correctly.
- Use a neutral zone (e.g. kidney dish) so sharps are never passed hand to hand.
- Have vaccinations against blood-borne viruses such as hepatitis B.
- Know the agency sharps policy and how to report a sharps-related injury.

ROUTINE ENVIRONMENTAL CLEANING

Infectious agents may be more easily transmitted if poor environmental hygiene occurs in the healthcare environment. All organisations must have regularly updated protocols covering cleanliness of the environment, equipment hygiene, sterile supplies, prevention of overcrowding or excessive transferring of clients between areas, disposal of clinical waste, managing accidents and spillages and post-exposure prophylaxis. All equipment should be decontaminated

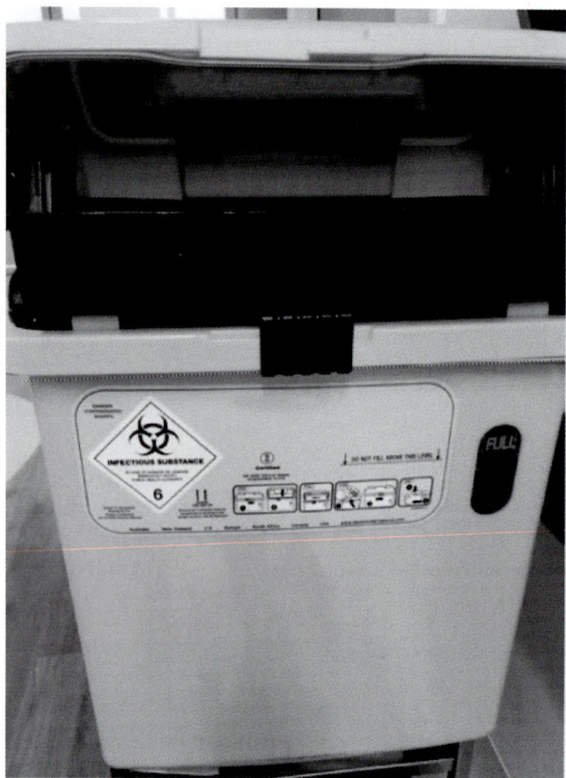

FIGURE 1.11 Sharps container.

correctly after use, and clinical waste disposed of properly in hospitals and at home.

Management of blood and body substance spills

Health facilities have specific protocols to manage spills that are similar to the following.

- Small spills (vomit, urine) should be cleaned promptly with a detergent solution.
- Large spills should be confined, visible organic matter removed, broken glass or sharps picked up with forceps, and excess liquid soaked up with paper towels or an absorbent agent.
- Appropriate PPE should be worn.
- Alcohol solutions should not be used to clean spillages.

Reprocessing of reusable equipment and instruments

Local organisation policies for cleaning, disinfection and sterilisation of equipment must meet the relevant Australian standards. Dry-packaged sterile instruments must be stored in a clean environment and protected from damage. Midwives must check that equipment or packaging is not damaged and the sterilisation or use-by date has not expired.

Aseptic technique

Aseptic technique is vital to protect women during clinical procedures and prevent transmission of pathogenic microorganisms and will be covered in Chapter 2.

TRANSMISSION-BASED PRECAUTIONS

Transmission-based precautions are the second tier of infection control and are implemented in addition to standard precautions when a patient is known to or is suspected to have an infection transmitted via airborne, droplet or contact routes. Transmission-based precautions target the infectious agent of concern. Midwives triaging women who present for care should be aware of the possibility of a potential infection and the risk of disease transmission. Rapid identification of conditions that can be transmitted to others is important to prevent the spread of infection and implement the appropriate transmission precautions (Zimmerman et al 2016). Several transmission-based precautions may need to be applied if the condition has multiple routes of transmission. A combination of measures is involved and includes:

- standard precautions
- use of PPE
- patient-dedicated or single-use equipment (blood pressure cuffs, nebulisers etc.)
- single room with en suite
- appropriate air-handling requirements
- focused environmental cleaning and disinfecting
- restriction of transfer between facilities.

The decision to use transmission-based precautions needs a multidisciplinary risk assessment. The person responsible for infection control needs to be contacted for implementation of transmission-based precautions including signs and equipment required for placement outside the patient's room. Ensure women and families are provided with the appropriate fact sheets that are available (e.g. MRSA, VRE and *C. difficile*). They can be obtained from the NHMRC and the Australian Commission on Safety and Quality in Health Care website.

Contact precautions

Contact precautions are initiated when there is a risk of infection transmission by direct contact with the patient or indirect contact with the patient care environment. Midwives working with students have a responsibility to model good infection control practices. An Australian study examining the knowledge level of third-year nursing students found knowledge of standard precautions was almost 90%, but only 27% of questions on transmission-based precautions were answered correctly (Mitchell et al 2014). Contact precautions are required for methicillin-resistant *S. aureus* (MRSA) (Fig 1.12), *C. difficile*, VRE

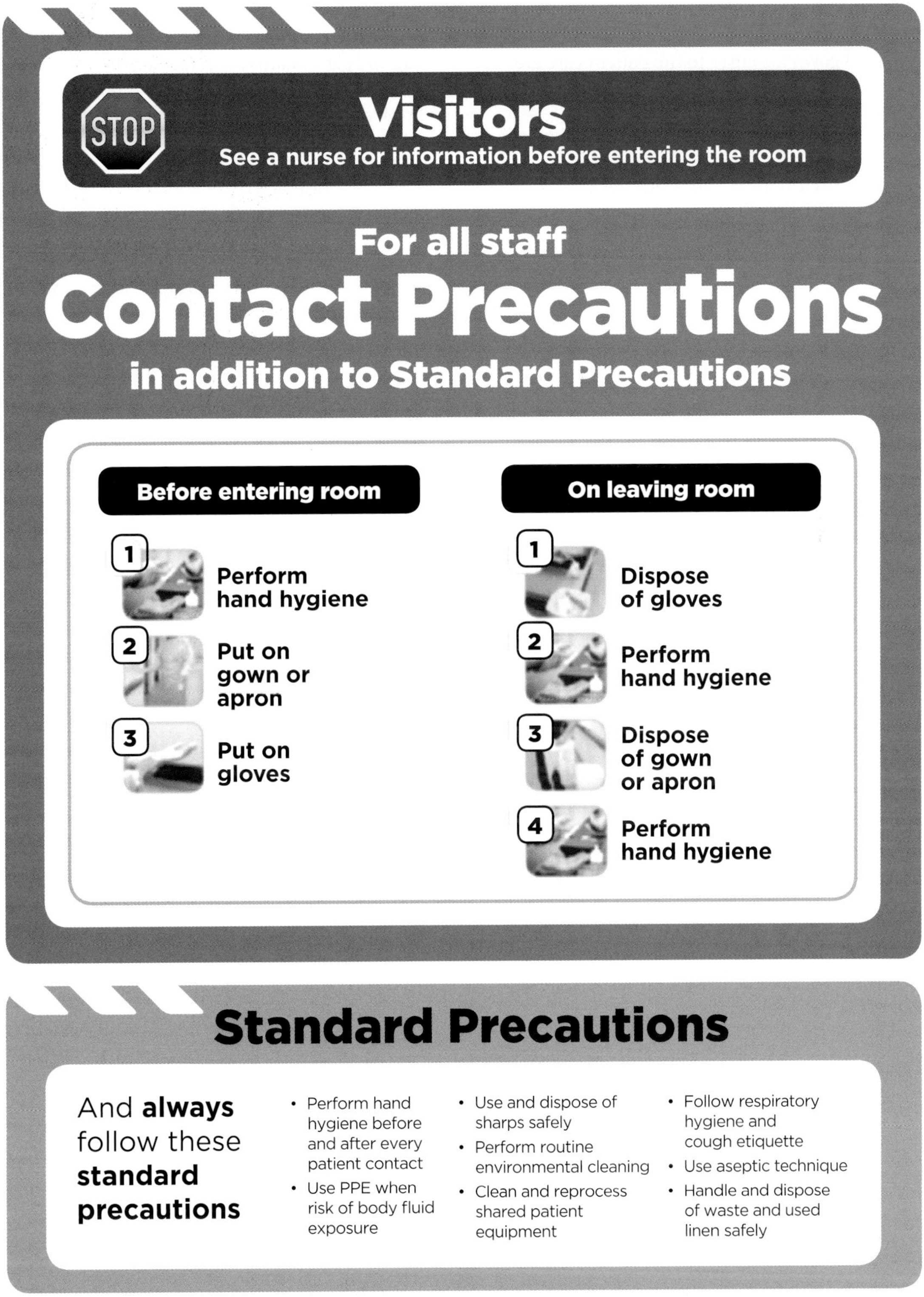

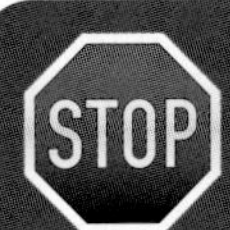

Visitors

See a nurse for information before entering the room

For all staff

Contact Precautions

in addition to Standard Precautions

Before entering room

1 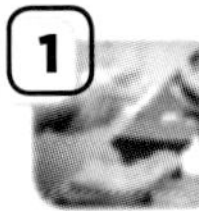 Perform hand hygiene

2 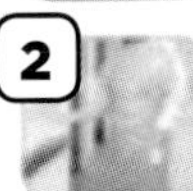 Put on gown or apron

3 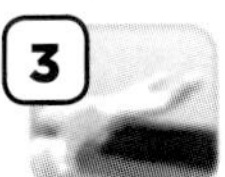 Put on gloves

On leaving room

1 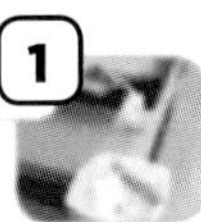 Dispose of gloves

2 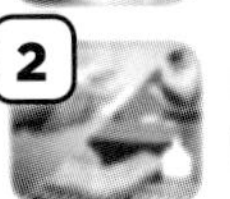 Perform hand hygiene

3 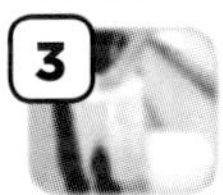 Dispose of gown or apron

4 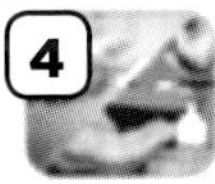 Perform hand hygiene

Standard Precautions

And **always** follow these **standard precautions**

- Perform hand hygiene before and after every patient contact
- Use PPE when risk of body fluid exposure
- Use and dispose of sharps safely
- Perform routine environmental cleaning
- Clean and reprocess shared patient equipment
- Follow respiratory hygiene and cough etiquette
- Use aseptic technique
- Handle and dispose of waste and used linen safely

AUSTRALIAN COMMISSION ON SAFETY AND QUALITY IN HEALTH CARE

FIGURE 1.12 Contact precautions.
Source: Reproduced with the permission of the Australian Commission on Safety and Quality in Health Care.

and norovirus (NHMRC 2019). Contact precautions include:

- hand hygiene
- gloves and gown for entry to the patient care area
- ensuring clothing and skin have no contact with potentially contaminated surfaces
- removing gown and gloves, perform hand hygiene before leaving the patient care area
- wearing a surgical mask and protective eyewear or face shield if there is the potential for splashes or sprays of body substances into the face and eyes.

Droplet precautions

Droplet precautions are instituted for infections transmitted through close respiratory or mucous membrane contact with respiratory secretions generated by coughing, sneezing and talking (respiratory syncytial virus, influenza, norovirus, meningococcus, pertussis, group A streptococcus). Protective eyewear is only recommended if the risk of splashes or spray exists.

Droplet precautions require:

- hand hygiene when entering and leaving room
- wearing a surgical mask when entering the room
- explanation of respiratory hygiene and cough etiquette (Fig 1.13).

Airborne precautions

Airborne precautions are required for infectious agents transmitted by small airborne droplet nuclei and small particles 'which remain infective over time and distance' (NHMRC 2019, p. 115). Airborne precautions are required for measles (rubeola), chickenpox (varicella) and *M. tuberculosis*. Airborne precautions are the same as for droplet precautions, except that an individually fitted P2 respirator is used instead of a surgical mask. P2 respirators meet Australian and New Zealand standards (AS/NZS1716) and are used to protect health workers from airborne respiratory infections. All hospitals require a respiratory isolation room that provides a negative pressure when compared to adjacent areas (Department of Health 2016) for airborne respiratory infections (Fig 1.14).

People placed under transmission-based precautions report fewer visitors, less care, less human interaction and less contact with health professionals, which can result in substandard care (Godsell et al 2013). Women subjected to transmission precautions may feel lonely and distressed with fewer opportunities to develop a relationship with carers or ask questions or feel understood.

General principles

- In a hospital environment, the use of a single room with en suite and an anteroom (if available) where necessary items can be stored.
- Notes and charts are kept outside the room.
- Doors remain closed.
- The room has a sign outside clearly indicating transmission precautions.
- The room should be equipped with all the essential but minimum materials required (e.g. sphygmomanometer, washing equipment, water jug and glass, sharps box, antibacterial soap and disposable towels, dissolvable linen sack for clinical waste, Pinard stethoscope, etc). The linen bag is sealed in the room and then removed, but otherwise none of the equipment is removed from the room until cleaned or disposed of appropriately after the woman's departure. Unnecessary furniture is removed.
- A transmission-precautions sign is placed on the door to remind all staff. Instructions should be given to friends and relatives on how to maintain transmission precautions.
- A trolley outside the room contains items that are needed when entering the room (e.g. gloves, disposable gowns, masks, goggles, overshoes, plastic aprons and ABHR).
- The midwife should recognise the value of the multidisciplinary team: the infection control nurse, microbiologist, obstetrician and midwife will all need to work in close communication and partnership to provide appropriate care for the woman. The woman may remain in her room for birth and additional precautions should be instigated accordingly.
- Ideally, specific members of staff may be assigned to care for infected women; they should then have restricted access to other women, especially any who may be considered vulnerable to infection.

PROTECTIVE ISOLATION

This involves protecting an individual from infection because they are in some way vulnerable or immunocompromised. The midwife is less likely to be involved in this type of care. All unnecessary visitors are prohibited and extreme care is taken to ensure no infection is taken into the room. A positive pressure environment is needed where clean air is drawn into the room from outside and forced out into the general ward area. Hands are decontaminated and protective clothing is applied before entering and removed after leaving the room.

Antimicrobial stewardship

Overuse and misuse of antibiotics has resulted in serious negative consequences such as the emergence of **multidrug-resistant organisms (MROs)**. Antimicrobial stewardship optimises the selection, dose, duration or route of administration of antimicrobial medications (Nagel et al 2016). New Zealand midwives and Australian midwives endorsed to prescribe, have a responsibility to prescribe antibiotics appropriately to minimise the consequences of inappropriate antibiotic administration. The threats from antibiotic resistance are recognised worldwide and resistance is increasing in New Zealand and Australia. The number of patients admitted to hospital with MROs is predicted to increase dramatically (Gray 2015).

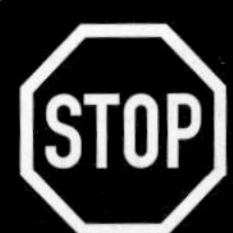

Visitors

See a nurse for information before entering the room

For all staff

Droplet Precautions

in addition to Standard Precautions

Before entering room	On leaving room
1 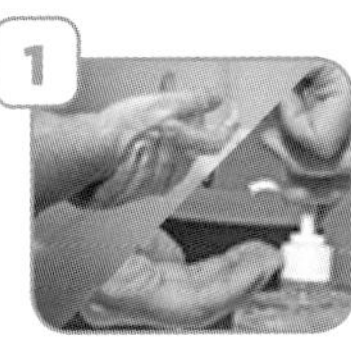 Perform hand hygiene	1 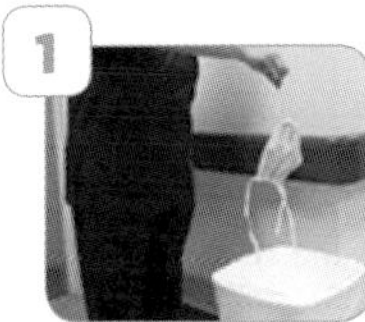 Dispose of mask
2 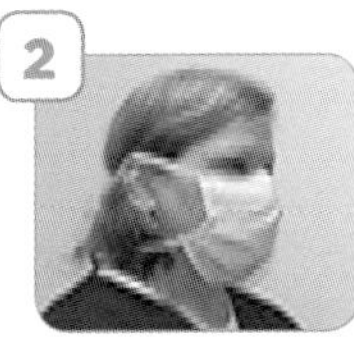 Put on a surgical mask	2 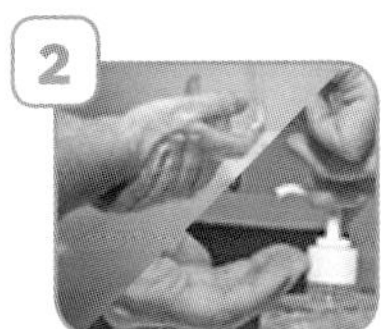 Perform hand hygiene

Standard Precautions

And **always** follow these **standard precautions**

- Perform hand hygiene before and after every patient contact
- Use PPE when risk of body fluid exposure
- Use and dispose of sharps safely
- Perform routine environmental cleaning
- Clean and reprocess shared patient equipment
- Follow respiratory hygiene and cough etiquette
- Use aseptic technique
- Handle and dispose of waste and used linen safely

AUSTRALIAN COMMISSION ON SAFETY AND QUALITY IN HEALTH CARE

FIGURE 1.13 **Droplet precautions.**
Source: Reproduced with the permission of the Australian Commission on Safety and Quality in Health Care.

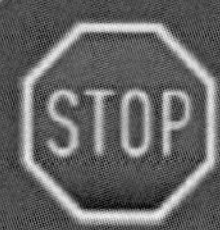

Visitors

See a nurse for information before entering the room

For all staff

Airborne Precautions

in addition to Standard Precautions

Before entering room

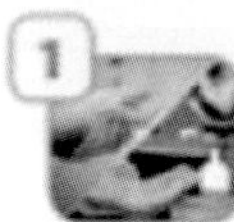

1. Perform hand hygiene

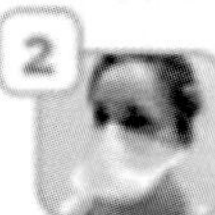

2. Put on N95 or P2 mask

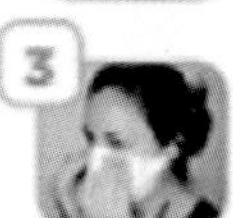

3. Perform a fit check of the mask

On leaving room

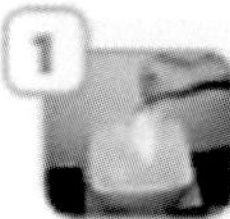

1. Dispose of mask

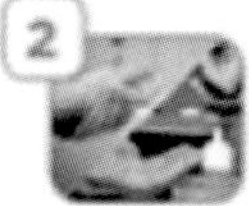

2. Perform hand hygiene

Keep door closed at all times

Standard Precautions

And **always** follow these **standard precautions**

- Perform hand hygiene before and after every patient contact
- Use PPE when risk of body fluid exposure
- Use and dispose of sharps safely
- Perform routine environmental cleaning
- Clean and reprocess shared patient equipment
- Follow respiratory hygiene and cough etiquette
- Use aseptic technique
- Handle and dispose of waste and used linen safely

AUSTRALIAN COMMISSION ON SAFETY AND QUALITY IN HEALTH CARE

FIGURE 1.14 **Airborne precautions.**
Source: Reproduced with the permission of the Australian Commission on Safety and Quality in Health Care.

SKILL 1.7 Entering, attending care and leaving the room

1. Gather any necessary additional equipment.
2. Wash and dry hands.
3. Put on an apron and any other protective clothing necessary for the procedure.
4. Use ABHR (apply gloves only if expecting to handle body fluids).
5. Knock, enter the room and close the door.
6. Complete the necessary care, containing all the tasks within the room.
   a. Crockery may be taken out of the room, providing it is to be decontaminated in a dishwasher.
   b. Domestic services are required to clean the room and bathroom daily using approved cleansers and including a thorough damp dusting; other spillages should be cleaned according to standard precaution guidelines.
   c. Cleaning cloths and similar items remain in the room for the duration of the stay and are only used in that room.
   d. Used linen should be placed in the dissolvable sack in the room. This must be sealed before leaving the room. Clinical waste is managed in the same way.
7. On preparing to leave the room, remove gloves (if worn) and apron and place in the clinical waste.
8. Decontaminate hands.
9. Close the door on leaving.
10. Use ABHR once outside the room. If an enteric (intestinal) infection such as *Escherichia coli* or *C. difficile* is present, use soap and water.
11. On discharge, thoroughly clean the room using approved solutions; steam cleaning may be required. Wash and dry all furniture and equipment, send curtains to the laundry; steam clean carpeted floor.

Role and responsibilities of the midwife

These can be summarised as:

- recognising the importance of correct hand hygiene
- following the principles of hand care
- recognising when and how hand hygiene should be undertaken
- reducing the risk of contamination to self and others through appropriate hand hygiene
- recognising the significance of standard precautions and PPE
- the need to be familiar with up-to-date reports and protocols
- the need to report and act on spillages or incidents.

SUMMARY

- Hand hygiene is an important means of infection control.
- Healthcare professionals involved in direct patient care should be 'bare below the elbows'.
- Alcohol-based hand rubs (ABHRs) remove almost all transient microorganisms and significantly reduce the number of resident microorganisms, but do not remove blood, body fluid, dirt and spores (e.g. from *C. difficile*).
- Standard precautions aim to protect all staff, women, babies and visitors from potentially serious infections by using a range of measures including hand hygiene and PPE.
- The midwife works with a high-risk client group and should include a risk assessment for standard precautions and PPE use in every clinical situation.
- Protective isolation prevents infection from entering the room by use of protective measures.

Self-assessment exercises

The answers to the following questions may be found in the text.

1. Why is hand hygiene important?
2. What are the general principles of hand care and why are they important?
3. In what situations would the midwife use an ABHR?
4. When should the midwife undertake hand hygiene?
5. What are the principles of hand hygiene?
6. Describe what constitutes standard precautions and transmission-based precautions.
7. Describe how to correctly don a gown for contact precautions.
8. Demonstrate how to remove soiled gloves, apron and goggles.

Resources

Australian Commission on Safety and Quality in Health Care has links to standards, publications and resources: www.safetyandquality.gov.au.

Australian Group on Antimicrobial Resistance (AGAR): www.agargroup.org.

Australasian College for Infection Prevention and Control (ACIPC): www.acipc.org.au.

Australian Government Department of Health provides current information on COVID-19: www.health.gov.au.

Australian Institute of Health and Welfare (AIHW) MyHospitals website has information on Australia's hospital system including the rate of bloodstream infections: aihw.gov.au/reports-data/myhospitals.

Australian Society of Antimicrobials: www.asainc.net.au.

Australasian Society for Infectious Diseases: www.asid.net.au.

Communicable Diseases Network of Australia: www.health.gov.au/internet/main/publishing.nsf/Content/cda-cdna-index.htm.

Hand Hygiene Australia: www.hha.org.au.

Hand Hygiene New Zealand: www.handhygiene.org.nz.

Ministry of Health of New Zealand provides current information on (COVID-19): www.health.govt.nz.

National Health and Medical Research Council (NHMRC): Australian guidelines for the prevention and control of infection in healthcare, 2019. www.nhmrc.gov.au/about-us/publications/australian-guidelines-prevention-and-control-infection-healthcare-2019.

National Health and Medical Research Council (NHMRC): Clinical educators guide for the prevention and control of infection in healthcare, 2019. Commonwealth of Australia. www.nhmrc.gov.au/sites/default/files/documents/attachments/Clinical-Educators-Guide-WEB.pdf.

Needlestick Injury Hotline: Provides information about what to do after a needlestick injury. Freecall 1800 804 823.

References

Accardi R, Castaldi S, Marzullo A, et al: Prevention of healthcare associated infections: a descriptive study, Annali di Igiene 29(2):101–115, 2017.

Australian Commission on Safety and Quality in Health Care (ACSQHC): Carbapenemase-producing Enterobacteriaceae (CPE)—Information for clinicians, 2020. Online 15 June 2021. Available: www.safetyandquality.gov.au/publications-and-resources/resource-library/carbapenemase-producing-enterobacteriaceae-cpe-information-clinicians.

Australian Commission on Safety and Quality in Health Care (ACSQHC): National hand hygiene initiative manual. 2019. Available: www.safetyandquality.gov.au/sites/default/files/2020-09/nhhi_user_manual_-_sep_2020_1.pdf.

Australian Commission on Safety and Quality in Health Care (ACSQHC): National safety and quality health service standards. 2nd ed.—version 2. 2021. Available: www.safetyandquality.gov.au/sites/default/files/2021-05/national_safety_and_quality_health_service_nsqhs_standards_second_edition_-_updated_may_2021.pdf.

Australian Institute of Health and Welfare (AIHW): Bloodstream infections associated with hospital care 2019–20. Cat. no. HSE 240. Sydney, 2021. Online 15 June 2021. Available: www.aihw.gov.au/reports/health-care-quality-performance/bloodstream-infections-associated-withhospital-ca.

Australian Nursing & Midwifery Federation (ANMF): Diligence in infection prevention, Australian Nursing & Midwifery Journal 23(8):7, 2016.

Carrico AR, Spoden M, Wallston KA, et al: The environmental cost of misinformation: why the recommendation to use elevated temperatures for handwashing is problematic, International Journal of Consumer Studies 37(4):433–441, 2013.

Centers for Disease Control and Prevention: Methicillin-resistant *Staphylococcus aureus* (MRSA), 2015. Online 2 Jan 2018. Available: www.cdc.gov/mrsa/healthcare/index.html.

Clinical Excellence Commission: COVID-19 infection prevention and control manual for acute and non-acute healthcare settings, Sydney, 2021.

Clinical Excellence Commission: Infection prevention and control practice handbook. Sydney, 2020. Online 8 January 2021. Available: www.cec.health.nsw.gov.au/__data/assets/pdf_file/0010/383239/IPC-Practice-Handbook-2020.PDF.

Criscitelli T: Fast facts for the operating room nurse: an orientation and care guide in a nutshell, Springer Publishing Company, New York, 2014.

Department of Health: Infection control guidelines for the management of patients with suspected or confirmed pulmonary tuberculosis in healthcare settings, Australian Government, 2016. Online 15 June 2021. Available: www.health.gov.au/internet/main/publishing.nsf/content/cda-cdi4003i.htm.

Foong YC, Green M, Zargari A, et al: Mobile phones as a potential vehicle of infection in a hospital setting, Journal of Occupational and Environmental Hygiene 12:D232–D325, 2015.

Freeman JT, Dawson L, Jowitt DM, et al: The impact of the Hand Hygiene New Zealand programme on hand hygiene practices in New Zealand's public hospitals, The New Zealand Medical Journal 129(1443), 2016.

Godsell M, Shaban RZ, Gamble J: 'Recognizing rapport': Health professionals' lived experience of caring for patients under transmission-based precautions in an Australian health care setting, American Journal of Infection Control 41:971–975, 2013.

Goldberg JL: Guideline implementation: hand hygiene, AORN Journal 105(2):203–212, 2017.

Goto M, Al-Hasan MN: Overall burden of bloodstream infection and nosocomial bloodstream infection in North America and Europe, Clinical Microbiology and Infection 19:501–509, 2013.

Gray J: Infection control: beyond the horizon, Journal of Hospital Infection 89:237–240, 2015.

Griffith R: Reducing injuries from health care sharps, British Journal of Midwifery 23(1):68–69, 2015.

Hand Hygiene Australia (HHA): What is hand hygiene? 2021. Online 15 June 2021. Available: www.hha.org.au.

Harper A: Sepsis. In: Saving mothers' lives: reviewing maternal deaths to make motherhood safer: 2006–08. The eighth report on confidential enquiries into maternal deaths in the United Kingdom, British Journal of Obstetrics and Gynaecology 118(Suppl 1):85–96, 2011.

Harris AD, Morgan DJ, Pineles L, et al: Deconstructing the relative benefits of a universal glove and gown intervention on MRSA acquisition, Journal of Hospital Infection 96(1):49–53, 2017.

Hewagama S, Spelman T, Woolley M, et al: The epidemiology of *Staphylococcus aureus* and Panton-Valentine Leucocidin (*pvl*) in Central Australia, 2006–2010, BMC Infectious Diseases 16:1–6, 2016.

Higgins CL, Palmer AM, Cahill JL, et al: Occupational skin disease among Australian healthcare workers: a retrospective analysis from an occupational dermatology clinic, 1993–2014, Contact Dermatitis 75(4):213–222, 2016.

Jian S, Chow B, Hanowski B, et al: Correlation between hand hygiene compliance and methicillin-resistant *Staphylococcus aureus* incidence, The Canadian Journal of Infection Control 31(4):215–220, 2016.

Kingston LM, O'Connell NH, Dunne CP: Survey of attitudes and practices of Irish nursing students towards hand hygiene, including handrubbing with alcohol-based hand rub, Nurse Education Today 52:57–62, 2017.

Kwiecinski JM, Horswill AR: *Staphylococcus aureus* bloodstream infections: pathogenesis and regulatory mechanisms. Current Opinion in Microbiology, 53, 51–60, 2020. doi:10.1016/j.mib.2020.02.005.

Loveday HP, Wilson JA, Pratt RJ, et al: epic3: National evidence-based guidelines for preventing healthcare-associated infections in NHS hospitals in England, Journal of Hospital Infection 86(Suppl 1):S1–S70, 2014.

Martirani R, Weaving AP: Infection prevention and control. In Dougherty L, Lister S, editors: The Royal Marsden Hospital Manual of clinical nursing procedures, 8th ed., Wiley-Blackwell, Oxford, 2011, pp. 93–154.

Mata G, Oliver K, Geale S, et al: Infection control: it's not just what you wear–it's how you take it off, Australian Nursing & Midwifery Journal 23(3):55, 2015.

Mitchell BG, Say R, Wells A, et al: Australian graduating nurses' knowledge, intentions and beliefs on infection prevention and control: a cross-sectional study, BMC Nursing 13(43): 2014.

Murphy C: The serious and ongoing issue of needlestick in Australian Healthcare settings, Collegian (Royal College of Nursing, Australia) 21:295–299, 2014.

Murphy CM, Di Ruscio F, Lynskey M, et al: Identification badge lanyards as infection control risk: a cross-sectional observation study with epidemiological analysis, Journal of Hospital Infection 96:63–66, 2017.

Nagel JL, Kaye KS, LaPlante KL, et al: Antimicrobial stewardship for the infection control practitioner, Infectious Disease Clinics of North America 30:771–784, 2016.

National Health and Medical Research Council: Australian guidelines for the prevention and control of infection in healthcare. Commonwealth of Australia, Canberra, 2019. Available: www.nhmrc.gov.au/about-us/publications/australian-guidelines-prevention-and-control-infection-healthcare-2019.

National Institute for Health and Care Excellence (NICE): Infection prevention and control Quality Standard 61, 2014. Online 15 May 2017. Available: www.nice.org.uk.

NSW Health: Work health and safety—blood and body substances occupational exposure prevention. GL2018_013, 2018. Online 15 June 2021. Available: www1.health.nsw.gov.au/pds/ActivePDSDocuments/GL2018_013.pdf.

Olson CK, Iwamoto M, Perkins KM, et al: Preventing transmission of Zika virus in labour and delivery settings through implementation of standard precautions—United States, 2016, MMWR. Morbidity and Mortality Weekly Report 65(11):290–292, 2016.

Oster AM, Russell K, Stryker JE, et al: Update: Interim guidance for prevention of sexual transmission of Zika virus—United States, 2016, MMWR. Morbidity and Mortality Weekly Report 65:323–325, 2016.

Public Health Surveillance NZ: Zika Virus infections weekly report, 2017. Online 15 May 2017. Available: surv.esr.cri.nz.

Standards Australia: Single-use sterile rubber surgical gloves—Specification (ISO 10282:2014, MOD), 2014. Online 15 June 2021. Available online: www.standards.org.au/standards-catalogue/sa-snz/health/he-013/as-slash-nzs—4179-colon-2014.

Storr J, Twyman A, Zingg W, et al, WHO Guidelines Development Group: Core components for effective infection prevention and control programmes: new WHO evidence-based recommendations, Antimicrobial Resistance and Infection Control 6:6, 2017.

Tomas ME, Kundrapu S, Thota P, et al: Contamination of health care personnel during removal of personal protective equipment, JAMA Internal Medicine 175(12):1904–1910, 2015.

Turienzo CF, Brown M: What should midwives know about Zika virus infection? British Journal of Midwifery 24(10):694–700, 2016.

Turner NA, Sharma-Kuinkel BK, Maskarinec SA et al.: Methicillin-resistant *Staphylococcus aureus*: an overview of basic and clinical research. Nature Reviews Microbiology 17:203–218, 2019.

Victoria State Government: Coronavirus (COVID-19) Infection prevention and control guideline 26 October 2020, version 5, 2020.

White KM, Jimmieson NL, Graves N, et al: Key beliefs of hospital nurses' hand-hygiene behaviour: protecting your peers and needing effective reminders, Health Promotion Journal of Australia 26(1):74–78, 2015.

Wilson J, Loveday H: Does glove use increase the risk of infection? Nursing Times 110(39):12–15, 2014.

Wilson J, Prieto J, Singleton J, et al. The misuse and overuse of non-sterile gloves: application of an audit tool to define the problem, Journal of Infection Prevention 16(1):24–31, 2015.

World Health Organization (WHO): Report on the burden of endemic health care-associated infection worldwide. Clean care is safter care. WHO, 2011. Online 12 May 2017. Available: apps.who.int/iris/bitstream/10665/80135/1/9789241501507_eng.pdf.

World Health Organization (WHO): Timeline: WHO's COVID-19 response. WHO, 2021. Online 15 June 2021. Available: www.who.int/emergencies/diseases/novel-coronavirus-2019/interactive-timeline/#!.

Zimmerman P-A, Mason M, Elder E: A healthy degree of suspicion: A discussion of the implementation of transmission-based precautions in the emergency department, Australasian Emergency Nursing Journal 19(3):149–152, 2016.

CHAPTER 2
ASEPSIS

Learning outcomes

Having read this chapter, the reader should be able to:

- discuss the principles of asepsis, including non-touch technique and establishing an aseptic field
- identify key sites and key parts
- summarise the role and responsibilities of the midwife.

ASEPSIS

Asepsis refers to being free of pathological organisms and the process of destroying or removing organisms to prevent transmission of infection. Aseptic technique is a critical component of midwifery care. The goal of aseptic technique is to prevent pathogenic organisms from being present in sufficient amounts to cause infection and avoid the introduction of pathogenic organisms to susceptible sites by contaminated hands, surfaces and equipment (National Health and Medical Research Council [NHMRC] 2019). The term *sterile technique* has been used in the past; however, in normal clinical practice it is impossible to create a sterile environment and the term asepsis is now preferred. Healthcare-associated infections (HAIs) are costly in monetary and human terms and are often preventable. Not only can an infection destroy the lives of those we care for, but it can also have personal and professional ramifications. Healthcare complaints from lapses in asepsis techniques can lead to litigation. Healthcare professionals have lost their registration after deaths from sepsis were traced back to poor aseptic technique. A systematic review found research on aseptic techniques was lacking and translation into practice was poor (Haesler et al 2016). Midwives must know the principles of aseptic non-touch technique, which should remain constant in the practice of all clinical procedures to protect women from HAI.

Vaginal birth carries a low risk of HAI, but the risk increases twofold for planned caesarean births and tenfold in the context of an emergency caesarean section (Gregor et al 2014). Puerperal sepsis continues to be a leading cause of maternal death globally (Greer et al 2020). Caesarean section is considered a risk factor for development of puerperal sepsis (Buddeberg & Aveling 2015). Puerperal sepsis was once known as childbed fever and prior to the introduction of antibiotics caused 20–50% of maternal mortality (Buddeberg & Aveling 2015). The Australian Institute of Health and Welfare (AIHW 2020) maternal mortality report states 23 maternal deaths resulted from sepsis from 2009 to 2018. Sepsis may be related to endometritis, chorioamnionitis, postpartum puerperal sepsis and sepsis following a caesarean section. The Perinatal and Maternal Mortality Review Committee (PMMRC 2019) report indicates the maternal mortality ratio in New Zealand decreased from 10 per 100,000 births in 2016 to 9 in 2017. From 2006 to 2017 pregnancy-related infection caused 5% of direct maternal deaths, and infection in the context of preexisting conditions exacerbated by pregnancy and birth caused 7% of direct maternal deaths (PMMRC 2019).

THE ANTT PRACTICE FRAMEWORK

The *Australian Guidelines for the Prevention and Control of Infection in Healthcare* (NHMRC 2019) describe **aseptic non-touch technique (ANTT)** as the framework for aseptic practice. ANTT provides a sequential, logical standardised and auditable approach to asepsis management. The ANTT framework is also used in New Zealand and has been widely adopted internationally. The United Kingdom's National Institute for Health and Care Excellence (NICE 2017) recently reviewed their evidence on ANTT. Preventing sepsis is a multi-faceted issue and occurs in the context of the whole-of-healthcare provision, including appropriate prescribing of antibiotics, use of personal protective equipment (PPE), safe sharps disposal, staff education and environmental hygiene. The ANTT framework provides a standardised approach to protecting women from the introduction of pathogens and utilises three strands: education, standardised guidelines and an audit component.

The core components of ANTT include risk assessment, hand hygiene, glove use and aseptic fields, in addition to using a non-touch technique where key parts are identified and not touched either directly or indirectly (Loveday et al 2014). ANTT utilises two aseptic fields: a general aseptic field to promote asepsis and a critical aseptic field to ensure asepsis.

ANTT principles

In clinical practice, ANTT uses the following principles.

1. ANTT is used for invasive procedures and to maintain asepsis when using medical devices.
2. To achieve asepsis, key parts and key sites are protected, hindering transfer of microorganisms from the healthcare worker and the environment.
3. ANTT aims to be both efficient and safe, with surgical ANTT used for complex procedures and standard ANTT used for uncomplicated procedures.
4. The choice of standard or surgical ANTT is based on risk assessment, paying attention to the technical difficulty of protecting key parts and key sites.

Risk assessment

ANTT risk assessment considers the risk of contamination, the technical difficulty, the length of procedure and if key parts and sites will be touched (Fig 2.1).

Key parts and key sites

ANTT is based on a concept of key part and key site protection for all invasive procedures involving a risk of infection for the woman.

- **Key parts** are the critical parts of the equipment used for a procedure; if they become contaminated they are likely to cause an infection. Key parts are any items (equipment or fluids) that have direct or indirect contact with the key sites; for example, the peripheral cannula and the insertion point of any connections into it are both key parts. Before and after accessing key parts, such as needleless injection ports, catheter hubs, bottle tops or sampling ports, they should be cleaned with a 70% alcohol swab or solution (using a scrubbing action) and allowed to air-dry for a minimum of 15 seconds (Cameron-Watson 2016). Around 50% of IV catheter colonisation occurs post-insertion, making it critical to understand and comply with proper care of key parts (Moureau & Flynn 2015) (Fig 2.2).

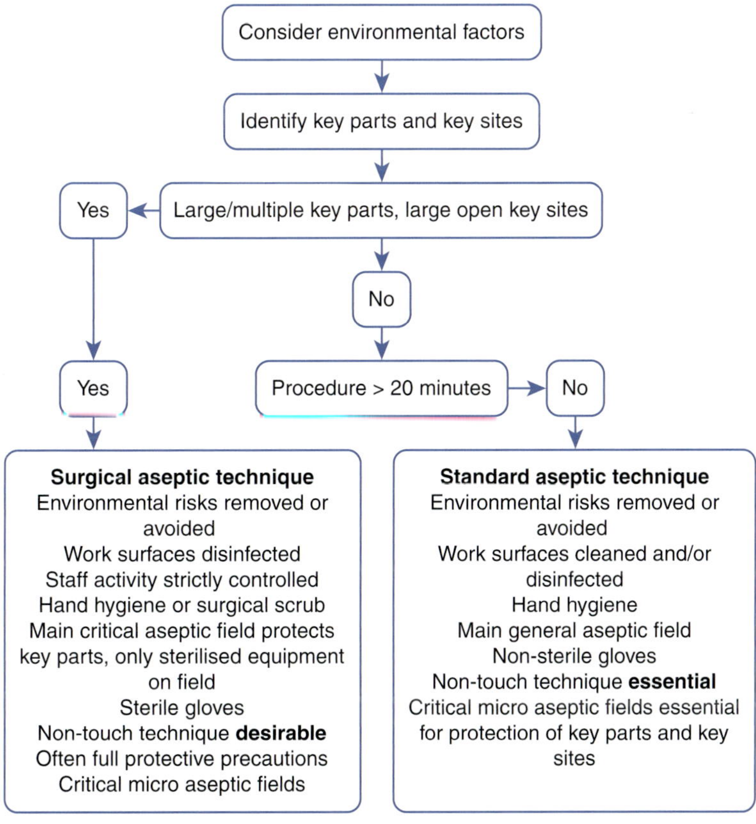

FIGURE 2.1 **Risk assessment flow chart.**

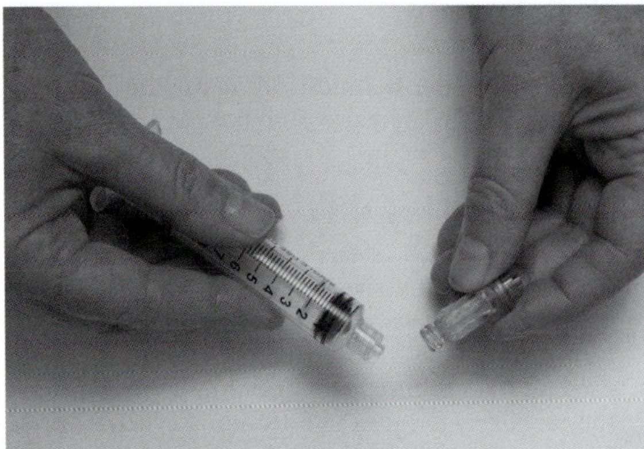

FIGURE 2.2 Examples of key parts: a syringe and a Luer lock connector.

- **Key sites** are any portal of entry on the woman that could be infected. This includes where medical devices access the body (e.g. insertion, puncture sites) (Fig 2.3) and open wounds (Rowley & Clare 2011). When inserting a urinary catheter, the key site is the urethra; if undertaking venepuncture, the key site is the skin/puncture site (Fig 2.3). Key sites require cleaning; for example, prior to venepuncture the skin should be cleaned for 30 seconds with 70% alcohol, 2% chlorhexidine (or locally approved cleanser), using the right-to-left and up-and-down approach.

STANDARD ANTT

A differentiation is made between standard ANTT and surgical ANTT. **Standard ANTT** generally uses a smaller general aseptic field and relies more heavily on a non-touch technique, and therefore may use non-sterile gloves. The midwife considers their level of competency and the technical difficulty of maintaining asepsis of key parts and key sites. If a procedure is likely to take 20 minutes or less and be technically simple due to involving few and relatively small key parts and key sites, then it is safe and efficient to use standard ANTT. The main aseptic field in standard ANTT is managed 'generally', and clean but not necessarily sterile equipment may be placed onto it. It is therefore promoting asepsis. On a general aseptic field, key parts are protected by individual caps and covers, which are said to be micro critical aseptic fields. The available equipment (e.g. plastic tray or dressings trolley) is cleaned using the locally approved cleanser. Sterile items, such as dressings pack, are then removed from their outer packaging and placed onto the cleansed area. Care is taken to open the pack using only the corners so that the inside of the pack remains an aseptic field. Other items are then added aseptically to the field. For some standard ANTT procedures sterile gloves are worn (e.g. urinary catheterisation, perineal repair, vaginal birth) and local protocols should be followed. Examples of standard ANTT include:

- venepuncture and peripheral cannulation
- urinary catheterisation

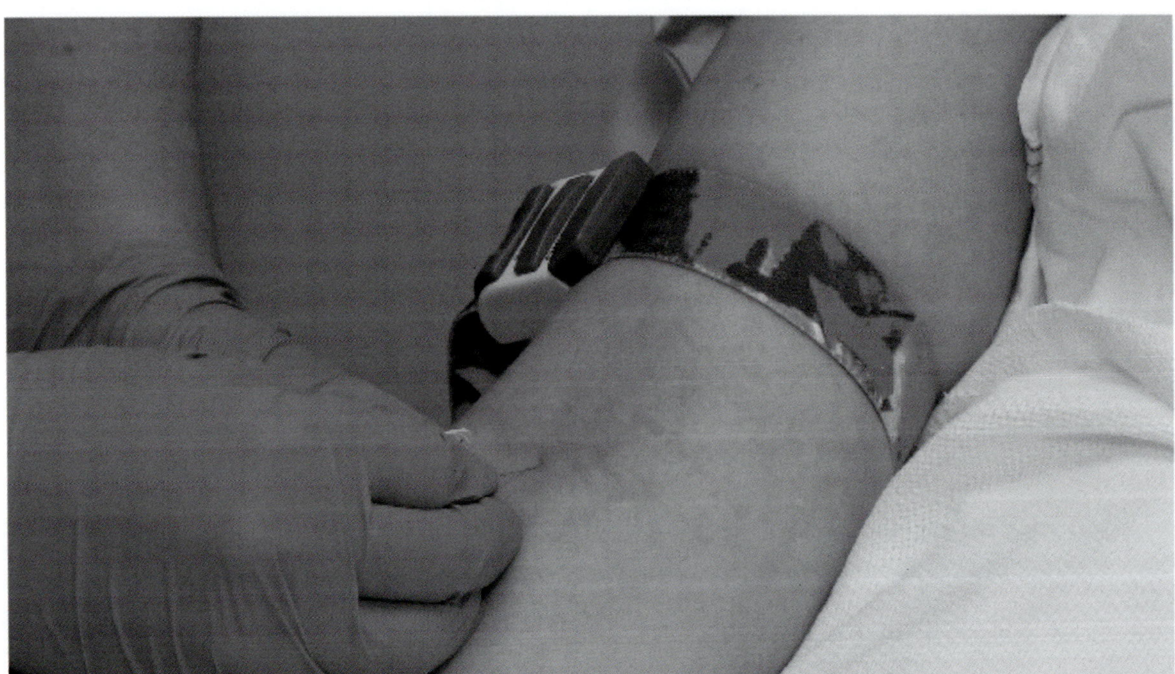

FIGURE 2.3 Key site venepuncture.

- examination per vaginam
- childbirth
- perineal suturing
- simple wound dressing.

Standard ANTT is used for birth; the equipment is opened onto a sterile field using a non-touch technique. Although the perineal area is not sterile and birth is not a sterile process, the midwife must avoid introducing contamination into the genital tract. Serious puerperal sepsis has been linked to a health professional who carried group A streptococcal bacteria in lesions on her hands (Palaniappan et al 2012).

SURGICAL ANTT

Surgical ANTT is used in operating theatres and consists of a surgical hand scrub, full protective gown and sterile gloves. Surgical ANTT uses a critical aseptic field managed as a key part, so only sterilised equipment and items can come into contact with it. Surgical ANTT is also used in other clinical settings for complicated invasive procedures, such as insertion of central lines and epidurals. Midwives frequently set up the equipment for insertion of an epidural and support the anaesthetist during the insertion process while continuing to attend to the woman's needs.

If the procedure is more complex, will take a long time or involves larger key sites or many key parts, then surgical ANTT is appropriate. Sometimes ANTT-specific risk assessment may determine that a procedure falls into either category due to the competency of the practitioner or the technical difficulty of maintaining key part/site protection. Whichever approach is used, the emphasis is on the *non-touching* of key sites and key parts. This is the case when surgical ANTT is used for:

- complex or large wound dressings
- peripherally inserted central venous catheter (PICC) or central venous catheter (CVC) insertion
- epidural insertion
- lower segment caesarean section.

Use a non-touch technique to protect key parts and key sites from contamination. Even when wearing sterile gloves, key parts should not be touched directly if possible. When establishing an aseptic field, avoid touching any materials as they are placed on the field.

Be aware of contributory factors (e.g. hand hygiene) and environmental conditions. The ANTT guidelines show clearly when hand hygiene should take place (see Resources for website address). This is always before commencing and after completing a procedure and may also be necessary during the procedure. For example, hand hygiene should be performed prior to assessing a site for cannulation and again before inserting the cannula. Before undertaking an aseptic procedure it is important to minimise possible environmental contamination, such as bed-making or people coughing nearby, as this can increase airborne pathogens.

Equipment

Centrally sterilised equipment is usually autoclaved. The colour change on the packet indicates sterility, but the pack should be inspected to ensure it has not been damaged or wet prior to use. Sterile items should be used before their expiry date. Sterile lotions, syringes, cannulas and so on are all supplied for single use only (unless otherwise stated) and are disposed of after use. Increasingly, a system operates that allows sterile packs to be traced through the system, from central sterilising through to which operator used them for which woman. A label (or something similar) is placed in the woman's record after the equipment has been used and the same verification returns to the sterile supplies department.

Use of an assistant

Frequently in practice the midwife will undertake aseptic procedures alone. However, the use of an assistant is helpful in maintaining the asepsis. The assistant needs to:

- perform hand hygiene
- handle and open the external wrappers and pass the sterile contents to the aseptic field or directly to the midwife (Fig 2.4) if asked
- aid the woman to be comfortable and 'uncovered' at the correct time
- take care not to contaminate the sterile field
- collect additional items if necessary.

SKILL 2.1 Aseptic procedure

1. Check the identity of the woman and ensure she has given consent and is in an appropriate place for the procedure.
2. Perform hand hygiene, locate a clean trolley and tray, and clean them with the locally approved wipes.
3. Gather the equipment needed, checking for sterility, expiry date and so on. Place on the lower shelf of the trolley.
4. Take the trolley to the woman and position her accordingly, keeping her covered until ready.
5. Perform hand hygiene and put on an apron.
6. Hold the outer wrapper of the sterile pack and open it carefully (not touching any part of the inner wrapper) onto the cleansed trolley top.
7. Open out the sterile inner wrapper by using only the corners or edges of the paper to create an aseptic field (Fig 2.5).

Continued

SKILL 2.1 Aseptic procedure—cont'd

8. Slide or 'drop' all other items needed onto the aseptic field without them touching anything else.
9. Use alcohol-based hand rub (ABHR) or wash hands with soap and water, then apply the chosen gloves.
10. Ensure the woman is comfortable and ask her to remove any covers. Establish an aseptic field around her, placing the drapes appropriately.
11. Undertake the procedure using a non-touch technique for all key sites and key parts.
12. Once this is completed and the woman is made comfortable, dispose of the equipment correctly. Dispose of the aseptic field by wrapping the remaining contents (if disposable) in the paper and placing them in a waste container.
13. Remove gloves and apron and put them into the clinical waste.
14. Clean the trolley using the locally agreed wipes.
15. Prepare non-disposable items for return to the sterile supplies department in the agreed format.
16. Perform hand hygiene and complete the woman's records.

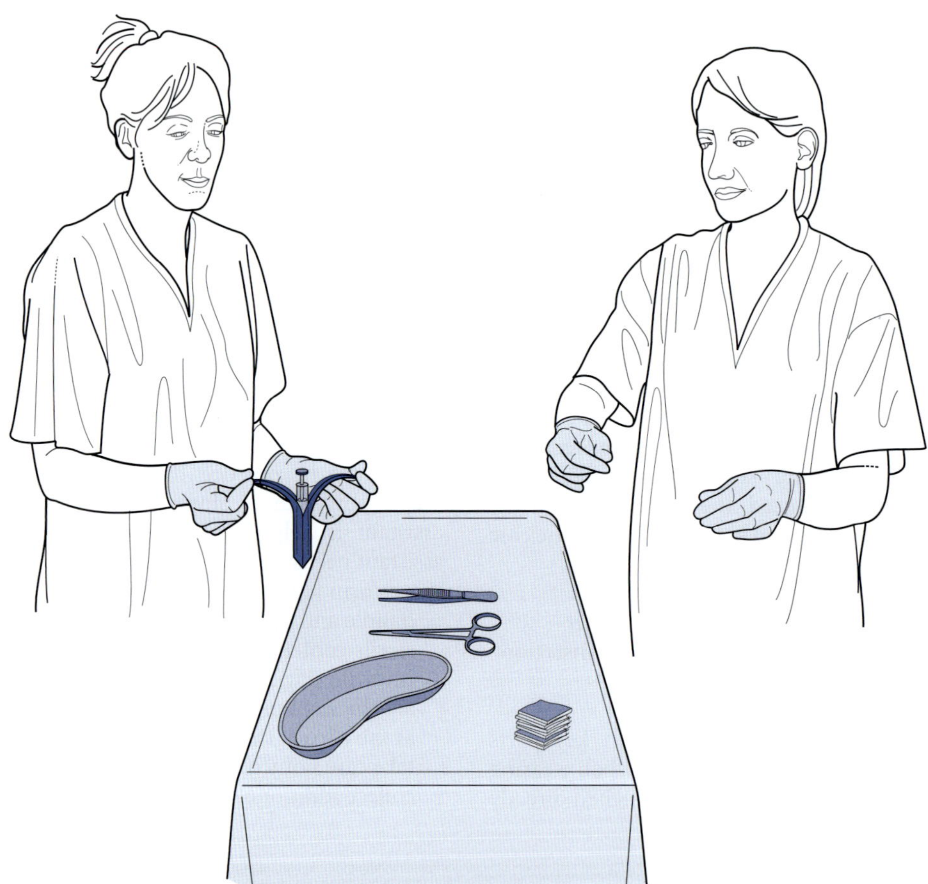

FIGURE 2.4 **Assistant passing items to maintain an aseptic field.** Source: Nicol M, Bavin C, Bedford-Turner S, et al: Essential nursing skills, 2nd ed, Mosby, Edinburgh, 2000.

Surgical scrub

This involves washing the hands and forearms to remove as many transient and resident microorganisms as possible and maintain the lowest possible microbial count throughout the surgical procedure. Washing should take at least 3–5 minutes (Australian College of Perioperative Nurses [ACORN] 2014). A surgical scrub requires a deep sink with automatic controls and an antimicrobial scrub solution. A surgical scrub brush (usually with a sponge on one side) and a nail pick are used as part of a surgical scrub.

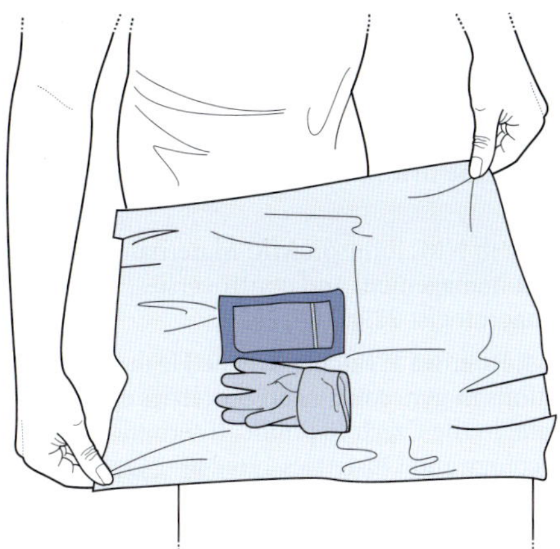

FIGURE 2.5 **Opening a sterile pack to create an aseptic field.**
Source: Nicol M, Bavin C, Bedford-Turner S, et al: Essential nursing skills, 2nd ed, Mosby, Edinburgh, 2000.

SKILL 2.2 Surgical scrub

1. Remove all jewellery and don protective equipment such as a surgical face mask.
2. Scrub all surfaces of the hands, beginning with the nails and fingers, and then wash the forearms. The first scrub of the day should take 5 minutes and subsequent scrubs 3 minutes (ACORN 2014).
3. Ensure fingernails are short and clean with no nail polish, fillers or artificial nails.
4. Check hands for damage such as lesions, abrasions or cuts.
5. Turn the taps on and adjust the water flow and temperature to lukewarm, taking care not to splash the water.
6. Start the timer, wet hands and forearms under running water and lather with antimicrobial solution to 5 cm below the elbows, keeping hands higher than elbows.
7. Under running water clean under nails with a bristled scrub brush or nail pick.
8. Rinse hands and arms under running water.
9. Wash arms with circular motion from hands to elbows without returning to hands; discard the brush.
10. Re-apply antimicrobial solution and wash all surfaces of hands, fingers and wrists. Wash arms using a circular motion from hands to elbows; do not return to hands.
11. Ensuring hands are above elbows, rinse hands and arms carefully under running water without touching taps.
12. Turn off taps using the electronic sensor or foot pedal. Shake off excess water, clasp hands and hold away from the body.
13. Walk carefully to the operating theatre to dry hands with a sterile towel and don sterile gown and gloves.

Role and responsibilities of the midwife

These can be summarised as:

- appreciating the significance and principles of aseptic practice and undertaking the procedure thoroughly and consistently; the ANTT framework uses a non-touch technique for all key sites on the woman and key parts of the equipment and fluids, so practice should be regularly updated and midwives should ensure they maintain competency
- working in a team, which allows the midwife to seek support if unsure and to challenge any examples of poor practice; staff should protect themselves as well as their clients
- documenting all care given contemporaneously
- in partnership with the woman and considering her wishes, discussing the best available evidence.

SUMMARY

- The principles of asepsis should be included (adapted if necessary) for every invasive procedure in which body defences are breached.
- ANTT offers a standardised technique. When undertaking an aseptic procedure, the midwife should not touch the key site or the key parts. These are different for each procedure.
- When touching key parts or key sites is unavoidable, sterile gloves should be used.
- The ANTT approach includes risk assessment, management of the environment, use of aseptic fields, non-touch technique and prevention of cross-infection.
- Effective hand hygiene is essential before and after every patient contact, and often during procedures.

Self-assessment exercises

The answers to the following questions may be found in the text.

1. Give four examples of the circumstances in which aseptic practice is indicated.
2. List examples of key parts and key sites.
3. Demonstrate opening a sterile pack, including preparation of the aseptic surface used.
4. Summarise the role and responsibilities of the midwife when undertaking an aseptic procedure.

Resources

AVATAR Group, Alliance for Vascular Access Teaching and Research: www.avatargroup.org.au.

Aseptic Non-Touch Technique (ANTT): www.antt.org.

Australian and New Zealand Audit of Surgical Mortality: National Report 2016, Adelaide, 2017. Online 3 July 2021. Available: www.surgeons.org/-/media/Project/

RACS/surgeons-org/files/surgical-mortality-audits/anzasm-reports/2017-10-05_rpt_racs_anzasm_national_report_2016.pdf.

Australian College of Perioperative Nurses (ACORN): www.acorn.org.au.

Australian Council on Healthcare Standards (ACHS): www.achs.org.au.

Bowden F: Golden staph: the deadly bug that wreaks havoc in hospitals. The Conversation, 2015. Online 3 July 2021. Available: theconversation.com/golden-staph-the-deadly-bug-that-wreaks-havoc-in-hospitals-39790.

Infection Prevention & Control Nurses College (IPCNC): www.infectioncontrol.co.nz.

MJA Podcasts: Episode 17. Antimicrobial resistances with Professor Cheryl Jones, 206(7), 2017. Online 3 July 2021. Available: www.mja.com.au/multimedia/podcasts?utm_source=mja&utm_medium=web&utm_campaign=related_content#2017-04-13T01_07_39-07_00.

National Health and Medical Research Council (NHMRC): Australian Guidelines for the Prevention and Control of Infection in Healthcare. 3.1.6 Aseptic technique. Commonwealth of Australia, Canberra, 2019. Online 13 March 2021. Available: www.nhmrc.gov.au/about-us/publications/australian-guidelines-prevention-and-control-infection-healthcare-2019.

National Institute for Health and Care Excellence (NICE): Infection evidence update September 2014. Evidence Update 64, 2014. Online 15 Jan 2018. Available: www.nice.org.uk/guidance/cg139/evidence/evidence-update-185182813.

NSW Government Health Care Complaints Commission: Annual Report 2019–20, 2020. Online 3 July 2021. Available: www.hccc.nsw.gov.au/Publications/Annual-Reports.

References

Australian College of Perioperative Nurses (ACORN): Aseptic non-touch technique (ANTT), 2014. Online 3 July 2021. Available: www.antt.org.

Australian Institute of Health and Welfare (AIHW): Maternal deaths in Australia. Cat. no. PER 99, AIHW, Canberra, 2020. Online 7 January 2021. Available: www.aihw.gov.au/reports/mothers-babies/maternal-deaths-in-australia.

Buddeberg BS, Aveling W: Puerperal sepsis in the 21st century: progress, new challenges and the situation worldwide, Postgraduate Medical Journal 91:572–578, 2015.

Cameron-Watson C: Port protectors in clinical practice: an audit, The British Journal of Nursing 25(8):S25–S31, 2016.

Greer O, Shah NM, Johnson MR: Maternal sepsis update: current management and controversies, The Obstetrician & Gynaecologist 22:45–55, 2020.

Gregor M, Paterová P, Buchta V, et al: Healthcare-associated infections in gynecology and obstetrics at a university hospital in the Czech Republic, International Journal of Gynecology and Obstetrics 126:240–243, 2014.

Haesler E, Thomas L, Morey P, et al: A systematic review of the literature addressing asepsis in wound management, Wound Practice & Research 24(4):208–216, 2016.

Loveday H, Wilson W, Pratt RJ, et al: Epic3: National evidence-based guidelines for preventing healthcare—associated infections in NHS hospitals in England, Journal of Hospital Infection 86(Suppl 1):S1–S70, 2014.

Moureau NL, Flynn J: Disinfection of needleless connector hubs: clinical evidence systematic review, Nursing Research and Practice Article ID:796762, 2015.

National Health and Medical Research Council (NHMRC): Australian Guidelines for the Prevention and Control of Infection in Healthcare, Canberra: Commonwealth of Australia. 2019. Online 13 March 2021. Available: www.nhmrc.gov.au/about-us/publications/australian-guidelines-prevention-and-control-infection-healthcare-2019.

National Institute for Health and Care Excellence (NICE): Surveillance report 2017—Health-care-associated infections (2012) NICE guideline CG139, 16 January 2017. Available: www.ncbi.nlm.nih.gov/books/NBK551731/.

Palaniappan N, Menezes M, Willson P: Group A streptococcal puerperal sepsis: management and prevention. Obstetrician & Gynaecologist 14:9–16, 2012.

Perinatal and Maternal Mortality Review Committee (PMMRC): Thirteenth annual report of the Perinatal and Maternal Mortality Review Committee: reporting mortality 2017, Health Quality & Safety Commission New Zealand, Wellington, 2019. Available: www.hqsc.govt.nz/assets/PMMRC/Publications/13thPMMRCreport/13thPMMRCAnnualReportWebFINAL.pdf.

Rowley S, Clare S: ANTT: A standard approach to aseptic technique, Nursing Times 107(36):12–14, 2011.

CHAPTER 3

PRINCIPLES OF HYGIENE NEEDS

Learning outcomes

Having read this chapter, the reader should be able to:

- discuss the ways in which the midwife facilitates personal hygiene
- describe perineal care
- identify the principles applied for the making of an occupied or unoccupied bed
- discuss the midwife's role and responsibilities in relation to each of these aspects of care.

This chapter considers the skills required to meet the complete range of hygiene needs of the woman. Cleanliness and attention to physical appearance can be significant in promoting psychological wellbeing, as well as physical health. The principles of bed-making are considered, as well as personal, perineal and oral hygiene.

PERSONAL HYGIENE

Cleanliness is a basic human right and can help people feel comfortable and well cared for. Maintaining personal hygiene needs to be tailored to a person's needs and abilities (Green 2014).

Midwives work with women who are generally able to care for their own hygiene needs. However, women may need assistance with personal hygiene in the following situations:

- immobility—epidural or spinal analgesia, surgery or existing mobility problem
- intensive or high-dependency care
- prescribed bed rest (e.g. antepartum haemorrhage)
- multiple pregnancy
- post-caesarean section or other surgery such as cerclage placement.

Maintaining personal hygiene improves wellbeing and self-image (Veje et al 2019). Psychologically most people feel 'better' when they can wash. The skin itself is the largest body organ and needs to be kept free from breaks and infection to protect the inner organs. When a wound does exist, good standards of hygiene help to prevent bacterial colonisation and aid healing (Powers & Fortney 2014). Perineal hygiene is important, particularly when perineal trauma is present. Pouring warm water over the perineum and patting the area dry from front to back will keep the area clean, and women should also be advised to change sanitary pads regularly (Hajjaj 2017). Pressure area care is an important aspect of care to help maintain skin integrity.

In ensuring the woman's hygiene needs are met, the midwife should consider facilitating as much independence as is possible. Many people will feel embarrassed to have someone else undertaking very personal aspects of care; mobility is also encouraged when appropriate to reduce the thromboembolic risks that accompany childbearing.

Personal hygiene needs can be met by:

- assisting a woman to sit with a bowl, or at a sink, with the midwife assisting as necessary
- assisting a woman into a shower, remaining with her or returning after a few minutes to assist as required.

When assisting a woman to facilitate her own needs, care should be taken to ensure she has everything she needs with her (clean clothes, toiletries, pads, towels, etc.) and she has access to assistance and a call bell. Following birth, a woman may become light-headed when she stands up and blood loss often increases. When a woman gets up for the first time it is important to progress slowly and check that she does not feel light-headed. It is preferable to have a person in the room the first time the woman has a shower or goes to the toilet. Women may need support with toileting and this is an important aspect of personal hygiene. The need for analgesia should be considered prior to showering or getting up after a caesarean section. Women may find it tiring getting up to go to the toilet, washing and dressing.

Assisting with hygiene needs necessitates risk assessment. The use of infection control strategies (standard precautions and personal protective equipment [PPE]) and moving and handling guidelines should be employed accordingly (Patrick 2016). Consideration should also be given to upholding individual wishes, cultural preferences, dignity and privacy.

BED BATHING

Bed bathing aims to meet the complete hygiene needs of a woman if she is confined to bed. If it is required, bed bathing can support psychological wellbeing by providing uninterrupted individualised care. Soap (or soap substitute) and water are equally effective cleansing agents for use during a bed bath (Groven et al 2017). It is also a time in which holistic care is completed. The following aspects of care should accompany a bed bath:

- observation of consciousness and levels of pain at rest and with movement
- observation of the skin, particularly areas of pressure inflammation, infection or allergy
- general health and nourishment, oral intake of diet and fluids
- ante- or postnatal examination
- assessment of vital signs
- wound care
- catheter or bladder care
- bowel care
- attention to circulation, passive or active exercises
- observations for varicosities or oedema
- prevention of complications associated with immobility
- care of intravenous infusion and fluid balance
- oral hygiene
- hair washing, pedicure or manicure
- therapeutic touch, communication, education
- attention to a safe and aesthetic environment, including changes of sheets and bedding.

SKILL 3.1 Bed bath

- Discuss the procedure and obtain informed consent.
- Offer analgesia as necessary.
- Conduct the procedure in a warm environment.
- Gather all necessary equipment (washbasin, washcloths, bath towels, bath blanket, clean nightclothes, linen bag) before commencing to reduce the risk of interruption.
- Use the woman's own or single-use toiletries.
- Ensure privacy by closing door or curtains.
- Perform hand hygiene and don disposable gloves; check the woman does not have a latex allergy if latex gloves are to be used.
- Provide a bedpan if necessary.
- Raise the bed to a comfortable height.
- Lower the closest side rail and help the woman into a comfortable position with correct body alignment.
- Loosen the covers at the foot of the bed and place a blanket over the top sheet, then fold the sheet and remove it from beneath the blanket.
- Remove gown or nightclothes (if IV is in situ remove clothing from the arm without an IV first, then slide clothing over the arm with IV tubing and remove).
- Put the side rail up and place the washbasin containing warm water on the side table.
- Place a towel under each area to be washed then expose the area; use a washcloth to clean each area then rinse each area and pat dry.
- Cleanse areas such as the perineum using disposable cloths or change the washcloth after use.
- Change water as necessary (e.g. after cleansing the perineum).
- Use a coordinated approach so there is minimal exposure of the body.
- Dress the woman in a clean gown or her own nightclothes.
- Dispose of soiled linen and equipment appropriately.
- Ensure the woman is in a comfortable position and has access to her call bell and anything else she may need.
- Remove gloves and perform hand hygiene.

SKILL 3.2 Modified bed bath and postoperative wash

A modified bed bath and postoperative wash follow the same procedure as a bed bath with the following modifications.

Modified bed bath

- Place the washbowl (containing warm water), toiletries, washcloth and towel on a tray in front of the woman.
- Allow the woman to wash and dry her face, chest, arms and other areas she wishes to bathe.
- Wash the woman's back or any areas which are difficult for her to access comfortably.

Postoperative wash

- Offer analgesia prior to commencing.
- Wash the woman's face, hands, arms, chest and abdomen.
- Provide perineal care, assess lochia and replace maternity pad if necessary.
- Roll the woman onto her side and wash her back.
- Change the underpad and drawsheet (plus sheet if soiled) by rolling up the drawsheet/sheet as for making an occupied bed.
- Remove the theatre gown and dress the woman in a clean gown or her own nightclothes.

After birth, all women, regardless of mode of birth, will have lochial loss and require good perineal hygiene to help prevent infection, promote healing and increase comfort. In 2018 approximately 22% of women who experienced an unassisted vaginal birth had an episiotomy and 78% with an instrumental birth received an episiotomy, while approximately 3% of women with a vaginal birth sustained a third- or fourth-degree tear (Australian Institute of Health and Welfare [AIHW] 2020). The midwife may perform perineal hygiene or support the woman to undertake it herself. Plain warm water is used as soaps and other substances can be irritants to the delicate tissues of the perineum. When a woman is sitting on the toilet (or bedpan) warm water can be poured over the genital area, followed by gently patting the area dry with disposable wipes.

SKILL 3.3 Care of the woman with perineal trauma

Women need to be assisted with evidence-based care of the perineum and be aware of the signs and symptoms of an infected perineal wound. For an extensive discussion of perineal care see Pairman and colleagues, *Midwifery: Preparation for Practice* (4th ed., 2018). Midwives need to understand the process of perineal wound healing, how to provide appropriate perineal wound care, assist with alleviating perineal pain and to ask women if they have any concerns (Steen & Diaz 2018). Women have indicated that they experience a lack of adequate information and support regarding perineal care (Lindberg et al 2020).

Perineal care includes:

- using maternity pads as they are softer and generate less friction (Bick & Bassett 2013)
- regularly changing sanitary pads and washing hands before and after changing pads
- regularly cleansing the perineum, bathing or showering at least daily, gently patting the area dry (Bick & Bassett 2013)
- treating pain with systemic analgesia such as paracetamol, rectal indomethacin suppository (Delaram et al 2015) or topical lignocaine (Delaram et al 2015) that does not contain steroids as they can lead to wound breakdown (Dahlen 2015)
- applying ice or gel packs, which can be used in the first 24–72 hours (de Souza Bosco Paiva et al 2016)
- following a careful diet (increase in protein, vitamins and fibre), as this can aid healing and prevent constipation
- recommencing pelvic floor muscle exercises, as this has been shown to decrease urinary incontinence episodes (Hall & Woodward 2015)
- being alert to signs of perineal infection, including persistent or increasing pain, oedema, delayed healing and discharge (Dalton & Castillo 2014)
- checking the area daily with a hand mirror
- supporting the perineal wound when coughing or defecating
- applying topical lavender, which may be soothing (Steen & Diaz 2018).

ORAL HYGIENE

Oral hygiene makes an important contribution to good health, and poor oral hygiene is associated with systemic diseases (Danckert et al 2016). Inadequate oral hygiene can result in gingivitis, cavities, halitosis, discomfort and pain (Bonetti et al 2015). The oral cavity houses over 500 species of bacteria, some of which may cause periodontal disease in susceptible women (Moore & Blair 2017).

Diabetes, malabsorption from coeliac disease, iron deficiency and inadequate plaque removal are associated with periodontal disease (Critchlow 2017). Other risk factors related to periodontal disease and dental decay include a diet high in refined carbohydrates and smoking. Dental decay is not just a localised problem but is associated with cardiovascular disease, diabetes and respiratory infection (Vamos et al 2015). Saliva is vital to maintain the health of the oral tissue and helps with digestion and mastication. Xerostomia (dry mouth) is a common medication side effect and causes discomfort, taste disturbances and difficulty with speaking (Critchlow 2017).

During pregnancy, increasing hormone levels can affect the host immune–inflammatory response to bacteria in the oral cavity, increasing inflammation and leading to red, tender and swollen gums (Moore & Blair 2017). Pregnancy also increases susceptibility to gingivitis (inflammation of soft tissue around the tooth) and periodontitis (inflammation which destroys supporting structures around the tooth). In addition, changes in saliva pH and fluid retention within the gums can predispose women to dental caries. C-reactive protein, a marker of inflammation, is higher when periodontal disease is present during pregnancy due to an increase in systemic inflammation. Periodontal pathogens and their by-products may spread, possibly triggering a placental/fetal inflammatory response which has been linked to adverse events such as premature birth, pre-eclampsia and low birth weight (Moore & Blair 2017). During pregnancy only one-third of women living in Australia consult a dentist (George et al 2012).

Oral hygiene involves assessing and keeping the oral cavity clean, moist and pathogen-free (Coke et al 2015). The oral cavity includes the gums, tongue, lips and teeth. Unfortunately, women's oral health is often neglected during pregnancy when swollen or bleeding gums may be present (Vamos et al 2015). A study in New South Wales found that while many midwives are interested in oral health during pregnancy, they do not provide information on oral health as they lack expertise and appropriate guidelines (George et al 2016). The majority of well women in the perinatal period can attend to their own oral hygiene without assistance. However, the hospital environment can have an impact on oral hygiene as women may not be able to clean their teeth without help and items such as a toothbrush may not be accessible (Danckert et al 2016). In hospitals patients often receive inadequate oral hygiene (Bruan-Wimmer & Ruiz-Skol 2012).

The oral mucosa and lips should remain soft, moist and damage-free, the teeth free from plaque and debris. These measures help prevent oral infection and discomfort. Good oral hygiene also helps prevent ventilator-associated pneumonia in those requiring intensive care (Kiyoshi-Teo & Blegen 2015).

Physically, an unclean mouth is unpleasant; it can also affect how the woman feels psychologically. If a woman is unable to attend to her own oral hygiene, for whatever reason, the midwife must carry out this aspect of care with her. Informed consent is gained.

Likely occasions when the midwife will need to assist include:

- when nil by mouth:
  - pre- or post-surgery
  - nasogastric tube in situ
  - unconscious, receiving intensive or high-dependency care
- nausea and vomiting
- oxygen therapy
- mouth breathing (e.g. labour)
- use of inhalational analgesia
- if affected by mouth-drying or unpleasant tasting medicines
- diabetes.

SKILL 3.4 Oral hygiene

For oral hygiene, essential equipment includes:

- a toothbrush, soft with a small head
- toothpaste, fluoride, pea-sized amount
- water for rinsing, paper towels for drying, receiver for spitting (if not at the sink)
- interdental brushes.

Depending on the woman's position and degree of alertness, covering for her clothing may be needed. Ideally the woman is in an upright position, but if this is not possible suction may be needed. The unconscious or semiconscious woman will benefit from the use of a specific suction toothbrush (Chick & Wynne 2020).

The toothbrush is held against the teeth with the bristles at a 45° angle (bristles pointing towards the roots of the teeth) (Jones 2014) and moved gently, slightly from side to side, systematically around the top and then the lower jaw, on all surfaces of the teeth. Electric toothbrushes should be held over the tooth being cleaned for 10 seconds, and then moved onto the next tooth. The need to 'scrub' the teeth is not necessary when the brushhead is revolving.

The tongue and gums can also be gently brushed (Wilson 2011), and the mouth should be rinsed thoroughly. Foam sticks are considered less effective than a toothbrush, but may be useful in situations where the mouth is sore. Mouthwash is also an alternative to brushing, but only on a short-term basis. Lip balm or moisturiser may be applied to dry, chapped lips.

If possible, the woman should rinse her mouth and spit the contents into a container. This aspect of care is documented at the same time, as for any other aspect of care.

BED-MAKING

Changing sheets or remaking a bed is indicated if the sheets are soiled, sweaty or dishevelled. The aim is to ensure the bed is crease-free to protect skin integrity and increase comfort. Standard precautions and correct disposal of used linen reduce the risk of infection transmission. The timing of bed-making should fit in with the needs of the woman and her infant. The infants of postnatal women also often have contact with the woman's bed clothes, such as using pillows when breastfeeding; this also necessitates frequent bed linen changes to minimise the infant's exposure to potential cross-infection.

SKILL 3.5 Bed-making

- Gather all equipment before commencing. The bed should be at a suitable working height for both practitioners and should be easily accessible.
- Clean the mattress according to the agreed protocol if it is contaminated in any way.
- Take care to ensure none of the bedding touches the floor, such as the pillows or other items that will be reapplied to the bed; these should be carefully stacked on a clean surface.
- Work in a coordinated way (e.g. lifting the mattress at the same time; this allows the sheets to be anchored correctly).
- Consider the woman's preference when deciding how many layers of bedding to add.
- Keep a linen skip close by so soiled linen can be disposed of immediately.

SKILL 3.6 Making an occupied bed

- Explain the procedure.
- Offer analgesia prior to making the bed if necessary.
- Ensure all catheters, drains and infusions are in a safe position and will not have traction applied.
- Maintain temperature by keeping the woman warm and covered.
- Maintain privacy by covering the woman with a sheet or blanket.
- Assist the woman to roll onto her side, facing the assistant.
- Untuck the old sheet and roll it up next to the woman's back (Fig 3.1).
- Tuck in the new sheet at the top, bottom and side of the bed and roll it up next to the woman's back.
- Assist the woman to roll over the 'lump' of linen to face the midwife on her other side.
- Remove old linen.
- The new sheet is pulled outwards and tucked in.
- Reposition the woman into a comfortable position.

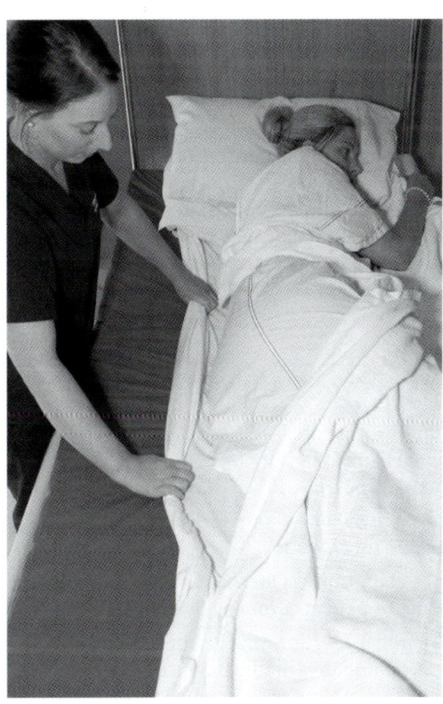

FIGURE 3.1 Making an occupied bed. Untucking the old sheet and rolling it up next to the woman's back.

Role and responsibilities of the midwife

These can be summarised as:

- completing the procedures safely with the maintenance of dignity and privacy, applying infection control, moving and handling protocols
- ensuring informed consent is gained and working within current evidence-based practice offering an individualised approach, encouraging independence and mobility where possible
- contemporaneous record keeping.

SUMMARY

- Attention to all types of hygiene benefits the physical and psychological wellbeing of the woman. Good hygiene reduces infection and improves wound healing.
- The midwife should adapt care according to the individual woman's needs and level of dependence.
- Perineal hygiene may be both cleansing and soothing, particularly after a vaginal birth.
- Inadequate oral hygiene can contribute to poor health.

Self-assessment exercises

The answers to the following questions may be found in the text.

1. Discuss the significance of personal hygiene.
2. Identify the ways in which a woman may be assisted to wash when her mobility is restricted.
3. Discuss the advice given to a woman regarding the care of her perineum.
4. Demonstrate bed-making—occupied and unoccupied.
5. Describe how to complete an oral toilet.
6. Summarise the midwife's responsibilities in relation to the complete hygiene needs of the woman.

References

Australian Institute of Health and Welfare (AIHW): National Core Maternity Indicators 2018: summary report, Cat. no. PER 109, AIHW, Canberra, 2020.

Bick D, Bassett S: How to provide postnatal perineal care, Midwives 16(2):34–35, 2013.

Bonetti D, Hampson V, Queen K, et al: Improving oral hygiene for patients, Nursing Standard 29:44–50, 2015.

Bruan-Wimmer JA, Ruiz-Skol P: Impact of an oral hygiene education initiative on the practice of oral care by unregulated care providers guided by registered nurses, Canadian Journal of Dental Hygiene 46:223–230, 2012.

Chick A, Wynne A: Introducing an oral care assessment tool with advanced cleaning products into a high-risk clinical setting. British Journal of Nursing 29(5):290–296, 2020.

Coke L, Otten K, Staffileno B, et al: The impact of an oral hygiene education module on patient practices and nursing documentation, Clinical Journal of Oncology Nursing 19:75–80, 2015.

Critchlow D: Part 3: Impact of systemic conditions and medications on oral health, British Journal of Community Nursing 22:181–190, 2017.

Dahlen H: Perineal care and repair. In Pairman S, Pincombe J, Thorogood C, et al, editors: Midwifery: preparation for practice, 3rd ed., Churchill Livingstone, Elsevier, Sydney, 2015.

Dalton E, Castillo E: Post partum infections: a review for the non-OBGYN, Obstetric Medicine (1753–495X) 7:98–102, 2014.

Danckert R, Ryan A, Plummer V, et al: Hospitalisation impacts on oral hygiene: an audit of oral hygiene in a metropolitan health service, Scandinavian Journal of Caring Sciences 30:129–134, 2016.

Delaram M, Dadkhah NK, Jafarzadeh L: Comparison of indomethacin suppository and lidocaine cream on post-episiotomy pain: a randomized trial, Iranian Journal of Nursing and Midwifery Research 20:450–453, 2015.

de Souza Bosco Paiva C, Junqueira Vasconcellos de Oliveira SM, Amorim Francisco A, et al: Length of perineal pain relief after ice pack application: a quasi-experimental study, Women and Birth: Journal of the Australian College of Midwives 29:117–122, 2016.

George A, Dahlen HG, Reath J, et al: What do antenatal care providers understand and do about oral health care during pregnancy? A cross-sectional survey in New South Wales, Australia, BMC Pregnancy and Childbirth 16:1–10, 2016.

George A, Johnson M, Blinkhorn A, et al: Views of pregnant women in South Western Sydney towards dental care and an oral-health program initiated by midwives, Health Promotion Journal of Australia 24:178–184, 2012.

Green D: Supporting an individual in maintaining personal hygiene, Nursing & Residential Care 16: 646–649, 2014.

Groven FMV, Zwakhalen SMG, Odekerken-Schröder G, et al: How does washing without water perform compared to the traditional bed bath? A systematic review, BMC Geriatrics 17:1–16, 2017.

Hajjaj JP: Clinical practice: perineal suturing, British Journal of Midwifery 25:297–300, 2017.

Hall B, Woodward S: Pelvic floor muscle training for urinary incontinence postpartum, British Journal of Nursing 24:576–579, 2015.

Jones ML: Oral hygiene: important yet often neglected, British Journal of Healthcare Assistants 8(10):479–481, 2014.

Kiyoshi-Teo H, Blegen M: Influence of institutional guidelines on oral hygiene practices in intensive care units, American Journal of Critical Care 24:309–317, 2015.

Moore J, Blair F: Periodontal health and pregnancy, British Journal of Midwifery 25:289–292, 2017.

Lindberg I, Persson, M, Nilsson M, et al: 'Taken by surprise'—women's experiences of the first eight weeks after a second-degree perineal tear at childbirth.

Midwifery 87:102748-102748, 2020. doi:10.1016/j.midw.2020.102748

Pairman S, Tracy S, Dahlen H, Dixon L: Midwifery: preparation for practice, 4th ed., Elsevier, 2018.

Patrick G: Risks of moving and handling, Nursing Standard 30(52):64–65, 2016.

Powers J, Fortney S: Bed baths: much more than a basic nursing task, Nursing 44:67–68, 2014.

Steen M, Diaz M, Perineal trauma: a women's health and wellbeing issue, British Journal of Midwifery 26(9): 574–584, 2018. doi:10.12968/bjom.2018.26.9.574

Vamos CA, Thompson EL, Avendano M, et al: Oral health promotion interventions during pregnancy: a systematic review, Community Dentistry & Oral Epidemiology 43:385–396, 2015.

Veje PL, Chen M, Jensen CS, et al: Bed bath with soap and water or disposable wet wipes: Patients' experiences and preferences, Journal of Clinical Nursing 28(11–12): 2235–2244, 2019. doi:10.1111/jocn.14825

Wilson A: How to provide effective oral care, Nursing Times 107(6):14–15, 2011.

SECTION 2

VITAL SIGNS

CHAPTER 4 TEMPERATURE

Learning outcomes

Having read this chapter, the reader should be able to:

- define normal body temperature for the childbearing woman and her infant
- describe factors influencing body temperature and the changes related to childbearing
- discuss the suitable sites for temperature measurement and equipment for each site
- describe types of thermometers and their correct use
- identify when and how temperature measurement should be undertaken
- demonstrate how to take a neonate's temperature
- discuss the midwife's role and responsibilities in relation to temperature measurement.

This chapter describes how to measure temperature as accurately as possible and discusses the different sites for assessing temperature and the equipment available for each site.

BODY TEMPERATURE

Body temperature is the balance between heat gain and heat loss. The hypothalamus acts as the body's thermostat by helping to balance heat loss and heat generation. Core body temperature refers to the temperature of the deeper tissues of the body; surface temperature refers to the peripheral or skin temperature (Cooper & Gosnell 2018). Humans are homeothermic, maintaining their core temperature within a relatively constant range: 37° Celsius (C) ± 1°C. Humans cannot tolerate extreme changes at either end of the temperature range. Hyperthermia is cytotoxic with endothermic damage occurring at 40°C and cell death at 41°C (Walter et al 2016). Temperatures above 41°C can lead to multi-organ failure, brain dysfunction, coma, cardiovascular collapse and death (Raukar et al 2017). Animal studies indicate hyperthermia during pregnancy can be teratogenic. Maternal hyperthermia is defined as a core temperature of ≥ 39.0°C (Ravanelli et al 2019). Body temperature less than 28°C results in uncoordinated muscle activity, fatigue, unconsciousness, cardiac arrhythmias and death.

Maintenance of body temperature within the individual's normal temperature range is essential to ensure optimal functioning of all cells. Rises in body temperature increase the demands for oxygen and therefore increase the heart rate. The physiological changes of pregnancy make women vulnerable to heat exposure and can challenge thermoregulation (Chersich et al 2020, Sun et al 2019). The nature of oxygen transfer to the fetus means it is more likely to be compromised if the mother is pyrexial. Recent research indicates an association between heat exposure and adverse pregnancy outcomes including preterm birth, decreased fetal growth and stillbirth, particularly late in pregnancy (Chersich et al 2020, Kanner et al 2020). Pre-eclampsia appears to be increased in 'warm' pregnancies and if conception occurred at a hotter time of year in some populations (Shashar et al 2020). The impact of ambient temperature on pregnancy is gaining increasing importance in the context of climate change and global warming. Peripheral temperatures reduce proportionally as distance increases from the core. Measurement of body temperature aims to detect alterations in core temperature (Sund-Levander & Grodzinsky 2013).

Elevations in temperature are described by the terms febrile, hyperthermia and pyrexia; low body temperature is called hypothermia. Signs and symptoms of elevated temperature include increased thirst, anorexia, flushed and warm skin, irritability, glassy eyes, photophobia, headache, increased pulse and respiration, restlessness or excessive sleepiness, increased perspiration and disorientation (Cooper & Gosnell 2018).

Normal values

Normal body temperature is considered to be from 36.1°C to 37.5°C. Different body temperature assessment sites have different normal values. These are usually determined according to the proximity of the site to a major blood vessel and the route it is taking to or from the heart. Each person has their own usual oral temperature set point within the normal temperature range. Most health services use an early warning observation chart which indicates escalation for vital signs outside the normal range.

Factors influencing body temperature

Sensitive neurons in the hypothalamus regulate body temperature to keep it at its 'set point'. If the hypothalamus detects a higher temperature in the blood than the set point, heat loss measures are employed (e.g. sweating). Heat generation mechanisms (e.g. shivering) commence when the body core temperature is approximately 1.5°C below the body's set point (Doyle & Schortgen 2016).

Body temperature is influenced by the following.

- Diurnal variations: Circadian rhythms influence both the core and peripheral temperature. Body temperature is lowest during the night and peaks in the late afternoon to early evening.
- Gender: Women have a higher body temperature than men. A fertile woman's body temperature is influenced by reproductive hormones, particularly oestradiol and progesterone (Webster & Smarr 2020), with body temperature being lower before ovulation (oestrogen effect) and 0.3–0.5°C higher following ovulation (progesterone effect). This rise in body temperature is maintained until progesterone levels decrease prior to the onset of menstruation.
- Age: The young and the old have more difficulty maintaining body temperature in response to environmental changes and illness.
- Digestion: A slight increase in temperature of 0.1–0.2°C has been noted to occur with normal digestion.
- Basal metabolic rate and resting metabolic rate: Heat is produced because of chemical reactions within the body. Resting metabolic rate (RMR) refers to energy expended by the body at rest. Basal metabolic rate (BMR) is similar but is measured in the morning following an overnight fast with no exercise in the previous 24 hours (McMurray et al 2014). BMR and RMR are lower in women, decrease with age and are lower in obese adults (McMurray et al 2014). Fever and disorders such as hyperthyroidism can increase BMR and RMR (McMurray et al 2014).
- Exercise: Body heat is increased by exercise; exertional heat stroke can occur in athletes (Walter et al 2016).
- Hot baths: These can raise the body temperature by 0.5–1.0°C for up to 45 minutes.
- Infection: Leucocytes release endogenous pyrogens in response to stimulation by pyrogenic substances such as bacterial, viral and protozoal infection and necrotic tissue. This causes the set point within the hypothalamus to be 'reset' at a higher level. The affected person feels cold and the body attempts to raise the temperature to maintain it within its higher 'normal' range. When the level of endogenous pyrogens decreases, the thermostat returns to its original setting. The person then feels hot, with the body attempting to lower the temperature to its normal setting. Shivering (the response to cold) and rigors (the response to pyrexia or hyperpyrexia) can appear the same clinically; in either instance body temperature should be carefully assessed (Grainger 2013). Other non-pyrogenic disorders can also cause pyrexia. These include malignancy, hyperthyroidism, drugs, allergies and central nervous system damage (e.g. stroke).
- General anaesthesia: Thermoregulation is impaired by general anaesthesia and the thresholds for vasoconstriction and shivering are reduced (Sessler 2016).
- Environment: Extremes of temperatures have the potential to raise or lower body temperature.
- Ingestion of hot substances: Drinking hot or cold liquids and eating hot or cold food can cause variations in oral temperature readings.

GUIDELINES DURING PREGNANCY

A recent systematic review indicated no pregnant women exceeded a core temperature of 39.0°C (during exercise on land, water immersion exercise, hot water bathing or sauna exposure) (Ravanelli et al 2019). According to Ravanelli and colleagues (2019) the following activities will not elevate core temperature beyond the teratogenic temperature threshold and are therefore considered safe for pregnant women:

- exercise for up to 35 minutes at 80–90% of maximum heart rate in 25°C and 45% relative humidity
- water immersion exercise for up to 45 minutes in water with a temperature ≤ 33.4°C
- sitting in a hot water bath of 40°C for up to 20 minutes
- sitting in a hot/dry sauna of up to 70°C for up to 20 minutes.

During pregnancy women's thermoregulatory capacity appears to be enhanced due to biophysical factors such as increased body mass and surface area, resulting in smaller changes in core temperature elevation during exercise and heat exposure as pregnancy advances (Ravanelli et al 2019).

Temperature changes related to childbirth

Pregnancy: maternal

During pregnancy, progesterone and a raised metabolic rate increase the amount of heat generated by 30–35%.

Although the body attempts to compensate for this by increasing heat loss mechanisms, the maternal temperature can increase by 0.5°C (Blackburn 2018).

Pregnancy: fetal

Intrauterine temperature is determined partly by maternal temperature and partly by the maternal–fetal gradient, as the fetus is unable to regulate its own temperature. Generally, the fetal temperature is approximately 0.8°C higher than the maternal temperature (Blackburn 2018). Maternal hyperthermia is generally considered to be ~2°C above normal temperature (or around 39°C). In the first trimester maternal hyperthermia is associated with an increased risk of fetal anomalies including structural and cardiovascular defects, oral clefts, ear defects, cataracts, hypospadias and renal anomalies (Graham 2020). Antipyretics may reduce with risk of fetal anomalies (Graham 2020). An elevated fetal temperature is associated with intrauterine hypoxia, fetal tachycardia and preterm labour (Blackburn 2018).

Labour

During labour, a rise in temperature can indicate infection, dehydration or increased muscular activity from uterine contractions. Use of epidural analgesia during labour is associated with an increase in maternal fever (Douma et al 2015) due to reduced heat dissipation (Blackburn 2018). Maternal hyperthermia is associated with fetal hypoxia, fetal tachycardia and an increased need to resuscitate the newborn infant (Blackburn 2018).

Caesarean section

It is important to maintain maternal temperature during caesarean section to prevent neonatal hypothermia at birth. Women who have a caesarean section are susceptible to a decline in core temperature related to epidural or spinal anaesthesia which exacerbates vasodilation, as does oxytocic administration; intrathecal morphine also increases hypothermia (Munday et al 2014).

Postnatal period: maternal

A transient rise in maternal temperature can occur within the first 24 hours following birth. This may result from the stress of labour and be related to dehydration. Blackburn (2018) suggests that up to 6.5% of women have a rise in temperature up to 38°C in the 24 hours following a vaginal birth. In the majority of cases, this is physiological and resolves spontaneously. An early warning system should still be used and action taken accordingly, particularly if the temperature rise was considered indicative of an infection (e.g. puerperal infection, mastitis, urinary tract infection) (see Chapter 6, Recognising and responding to clinical deterioration using early warning systems). An inflammatory response, such as the development of a deep venous thrombosis, would also be considered. The temperature may also rise physiologically in breastfeeding women around the second to third day when lactogenesis occurs. This will resolve spontaneously once lactation is established, although it can take several days.

Postnatal period: neonate

Neonates emerge from the warmth of the uterus (37°C+) to an environment of approximately 21°C, and need to establish several adaptations to extrauterine life simultaneously. Thermoregulation is difficult for the adapting neonate and is further affected by the following.

- The large ratio of surface area to body mass with thin layers of insulating subcutaneous fat creates an increased opportunity to lose body heat, especially from the head.
- The temperature drops significantly at birth when the baby leaves the warm intrauterine environmental and encounters a lower ambient temperature (avoid open doors or windows, fans, cold mattresses, etc.).
- Neonates are born wet from amniotic fluid with evaporative heat loss occurring at around 0.58 kcal per mL^{-1} of fluid evaporated (Lubkowska et al 2019).
- Certain factors can affect thermoregulation, such as being predisposed to problematic thermoregulation (e.g. prematurity), being small for gestational age, delivery by caesarean section, hypoxia, sedation (e.g. maternal use of opioids in labour) and congenital anomaly.

Heat production comes mainly from metabolic processes, with moving and shivering both being limited activities for neonates. In a full-term neonate brown adipose tissue constitutes approximately 10% of body weight—the breakdown of brown adipose tissue generates heat (Lubkowska et al 2019). Warmed external clothing helps, while the stores of brown fat are utilised, along with calories from milk. Metabolism requires both glucose and oxygen; a cold neonate rapidly becomes hypoxic and hypoglycaemic and develops serious metabolic acidosis. The problems are compounded significantly if the neonate is preterm or small for gestational age. Both hypothermia and hyperthermia increase the neonate's demand for oxygen by increasing metabolic demands. Dehydration and brain damage can occur. Hypothermia in preterm infants is reduced by taking measures to reduce convective and conductive heat loss (Bowman & LiVolsi 2015).

Controlled cooling may take place in neonatal intensive care units as part of the treatment to reduce hypoxic ischaemic encephalopathy. Careful temperature assessment is undertaken in each stage of the process: reducing, cooling and rewarming.

Educating parents to understand the significance of avoiding hypothermia and hyperthermia in the newborn and neonate is also an important part of the midwife's role. Neonatal thermoregulation is essential for survival and all necessary measures to maintain it should be taken (Blackburn 2018).

ADULT TEMPERATURE ASSESSMENT

The gold standard for measurement of core body temperature is the pulmonary artery catheter; however, this method is invasive and impractical in normal clinical care (Iden et al 2015). Accurate measurement of body temperature is important to detect alterations in neonates and women. Temperature measurement is part of routine clinical assessment and altered temperature may indicate the need for further clinical investigation, such as swabs or urine tests. Temperature is assessed in women with antenatal conditions, during labour and postpartum. Temperature assessment may be required more frequently if a woman appears unwell. Other reasons for more frequent temperature assessment include prelabour ruptured membranes, prostaglandin use, the presence of certain conditions (e.g. pre-eclampsia, haemorrhage or sepsis) and if an iron or blood transfusion is being administered. Sepsis may be associated with hypothermia, and hyperthermia may be disguised by paracetamol or other antipyretics.

Temperature recording sites

Ideally a site would be convenient, pain-free, sensitive and responsive, defined by a normal temperature range, independent of external effects (Davie & Amoore 2010). Choice of thermometer depends on the accuracy and availability of the equipment, safety and the ability to access the appropriate site. In all circumstances the midwife should be fully trained to competently use the equipment available and be up to date with current research. Equipment must always be used according to the manufacturer's instructions. Recent technological advances include wearable technology with the ability to continuously record body temperature and transfer it to a paired smart phone (Aptekar et al 2016). Wearable technology can monitor wrist temperature and other physiological parameters to detect ovulation and enhance fertility awareness (Goodale et al 2019).

Oral (mouth)

The thermometer is placed in the **sublingual pockets**, located on either side of the tongue (Fig 4.1). The **sublingual artery**, a branch of the carotid artery, runs below the sublingual pockets. Oral temperatures are usually 0.5°C lower than rectal temperature readings (Tollefson & Hillman 2019). Electronic thermometers (Fig 4.2A, B) are commonly used as they are easy to read.

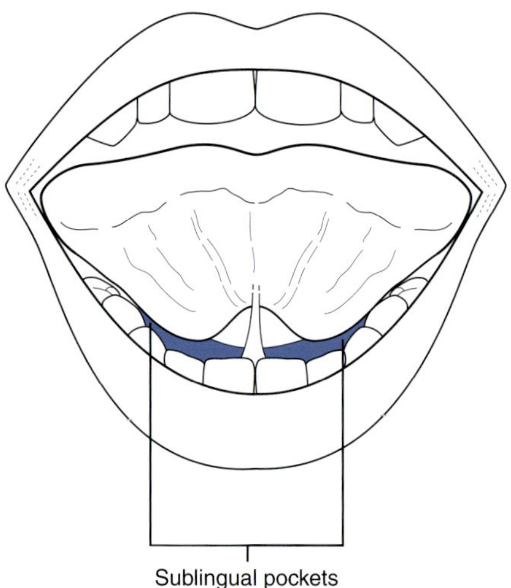

FIGURE 4.1 **Sublingual pockets of the mouth.**
Source: Johnson R, Taylor W: Skills for midwifery practice, ed 4, London, 2016, Elsevier.

Advantages	Disadvantages	Suitable thermometers
Easy access, fast, accurate, most accurate when thermometer placed in posterior sublingual pocket, easy to read. Suitable for adults and older children.	Affected by hot or cold substances, smoking, mouth breathing, tachypnoea. Not safe for infants, young children or unconscious or delirious patients.	• Electronic thermometer/ digital probe thermometer • Disposable thermometer

Forehead (temporal artery)

Measures temperature at the superficial **temporal artery**, which is approximately 1 mm beneath the skin of the forehead.

Advantages	Disadvantages	Types
Easy access, fast, easy to read. Can be used for children over 3 months of age (Hurwitz et al 2015).	Not recommended due to low accuracy (Kiekkas et al 2016). Affected by variations in skin temperature, sweat and make-up. Does not measure core temperature; impacted by local blood flow, room temperature, device placement, physical activity and amount of subcutaneous fat (Robertson & Hill 2019).	• Temporal artery (infrared heat scanner) • Disposable liquid crystal thermometer • Forehead chemical dot thermometers are unreliable and should not be used by health professionals (NICE 2019)

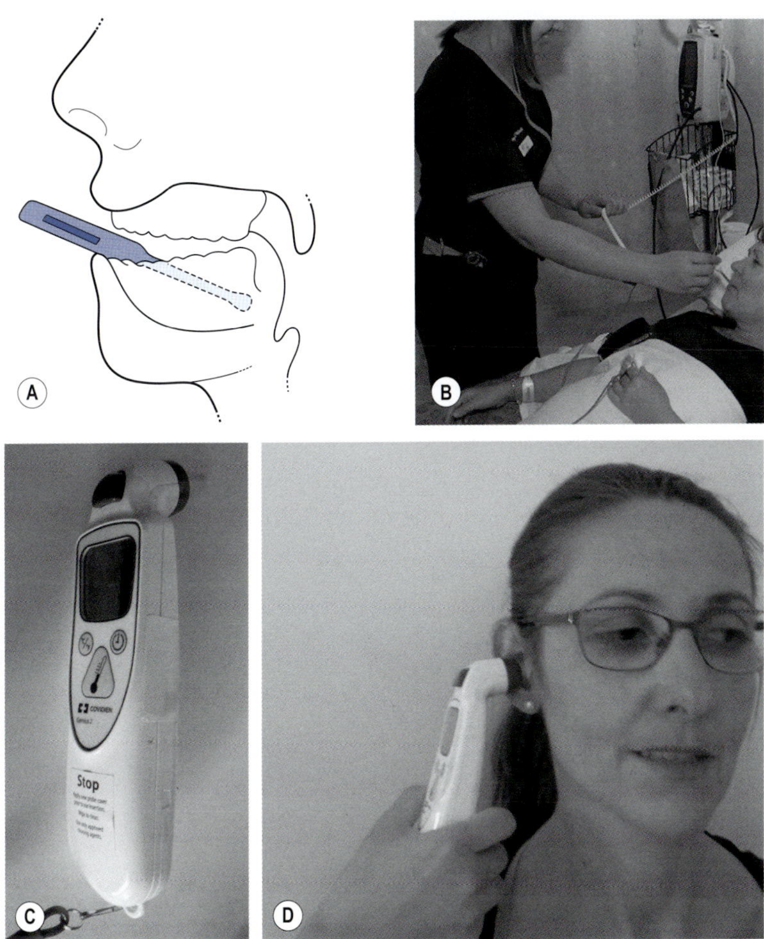

FIGURE 4.2 A, B, Electronic thermometer. C, D, Tympanic thermometer.
Source: Jamieson EM, McCall JM, Blythe R, et al: Clinical nursing practices, 3rd ed., Churchill Livingstone, Edinburgh, 1997.

Axilla

Measures temperature in the skin folds of the axilla (armpit) (Fig 4.3).

Advantages	Disadvantages	Types
Easy area to access, may require removal of clothes, easy to read. Suitable for newborns, infants and children.	Affected by ambient temperatures and vasomotor activity. Low accuracy, slow.	• Electronic • Disposable chemical dot thermometer can be used to measure axillary temperature of children over 4 weeks of age (El-Radhi 2014)

Ear (tympanic membrane)

Measures the temperature of the tympanic membrane (Fig 4.2C, D); the internal and external carotid arteries and the hypothalamus are in close proximity to the tympanic membrane.

Advantages	Disadvantages	Types
Easy area to access, fast (< 3 seconds), easy to read, high accuracy when used correctly. Suitable for children over 2 years of age.	Affected by incorrect placement or poor technique, moisture, presence of hearing aid within the last 20 minutes, excessive ear wax, otitis media, recent ear surgery, raised ambient air temperature (e.g. an incubator), dirty or moist lens on the equipment.	Tympanic thermometer

Rectal

Measures the temperature of the rectum.

Advantages	Disadvantages	Types
High accuracy, fast.	Invasive, poorly tolerated due to discomfort and embarrassment, not suitable with diarrhoea, rectal surgery, neutropenia, quadriplegics (may cause vagal stimulation leading to bradycardia and syncope). Potential to damage rectal mucosa.	• Electronic thermometer • Disposable thermometer

Oesophagus and pulmonary artery

Measures the core body temperature at the oesophagus and pulmonary artery.

Advantages	Disadvantages	Types
High accuracy	Invasive, only accessible in high dependency/ intensive care	Pulmonary artery catheter

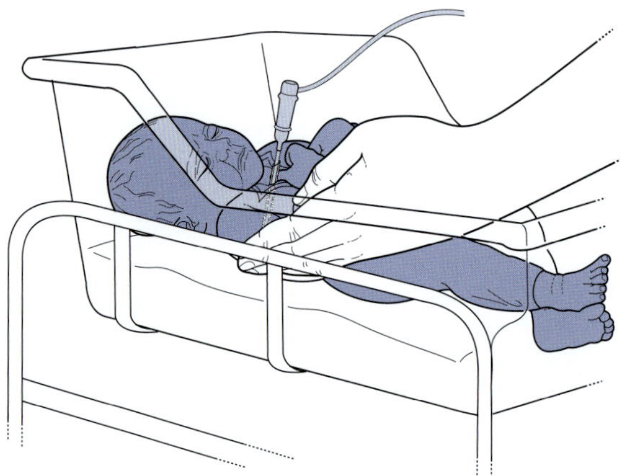

FIGURE 4.3 **Taking a neonate's temperature: axillary site using electronic thermometer.**
Source: Johnson R, Taylor W: Skills for midwifery practice, ed 4, London, 2016, Elsevier.

SKILL 4.1 Recording adult temperature

General instructions for all devices

1. Gain informed consent.
2. Perform hand hygiene.
3. Gather equipment, thermometer and disposable cover (to prevent cross-infection), observation chart, pen.
4. Clarify if environmental factors exist (e.g. recent hot drink for oral temperature, perspiration on forehead for temporal temperature).
5. Apply disposable cover and switch on thermometer.

Oral temperature

- Place covered electronic thermometer in posterior sublingual pocket, lateral to centre of jaw; mouth is then closed.

Axillary temperature

- Remove thermometer from cover and place securely in the axilla (armpit) while arm is held against the body.
- Explain procedure and gain informed consent.

Tympanic temperature

- Insert covered speculum of tympanic thermometer into ear canal, press the scan button and hold in position.

Temporal artery temperature

- Position sensor on the centre of the forehead, press the scan button and lightly slide the thermometer to the patient's right in a horizontal line. Release the scan button. Some temporal artery thermometers do not touch the skin.

After taking the temperature

1. Remove the thermometer when the alarm sounds and check the reading.
2. Dispose of the thermometer cover.
3. Clean the thermometer and return it to the unit.
4. Discuss the findings with the woman.
5. Perform hand hygiene.
6. Document observations and report any abnormal findings.

NEONATAL TEMPERATURE ASSESSMENT

The axilla is commonly used for temperature measurement. The normal values for a neonatal axilla recording are between 36.5°C and 37.5°C. Tympanic and temporal thermometers are considered less accurate in neonates and are not generally used. Disposable chemical dot thermometers should be avoided. Skin sensors are part of the newborn resuscitation trolley and are also used to monitor temperature in the neonate. Appropriate placement of the skin probe is important for accurate measurement of temperature. Dorsal, thoracic or axillary positions are considered suitable (Bensouda et al 2018). Skin probes should not be situated over brown fat areas as the temperature measurement may be falsely elevated.

Indications for temperature monitoring in the neonate are: following birth, any complications such as meconium aspiration, active resuscitation, prolonged rupture of membranes, maternal pyrexia, prematurity, being small for gestational age and feeding poorly; phototherapy; any time the neonate looks unwell, feels cool, feels hot or looks red, pale, sweaty or jittery. The local protocol for observations should be followed. If the temperature is abnormal it would generally be recorded hourly for 4 hours and then ceased when stable.

SKILL 4.2 Recording newborn temperature

1. Ideally, parents are present and their informed consent has been gained.
2. Perform hand hygiene.
3. Observe the neonate generally, particularly noting colour, behaviour and other clinical indicators.
4. Gather equipment: thermometer and disposable cover (to prevent cross-infection), observation chart and pen.
5. Place the neonate in a safe and warm environment (e.g. in the cot or in the mother's arms).
6. Loosen clothing so the axilla is accessible; if respiration is being counted at the same time then the chest may be exposed.
7. Place the covered thermometer in the axilla and hold the arm gently across the chest to keep the thermometer secure (Fig 4.3).
8. Remove the thermometer when the alarm sounds and check the reading.
9. Dispose of the thermometer cover.
10. Replace the neonate's clothing and return the neonate to their parents or cot.
11. Perform hand hygiene.
12. Document findings and take any action required in response to the assessment.

Role and responsibilities of the midwife

These can be summarised as:

- recognising the significance of an accurate temperature measurement and when to undertake it
- the use of appropriate equipment in the correct sites, recognising the need for consistency and to reduce user error
- referral or further action, if indicated
- contemporaneous record keeping
- appropriate communication, including patient education, in gaining informed consent.

SUMMARY

- The body temperature should remain within a relatively constant range.
- Maintaining normal temperature is essential for optimal body functioning.
- Hyperthermia and hypothermia can have detrimental effects.
- Monitoring temperature is important for detection and treatment of abnormal temperature.

Self-assessment exercises

The answers to the following questions may be found in the text.

1. Discuss the factors that influence body temperature.
2. What is the normal temperature range for the woman and how does this alter during the ante-, intra- and postpartum periods?
3. List the occasions when temperature assessment is undertaken for a childbearing woman and a newborn.
4. Discuss the advantages and disadvantages of each of the sites for temperature assessment.
5. Demonstrate taking a woman's temperature using a tympanic thermometer.
6. Demonstrate taking a neonate's temperature using the axillary site.
7. Summarise the role and responsibilities of the midwife when undertaking temperature assessment.

References

Aptekar D, Costantini L, Katilius J, Webster W: Continuous, passive personal wearable sensor to predict ovulation [21G]. Obstetrics & Gynecology 127:64S, 2016. Available: https://doi.org/10.1097/01.AOG.0000483905.29999.b1.

Bensouda B, Mandel R, Mejri A, et al: Temperature probe placement during preterm infant resuscitation: a randomised trial, Neonatology 113(1):27–32, 2018.

Blackburn ST: Maternal, fetal and neonatal physiology: a clinical perspective, 4th ed., Elsevier Saunders, Maryland Heights, 2018.

Bowman DS, LiVolsi K: Improvement in rates of preterm infant hypothermia by the implementation of a best practice bundle, Journal of Obstetric, Gynecologic & Neonatal Nursing 44:S54, 2015.

Chersich P: Associations between high temperatures in pregnancy and risk of preterm birth, low birth weight, and stillbirths: systematic review and meta-analysis BMJ 371:m3811–m3811, 2020. Available: https://doi.org/10.1136/bmj.m3811.

Cooper K, Gosnell K: Foundations and adult health nursing, Elsevier Mosby, St Louis, 2018.

Davie A, Amoore J: Best practice in the measurement of body temperature, Nursing Standard 24(42):42–49, 2010.

Douma MR, Stienstra R, Middeldorp JM, et al: Differences in maternal temperature during labour with Remifentanil patient-controlled analgesia or epidural analgesia: a randomised controlled trial, International Journal of Obstetric Anesthesia 24:313–322, 2015.

Doyle JF, Schortgen F: Should we treat pyrexia? And how do we do it? Critical Care 20:303, 2016.

El-Radhi AS: Determining fever in children: the search for an ideal thermometer, British Journal of Nursing 23(2):91–94, 2014. Available: https://doi.org/10.12968/bjon.2014.23.2.91

Goodale BM, Shilaih M, Falco L et al: Wearable sensors reveal menses-driven changes in physiology and enable prediction of the fertile window: observational study, Journal of Medical Internet Research 21(4):e13404–e13404, 2019. doi:10.2196/13404.

Graham JM: Update on the gestational effects of maternal hyperthermia. Birth Defects Research 112(12):943–952, 2020.

Grainger A: Principles of temperature monitoring, Nursing Standard 27(50):48–55, 2013.

Hurwitz B, Brown J, Altmiller G: Improving pediatric temperature measurement in the ED, American Journal of Nursing 115(9):48–55, 2015.

Iden T, Horn E-P, Bein B, et al: Intraoperative temperature monitoring with zero heat flux technology (3M SpotOn sensor) in comparison with sublingual and nasopharyngeal temperature: an observational study, European Journal of Anaesthesiology 32:387–391, 2015.

Kanner J, Williams AD, Nobles C et al: Ambient temperature and stillbirth: risks associated with chronic extreme temperature and acute temperature change Environmental Research 189:109958–109958, 2020. doi:10.1016/j.envres.2020.109958.

Kiekkas P, Stefanopoulos N, Bakalis N, et al: Agreement of infrared temporal artery thermometry with other thermometry methods in adults: systematic review, Journal of Clinical Nursing 25:894–905, 2016.

Lubkowska A, Szymański S, Chudecka M: Surface body temperature of full-term healthy newborns immediately after birth-pilot study, International Journal of Environmental Research and Public Health 16(8):1312, 2019. doi:10.3390/ijerph16081312.

McMurray RG, Soares J, Caspersen CJ, et al: Examining variations of resting metabolic rate of adults: a public health perspective, Medicine & Science in Sports & Exercise 46:1352–1358, 2014.

Munday J, Hines S, Wallace K, et al: A systematic review of the effectiveness of warming interventions for women undergoing cesarean section, Worldviews on Evidence-based Nursing 11:383–393, 2014.

National Institute for Health and Care Excellence (NICE): Fever in under 5s: assessment and initial management, NICE Guideline, No. 143. London, 2019. Online 4 July 2021. Available: www.nice.org.uk/guidance/ng143 .

Raukar N, Lemieux RS, Casa DJ, et al: Identification and treatment of exertional heat stroke in the prehospital setting, Journal of Emergency Medical Services 2017. 9 May. Online 4 July 2021. Available: www.jems.com/patient-care/identification-and-treatment-of-exertional-heat-stroke-in-the-prehospital-setting/.

Ravanelli N, Casasola W, English T et al: Heat stress and fetal risk. Environmental limits for exercise and passive heat stress during pregnancy: a systematic review with best evidence synthesis. British Journal of Sports Medicine 53(13):799–805, 2019. doi:10.1136/bjsports-2017-097914.

Robertson M, Hill B: Monitoring temperature. British Journal of Nursing 28(6):344–347, 2019.

Sessler DI: Perioperative thermoregulation and heat balance, Lancet 387:2655–2664, 2016.

Shashar S, Kloog I, Erez O et al: Temperature and preeclampsia: Epidemiological evidence that perturbation in maternal heat homeostasis affects pregnancy outcome PLOS ONE 15(5):e0232877, 2020. doi:10.1371/journal.pone.0232877.

Sun S, Spangler KR, Weinberger KR et al: Ambient temperature and markers of fetal growth: a retrospective observational study of 29 million US singleton births. Environmental Health Perspectives 127(6):67005, 2019. doi:10.1289/EHP4648.

Sund-Levander M, Grodzinsky E: Assessment of body temperature measurement options, British Journal of Nursing 22(15):880–888, 2013.

Tollefson J, Hillman E: Clinical psychomotor skills, 7th ed., Cengage, South Melbourne, 2019.

Walter EJ, Hanna-Jumma S, Carraretto M, et al: The pathophysiological basis and consequences of fever, Critical Care 20:1–10, 2016.

Webster WW, Smarr B: Using circadian rhythm patterns of continuous core body temperature to improve fertility and pregnancy planning. Journal of Circadian Rhythms 18(1):5, 2020. Available: http://doi.org/10.5334/jcr.200.

CHAPTER 5 PULSE

Learning outcomes

Having read this chapter, the reader should be able to:

- discuss factors influencing the heart rate
- discuss the significance of an abnormal rate, rhythm and/or amplitude for the woman
- identify the normal range for the childbearing woman and the neonate
- discuss the midwife's role and responsibilities in relation to pulse assessment, identifying when, where and how it is undertaken
- discuss why manual assessment of the pulse is important.

DEFINITION

A pulse is initiated as the left ventricle of the heart contracts, producing rhythmic expansion and contraction of arteries as blood enters the circulation. The pulse can be felt by compressing an artery against a bone or firm tissue and then be assessed for rate, rhythm and amplitude (volume).

The pulse is a direct indicator of the action of the heart and provides information about cardiac function and peripheral perfusion (Khan 2021). Assessment of cardiovascular function includes observing general appearance and looking for signs and symptoms of dysfunction; for example, cyanosis, pallor, cool skin and temperature (Khan 2021). Clinical observation and alterations in the pulse provide information on a woman's cardiovascular state. Signs of a postpartum haemorrhage include pallor and a rapid thready pulse as the heart rate increases in an attempt to maintain cardiac output.

The pulse rate is visually displayed on electronic equipment such as blood pressure machines and oxygen saturation monitors. However, these displays do not take the place of regular manual assessment of the pulse as they do not provide information on rhythm or amplitude.

FACTORS THAT INFLUENCE THE MATERNAL HEART RATE

The pulse rate is controlled by the heart's conducting system and the autonomic nervous system. The sinoatrial node within the heart initiates impulses that spread across the conducting system to all areas of cardiac muscle, causing atrial and subsequently ventricular contraction. The parasympathetic nerve fibres—primarily the vagus nerve—reduce the heart rate, while the sympathetic nerve fibres increase the heart rate. Low-intensity stretching exercises during pregnancy have been shown to result in a small decrease in the maternal heart rate, which may have beneficial effects on health (Logan & SeonAe 2017).

Cardiac activity is also affected by chemicals and ions; for example, adrenaline increases the heart rate and excess potassium (hyperkalaemia) can cause bradycardia.

Factors that increase the heart rate

- Anaemia
- Anaphylaxis: causes weak thready pulse, tachycardia, irregular pulse
- Changes in position (e.g. from sitting to standing)
- Dehydration
- Disease (e.g. hyperthyroidism, pulmonary embolism)
- Emotions: stress, anxiety, nervousness, fear, excitement
- Exercise
- Gender: females have a slightly higher pulse rate than males
- Haemorrhage
- Hyperventilation
- Hypovolaemic shock
- Illicit drugs such as amphetamines and cocaine
- Infection (with or without changes to other vital signs)

- Medications (e.g. salbutamol)
- Pain
- Pregnancy and labour
- Pulmonary conditions causing poor oxygenation
- Pyrexia—the pulse can increase 7–10 beats per minute (bpm) with each degree of temperature increase
- Sepsis

Factors that decrease the heart rate

- Age: heart rate decreases with age
- Athleticism
- Disease (e.g. hypothyroidism)
- Electrolyte imbalance
- Good exercise tolerance (e.g. athletes)
- Hyperglycaemia
- Hypothermia
- Hypoxia
- Increased intracranial pressure
- Increased vagal tone
- Insult or injury: myocardial infarction or other injury may cause the heart to slow or stop
- Medications (e.g. beta blockers)
- Rest and relaxation: calm, controlled breathing
- Sleep

NORMAL VALUES

A healthy non-pregnant adult female has a heart rate of approximately 60–100 bpm with an average of 80 bpm (Hill & Miller-Rosser 2014). During pregnancy the heart rate increases by 15–20 bpm, blood volume by 40–45% and cardiac output by 40%; peripheral vasodilation, stroke volume and heart size also increase (Hill & Miller-Rosser 2014).

Tachycardia refers to an abnormally fast pulse rate (above 100 bpm). Tachycardia is often one of the first signs of maternal haemorrhage (Dennis et al 2016). Sustained tachycardia combined with pyrexia, tachypnoea or new onset confusion, or a heart rate >130 bpm regardless of other signs, is a red flag and warrants prompt referral of the woman for hospital assessment (or urgent investigation if she is already an inpatient), due to the association with sepsis (Churchill et al, 2014).

Bradycardia is a slow heart rate, generally considered to be below 60 bpm (Hill & Miller-Rosser 2014). However, women who have a high level of physical fitness may have a resting heart rate below 60. Bradycardia can result in impaired blood flow to the brain, syncope and may be a sign of poor perfusion.

Arrhythmia is an irregular pulse (the normal pulse is regular). Arrhythmia reflects an irregular pumping action of the heart which may be due to an electrolyte imbalance or damaged cardiac tissue (Khan 2021).

Amplitude indicates changes in the volume of blood being pumped around the body, the pulse strength and elasticity of the arterial wall. It is subjectively described as strong, bounding, normal, weak, thready or imperceptible. A decrease in pulse amplitude is indicative of poor cardiac output, which may be due to hypovolaemia resulting from shock, haemorrhage or cardiac tissue damage. A rapid, full or bounding pulse may be due to infection, hypertension, strenuous exercise or strong emotions (Khan 2021).

CHANGES RELATED TO CHILDBIRTH

Pregnancy

Normal pregnancy is associated with marked changes in the heart rate which commence as early as 5 weeks gestation (Pollock & Kingwell 2015). Therefore, the pulse baseline from the first trimester may underestimate the full extent of changes related to pregnancy (Mahendru et al 2014). Increased blood flow during pregnancy necessitates higher cardiac output, which is achieved by an increased heart rate and stroke volume. The maternal heart rate increases gradually as pregnancy progresses and by 32 weeks is 10–20 bpm higher than the pre-conception pulse (Iacobaeus et al 2017) or 15–20 bpm higher according to Durham and Chapman (2014). The maximum heart rate is reached in the third trimester (Mahendru et al 2014). The normal heart rate range at term is 64–104 bpm with an average of 84 bpm (Dennis et al 2016). The increase in maternal heart rate during pregnancy is estimated to be approximately 20% above the pre-conception baseline by the third trimester of pregnancy (Samways et al 2016).

During pregnancy, uterine activity gradually increases in frequency and intensity with moderate to strong Braxton Hicks contractions increasing the maternal and fetal heart rate as gestation progresses (Sletten et al 2016). In over 90% of women, there is a correlation between maternal and fetal heart rate, with both exhibiting a diurnal pattern of lower heart rates at night and higher heart rates in the afternoon (Sletten et al 2016). Healthy pregnant women seem to have limited preload reserve and decreased cardiac contractility, particularly in the third trimester, leading to increased vulnerability to fluid overload and cardiac failure (Vårtun et al 2015). As gestation proceeds, cardiac parasympathetic tone decreases and cardiac sympathetic tone increases (Carpenter et al 2017).

The QT interval (reflecting cardiac depolarisation and repolarisation) becomes shorter and has increased variability during the second half of pregnancy as the heart rate increases. These factors are associated with an increased risk of arrhythmia (Carpenter et al 2017). Mild cardiac arrhythmias (generally ventricular and atrial ectopics) and heart murmurs may occur during pregnancy and are usually benign, but warrant further investigation (Blackburn 2018). The number of women with more serious arrythmias is increasing, with atrial fibrillation the most common (MacIntyre et al 2018).

More women with cardiovascular disease are becoming pregnant and preexisting cardiac disease places additional stress on the cardiovascular system during pregnancy. In Australia and New Zealand, cardiovascular disease is a major cause of indirect maternal mortality. In 2018, cardiovascular disease was the most common cause of maternal mortality in Australia (Australian Institute of Health and Welfare [AIHW] 2020). Women with existing cardiac problems or any presenting cardiac symptoms need obstetric and cardiac care from doctors with expertise in cardiac disease related to pregnancy.

Labour

During labour, each contraction returns 300–500 mL of blood to the circulation (increasing cardiac output and heart rate) as blood is squeezed out of the uterus (Söhnchen et al 2011). In a non-pregnant woman the cardiac output is approximately 5 L/minute; during labour this increases to around 10.5 L/minute. In the first stage of labour the average heart rate is around 88 bpm, increasing to 96 bpm during contractions; during active pushing the maternal heart rate increases to an average of 157 ± 21 bpm and in 50% of women, reaches over 70% of heart rate reserve, which is equivalent to 172 ± 14 bpm (Söhnchen et al 2011). Recent research using continuous measurement indicates baseline hemodynamic status remains similar during the first and second stage of labour with an increase in haemodynamic stress during contractions (Bijl et al 2019). The changes in heart rate during pushing are similar to changes from physical exercise such as cycling or running, with higher heart rates seen in women with a low level of physical fitness (Söhnchen et al 2011). According to Towers and colleagues (2019) tachycardia is common during the second stage of labour with approximately one-third of women recording a sustained heart rate ≥ 100 bpm, over 18% of women had a heart rate ≥ 110 and over 9% a heart rate ≥ 120 bpm. The average mean heart rate in second stage was 93.8 ± 17.9 bpm (Towers et al 2019).

Intravenous oxytocin during labour greatly amplifies the normal increase in heart rate and exacerbates cardiovascular risk by decreasing peripheral arterial resistance, thereby increasing stroke volume, heart rate and cardiac output (Söhnchen et al 2011). An increase in the number and variety of arrhythmias may also be seen during labour (Blackburn 2018).

Postnatal maternal

During the puerperium the cardiovascular system reverts to its pre-pregnant state, with the heart rate generally reaching its pre-pregnancy rate by 12 weeks postpartum (Carpenter et al 2017). A study on healthy postnatal women with no evidence of sepsis, anaemia or significant haemorrhage found women's heart rates were lower following normal vaginal birth than instrumental or caesarean birth, possibly due to less blood loss following normal birth (Samways et al 2016). This study examined almost 17,000 postpartum heart rate readings and identified the mean and upper thresholds of normal (Table 5.1).

TABLE 5.1 POSTPARTUM MATERNAL HEART RATE

Hours postpartum	Mean heart rate (bpm)	Upper limit (mean + 2 standard deviations) (bpm)
6	83.6	108.2
12	84.5	109.4
24	85.4	110.4
48	84.3	109.7

Source: Adapted from Samways JW, Vause S, Kontopantelis E, et al: Maternal heart rate during the first 48h postpartum: a retrospective cross-sectional study, European Journal of Obstetrics, Gynecology and Reproductive Biology 206:41–47, 2016.

Establishing normal postpartum heart rate parameters ensures deviations can be detected in the first 48 hours when maternal morbidity and mortality are higher. Unexplained tachycardia (occurring in the absence of sepsis, haemorrhage or anaemia) should alert midwives to the possibility of other causes, including occult bleeding, cardiac disorders and pulmonary embolism.

SITES FOR PULSE MEASUREMENT

A pulse can be felt anywhere in the body where an artery near to the surface can be palpated against something firm, usually bone or tendon. The heart rate can also be heard by auscultating the apical pulse using a stethoscope. The most commonly used site in the adult is the radial artery, being readily accessible; other sites are indicated in Figure 5.1.

The **radial pulse** of the right wrist is best palpated by the midwife's left hand, and vice versa. The radial pulse can be used to assess rate and rhythm; however, it is a peripheral pulse and further from the heart, making it less accurate in assessing amplitude (Nicholson 2014). To find the radial pulse, place the index and middle finger gently in the groove of the woman's wrist that lies beneath the thumb. If a pulsation cannot be felt, the fingers should be moved gently along the groove until the pulse is located. If the pulse is difficult to palpate, exert more pressure from the middle finger as this can amplify the pulse wave against the index finger. The amount of pressure applied may need to be increased or decreased. The thumb should not be used to feel for the pulse as the thumb has a strong pulse of its own which can be mistaken for the woman's pulse (deWit & O'Neill 2014).

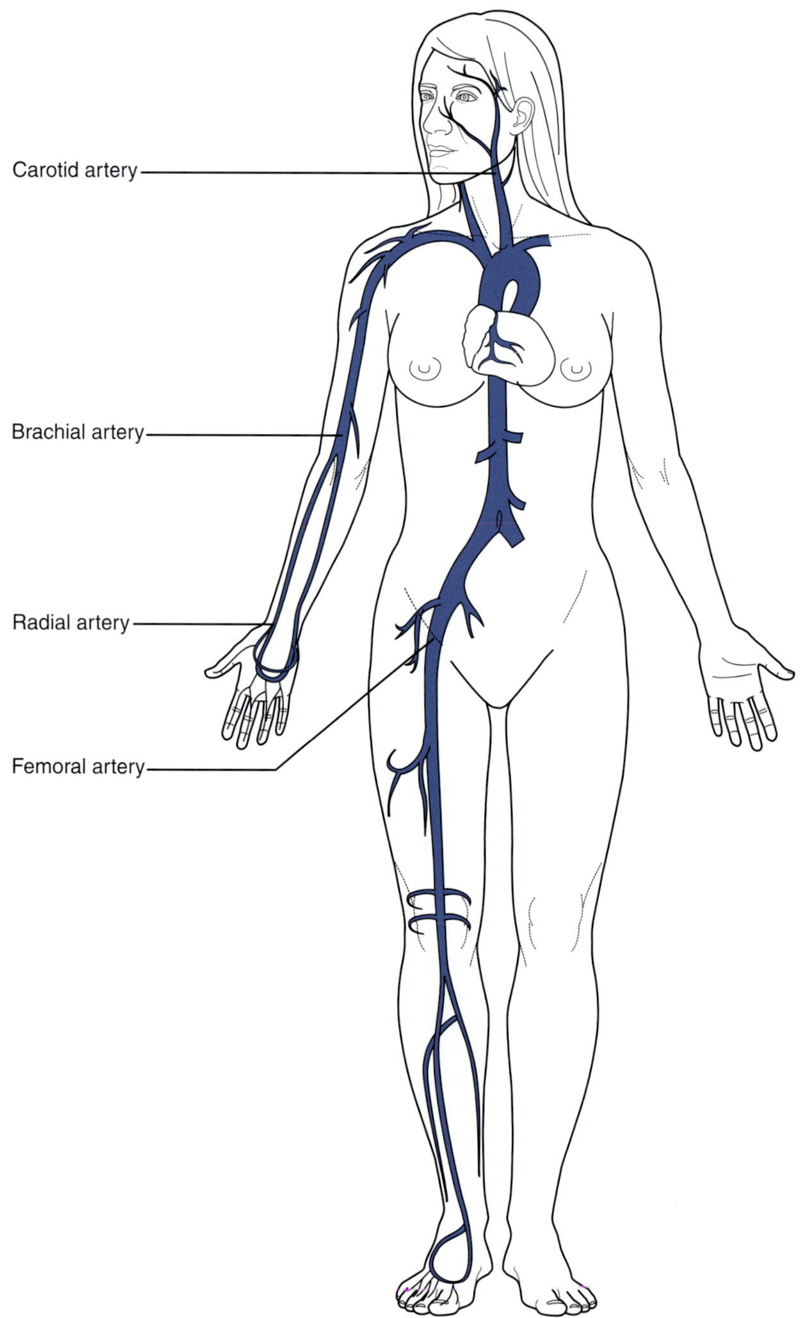

FIGURE 5.1 **Main sites for adult pulse assessment.**
Source: Adapted with kind permission from Thibodeau G, Patton K: Structure and function of the body, 14th ed., Elsevier Mosby, St Louis, 2012.

The **brachial pulse** is used in the measurement of blood pressure and is located in the antecubital fossa (triangular area anterior to the elbow). The brachial pulse is less superficial and can be more difficult to palpate than the radial pulse. The woman should have her arm slightly bent with the palm uppermost and the midwife places her index and middle finger on the inner side of the crease of the elbow. Apply firm pressure for 5 seconds; if no pulsation is felt, begin again in the centre of the crease, moving the fingers towards the woman's body.

The **carotid pulse** is found by placing three to four fingertips against the larynx (at the top of the neck just under the jaw, midpoint between the chin and earlobe), using gentle pressure on one side only. If both sides are compressed the arterial circulation to the brain can be disrupted. The carotid artery is palpated when peripheral circulation is compromised and the radial pulse is unobtainable due to collapse or serious clinical deterioration.

The **femoral pulse** is located in the groin and is most easily accessed when the woman is lying flat. Three fingers are placed over the superior pubic ramus (near the crease of the groin) and direct downward pressure is applied (this may be quite deep) to feel the pulsation. Palpation of the femoral arteries in the neonate is also part of the neonatal examination.

Pulse deficit occurs when there is difference between the apical and radial pulse, which should be identical. To check the pulse deficit, the apex beat and radial pulse are counted simultaneously. One midwife counts the apical pulse using the diaphragm side of the stethoscope, placing it in the midline on the left side of the chest between the fifth and sixth ribs. The second midwife counts the radial pulse, with both midwives using the same watch to commence and finish recording the heart rate over a minute (Cooper & Gosnell 2018). Both readings are recorded using different coloured inks. If the stethoscope being used does not belong to the midwife, the earpieces should be disinfected before and after use; for example, with an alcohol-impregnated swab (Lippincott et al 2015). The diaphragm and bell should also be disinfected before and after use to reduce the effect of cross-contamination (Campos-Murguia, Leon-Lara, Munoz et al 2014).

INDICATIONS

While care should be individual and according to need, indications for maternal pulse assessment are:

- on admission
- where there is any deviation from normal, where the vital signs are abnormal or outside the parameters of the institution's early warning system which triggers repeating vital signs and further investigation
- prior to blood pressure measurement, especially when using an electronic sphygmomanometer, as an irregular pulse or compromised cardiac output increases inaccuracy of readings and manual palpation is necessary to detect arrhythmias (Nicholson 2014)
- when auscultating the fetal heart, including when applying a cardiotocograph (see Chapters 27 and 33)
- during labour—hourly (but not during a contraction)—and prior to transfer of care following labour (NICE 2017); local protocols may vary
- following caesarean section the pulse should be recorded every 15 minutes until vital signs are stable and then every 30 minutes for at least 2 hours, progressing to hourly and then 4-hourly provided the observations are stable (Tracy & Hartz 2015); local guidelines and protocols should be followed
- during postnatal assessment, if indicated
- during prelabour spontaneous rupture of membranes
- during treatment for preterm labour using tocolytic drugs
- following intrathecal administration (medication reaches the cerebrospinal fluid) or with patient-controlled anaesthesia (PCA) opioid use (according to local protocol)
- before, during and after a blood or iron transfusion.

SKILL 5.1 Adult radial pulse

1. Obtain informed consent.
2. Ensure the woman is comfortable and, if possible, in the same position as for the previous assessment.
3. Perform hand hygiene.
4. Locate the radial artery, pressing down using moderate pressure and supporting the woman's wrist and arm across her chest (if the wrist is held too firmly the pulse may be occluded; if held too lightly it is difficult to count).
5. Count the pulse for 30 seconds if it is regular, then double it; or 60 seconds if it is irregular or slow, noting also the rhythm and amplitude.
6. Undertake respiration assessment (see Chapter 6) if necessary.
7. Discuss the results with the woman, explaining whether and when it will be necessary to reassess the pulse.
8. Perform hand hygiene.
9. Document the findings and act accordingly.

ASSESSING HEART RATE IN THE NEONATE

In the neonate the heart rate is usually recorded from the apical site by auscultation using a stethoscope or palpated. The apex beat is preferred as it is the most reliable. If the apical site is not accessible, the brachial or femoral pulses can be used (Fig 5.2). Immediately after birth the pulse can be felt at the base of the umbilical cord. Heart rate can also be obtained using a pulse oximeter or placing electrocardiography (ECG) electrodes on the chest.

The normal heart rate for a newborn has been reported as 100–160 bpm (England 2014). In Australia, 110–160 bpm is generally considered normal. In the first seconds of life the newborn heart rate is around 120 bpm, increasing significantly during the first

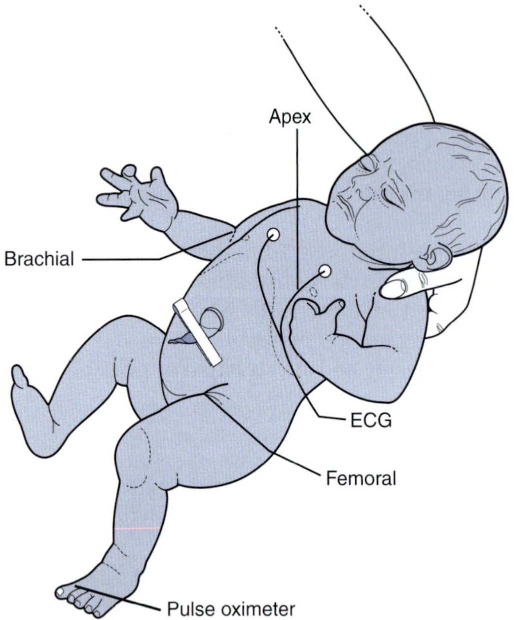

FIGURE 5.2 **Main sites for neonatal pulse assessment.**
Source: Johnson R, Taylor W: Skills for midwifery practice, 4th ed., Elsevier, London, 2016.

60 seconds until it stabilises in the 130s (Linde et al 2016). According to Bancalari and colleagues (2016), the average heart rate 1 minute after birth is 150 bpm, increasing to 161 at 7 minutes and decreasing to a mean of 135 bpm at 24 hours. The newborn's heart rate varies noticeably with respiration and should be counted for 1 minute. Approximately 1–5% of neonates have an arrhythmia and for the majority it will disappear during the first month (Silva et al 2016). If an irregular heartbeat is heard on auscultation the neonate should be referred to a neonatologist or paediatrician.

Indications for assessing the newborn heart rate

- At birth as part of Apgar scoring and resuscitation (see Chapter 48 for both)
- When there are any signs of cyanosis, irritability or illness
- As part of vital sign observations for suspected or potential infection (e.g. prolonged rupture of membranes, known maternal Group B streptococcus, meconium aspiration)

SKILL 5.2 Assessing newborn heart rate

The neonate should be peaceful and not crying when undergoing pulse assessment. When using a stethoscope, the bell and/or diaphragm and earpieces should be cleaned before and after use (Campos-Murguia et al 2014).

1. Obtain informed consent from the parents, expecting at least one parent to be present throughout.
2. Perform hand hygiene.
3. Loosen the clothing and access the chosen site.
4. Place a warmed stethoscope over the apex of the heart (midline, left side of the chest); *or* place index and middle fingers over the apex; *or* place the index and middle fingers over the brachial artery. Count the pulse for 60 seconds, noting amplitude and rhythm.
5. Observe the colour, behaviour and general condition of the neonate at the same time. Other vital sign observations may also be undertaken (e.g. temperature, respiratory assessment).
6. Replace the clothing and ensure comfort.
7. Discuss the results with the neonate's parents.
8. Perform hand hygiene and clean the stethoscope if used.
9. Document the findings and act on any deviations from normal.

SKILL 5.3 Other means of pulse measurement

- ECG monitors give a continuous or single reading, or printout of the heart rate and pattern.
- Automated blood pressure machines may provide a single heart rate reading.
- Pulse oximeters (see Chapter 6) also give a continuous heart rate reading, as do cardiotocograph machines for fetal heart assessment when the finger probe is attached.

Electronic equipment relies on oscillation where changes in the pulse waveform are converted to an electronic format. They are unable to provide information on the regularity and amplitude of the pulse (Nicholson 2014). Pulse oximeters work on changes in light absorption and blood flow.

Documentation

Pulse assessment can be written in the records of the woman/neonate as prose. However, if repeated observations are undertaken, an overall picture is best obtained if the findings are recorded pictorially on an observations chart. This will show at a glance if there is a pattern emerging or if the condition is changing and triggering the need for further investigation or actions.

Role and responsibilities of the midwife

These can be summarised as:

- recognising the normal pulse characteristics, including rate, rhythm and amplitude and identifying any deviation from normal
- recognising when assessment of the pulse is indicated
- undertaking the assessment correctly
- escalating and referring as indicated when deviations from normal are detected
- contemporaneous record keeping.

SUMMARY

- Pulse assessment is a straightforward, non-invasive skill of considerable importance.
- An accurate assessment includes the rate, rhythm and amplitude of the pulse.
- Assessment of the general condition of the woman or neonate is made simultaneously.

Self-assessment exercises

The answers to the following questions can be found in the text.

1. Discuss the significance of pulse assessment and when it should be undertaken during pregnancy or postpartum.
2. What changes occur to the heart rate during pregnancy and labour and why do they occur?
3. Discuss the factors that increase the heart rate.
4. Summarise the role and responsibilities of the midwife when undertaking pulse assessment.

References

Australian Institute of Health and Welfare (AIHW) 2020. Maternal deaths in Australia. Cat. no. PER 99. Canberra: AIHW. Online 13 March 2020. Available: www.aihw.gov.au/reports/mothers-babies/maternal-deaths-in-australia.

Bancalari A, Araneda H, Echeverría P, et al: Arterial oxygen saturation and heart rate after birth in newborns with and without maternal bonding, Pediatrics International 58:993–997, 2016.

Bijl RC, Valensise H, Novelli GP et al: Methods and considerations concerning cardiac output measurement in pregnant women: recommendations of the International Working Group on Maternal Hemodynamics. Ultrasound in Obstetrics & Gynecology 54(1):35–50, 2019.

Blackburn S: Maternal, fetal and neonatal physiology: a clinical perspective, 5th ed., Elsevier, St Louis, 2018.

Campos-Murguia A, Leon-Lara X, Munoz J, et al: Stethoscopes as potential intrahospital carriers of pathogenic microorganisms, American Journal of Infection Control 42(1):82–83, 2014.

Carpenter RE, Emery SJ, Uzun O, et al: Influence of antenatal physical exercise on heart rate variability and QT variability, The Journal of Maternal-Fetal & Neonatal Medicine 30:79–84, 2017.

Churchill D, Rodger A, Clift J, et al: Think sepsis. In Knight M, Kenyon S, Brocklehurst P, et al, editors: Saving lives, improving mothers' care: lessons learned to inform future maternity care from the UK and Ireland Confidential Enquiries into Maternal Deaths and Morbidity 2009–12, Oxford, 2014, on behalf of MBRRACE-UK, National Perinatal Epidemiology Unit, pp. 27–43.

Cooper K, Gosnell K: Foundations and adult health nursing, 8th ed., Elsevier Mosby, St Louis, 2018.

Dennis AT, Hardy L, Dennis A: Defining a reference range for vital signs in healthy term pregnant women undergoing caesarean section, Anaesthesia and Intensive Care 44:752–757, 2016.

deWit S, O'Neill P: Fundamental concepts and skills for nursing, 4th ed., Elsevier, St Louis, 2014.

Durham RF, Chapman L: Maternal-newborn nursing: the critical components of nursing care, 2nd ed., FA Davis, Philadelphia, 2014.

England C: Recognising the healthy baby at term through examination of the newborn screening. In Marshall J, Raynor M, editors: Myles textbook for midwives, 16th ed., Elsevier, Edinburgh, 2014, pp. 591–610.

Hill R, Miller-Rosser K: Vital signs. In Dempsey J, Hillege S, Hill R, editors: Fundamentals of nursing and midwifery: a person-centred approach to care, 2nd ed., Lippincott, Williams and Wilkins, Sydney, 2014.

Iacobaeus C, Andolf E, Thorsell M, et al: Longitudinal study of vascular structure and function during normal pregnancy, Ultrasound in Obstetrics & Gynecology: The Official Journal of the International Society of Ultrasound in Obstetrics and Gynecology 49(1): 46–53, 2017.

Khan R: Vital signs. In Koutoukidis G, Stainton K, editors: Tabbner's nursing care, 8th ed., Elsevier Australia, Chatswood, 2021. Chapter 20: Vital sign assessment.

Linde JE, Øymar K, Schulz J, et al: Normal newborn heart rate in the first five minutes of life assessed by dry-electrode electrocardiography, Neonatology (16617800) 110:231–237, 2016.

Lippincott, Williams & Wilkins: Lippincott nursing procedures, 7th ed., Wolters Kluwer, Philadelphia, 2015, pp. 614–616.

Logan JG, SeonAe S: Effects of stretching exercise on heart rate variability during pregnancy, The Journal of Cardiovascular Nursing 32:107–111, 2017.

MacIntyre C, Iwuala C, Parkash R: Cardiac Arrhythmias and Pregnancy. Current Treatment Options in Cardiovascular Medicine, 20(8):1–13, 2018.

Mahendru AA, Everett TR, Wilkinson IB, et al: A longitudinal study of maternal cardiovascular function from preconception to the postpartum period, Journal of Hypertension 32:849–856, 2014.

National Institute for Health and Care Excellence (NICE): CG55 Intrapartum care for healthy women and babies, 2017. Online 27 March 2021. Available: www.nice.org.uk.

Nicholson C: Advanced cardiac examination: the arterial pulse, Nursing Standard 28:50–59, 2014.

Pollock W, Kingwell A: Pregnancy and postpartum considerations. In Aitken L, Marshall A, Chaboyer W, editors: ACCCN's critical care nursing, 3rd ed., Elsevier, Sydney, 2015.

Samways JW, Vause S, Kontopantelis E, et al: Maternal heart rate during the first 48h postpartum: a retrospective cross-sectional study, European Journal of Obstetrics, Gynecology and Reproductive Biology 206:41–47, 2016.

Silva A, Soares P, Flor-de-Lima F, et al: Neonatal arrhythmias—morbidity and mortality at discharge, Journal of Pediatric and Neonatal Individualized Medicine 5(2):E050212, 2016.

Sletten J, Kiserud T, Kessler J, et al: Effect of uterine contractions on fetal heart rate in pregnancy: a prospective observational study, Acta Obstetricia et Gynecologica Scandinavica 95:1129–1135, 2016.

Söhnchen N, Melzer K, Tejada BM, et al: Maternal heart rate changes during labour, European Journal of Obstetrics, Gynecology and Reproductive Biology 158:173–178, 2011.

Towers CV, Trussell J, Heidel RE et al: Incidence of maternal tachycardia during the second stage of labor: a prospective observational cohort study. The Journal of Maternal-Fetal & Neonatal Medicine 32(10):1615–1619, 2019.

Tracy SK, Hartz D: Interventions in pregnancy, labour and birth. In Pairman S, Pincombe J, Thorogood C, et al, editors: Midwifery: preparation for practice, 3rd ed., Churchill Livingstone, Elsevier, Sydney, 2015.

Vårtun Å, Flo K, Wilsgaard T, et al: Maternal functional hemodynamics in the second half of pregnancy: a longitudinal study, PLoS ONE 10:1–15, 2015.

CHAPTER 6 RESPIRATION

Learning outcomes

Having read this chapter, the reader should be able to:

- define external respiration, identifying the normal ranges for mother and neonate
- discuss when respiration should be assessed and the factors influencing respiration
- undertake assessment of respiration accurately
- recognise an abnormal respiratory rate, pattern and sounds
- discuss the safe and accurate use of pulse oximetry
- discuss when and why an early warning observation chart should be used.

RESPIRATORY ASSESSMENT

Changes in the physiology of respiratory rate occur during pregnancy. The respiratory rate is one of the more sensitive markers for identifying patients at risk of clinical deterioration (Kellet & Sebat 2017; Flenady et al 2017) with higher respiratory rates predicting increased risk (Mora et al 2016). A respiratory rate over 20 breaths per minute is an important sign of respiratory distress, hypoxia and acidosis (Flenady et al 2017). A retrospective audit in Australia found the respiratory rate was the most frequently omitted vital sign (Kellet & Sebat 2017). In women who died from sepsis, the respiratory rate was often not recorded (Churchill et al 2014).

Respiration assessment is important for both the woman and the neonate—it is one of the core physiological observations necessary to detect clinical deterioration and is part of early warning observation charts (Australian Commission on Safety and Quality in Health Care [ACSQHC] 2017, Health Quality & Safety Commission New Zealand 2016).

This chapter considers the effects of childbirth on the respiratory system, other factors affecting respiration and the midwife's role and responsibilities in completing the observation correctly. Pulse oximetry is also discussed.

DEFINITION

External respiration refers to the breathing movements observed during inspiration (when the body gains oxygen) and expiration (as carbon dioxide is excreted). Internal respiration is the exchange of gases in the alveoli and at tissue level (Bullock & Hales 2018). Assessment of respiration includes observation of the rate (number per minute), depth, quality and regularity of breaths and any associated signs (e.g. skin colour). Breath sounds may also be heard, or the rise and fall of the chest can be felt or visually observed. Respiration can be consciously controlled (e.g. for swimming, singing), but is unconsciously determined by definite and precise mechanisms. Control of the respiratory rate is complex and includes the brainstem (medulla oblongata and pons) (Bullock & Hales 2018).

Eupnoea is normal breathing at rest. Normal respirations are regular with an expiratory phase which is slightly longer than the inspiratory phase with a ratio of 1:1.5 or 1:2 (Bullock & Hales 2018). The diaphragm flattens during inspiration and the intercostal muscles pull the ribs upwards and outwards increasing the intrathoracic volume and pulling approximately 500 mL of air into the lungs (Schoenwald & Douglas 2017). The longer expiration allows a conversation to be held. A quick assessment of respiratory impairment is to ask the woman a question—if she can only speak in short sentences, there is a degree of respiratory distress. Posture such as sitting up or leaning forwards enhances the mechanics of breathing by increasing involvement of accessory inspiratory muscles (Mesquita Montes et al 2018).

NORMAL VALUES

Automatic control of breathing occurs within the respiratory centres in the medulla oblongata and pons which regulate breathing according to reflex responses and chemical signals, mainly carbon dioxide in the blood (Bullock & Hales 2018). For example, an excessive carbon dioxide level in the blood (hypercapnia) will cause respirations to increase until the carbon dioxide level returns to normal (Porrit 2021).

The normal respiratory rate for a healthy adult at rest is 12–20 breaths per minute (Bullock & Hales 2018, Cooper & Gosnell 2018). A large study aiming to determine normal vital signs in a term pregnancy found the average respiratory rate was 18 ± 1.5 breaths per minute with a reference range of 15–21 breaths per minute (Dennis et al 2016). When a woman's respiratory rate is > 25 breaths per minute a clinical review is triggered and if > 30, the rapid response protocol is initiated (Clinical Excellence Commission 2021).

Tachypnoea is an increased respiratory rate above 20 breaths per minute (Churchill et al 2014). Rapid, shallow breathing can occur in response to metabolic acidosis, exercise, fear, pain and fever (the rate rises approximately 4 breaths/minute for each degree the temperature increases). Tachypnoea is the most sensitive indicator of an impending adverse event. The Australian Sepsis Network (2021) advises that a respiratory rate ≥ 25 is a red flag and when combined with another abnormal vital sign, such as temperature > 38.5°C or < 35.5°C, and tachycardia is suggestive of sepsis. Women with suspected sepsis have a high risk of deterioration and observations should be recorded at least every 30 minutes for 2 hours, then hourly for 4 hours. Signs of deterioration in cases of suspected sepsis include a respiratory rate ≥ 25 (Bowyer et al 2017).

Early warning systems, such as Between the Flags (in New South Wales) and Track and Trigger (in Victoria), indicate that a respiratory rate > 25 must trigger action regardless of other observations.

Bradypnoea refers to a decreased respiratory rate of less than 10 breaths per minute (Cooper & Gosnell 2018). Bradypnoea may be a sign of impending respiratory arrest.

Dyspnoea denotes difficulty with breathing and the woman may be seen to use some accessory muscles of respiration (e.g. sternomastoid, scalene, abdominal) and have nasal flaring. Breathlessness (dyspnoea) during normal activity is reported by approximately 70% of healthy pregnant women and can be present from the first trimester (LoMauro & Aliverti 2015). Dyspnoea may be present in women with underlying conditions such as asthma or cardiac disease.

Apnoea is an absence of respiration for a period of 20 seconds or longer.

Breathing is usually silent; when sounds are present, they are usually the result of narrowed airways or moisture within, or inflammation of, the lungs or pleura.

- *Stertorous* breathing occurs when respiration is laboured and a snoring sound is heard due to an obstructed airway (e.g. from tracheal secretions).
- *Wheezing* is due to narrowed airways, particularly the smaller bronchi and bronchioles (e.g. in asthma), and is heard as a high-pitched, squeaking sound.
- *Bubbling* or gurgling sounds occur as air passes through moist secretions within the respiratory tract.
- *Crackles* are an abnormal non-musical sound heard on auscultation during inspiration and sound like hair rubbed together close to the ear.
- *Stridor* occurs when there is an obstruction or spasm within the trachea or larynx and is heard as a high-pitched musical sound, especially during inspiration (Khan 2021).

CHANGES RELATED TO CHILDBIRTH

Pregnancy

During pregnancy the function and anatomy of the respiratory tract change due to hormonal and biochemical alterations, along with mechanical changes due to the enlarging uterus. To support the fetus and uterus, oxygen demands increase, with oxygen consumption 20–30% above the non-pregnant baseline by the third trimester (Lapinsky 2017). Breathing shifts from abdominal to thoracic as the uterus enlarges. The diaphragm is displaced up to 4 cm higher as the lower ribs flare and the transverse diameter of the chest increases up to 6 cm from widened subcostal angles, countering the effect of the enlarging uterus and elevated diaphragm (Durham & Chapman 2014). Minute ventilation increases up to 48% in the first trimester due to increased tidal volume, leaving the respiratory rate barely altered, although pulmonary physiology has changed (LoMauro & Aliverti 2015).

Labour

During labour the respiratory rate increases as women work with their contractions (Marshall & Raynor 2020). Oxygen consumption increases 40–60% and inadequate oxygenation can increase the severity of pain, which in turn can result in hyperventilation. The number and strength of contractions affect the pattern and depth of respiration during labour. Breath-holding should be discouraged as it increases $PaCO_2$ levels, which in turn results in compensatory hyperventilation in an effort to lower $PaCO_2$ levels. Maternal hyperventilation can also lead to dizziness, tingling and decreased fetal oxygenation (Blackburn 2018). Deep, slow breathing between contractions should be encouraged to maintain oxygenation amid considerable muscular activity.

Postnatal period

Respiration returns swiftly to its pre-pregnancy rate, volume and pattern once labour is completed. This is due to the decrease in intra-abdominal pressure that allows increased movement of the diaphragm and the decrease in progesterone. Anatomical changes revert to their pre-pregnant state by 24 weeks post-birth (Blackburn 2018).

FACTORS INCREASING RESPIRATORY RATE

- The respiration rate and depth can be consciously controlled, which can be useful (e.g. breathing patterns in labour). If acidosis or alkalosis occurs, respiration adjusts automatically to maintain acid–base balance in conjunction with other body systems.
- Acidosis.
- Anxiety, nervousness, stress, excitement, fear and other emotions can affect respiration.
- Caffeine.
- Disease: lung or cardiac.
- Exercise/exertion: an increase in oxygen demand causes an increase in respiration.
- Fever increases the body's oxygen demands.
- Haemorrhage/anaemia reduces red blood cells, decreasing the oxygen-carrying capacity of the blood. To overcome this hypoxia, the respiration rate increases to supply the body with extra oxygen.
- High altitude reduces the amount of saturated haemoglobin in the blood.
- Hypercapnia (also known as hypercarbia) is an increased level of carbon dioxide in the blood leading to respiratory acidosis. The respiratory rate increases in an attempt to remove the excess carbon dioxide. Causes are related to a failure to eliminate carbon dioxide and include anaesthesia, sedatives, narcotics, trauma and some neuromuscular disorders such as myasthenia gravis and Guillain-Barré syndrome (Kacmarek et al 2020).
- Hypocapnia (also known as hypocarbia) is a reduced level of carbon dioxide in the blood leading to respiratory alkalosis. The most common cause is hyperventilation from anxiety. Other possible causes of hyperventilation are hypoxia, pulmonary embolism, anaemia and asthma. Hyperventilation causes excessive carbon dioxide loss (Cooper & Gosnell 2018).
- Hypotension.
- Medications, salbutamol, amphetamines, cocaine.
- Infection can impair lung function—the lungs work harder to oxygenate the body.
- Smoking causes long-term changes in the lungs which increase the respiratory rate.
- Pain: hyperventilation is a physiological response to pain.
- Young age: lung capacity increases from infancy to adulthood, which decreases the respiratory rate.

FACTORS DECREASING RESPIRATORY RATE

- Alcohol
- General anaesthetic: the woman will require mechanical ventilation as paralysis of her respiratory function is induced
- Hypothermia: initially the respiratory system is stimulated by exposure to cold; as hypothermia persists, the respiratory rate decreases significantly
- Increased intracranial pressure
- Insult or injury: complications such as pulmonary embolism can cause infarction of lung tissue and respiration may cease
- Medications; for example, bronchodilators dilate the airways decreasing the respiratory rate
- Narcotics: opioids depress respiration; they are unlikely to have this effect in a healthy woman receiving small doses, but transplacental passage of the opioid occurs and there is a risk of respiratory depression for the neonate at birth
- Position: a slumped or stooped position may impair depth of respiration
- Rest/sleep decreases both rate and depth of respiration

INDICATIONS FOR MATERNAL RESPIRATORY ASSESSMENT

- As part of baseline observations
- Whenever other vital signs are recorded, particularly when completing a set of observations
- Admission to hospital, particularly with any respiratory complaint (e.g. asthma, chest infection), chest pain, breathlessness, cyanosis, after a road traffic accident or with any serious disorder (e.g. haemorrhage, thromboembolism)
- Prior to commencing resuscitation
- After recovery from anaesthesia
- Following intrathecal opioids
- Patient-controlled analgesia or epidural with opioids
- Any signs of altered breathing pattern

SKILL 6.1 Assessment of maternal respiration

1. Obtain general consent to complete observations. If a woman is aware her respirations are being counted, she may begin to think about them, which may alter the reading.
2. Perform hand hygiene.
3. Ensure the woman is in a comfortable sitting position.
4. Observe her ability to speak and cough.

Continued

SKILL 6.1 Assessment of maternal respiration—cont'd

5. Note any signs of increased respiratory effort: nasal flaring, pursed lips, use of accessory muscles (e.g. shoulder/neck) and any audible cough/wheeze or grunting sound.
6. Note sound, depth, regularity and symmetry (both sides of the chest rise evenly) of respiration (Sunhill et al 2018).
7. Observe the woman's colour, behaviour (shortage of oxygen can result in confused behaviour and speech), level of consciousness and condition. Central cyanosis (due to prolonged hypoxia) might be seen in the mucous membranes (e.g. lips, tongue, nail beds); peripheral cyanosis usually results from vasoconstriction occurring from a physiological response to a cold environment or a pathological cause (e.g. hypovolaemia).
8. Count respiratory rate (one inhalation and one exhalation = one respiration) by watching the rise and fall of the chest; this can be done immediately after counting the pulse or while measuring peripheral oxygen saturation. The respiration rate should be counted for 60 seconds if irregular, otherwise for 30 seconds, then doubled (Rebeiro et al 2017).
9. Document all findings and act on any deviations from normal. The findings can be recorded pictorially on an observations chart or written in prose. Discuss the findings with the woman.

THE NEONATE

The newborn neonate has an erratic periodic breathing pattern which is interspersed with periods of apnoea (10–15 seconds) with a respiratory rate of 30–40 breaths per minute that can increase to 60 (Ransome & Marshall 2020). Due to the weakness of the intercostal muscles, the neonate may appear to be breathing abdominally as the diaphragm is used extensively (Blackburn 2018).

Tachypnoea in the newborn (above 60 breaths per minute) is the earliest sign of respiratory disease and may also indicate other illnesses (e.g. cardiac, metabolic or infectious) (Marshall & Raynor 2020). The neonate may show other signs of respiratory difficulty when tachypnoeic, such as: nasal flaring where the nares increase in size to decrease the airway resistance up to 40%; grunting from forced expiration through a partially closed glottis (Gardner et al 2016); and using accessory muscles of respiration (the thin chest walls are pulled inwards on inspiration—recession/retraction, usually seen around the sternum, intercostal, subcostal and supracostal muscles) Grunting occurs during expiration as the glottis abruptly closes to increase airway pressure and the functional residual capacity of the lungs (Pramanik et al 2015, Reuter et al 2014).

Neonates are mainly diaphragmatic breathers, which means their diaphragm moves symmetrically with each breath. Asymmetrical breathing should be investigated, particularly following shoulder dystocia, as damage to the neonate's phrenic nerve may have resulted, and can cause asymmetrical breathing movement. The preterm infant may have an immature respiration centre in the brain or structural/physiological deficiencies (e.g. lack of surfactant).

NEONATAL RESPIRATION AT BIRTH

In the fetus terminal air sacs appear from 24 weeks and develop into alveoli, with lung development continuing during early childhood (Pschirrer & Little 2020).

Surfactant levels increase significantly after 30 weeks (Coad et al 2020). Therefore, a neonate born preterm is likely to experience respiratory difficulties. In addition, the neonate's lungs are fluid-filled, and the fluid must be removed at birth and replaced with air for effective ventilation to occur.

Respiration is initiated as the neonate is born and the fetal circulation adapts to the extrauterine circulation, but the process begins before birth. Lung fluid absorption begins during early labour and fluid is expelled through the neonate's nose and mouth as the thorax is squeezed during the neonate's journey through the birth canal. At birth, approximately 35% of the original lung fluid volume remains and must be removed (Blackburn 2018). During birth by caesarean section the fetus does not have the pressure on the thorax and may retain more lung fluid. Neonates born by caesarean section have increased risk of transient tachypnoea of the newborn and persistent pulmonary hypertension.

The first diaphragmatic breath occurs within 9 seconds of birth and generates high positive intrathoracic pressures (70 cmH_2O). As the pressure begins to decrease (30–40 cmH_2O), air enters the lungs. Subsequent breaths require less pressure as the smaller airways and alveoli remain open due to the action of surfactant.

Respiration is initiated by several factors:

- stimulation (light, tactile and temperature)
- compression and decompression of the chest as it passes through the vagina
- stimulation of chemoreceptors

- hypoxaemia and hypercapnia
- changes within the cardiovascular system to perfuse the lungs.

INDICATIONS FOR NEWBORN RESPIRATORY ASSESSMENT

- At birth, as part of the Apgar score
- Whenever vital signs are being recorded (e.g. after meconium-stained amniotic fluid, maternal prolonged rupture of membranes, known maternal Group B streptococcus, hypothermia and hypoglycaemia)
- Any signs of cyanosis, sternal recession, nasal flaring, noisy breathing (e.g. grunting) or increased work of breathing, where the neonate is using more energy to breathe (Sinha et al 2018)
- During resuscitation (see Chapter 42)

SKILL 6.2 Assessment of neonate's respiration

1. Informed consent must be gained from the parent(s).
2. Calm a crying or excited neonate so respiration can be counted accurately.
3. Expose the chest and abdomen.
4. Count the respiratory rate for 1 minute by observing, feeling or listening with a stethoscope. Count for 1 minute to increase accuracy as the newborn's respiratory rate is often irregular.
5. Note any signs of increased respiratory effort: nasal flaring, grunting, sternal, subcostal or supracostal recession/retraction.
6. Record findings, discuss them with the neonate's parent(s) and act on the findings accordingly.

PULSE OXIMETRY

Definition

Pulse oximetry is a non-invasive method of monitoring arterial oxygen saturation (referred to as SpO_2) and is used in conjunction with respiration assessment. Pulse oximetry can provide an early warning of hypoxaemia before visible cyanosis is evident, which may not occur until the SpO_2 is < 80% (Frank et al 2013).

Approximately 98–99% of the oxygen breathed in is carried by the haemoglobin in the blood to the body tissues and organs (arterial haemoglobin saturation: SaO_2). The other 1–2% is dissolved in the plasma and is known as the partial pressure of oxygen (PaO_2).

Pulse oximetry compares changes in the light absorption of oxygenated and deoxygenated blood (Myatt 2017).

Oxygenated blood absorbs red light at a wavelength of 640 nm and deoxygenated blood absorbs infrared light at 940 nm. The ratio of oxygenated haemoglobin (arterial, bright red blood) and deoxygenated haemoglobin (venous, dark red blood) is calculated and converted to a percentage to give the saturation reading (Myatt 2017).

Pulse oximeters are accurate to within 2–4% of oxyhaemoglobin levels measured in arterial blood gas samples but are less accurate for SpO_2 values < 80% (Kacmarek et al 2020). Pulse oximetry has rapidly gained acceptance because it is easy to use and non-invasive.

Normal values

Normal arterial oxygen saturation (SpO_2) in an adult is 95–100% (World Health Organization [WHO] 2011). The average SpO_2 for pregnant women at term is 99% ± 1.0% according to Dennis and colleagues (2016).

Babies have lower saturation levels at birth and should not receive supplemental oxygen unless they do not meet the lower limit of normal. The Australian and New Zealand Committee on Resuscitation (ANZCOR) developed the recommendations used in the Australian Resuscitation Council Guidelines (2016) for newborn SpO_2 levels. The targeted preductal SpO_2 readings in the first 10 minutes after birth are as follows.

- 1 minute: 60–70%
- 2 minutes: 65–85%
- 3 minutes: 70–90%
- 4 minutes: 75–90%
- 5 minutes: 80–90%
- 10 minutes: 85–90%

FACTORS AFFECTING ACCURACY OF PULSE OXIMETER READINGS:

- Anaemia: the SpO_2 may be normal despite a lowered potential to carry oxygen (Khan 2021).
- Bright or fluorescent lighting has minimal effect.
- Hypoxemia: In the context of hypoxemia the SaO_2 reading is frequently overestimated in infants and children (Ross et al 2014).
- Inaccurately sized, poorly fitting probe.
- Intravenous dyes, such as methylene blue, are used for diagnosis and may lead to falsely low readings.
- Jaundice: This does not appear to effect results (McGee 2018). A wearable transcutaneous bilirubinometer has been developed with the ability to measure oxygen saturation and heart rate (Inamori et al 2021).
- Low perfusion (decreased cardiac output, vasoconstriction, hypothermia).
- Movement causes motion artifact (e.g. shivering/tremors/seizures).
- Nail polish: Early studies found nail polish and artificial nails lowered readings (Kacmarek et al 2020). Some research indicates nail polish and

acrylic nails do not cause inaccurate results due to the increased sensitivity of the LED component (Kacmarek et al 2020, Purcell & Mannion 2018). However, other literature has found nail polish and artificial nails can impact accuracy (McGee 2018, Pilcher et al 2020, Villaflor et al 2013).

- Neonatal probes are supplied with their fixative tape; applying additional tape can affect the results.
- Supplemental oxygen: Hypoventilation will not be reliably detected when supplemental oxygen is being administered (Iscoe et al 2011).
- The darkness or lightness of skin pigment in neonates has minimal impact on accuracy (Foglia et al 2017). In adults, darker skin pigment may alter readings (Sjoding et al 2020).
- The right type of probe must be applied correctly by following the manufacturer's instructions.

SKILL 6.3 Assessment: maternal pulse oximetry

1. Explain the purpose of the procedure and obtain informed consent.
2. Perform hand hygiene.
3. Assess the appropriate monitoring site (Fig 6.1). Ensure there is adequate circulation at the site; if the woman's finger is used, remove any nail polish (as a precaution) and avoid oedematous sites. Remove earring if earlobe is used.
4. Attach the pulse oximeter sensor probe to the monitoring site (finger, toe or earlobe). The light should pass from the top to the bottom of the probe.
5. Ask the woman to remain still during the assessment as movement can affect accuracy.
6. Turn on the oximeter and observe the pulse waveform/intensity on the display. Check the pulse rate on the oximeter display matches the woman's radial pulse. If the pulses are different, the oximeter reading may be inaccurate.
7. Leave the probe in place until a constant value is reached.
8. Continuous monitoring will require alarms to be activated and set to detect alterations in the woman's condition. Ensure the woman's skin integrity by relocating the sensor every 2–4 hours.
9. Perform hand hygiene.
10. Document SpO_2 readings on the observations chart pictorially and in the notes if necessary.
11. Report any abnormal findings and take action if required.
12. Discuss the findings with the woman.

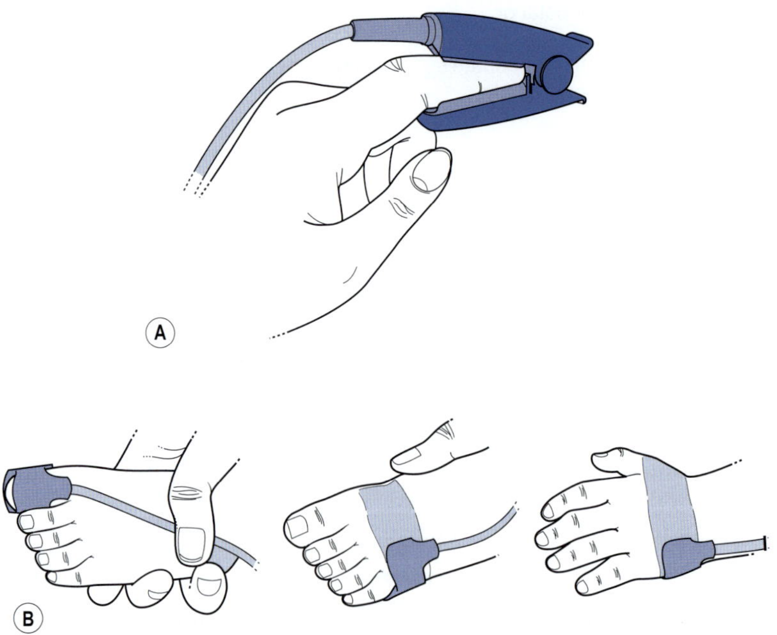

FIGURE 6.1 **A, Adult pulse oximetry probe. B, Neonatal pulse oximetry probe.**
Source: Adapted with kind permission from Jamieson EM, McCall J, Whyte L: Clinical nursing practices, 4th ed., Churchill Livingstone, Edinburgh, 2002.

SKILL 6.4 Assessment: newborn pulse oximetry

1. Informed consent must be gained from the parent(s).
2. Perform hand hygiene.
3. Ensure the neonate is in a quiet, alert state (McVea et al 2019). During crying, feeding and sleeping, the neonate can have periods of desaturation < 95%; when the neonate is in the active, alert state, motion artifact can create falsely low readings.
4. Ensure the monitoring site is not cold.
5. Place the oximeter sensor on the hand, wrist or foot; the light should pass from the top to the bottom of the probe.
6. Leave the probe in place until a constant value is reached.
7. Continuous monitoring will require alarms to be activated and set to detect alterations in the newborn's condition. Ensure skin integrity by relocating the sensor every 2–4 hours.

SKILL 6.5 Assessment: pulse oximetry screening for congenital heart disease

Pulse oximetry is increasingly used for early detection of critical congenital heart disease (CCHD) in neonates and is undertaken at 24–48 hours of age or close to discharge if less than 24 hours old (Andrews et al 2014). Early detection improves outcomes and is important as neonates with CCHD can deteriorate suddenly, making treatment more difficult (Cloete et al 2020). Although false positives and negatives occur, it is generally viewed as a useful screening tool—the routine newborn examination does not usually detect CCHD as the neonates rarely exhibit signs at this time (Ewer 2019). A failed pulse oximeter screen frequently results from non-CCHD causes including infection, respiratory problems or congenital anomalies (Hom & Martin 2016).

Follow the steps for pulse oximetry (Skill 6.4), and in addition:

- take a reading from the right hand (preductal) and either foot (postductal)
- allow 3–4 minutes for the screening
- if both are ≥ 95% or the difference is ≤ 3%, the screen is negative (normal)
- if both are < 90%, the screen is positive (abnormal) and the neonate requires medical review and referral for further testing
- if the readings are 90–94% or the difference is > 3%, the screen is considered borderline; if the neonate appears well and has a normal examination, the screen should be repeated in 1 hour (local protocols may vary); if the screening is not in the normal range after being repeated twice, the neonate requires a medical review and possibly referral to a specialist.

Thermal damage, which can cause necrosis, may occur in the neonate if a probe is left in one position for too long. It is therefore advisable to re-site the probe every 4 hours.

The midwife must be familiar with the equipment, noting correct storage, use and maintenance, and knowing when to refer.

Pulse oximetry use and findings must be documented.

RECOGNISING AND RESPONDING TO CLINICAL DETERIORATION USING EARLY WARNING SYSTEMS

The Australian Commission on Safety and Quality in Health Care (ACSQHC 2021) has developed a national consensus statement outlining the essential elements for recognising and responding to clinical deterioration. In the *National Safety and Quality Health Service (NSQHS) Standards* (2017), standard 8 is titled 'Recognising and responding to acute deterioration'.

Early warning systems have been introduced in Australia and New Zealand. The New Zealand Early Warning Score (NZEWS) is used for non-pregnant adults and a Maternity Early Warning System (MEWS) has been developed for childbearing women. Specialised maternity early warning systems account for the physiological changes of pregnancy. In Australia, each state/territory has an early warning system: Between the Flags (New South Wales), Queensland Adult Deterioration Detection System (Q-ADDS) (Queensland), Maternity Observation and Response Chart (MORC) (Western Australia), Modified Early Warning Score (MEWS) (Australian Capital Territory), Rapid Detection and Response Maternal Observation Chart (South Australia) and Modified Early Warning Score (MEWS) (Victoria).

The ACSQHC's *A Guide to Support Implementation of the National Consensus Statement* (2011) indicates that the following observations are important for recognising clinical deterioration: respiratory rate, oxygen saturation, heart rate, blood pressure, temperature and level of consciousness. A full set of vital signs should be taken; however, when compliance has been monitored, only 21% of vital signs involve a full set of measurements (Cardona-Morrell et al 2016).

Early warning systems chart each vital sign separately, making graphical trends easier to recognise. The vital signs are colour-coded with white as normal and other colours such as yellow and orange indicating increasing severity. Each chart contains information on the pathway the midwife should follow if observations are outside the normal zone. The pathways include notifying the midwife in charge, clinical review or initiation of a rapid response (e.g. calling the medical emergency team, commonly known as a MET call).

Although the respiratory rate is important for assessing clinical condition, it is the least recorded (Kellet & Sebat 2017).

Maternal early warning charts can be used for pregnant women from 20 weeks gestation and can be modified to include postnatal factors up to 6 weeks (Cole 2014) and PV loss.

Role and responsibilities of the midwife

These can be summarised as:

- recognising the significance of respiration assessment, when it is indicated and when other interventions such as pulse oximetry are required
- recognising normal respiration rates, depth, patterns and sounds, and identifying deviations from normal for both the woman and the neonate
- undertaking the assessment correctly
- using pulse oximetry appropriately
- completing the early warning observation chart accurately, identifying and acting on any triggers found.

SUMMARY

- Assessing respiration in an adult should be undertaken discreetly.
- A neonate's respiratory rate can be observed or felt and should be counted for 60 seconds.
- Respiration assessment includes rate, depth, regularity, sound and posture.
- The general condition of the woman or neonate is assessed simultaneously.
- Pulse oximetry is an accurate, non-invasive technique that measures oxygen saturation via a correctly fitted peripheral probe and can be used as a screening tool for critical congenital heart disease in the newborn.
- An early warning observation chart should be used for pregnant and postnatal women who have or are at risk of developing deviations from the normal.

Self-assessment exercises

The answers to the following questions may be found in the text.

1. Discuss how pregnancy, labour and the puerperium affect respiration. What would be the accepted normal values during these times?
2. Identify five factors that may increase respiration.
3. Why is a preterm neonate more likely to develop respiratory problems than a term neonate?
4. Describe when the midwife is likely to complete a respiration assessment:
   a. for a woman
   b. for a neonate.
5. Which factors affect the accuracy of pulse oximetry?
6. Summarise the role and responsibilities of the midwife when undertaking respiration assessment.
7. What is an early warning chart and why should it be used for a woman following a caesarean section?

Resources

Australian Commission on Safety and Quality in Health Care: Quick-start guide to the implementation of essential element 1: measurement and documentation of observations. ACSQHC, Sydney, 2012. Available: www.safetyandquality.gov.au/sites/default/files/migrated/Quick-start-guide-to-essential-element-1.pdf.

Australian Sepsis Network: Recognising sepsis. Online. Available: www.australiansepsisnetwork.net.au.

Clinical Excellence Commission—Between the flags, standard calling criteria. Online. Available: www.cec.health.nsw.gov.au/keep-patients-safe/deteriorating-patient-program/between-the-flags/standard-calling-criteria.

Health Quality & Safety Commission New Zealand: Deteriorating adult patient evidence summary, 2016. Online. Available: www.hqsc.govt.nz.

References

Andrews J, Ross A, Salazar M, et al: Smooth implementation of critical congenital heart defect screening in a newborn nursery, Clinical Paediatrics 53(2):173–176, 2014.

Australian Commission on Safety and Quality in Health Care (ACSQHC): National consensus statement: essential elements for recognising and responding to acute physiological deterioration second edition. ACSQHC, Sydney, January 2017. Online 14 March 2021. Available: www.safetyandquality.gov.au/sites/default/files/migrated/National-Consensus-Statement-clinical-deterioration_2017.pdf

Australian Commission on Safety and Quality in Health Care (ACSQHC): National safety and quality health service standards, 2nd ed.—version 2, ACSQHC, Sydney, 2021. Online 16 March 2021. Available: www.safetyandquality.gov.au/sites/default/files/2021-05/national_safety_and_quality_health_service_nsqhs_standards_second_edition_-_updated_may_2021.pdf.

Australian Commission on Safety and Quality in Health Care (ACSQHC): A guide to support implementation of the national consensus statement: essential elements for recognising and responding to clinical deterioration, Sydney, 2011, ACSQHC. Online 20 March 2021. Available: www.safetyandquality.gov.au/wp-content/uploads/2012/02/Nat-Consensus-Statement-PDF-Complete-Guide.pdf.

Australian Resuscitation Council (ARC): The ARC guidelines, 2016. Online 16 March 2021. Available: https://resus.org.au/guidelines/.

Australian Sepsis Network: Recognising sepsis, 2021. Online 16 March 2021. Available: www.australiansepsisnetwork.net.au/healthcare-providers/recognising-sepsis.

Blackburn ST: Maternal, fetal and neonatal physiology: a clinical perspective, 5th ed., Elsevier, St Louis, 2018.

Bowyer L, Robinson H, Barrett H, et al: SOMANZ Guidelines for sepsis in pregnancy. Society of Obstetric Medicine Australia and New Zealand, 2017.

Bullock S, Hales M: Principles of pathophysiology, 2nd ed., Pearson Australia, Melbourne, 2018.

Cardona-Morrell N, Prgomet M, Lake R, et al: Vital signs monitoring and nurse–patient interaction: a qualitative observational study of hospital practice, International Journal Nursing Studies 56:9–16, 2016.

Churchill D, Rodger A, Clift J, et al: Think sepsis. In Knight M, Kenyon S, Brocklehurst P, et al, editors: Saving lives, improving mothers' care—lessons learned to inform future maternity care from the UK and Ireland confidential enquiries into maternal deaths and morbidity 2009–12, MBRRACE-UK. National Perinatal Epidemiology Unit, Oxford, 2014, pp. 27–44.

Clinical Excellence Commission: Between the flags, 2021. Online 16 March 2021. Available: www.cec.health.nsw.gov.au/keep-patients-safe/deteriorating-patient-program/between-the-flags

Cloete E, Gentles TL, Webster DR et al: Pulse oximetry screening in a midwifery-led maternity setting with high antenatal detection of congenital heart disease. Acta Paediatrica 109(1):100–108, 2020.

Coad J, Pedley K, Dunstall M: Anatomy and physiology for midwives, 4th ed., Elsevier, Edinburgh, 2020.

Cole MF: A modified early obstetric warning system, British Journal of Midwifery 22(12):862–868, 2014.

Cooper K, Gosnell K: Foundations and adult health nursing, Mosby Elsevier, St Louis, 2018.

Dennis AT, Hardy L, Dennis A: Defining a reference range for vital signs in healthy term pregnant women undergoing caesarean section, Anaesthesia & Intensive Care 44:752–757, 2016.

Durham R, Chapman L: Maternal–newborn nursing: the critical components of nursing care, 2nd ed., F.A. Davis, Philadelphia, 2014.

Ewer A: Neonatal screening for critical congenital heart defects, Multidisciplinary Digital Publishing Institute (MDPI), 2019.

Flenady T, Dwyer T, Applegarth J: Accurate respiratory rates count: so should you! Australasian Emergency Nursing Journal 20(1):45–47, 2017.

Foglia E, Whyte R, Chaudhary A, et al: The effect of skin pigmentation on the accuracy of pulse oximetry in infants with hypoxemia, The Journal of Pediatrics 182:375–377, 2017.

Frank L, Bradshaw E, Beekman R, et al: Screening for critical congenital heart disease using pulse oximetry, Journal of Pediatrics 162(3):445–453, 2013.

Gardner SL, Enzman-Hines M, Nyp M: Respiratory diseases. In Gardner SL, Carter BS, Enzman-Hines M et al, editors: Merenstein & Gardner's handbook of neonatal intensive care, 7th ed., Mosby, St Louis, 2016, pp. 565–643.

Health Quality & Safety Commission New Zealand: Deteriorating adult patient evidence summary, 2016. Online 8 Jan 2021. Available: www.hqsc.govt.nz.

Hom LA, Martin GR: Newborn critical congenital heart disease screening using pulse oximetry: nursing aspects, American Journal of Perinatology 33:1072–1075, 2016.

Inamori G, Kamoto U, Nakamura F, et al: Neonatal wearable device for colorimetry-based real-time detection of jaundice with simultaneous sensing of vitals. Science Advances 7(10):eabe3793, 2021.

Iscoe S, Beasley R, Fisher A: Supplementary oxygen for nonhypoxemic patients: O_2 much of a good thing? Critical Care 15:305, 2011.

Kacmarek RM, Stoller JK, Heuer A: Egan's fundamentals of respiratory care. Elsevier, St Louis, 2020.

Kellett J, Sebat F: (2017). Make vital signs great again—a call for action, European Journal of Internal Medicine 45:13–19.

Khan R: Vital signs. Ch 20: Vital sign assessment. In Koutoukidis G, Stainton K, editors: Tabbner's nursing care, 8th ed., Elsevier Australia, Sydney, 2021.

Lapinsky SE: Management of acute respiratory failure in pregnancy, Seminars in Respiratory Critical Care Medicine 38(2):201–207, 2017.

LoMauro A, Aliverti A: Respiratory physiology of pregnancy, Breathe 11:297–301, 2015.

Marshall J, Raynor M: Myles textbook for midwives, 17th ed., Churchill Livingstone, Elsevier, Edinburgh, 2020.

McGee S: Cyanosis. In Evidence-based physical diagnosis, 4th ed., Elsevier 2018, pp. 69–72.e1.

McVea S, McGowan M, Rao B: How to use saturation monitoring in newborns. Archives of disease in childhood. Education and practice edition 104(1), 2019.

Mesquita Montes A, Tam C, Crasto C et al: Forward trunk lean with arm support affects the activity of accessory respiratory muscles and thoracoabdominal movement in healthy individuals. Human movement science 61:167–176, 2018.

Mora JC, Schneider A, Robbins R, et al: Epidemiology of early rapid response team activation after emergency department admission, Australasian Emergency Nursing Journal 19:54–61, 2016.

Myatt R: Pulse oximetry: what the nurse needs to know. Nursing Standard 31(31):42–45, 2017.

Pilcher J, Ploen L, McKinstry S, et al: A multicentre prospective observational study comparing arterial blood gas values to those obtained by pulse oximeters used in adult patients attending Australian and New Zealand hospitals, BMC Pulmonary Medicine 20(1):7–7, 2020. Available: https://doi.org/10.1186/s12890-019-1007-3

Porritt K: Vital signs. Ch 25 Nursing care of an individual: cardiovascular and respiratory. In Koutoukidis G, Stainton K, editors: Tabbner's nursing care, 8th ed., Elsevier Australia, Sydney, 2021.

Pschirrer R, Little GA: Part 1. In Campbell, D. Neonatology for primary care, 2nd ed., American Academy of Pediatrics, Itasca, Illinois, 2020, pp. 3–58.

Pramanik AK, Rangaswamy N, Gates T: Neonatal respiratory distress: a practical approach to its diagnosis and management. Pediatric Clinics of North America 62(2):453–469, 2015.

Purcell J, Mannion S: Medical fashion victims? Do nail polishes and acrylic nails affect digital pulse oximetry and patient management in the clinical setting? Euroanaesthesia 2018, The European Anaesthesiology Congress, Abstracts Programme Berlin, Germany, 30 May – 2 June 2018.

Ransome H, Marshall E: Recognising the healthy baby at term through examination of the newborn screening. In Marshall J, Raynor M, editors: 2020. Myles textbook for midwives, 17th ed., Elsevier, Edinburgh, 2017, pp. 814–847.

Rebeiro G, Wilson D, Scully N, et al: Fundamentals of nursing. Clinical skills workbook, 3rd ed., Elsevier, Sydney, 2017.

Ross P, Newth C, Khemani R: Accuracy of pulse oximetry in children, Pediatrics 133(1):22–29, 2014.

Reuter S., Moser C., Baack M. Respiratory distress in the newborn. Pediatrics in Review 2014;35(10):417–428.

Schoenwald & Douglas, Part 6. In Crisp J, Douglas C, Rebeiro G, Waters D: Potter & Perry's fundamentals of nursing 5th Australia and New Zealand edition, Elsevier, Sydney, 2017.

Sinha S, Miall L, Jardine L: Essential neonatal medicine, 6th ed., John Wiley & Sons, Hoboken, New Jersey, 2018.

Sjoding MW, Dickson RP, Iwashyna TJ, et al: Racial bias in pulse oximetry measurement. New England Journal of Medicine 383:2477–2478, 2020. doi:10.1056/NEJMc2029240

Villaflor C, Morean C, Lim N, et al: Effect of acrylic gel nail art on pulse oximetry readings, Singapore Nursing Journal 40(4):38–41, 2013.

World Health Organization (WHO): Pulse oximetry training manual, 2011. Online 14 March 2021. Available: www.who.int/patientsafety/safesurgery/pulse_oximetry/who_ps_pulse_oxymetry_training_manual_en.pdf.

CHAPTER 7
BLOOD PRESSURE

Learning outcomes

Having read this chapter, the reader should be able to:

- define blood pressure, identifying the difference between systolic and diastolic pressure and the normal range for the childbearing woman and neonate
- discuss the midwife's role and responsibilities in relation to the measurement of blood pressure, identifying when and how it is undertaken
- discuss the factors that influence blood pressure, including the changes relating to childbearing
- discuss factors influencing the accuracy of blood pressure measurement and how the midwife can minimise these
- describe how central venous pressure is measured using a manual manometer.

HYPERTENSIVE DISORDERS

Hypertensive (raised blood pressure) disorders are one of the most common pregnancy complications. In Australia between 2009 and 2018 there were 10 direct maternal deaths related to the effects of pre-eclampsia, eclampsia and other disorders of hypertension in pregnancy (AIHW 2020). The maternal mortality rate for hypertensive disorders from 2009 to 2018 was 0.3 per 100,000 women who gave birth in Australia (AIHW 2020). In New Zealand there were four maternal deaths (0.58 per 100,000 births at or over 20 weeks with a weight of at least 400 g if gestation is unknown) directly related to hypertensive disorders from 2006 to 2016 (Perinatal and Maternal Mortality Review Committee [PMMRC] 2018). Over this 10-year period 63 maternal deaths directly related to obstetric causes occurred, with 3.7% of these deaths related to hypertension (PMMRC 2018).

Hypertension during pregnancy is one of the four leading causes of maternal mortality globally (WHO 2019). Hypertensive disorders have long-term impacts. Women with chronic hypertension have increased rates (24%) of infants that are small for gestational age (SGA), defined as a birth weight below the 10th percentile (Morgan et al 2016), lower gestational ages at birth (Andreas et al 2016) and increased rates of neonatal unit admission and perinatal mortality (Agrawal & Wenger 2020). Increased blood pressures in early pregnancy are associated with pre-eclampsia later in pregnancy (Morgan et al 2016).

Hypertension is one of the common disorders of pregnancy with around 5–10% of women diagnosed (Agrawal & Wenger 2020). In Australia and New Zealand the number is estimated to be 9.2% (Helou et al 2017). The midwife is ideally placed to measure blood pressure in childbearing women, confirming normality, detecting deviations from normal and referring the woman for further assessment. It is crucial the midwife carries out this procedure accurately as changes in blood pressure can have serious consequences for both the woman and the fetus/neonate.

This chapter considers the issues surrounding the accurate measurement of arterial blood pressure, physiology, influencing factors and changes that occur during childbirth. The equipment used, technique of blood pressure measurement and factors influencing the accuracy of the recording are discussed. The chapter concludes with a discussion of venous blood pressure measurement.

DEFINITION

Blood pressure is the force exerted by the blood on the blood vessel walls. It varies within the different blood vessels, being highest in the large arteries closest to the heart and decreasing gradually within the smaller arteries, arterioles and capillaries. Blood pressure continues to reduce as blood returns to the heart via the venules and veins. Blood pressure measurement usually reflects the arterial blood pressure, although venous pressure may also be measured. The brachial artery is generally used to measure blood pressure in the adult (Fig 7.1).

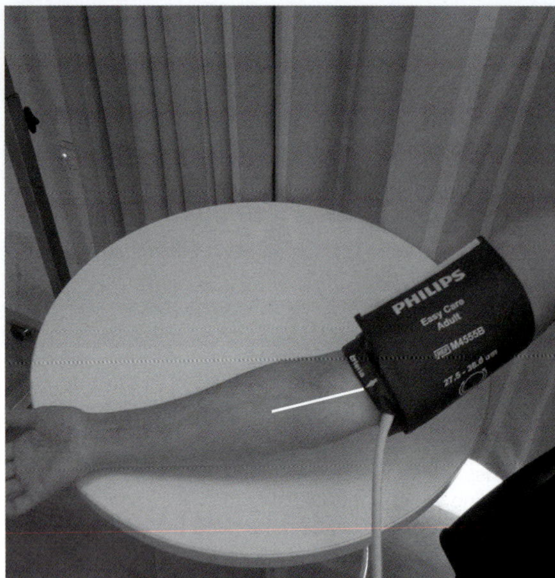

FIGURE 7.1 Brachial artery.

MEASURING BLOOD PRESSURE

Arterial blood pressure

Arterial blood pressure (ABP) is the pressure exerted on the arterial walls to facilitate blood flow around the body to ensure adequate oxygenation of the tissues and vital organs. It is not constant, increasing during ventricular contraction (systole) and decreasing when the ventricles relax (diastole). When recording blood pressure it is important to assess both the highest and lowest levels of pressure as these reflect differing physiological responses of the cardiac cycle. The ABP measurement is documented numerically in millimetres of mercury (e.g. systole 130 mmHg and diastole 80 mmHg, recorded as 130 over 80).

Systolic blood pressure

Systolic blood pressure (SBP) is the pressure exerted on the blood vessel walls following ventricular systole when the arteries contain the most blood and is the time of maximal pressure. SBP is determined by the:

- amount of blood ejected in the arteries (stroke volume)
- force of the contraction
- dispensability of the arterial wall.

An increase in the first two factors or a decrease in the third factor raises SBP and vice versa.

Diastolic blood pressure

Diastolic blood pressure (DBP) is the pressure exerted on the blood vessel walls during ventricular diastole when the arteries contain the least amount of blood, resulting in the least pressure being exerted on the blood vessel walls. DBP is influenced by the:

- degree of peripheral resistance
- systolic pressure
- cardiac output.

DBP is lower when these are reduced, particularly when the heart rate is slower, as there is less blood remaining in the arteries.

Mean arterial pressure

The **mean arterial pressure (MAP)** is the average pressure required to push the blood through the circulatory system. MAP remains relatively constant during normal pregnancy (Meah et al 2016). A low MAP is associated with decreased organ perfusion and a high MAP is associated with increased cardiac workload; therefore, MAP can indicate acute alterations in perfusion. A MAP > 60 is required for adequate perfusion (DeMers & Wachs 2020). Severe shock is defined as a MAP < 60 (El Ayadi et al 2016). A MAP < 50 is considered critical as cerebral blood flow is impaired (Russell 2014). A significant drop in blood volume due to haemorrhage or profound vasodilation caused by septic shock is associated with a decrease in the MAP (Ward & Linden 2017). When sepsis is present the target MAP is > 65 (Russell 2014).

Women with chronic hypertension who develop pre-eclampsia were found to have higher MAP when they commenced prenatal care, and women with preterm birth prior to 34 weeks had a significantly higher MAP (Morgan et al 2016). MAP was increased in women with high-risk pregnancy (Stott et al 2017). An elevated MAP at 11–13 weeks' gestation is associated with an increased incidence of SGA infants and maternal pre-eclampsia, particularly in women with chronic hypertension (Panaitescu et al 2017).

MAP decreases in the first and second trimester and increases in the third trimester (Melchiorre et al 2016). MAP is affected by the gestation of the pregnancy, the mother's age, body mass index (BMI), racial origin, history of chronic hypertension and diabetes (Wright et al 2015). Maternal obesity also increases MAP (Guy et al 2017, Vinayagam et al 2016). Maternal characteristics in combination with MAP detected 67% of women who developed pre-eclampsia resulting in a preterm birth (Silveira Rocha et al 2017). The MAP assists with interpreting changes occurring in blood pressure measurements when the systolic and diastolic pressures alter at different rates. It can be estimated electronically or mathematically using the formula:

Mean arterial pressure $= \frac{1}{3}$ systolic pressure $+ \frac{2}{3}$ diastolic pressure

Alternatively, it can be calculated by doubling the diastolic pressure reading, adding it to the systolic reading and dividing the total by three. Thus, a blood pressure of 110/65 mmHg has a MAP of 80 mmHg, while a blood pressure of 150/90 mmHg has a MAP of 110 mmHg. MAP ranges are listed (Tables 7.1 and 7.2).

TABLE 7.1 MEAN ARTERIAL PRESSURE (MAP) IN PREGNANCY

Parameter	Non-pregnant control	Trimester 1	Trimester 2	Trimester 3	Term	Postpartum control	*P* value
MAP mmHg	83 (IQR 71–90)	77 (IQR 70–83)	79 (IQR 73–83)	83 (IQR 73–87)	83 (IQR 74–90)	83 (IQR 77–93)	< 0.001

Note: Interquartile range (IQR) indicates the middle 50% of values.
Source: Melchiorre K, Sharma R, Khalil A, et al: Maternal cardiovascular function in normal pregnancy, Hypertension 67:754–762, 2016.

TABLE 7.2 NORMAL MEAN ARTERIAL PRESSURE (MAP) IN NORMOTENSIVE PREGNANCY AND PREGNANCY WITH GESTATIONAL HYPERTENSION

	Normotensive pregnancies	Gestational hypertension	P value
MAP (mmHg) at 12 weeks	85 (IQR 81–91)	92 (IQR 88–102.5)	0.0001
MAP (mmHg) at 20 weeks	83 (IQR 78–88)	92 (IQR 87–99)	0.0001

Note: Interquartile range (IQR) indicates the middle 50% of values.
Source: Vonck S, Staelens AS, Bollen I, et al: Why non-invasive maternal hemodynamics assessment is clinically relevant in early pregnancy: a literature review, BMC Pregnancy and Childbirth 16:27–35, 2016.

Pulse pressure

Pulse pressure (PP) is the difference between SBP and DBP; a normal SBP is around 40 mmHg higher than DBP (Lippincott et al 2015). PP normally decreases during pregnancy (Iacobaeus et al 2017). A rise in PP results from an increased SBP and/or a decrease in DBP due to increased stroke volume, decreased peripheral resistance or both, and is associated with infection, pyrexia, exercise and bradycardia. A decrease in PP is due to a decrease in SBP and/or an increase in DBP resulting from decreased stroke volume, increased peripheral resistance or both, and can result from hypovolaemia (e.g. shock and haemorrhage). A narrowing PP can indicate increasing blood loss (Priestley et al 2019). PP is also an indicator of the elasticity of blood vessels, with increased PP associated with stiffer, less-elastic vessels (Iacobaeus et al 2017). Women who develop complicated hypertension during pregnancy were found to have higher PP prior to pregnancy (Hale et al 2010).

Venous blood pressure

Venous blood pressure is the pressure exerted on the walls of the veins, reflecting venous flow to the heart (particularly circulating blood volume) and cardiac function. Central venous pressure (CVP) measures the pressure within the right atrium and is determined by:

- the volume of blood entering the right atrium (venous return)
- right ventricular function
- venous tone
- intrathoracic pressure.

NORMAL MATERNAL ARTERIAL BLOOD PRESSURE VALUES

The National Heart Foundation of Australia (NHFA) (2016) has developed guidelines for classification of blood pressure in adults. An optimal blood pressure is considered to be a systolic BP < 120 mmHg and a diastolic < 80 mmHg, with a systolic of 120–129 and a diastolic of 80–84 considered normal. Hypertension is defined as a blood pressure ≥ 140/90 mmHg (NHFA 2016). This is consistent with the National Institute for Health and Care Excellence (NICE) (2019) and the WHO (2021) definition of hypertension as a SBP ≥ 140 mmHg and a DBP ≥ 90 mmHg (Table 7.3).

TABLE 7.3 CLASSIFICATION OF CLINICAL BLOOD PRESSURE LEVELS IN ADULTS

Diagnostic category*	Systolic (mmHg)	Diastolic (mmHg)
Optimal	< 120 and	< 80
Normal	120–129 and/or	80–84
Grade 1 mild hypertension	140–159 and/or	90–99
Grade 2 moderate hypertension	160–179 and/or	100–109
Grade 3 severe hypertension	≥ 180 and/or	≥ 110
Isolated systolic hypertension	> 140 and	< 90
Pregnancy	≥ 140	≥ 90

*When the systolic and diastolic blood pressure levels fall into different categories, the higher diagnostic category applies.
Source: National Heart Foundation of Australia: Guideline for the diagnosis and management of hypertension in adults, 2016. Melbourne. Accessed 20 October 2017. Online 5 July 2021. Available: https://www.heartfoundation.org.au/conditions/hypertension. Reproduced with permission from Guideline for the diagnosis and management of hypertension in adults 2016. © 2016 National Heart Foundation of Australia.

Blood pressure varies according to age, lifestyle and other variables. In 2017–18, hypertension was present in 20% of Australian women over 18 years (AIHW 2019). The incidence of hypertension is rising in New Zealand and now affects more than one in five adult women (Health Navigator New Zealand 2015). Higher rates of hypertension occur in Indigenous Australians (Duffy et al 2016) and Māori communities (Oetzel et al 2017). Chronic hypertension prior to pregnancy increases the risk of pre-eclampsia, impaired fetal growth and other complications of pregnancy.

The Society of Obstetric Medicine of Australia and New Zealand (SOMANZ) (Lowe et al 2015) defines hypertension in pregnancy as:

- systolic blood pressure ≥ 140 mmHg and/or
- diastolic blood pressure ≥ 90 mmHg (Korotkoff V).

The Australian *Clinical Practice Guidelines: Pregnancy Care* indicate that women with a single DBP measurement of ≥ 110 mmHg or more, or two consecutive readings of 90 mmHg or more at least 4 hours apart (or proteinuria > 1+) should have increased monitoring and treatment needs to be considered (Department of Health 2020). Women with a SBP ≥ 140 mmHg on two consecutive readings at least 4 hours apart should also be subject to increased monitoring and possible treatment (Table 7.4).

For home monitoring of blood pressure an average BP measurement of ≥ 135/85 mmHg is used for diagnosis of hypertension (Sharman et al 2016). The Royal Australian College of General Practitioners has a Microsoft Excel spreadsheet available for recording and averaging BP values (see Resources at the end of the chapter).

The SOMNAZ guidelines recommend antihypertensive treatment during pregnancy for all women with SBP ≥ 160 mmHg or diastolic ≥ 110 mmHg. SBP ≥ 170 mmHg with or without diastolic ≥ 110 mmHg is classified as severe hypertension and warrants urgent treatment due to increased risk of maternal morbidity and mortality (Lowe et al 2015).

Hypotension (low blood pressure) is defined as SBP of < 90 mmHg (Bishop et al 2017, Sharma et al 2016) or a single episode of hypotension below 80% of the baseline value (Loubert et al 2017). Some studies use < 90 mmHg or ≥ 30% reduction in baseline SBP to define hypotension (Sharma et al 2016). The SOMNAZ guidelines for the investigation and management of sepsis in pregnancy indicate a SBP < 90 mmHg is indicative of sepsis until proven otherwise (Bowyer et al 2017). Hypotension is not the first indicator of haemorrhage as healthy women can lose up to 30% of their blood volume before their SBP decreases (Nathan, El Ayadi, Hezelgrave et al 2015).

When women are in the supine position after 33 weeks gestation, cardiac output is significantly reduced (Andreas et al 2016). Reduced maternal cardiac output can decrease uteroplacental blood flow and result in fetal compromise (Soma-Pillay et al 2016). Supine hypotension results from the pressure of the gravid uterus on the inferior vena cava and abdominal aorta leading to a reduction in venous return and stroke volume, which may decrease cardiac output by up to 25% (Soma-Pillay et al 2016). However, a study using MRI to examine the effects of position on maternal haemodynamics found the supine position resulted in a significant difference in cardiac output, beginning at 26–30 weeks in normal weight women but not in overweight/obese women (Nelson et al 2015).

TABLE 7.4 CLASSIFICATION OF HYPERTENSION IN PREGNANCY

Classification	Definition
Hypertension in pregnancy	≥ 140 mmHg and/or ≥ 90 mmHg (Korotkoff V).
Pre-eclampsia	Hypertension plus one or more of the following signs: • pulmonary oedema • renal, haematological, liver or neurological involvement • fetal growth restriction
Gestational hypertension	New onset of hypertension after 20 weeks gestation with no maternal or fetal features of pre-eclampsia with return to normal blood pressure within 3 months postpartum
Chronic hypertension 1. Essential hypertension 2. Secondary hypertension	 Essential hypertension is blood pressure ≥ 140/90 before pregnancy or before 20 completed weeks gestation with no known cause Secondary hypertension is due to another cause such as chronic kidney disease
White-coat hypertension	Blood pressure elevated in presence of a health professional but normal when assessed at home or with ambulatory blood pressure monitoring
Pre-eclampsia superimposed on chronic hypertension	Diagnosed when a woman with chronic hypertension develops symptoms of pre-eclampsia after 20 weeks gestation

Source: Lowe SA, Bowyer L, Lust K et al: The SOMANZ guideline for the management of hypertensive disorders of pregnancy, Australian and New Zealand Journal of Obstetrics and Gynaecology 55(1):11–16, 2015.

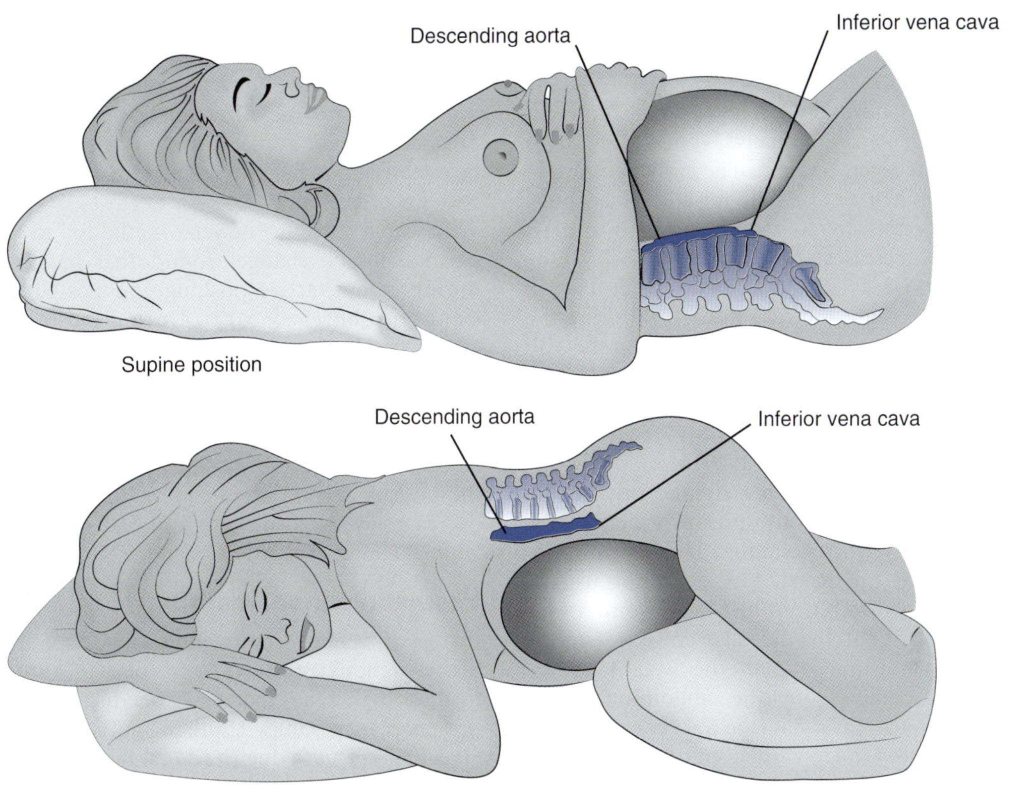

FIGURE 7.2 **Supine hypotension, relieved by right or left lateral position.**

The mechanism for reduction in supine hypotension with increased maternal body habitus may be related to extra adipose tissue cushioning the pregnant uterus, preventing compression of the aorta and inferior vena cava (Nelson et al 2015) (Fig 7.2).

Severe pre-eclampsia, preterm birth prior to 34 weeks and SGA infants have been associated with a blood pressure nadir (lowest blood pressure reading) at an earlier gestational age (Morgan et al 2016).

Blood pressure should be measured on both arms at the first assessment as blood pressure may vary between the right and left arm. A difference of 1–2 mmHg is normal; however, if there is an inter-arm difference of > 20 mmHg, the measurement should be repeated and, if the difference remains > 20 mmHg, the arm with the highest reading should be used for all subsequent measurements (NICE 2019). An inter-arm difference > 10 mmHg is associated with an increased risk of cardiovascular events (Schwartz et al 2017) and may indicate atherosclerotic plaques or other vascular occlusive diseases which are associated with increased cardiovascular risk (Sharma & Ramawat 2016). Failure to recognise an inter-arm difference can result in underestimation and under-treatment of raised blood pressure, which can have serious consequences for the woman and her fetus. If a woman has had a mastectomy, blood pressure should be taken on the arm on the opposite side to avoid causing oedema or further damage to lymphatic circulation (Lippincott et al 2015).

BLOOD PRESSURE CHANGES RELATED TO CHILDBIRTH

Pregnancy

Profound haemodynamic changes occur during pregnancy to support the growing fetus. These changes are primarily the result of hormonal and anatomical changes, resulting in increased blood volume, cardiac output and heart rate. In the non-pregnant individual this would result in an increase in blood pressure; however, during pregnancy these changes are counterbalanced by the hormonal effects (e.g. progesterone, prostaglandin) on the blood vessel walls, resulting in decreased peripheral resistance. The cardiovascular changes in pregnancy present a hyperdynamic, high-volume state with low resistance and are considered to be a response to the state of volume overload with improved myocardial and ventricular function in the first two trimesters, followed by a decline in function in the third trimester (Melchiorre et al 2016).

SBP and DBP normally decrease until 24 weeks gestation and then rise gradually (Vonck et al 2016) to pre-pregnancy levels by term. The early decrease in blood pressure is less for SBP than for DBP (Blackburn 2018). SBP decreases by an average of 5–10 mmHg, whereas DBP decreases 10–15 mmHg below the baseline by 24 weeks gestation (Murray & Hassell 2014). There is a slight increase in the PP during the third trimester due to the differences between the SBP and DBP.

Peak cardiac output occurs early in the third trimester and is 31% greater than non-pregnant values and then declines (Boardman et al 2016).

Venous pressures do not alter significantly during pregnancy, although venous pressure below the uterus does increase with gestation. This may impede venous return to the heart, but does not usually create problems. However, up to 8% of women may experience a transient hypotensive episode (supine hypotension syndrome) due to the weight of the gravid uterus compressing the abdominal aorta and inferior vena cava (aortocaval compression) decreasing venous return, cardiac output and stroke volume (Ayres-de Campos 2016). To avoid supine hypotension it is advisable that women are not laid flat on their back during the second half of pregnancy. Supine hypotension is rectified by changing to a lateral or semi-recumbent position. If required, a wedge can be placed under the woman's right side and hip to provide a lateral tilt (see Fig 7.2).

Labour

During labour increased anxiety and pain levels have been reported to result in a rise in blood pressure, especially in the primiparous woman (Blackburn 2018). Additionally, both systolic and DBPs increase during uterine contractions by up to 35 mmHg and 25 mmHg, respectively, as the circulation increases by 300–500 mL during a contraction with a resultant increase in cardiac output. During the first stage of labour cardiac output can increase by 10–15% (Blackburn 2018) or by 10–25% (Chestnut et al 2014) and by up to 50% during the second stage (Blackburn 2018) or 40% according to Chestnut and colleagues (2014). These increases return to the baseline level once the contraction is over; however, according to Chestnut and colleagues (2014), the increased cardiac output occurs between uterine contractions. Blood pressure is normally measured between contractions.

Recent technological advances in measuring cardiac output are challenging the accepted views on maternal haemodynamics outlined above. Cardiac function can now be measured by Ultrasound Cardiac Output (USCOM®) and the Non-invasive Cardiac Output Monitor (NICOM®), which have been validated against echocardiography and pulmonary artery catheterisation (Ghossein-Doha et al 2017). However, McLaughlin and colleagues (2017) note a gold standard measurement for cardiac output in pregnancy is not available and normal values need to be established in healthy pregnant women and women with hypertension.

Research using newer methods to evaluate haemodynamic changes found that baseline values during labour, active pushing and postpartum were similar (Kuhn et al 2017). During the first stage of labour, cardiac output increased for the majority of women, but also decreased in some women; however, heart rate and systolic arterial pressure increased in all women (Kuhn et al 2017). Late in the first stage of labour, heart rate and cardiac output increased and at the peak of second stage contractions cardiac output decreased while heart rate and SBP increased in all women (Kuhn et al 2017).

Postnatal period: maternal

Increased venous return following birth results in higher venous pressures, and cardiac output is up to 80% higher immediately after birth compared to pre-pregnancy values (Nathan, de Greef, Hezelgrave et al 2015). This is due to several factors: compression on the vena cava is relieved, lower extremity venous pressure declines, the 300–500 mL previously directed to the intervillous space of the placenta ceases after the cord is clamped resulting in autotransfusion of blood back into the central circulation, leading to increased circulating blood volume resulting in higher CVP, stroke volume and cardiac output (Chestnut et al 2014). The amount of blood returned to the circulation generally exceeds the normal blood loss associated with birth. Cardiac output declines sharply after birth due to decreased maternal cardiovascular demand and returns to pre-pregnancy values early in the postpartum period prior to a slight increase during the extended postpartum period (Meah et al 2016). Factors such as breastfeeding and physical activity following birth may account for variability between women (Meah et al 2016).

According to Blackburn (2018), the decline in cardiac output occurs in the 10–15 minutes after birth and stabilises around 1 hour after birth. The increased venous return to the heart also results in an increase in the size of the left atria for the first 3 days, increasing CVP (Blackburn 2018). In the 24 hours following birth, cardiac output decreases to slightly below pre-labour values, with a return to pre-pregnancy levels between 12 to 24 weeks postpartum (Chestnut et al 2014).

The increase in cardiac output immediately after birth has been questioned by research using minimally invasive devices which collect continuous data on haemodynamic parameters. Kuhn and colleagues (2017) found cardiac output did not increase significantly in the immediate postpartum period. The theory of autotransfusion occurring immediately after birth is based on studies which are now around 50 years old and may be less reliable (Kuhn et al 2017).

As the blood volume and physiological effects of pregnancy decrease, blood pressure returns to pre-pregnancy levels. In healthy women cardiovascular changes induced by pregnancy result in a slower pulse wave velocity and lower blood pressure 2 years postpartum, although these adaptations are likely to regress over time (Morris et al 2017). Women with pre-eclampsia have an increased risk of hypertension and cardiovascular disease as early as 10 years after pregnancy (Gomez et al 2016). At the end of pregnancy 17.9% of women have diastolic dysfunction and 28.4% have impaired myocardial relaxation, but all women recovered full cardiac function by 1 year postpartum (Melchiorre et al 2016) (Table 7.5).

FACTORS INFLUENCING ARTERIAL BLOOD PRESSURE

Accurate measurement of blood pressure is essential for diagnosis and treatment—ideally a woman is able to sit comfortably without stimulation for 5 minutes prior to blood pressure assessment (Levy et al 2016).

A variety of factors influence ABP, including the following.

- *Age:* Blood pressure increases with age due to loss of elasticity of the arterial walls.
- *Alcohol:* The majority of studies found all significant increases in blood pressure occurred within 60 minutes of ingestion and all significant

TABLE 7.5 MATERNAL HAEMODYNAMIC CHANGES

	Early first stage (3–7 cm) Mean (95% CI)	Late first stage (8–10 cm) Mean (95% CI)	Second stage Mean (95% CI)	Birth (10 cm and bearing down effort) Mean (95% CI)	Early postpartum (up to 15 minutes after birth) Mean (95% CI)
CARDIAC OUTPUT (L/min)					
Baseline	6.3 (5.7–6.9)	6.5 (6.1–6.9)	6.6 (6.1–7.1)	4.6 (4.1–5.1)	6.3 (5.6–7.0)
During contractions minimum	6.0 (5.3–6.7)	5.8 (5.4–6.2)	4.5 (4.0–5.1)	11.1 (10.3–11.8)	
During contractions maximum	9.2 (7.9–10.4)	9.9 (9.3–10.6)	10.6 (10.2–11.2)		
HEART RATE (BEATS/min)					
Baseline	82 (78–85)	83 (79–86)	86 (82–90)	79 (73–84)	86 (79–92)
During contractions minimum	67 (61–72)	67 (63–72)	70 (65–76)	141 (134–149)	
During contractions maximum	102 (95–110)	115 (104–126)	131 (124–137)		
SYSTOLIC ARTERIAL PRESSURE (mmHg)					
Baseline	134 (126–141)	136 (132–141)	136 (130–142)	116 (112–121)	129 (122–136)
During contractions minimum	130 (122–137)	124 (118–130)	118 (114–122)	179 (172–187)	
During contractions maximum	164 (154–174)	171 (164–178)	185 (179–191)		

Notes:
- Each baseline represents the mean value from one individual 30-second period between contractions (during labour) or without contractions (postpartum).
- For contractions, each observation indicates the minimum/maximum during one individual contraction.

Source: Adapted from Kuhn JC, Falk RS, Langesæter E: Haemodynamic changes during labour: continuous minimally invasive monitoring in 20 healthy parturients, International Journal of Obstetric Anesthesia 31:74–83, 2017.

decreases occurred from 60 minutes to 4 hours post ingestion (Kallioinen et al 2017). A consistently high alcohol intake is associated with higher blood pressure, although alcohol may also lower blood pressure by inhibiting the effects of antidiuretic hormone, resulting in vasodilatation and decreased blood volume.

- *Bladder:* An over-distended bladder with overwhelming urge to void can increase blood pressure (Kallioinen et al 2017).
- *Blood volume:* A reduction in circulating blood volume (e.g. haemorrhage, shock) results in a decrease in both SBP and DBP.
- *Caffeine:* Small to moderate increases in blood pressure occur for up to 180 minutes after ingestion of more than 200 mg of caffeine (Kallioinen et al 2017).
- *Cold:* Exposure to cold causes moderate to large increases in SBP and small to large increases in DBP (Kallioinen et al 2017).
- *Deep breathing:* Can reduce blood pressure by almost 5 mmHg (Zheng et al 2012).
- *Disease:* Any disease process affecting stroke volume, blood vessel diameter, peripheral resistance or respiration will alter blood pressure.
- *Diurnal variations:* SBP is highest in the evening, lowest in the morning and changes during rest and sleep periods.
- *Eating:* It was found that a light breakfast did not affect SBP and slightly decreased DBP in the 120 minutes following ingestion; a mixed meal had no effect after 60 minutes and moderate decreases in both SBP and DBP were seen at 180 minutes (Kallioinen et al 2017).
- *Exercise:* Increases blood pressure, with effects lasting 30–60 minutes.
- *Heart rate:* Blood pressure increases with an increasing heart rate, providing the circulating blood volume is unaltered.
- *Hereditary factors:* Some people have an inherited predisposition to raised blood pressure; 280 genetic variants have been associated with hypertension (Patel et al 2017). The strongest heredity risk factor is a family history of hypertension that developed prior to the age of 55 years (Patel et al 2017).
- *Position of arm:* During measurement, an unsupported arm can result in DBP increasing by 10%. Not having the arm at the level of the heart can vary blood pressure by 10 mmHg.
- *Position of body:* Blood pressure is about 10 mmHg higher in standing or sitting positions compared to left lateral, recumbent or supine positions (Blackburn 2018).
- *Renin:* High renin levels cause vasoconstriction, and an increase in blood volume (due to increased salt and fluid retention within the kidneys) will result in a rise in blood pressure.
- *Rest period:* Checking blood pressure after 5–10 minutes rest is recommended (Khan 2021, Nikolic et al 2014).
- *Smoking:* Stimulates sympathetic activity resulting in vasoconstriction and the release of norepinephrine and epinephrine, which increase SBP and DBP, with effects lasting up to 30–60 minutes.
- *Stress, fear, anxiety and pain:* These can all raise blood pressure by stimulating the sympathetic nervous system. 'White-coat' hypertension refers to anxiety-related hypertension resulting from attending a healthcare setting and may increase SBP > 20 mmHg and DBP > 10 mmHg (Vestgaard et al 2019). White-coat effect is more common in women (Kario et al 2019) with approximately 70% of healthy pregnant women having white-coat hypertension (Vestgaard et al 2019). Women with white-coat hypertension tend to have higher pre-pregnancy BMI and a higher prevalence of type 2 diabetes.
- *Talking:* If the woman talks while having her blood pressure measured, the DBP can increase by 5.3 mmHg and SBP by 6.2 mmHg (Zheng et al 2012).
- *Weight:* Overweight or obese women tend to have higher blood pressure.

INDICATIONS

Blood pressure is recorded throughout pregnancy, labour and the postnatal period. In Australia the *Clinical practice guidelines: pregnancy care* (Department of Health 2020) provides recommendations. The circumstances determining the frequency of blood pressure measurement vary. They include:

- the initial booking history to establish a baseline and identify existing hypertension (Department of Health 2020)
- at each antenatal visit (Department of Health 2020)
- during labour, initially and then 4-hourly (NICE 2017)
- following each epidural bolus (see Chapter 38)
- postnatally (Ministry of Health Manatū Hauora 2012)
- as the clinical condition dictates (e.g. shock and haemorrhage; symptoms such as headaches, visual disturbances or proteinuria; or when the early warning system (see Chapter 6) triggers further investigation and repeat of vital signs)
- hypertension of any cause
- preterm or sick neonate
- before, during and following a blood transfusion (see Chapter 24)
- following recovery from anaesthesia: with other vital sign observations, it should be taken every 30 minutes for 2 hours and then hourly until stable (NICE 2021).

EQUIPMENT

Sphygmomanometers

A **sphygmomanometer** is a device used to measure blood pressure and works by exerting a measured pressure on an artery. It consists of a manometer (pressure gauge), a cuff and a bulb for inflating the cuff. As the cuff inflates, the blood flow is occluded; as the pressure is released, blood begins to pulsate and flow through the artery, which can be detected via a pressure sensor in the cuff (oscillatory), or the resulting blood flow (Korotkoff sounds) can be heard through a stethoscope (auscultatory).

Manual auscultatory sphygmomanometers are classified as mercury (column) or aneroid (dial). The mercury-based auscultatory sphygmomanometer is considered the gold standard for blood pressure measurement (Lowe et al 2015, Tranquilli et al 2014). Currently, the SOMNAZ guidelines (Lowe et al 2015) recommend that a mercury sphygmomanometer should be used to validate automated and aneroid devices. However, mercury is highly toxic and can result in serious adverse health impacts (Department of Agriculture, Water and the Environment 2020). As a result, the use of mercury-based medical equipment is declining globally. Australia and New Zealand are both signatories to the Minamata Convention (United Nations 2013), which aims to reduce the adverse heath and environmental effects of mercury. Many health services in Australia and New Zealand are already phasing out medical devices containing mercury.

Aneroid manometers

Aneroid means without fluid. This type of manometer has a circular gauge encased in glass, with a needle that points to numbers (Fig 7.3). Pressure variations within the inflated cuff cause metal bellows within the gauge to expand and collapse, moving the needle up and down the gauge. Prior to use, the needle should be set at zero. These devices are lightweight, compact and portable but less accurate than mercury column manometers as the metal parts are liable to expand and contract with temperature changes. Aneroid manometers should undergo biomedical calibration on a regular basis to ensure accuracy. Aneroid manometers tend to underestimate SBP and overestimate DBP (Kallioinen et al 2017). A study comparing the accuracy of aneroid manometers with mercury manometers found they met the accepted standard of + or – 5 mmHg (Shahbabu et al 2016).

Mercury column manometers

These have mercury contained within a glass column, with ascending numbers on either side of the column. The mercury should be clearly visible, have no gaps and rest at the zero level. If the mercury is below zero, the reservoir can be topped up. The column of mercury needs to be upright and the mercury should be read at eye level, as looking up or down at the mercury

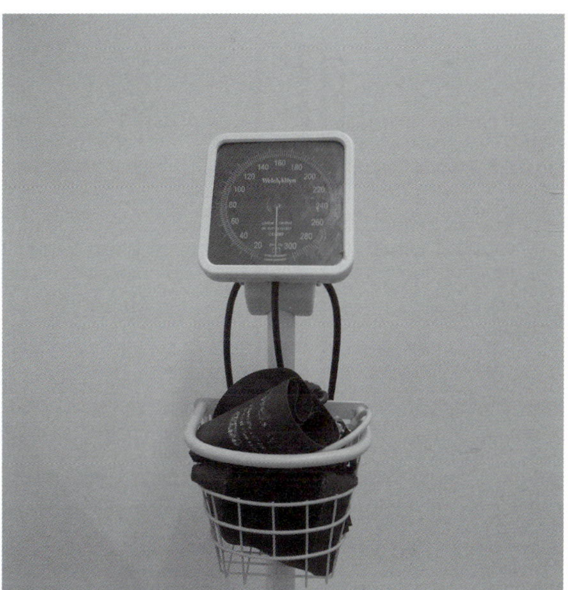

FIGURE 7.3 Aneroid manometer.

can result in distorted readings. When examining the manometer, ensure the air vent or filter at the top of the column is clear and clean (oxidation of mercury can make it appear dirty and difficult to read, so columns should be cleaned every year). If mercury spillage occurs, the safety data sheet (SDS) instructions should be followed to minimise risks of contamination (SafeWork Australia 2016, Worksafe New Zealand 2017) (Fig 7.4).

Oscillatory (automated or digital) manometers

Oscillatory manometers are electronic devices that calculate blood pressure automatically by measuring the vibration of the blood as it travels through the arteries and converting it into a digital reading. Following detection of the oscillometric pulse, the amplitude is analysed and a proprietary algorithm is used to calculate SBP and DBP (Alpert et al 2014). A cuff is placed around the arm and tubing is attached to the machine. The machine can be set to record blood pressure on a regular basis, inflating and deflating the cuff at the desired time interval. A stethoscope is not required as the systolic and diastolic pressures are displayed. The pulse is often counted and recorded at the same time.

Oscillatory manometers are commonly used in clinical practice and by pregnant women at home (Fig 7.5).

Oscillatory manometers can reduce the errors associated with auscultatory sphygmomanometers (e.g. observer bias, end/terminal digit preference, threshold avoidance), and do not require hearing

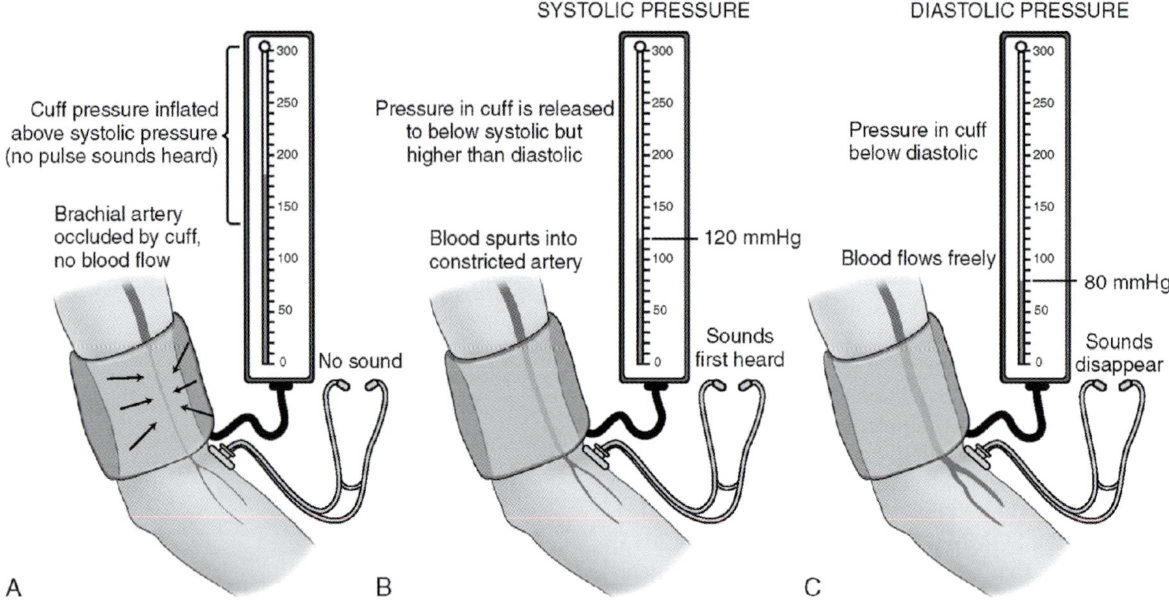

FIGURE 7.4 **Mercury column manometer.**
Source: Leonard P: Building a medical vocabulary with Spanish translations, Saunders, 2012.

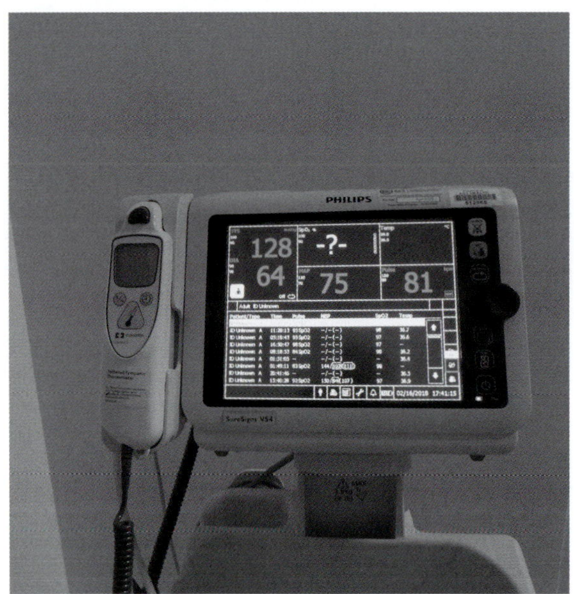

FIGURE 7.5 **Oscillatory manometer.**

sounds; therefore, they are suitable for people with hearing impairment. The *Guideline for the diagnosis and management of hypertension in adults—2016* now recommends the use of correctly maintained and validated non-mercury sphygmomanometers for blood pressure measurement (Gabb et al 2016). However, concern has been expressed regarding the accuracy of oscillometric blood pressure devices during pregnancy, with some devices failing to pass validation procedures (Hay et al 2016).

Inaccuracies are more apparent in women of more advanced maternal age and also women with a large arm circumference (Hay et al 2016). Oscillometry depends on arterial wall compliance which may be altered during hypotension; therefore, oscillometric devices need to be validated for accuracy in women with serious conditions such as haemorrhagic shock (Nathan et al 2016). Oscillatory devices are not accurate if cardiac arrhythmias are present (Davis et al 2015). Therefore, the radial or brachial pulse should be palpated prior to measuring blood pressure to ensure the most appropriate equipment is used.

Only oscillatory devices validated for pregnancy should be used (Bello et al 2018). If a woman has elevated blood pressure, it is good practice to estimate her blood pressure manually. Blood pressure is not significantly different when using an automated machine on bare and sleeved arms (Tuğrul & Karaçam 2020).

To ensure accuracy, automated devices should only be used if they have been validated, calibrated and maintained following the recommendations of the British and Irish Hypertensive Society (BIHS) (Lowe et al 2015). The society has a list of validated devices on their website (see Resources at the end of the chapter). To ensure accurate blood pressure comparisons between different recordings, measurements should be undertaken on similar equipment and the type of sphygmomanometer recorded.

Twenty-four hour ambulatory blood pressure monitoring

Twenty-four hour ambulatory blood pressure monitoring (ABPM) involves a woman wearing a portable device which monitors her blood pressure every 15–30 minutes during the day and every 30–60 minutes at night (Head et al 2012). The *Guideline for the diagnosis and management of hypertension in adults—2016* now recommends adults with a measured blood pressure in the clinic of ≥ 140/90 mmHg benefit from ambulatory or at home BP monitoring, as prediction of outcome is improved (Gabb et al 2016). ABPM is considered the gold standard for detecting white-coat hypertension (Sharman et al 2015) and is a stronger predictor of adverse pregnancy outcome than conventional blood pressure (Dorogova & Panina 2015). ABPM is useful for identifying women with suspected white-coat hypertension, particularly in the first half of pregnancy (Head et al 2012) (Table 7.6).

Home blood pressure monitoring

Home blood pressure monitors are widely available and can provide a reliable assessment of blood pressure (Sharman et al 2016) (Fig 7.6). Home blood pressure monitoring can be used to identify white-coat hypertension. Women are able to monitor their blood pressure at home and this can help with management and recognition of hypertension (Brown 2014). Memory storage is available and validated devices are accessible.

Before measuring their blood pressure at home, women are advised to:

- sit quietly for 5 minutes
- have feet flat on the floor, legs uncrossed
- have the back and arm supported, with the cuff at heart level
- take two measurements, 1 minute apart
- record measurements on paper or electronically
- take a copy of the blood pressure readings to their appointment
- avoid smoking or drinking caffeine in the 30 minutes before measurement

TABLE 7.6 NORMAL AMBULATORY BLOOD PRESSURE (ABP) IN PREGNANCY

Gestation	Normal mean daytime ABPs
Up to 22 weeks gestation	< 132/79 mmHg
At 26–30 weeks gestation	< 133/81 mmHg
At more than 30 weeks gestation	< 135/86 mmHg

Source: Head GA, McGrath BP, Mihailidou AS, et al: Ambulatory blood pressure monitoring in Australia: 2011 consensus position statement, Journal of Hypertension 30(2):253–256, 2012.

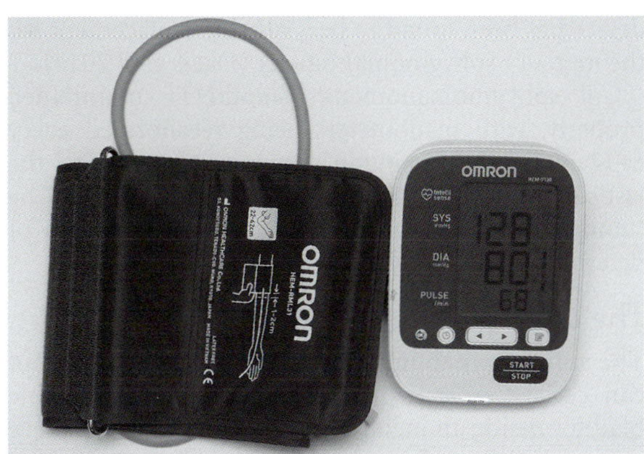

FIGURE 7.6 Home blood pressure monitor.

- avoid measuring if stressed or in pain (Sharma et al 2016)
- take blood pressure after voiding and before eating food or vigorous exercise
- avoid caffeine and cigarettes and do not take blood pressure until at least 30 minutes after use (Sharman et al 2015).

It is important to provide women with instructions on how to monitor their blood pressure at home to ensure readings are accurate. Levy and colleagues (2016) reported only 21% of patients were instructed to wait before taking their blood pressure.

When the home blood pressure monitor is turned on, it should register zero and the air valve should have a deflation rate of 2–3 mmHg per second (Khan 2021). A 2016 study found that although most home blood pressure monitors has a minimal difference (< 5 mmHg), in comparison with a mercury sphygmomanometer a significant proportion were inaccurate (Ruzicka et al 2016).

Validation protocols have been published by the Association for the Advancement of Medical Instrumentation (AAMI), the BIHS and the European Society of Hypertension.

Hybrid manometers

A third type of sphygmomanometer has been developed to improve accuracy and replace the mercury sphygmomanometer. The hybrid sphygmomanometer has both automated oscillometric and manual auscultatory features. A liquid crystal vertical display column is substituted for the mercury column and connects to a standard cuff range (Davis et al 2015). The device also has a digital display and four operational modes (Davis et al 2015). Although similarities with the mercury thermometer are present, the device must be turned on and cuff deflation needs to be slow to avoid variations in the liquid crystal during cuff deflation. For women with hypertension or pre-eclampsia the hybrid device has been found to be a suitable replacement for the mercury sphygmomanometer (Davis et al 2015).

All sphygmomanometers should be maintained properly, with manometers being recalibrated every 6–12 months to maintain accuracy. The date of the last calibration should be marked on the machine. The tubing should also be checked regularly for signs of deterioration and replaced accordingly.

The cuff

The sphygmomanometer cuff encircles the arm and can consist of a two-piece cuff with a removable bladder inside an inelastic fabric shell or a one-piece cuff consisting of a potential space inside a fabric shell (Fig 7.7) (Ringrose et al 2016). One-piece cuffs require less pressure for inflation as there is no extra air space between the shell and the bladder. The cuff is placed around the upper part of the arm, with the lower edge of the cuff positioned 2–3 cm above the point of brachial artery pulsation (Fig 7.8) or occasionally around the forearm or lower thigh. When the cuff is inflated to a pressure higher than the pressure within the artery, the artery is occluded. At this point, blood flow ceases and the pulse is no longer palpable. The cuff is held in place by Velcro fastenings and should be secure, as a loose cuff can distort the reading. A bulb is attached to the cuff by tubing and is squeezed to inflate the bladder. The cuff should be placed with the rubber tubing positioned superiorly and in line with the brachial artery. For cuffs attached to manual sphygmomanometers, a valve on the bulb controls the pressure within the cuff. Placing the cuff over clothing does not appear to affect the blood pressure reading (Kallioinen et al 2017). A one-piece cuff leads to lower blood pressure measurements, particularly with oscillometric manometers (Ringrose et al 2016).

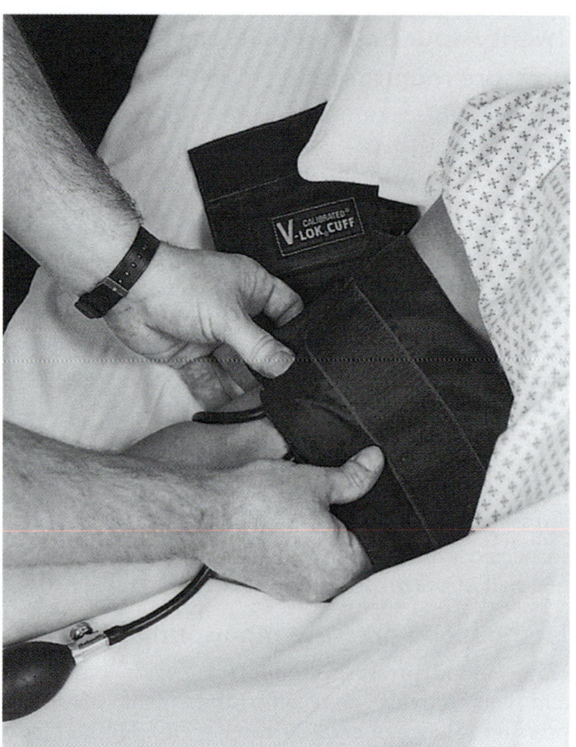

FIGURE 7.8 **Correct placement of cuff.**
Source: Christensen B, Kockrow EO: Foundations of nursing, Mosby, 2011.

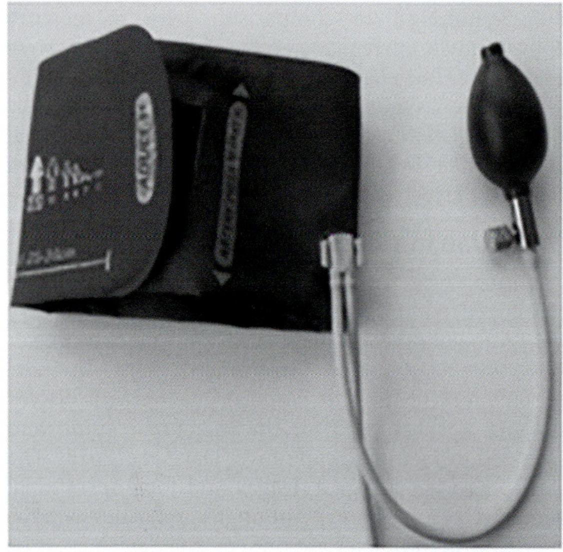

FIGURE 7.7 **Bladderless blood pressure cuff.**

If the upper arm cannot be used, the lower arm can be used by placing an appropriately sized cuff centrally above the radial artery, or the lower third of the thigh with the cuff placed above the posterior popliteal artery. Systolic pressure is 20–30 mmHg higher in the leg than in the arm. The lower arm and leg are rarely used in midwifery.

It is important to use the correct cuff size. A cuff that is too small in length or depth can give falsely high readings (cuff hypertension); conversely, a cuff that is too large can give falsely low readings (Sharman et al 2016). The length of the bladder should be at least 80% of the arm circumference, but not over 100% (BIHS 2017). Cuff lengths vary from 22 to 36 cm. The woman should have her mid-arm circumference (MAC) measured at the first visit to ensure the correct size cuff is used. Hogan and colleagues (2011) suggest that women with a BMI > 34.9 should be assigned a large cuff. If the BMI is 29.9–34.9 the MAC should be measured, as 44% of these women will require a large cuff. Eley and colleagues (2018) recommend the following cuff bladder sizes in relation to MAC:

- 22–26 cm small cuff (22 cm length × 12 cm width)
- 27–34 cm standard cuff (30 cm length × 16 cm width)
- 35–44 cm large cuff (36 cm length × 16 cm width).

Stethoscope

By placing a stethoscope over the artery the sounds of the blood flow and vibrations in the surrounding tissues can be heard. The level at which the artery is occluded and no sounds heard is equal to the systolic pressure. As the cuff is deflated, the pulse reappears and pulsating sounds are heard with each beat of the heart.

The stethoscope head may be in two parts, with a bell-shaped end and a flat diaphragm side, or it might have only the diaphragm shape (Fig 7.9). Either side of the stethoscope head can be used for auscultation as similar results are obtained with a slight increase in DBP with the bell in comparison with the diaphragm (Chengyu et al 2016). The diaphragm transmits a higher frequency and the bell a lower frequency. Although Korotkoff sounds are a lower frequency, the diaphragm covers a larger area and is recommended for manual blood pressure measurement (Fallon 2015). Care should be taken not to press too hard on the stethoscope head as this compresses the brachial artery, resulting in a misleading murmur and possibly lowering the DBP reading. The stethoscope should not be under the cuff edge as this can result in increases in DBP (Kallioinen et al 2017). The stethoscope can be used over clothing up to a thickness of 2 mm with no effect on blood pressure (Pinar et al 2010, Tuğrul & Karaçam 2020). However, a rolled-up sleeve causes a higher systolic and diastolic reading (Tuğrul & Karaçam 2020).

The stethoscope should be in good condition, particularly the earpiece, which should be clean and well fitting. The ear tips should be angled forwards into the external auditory canal as this maximises hearing (Alexis 2009). Before and following the procedure, the earpieces and diaphragm/bell of the stethoscope should be cleaned, as they can carry microorganisms, possibly resulting in cross-contamination to other women or midwives (Campos-Murguia et al 2014).

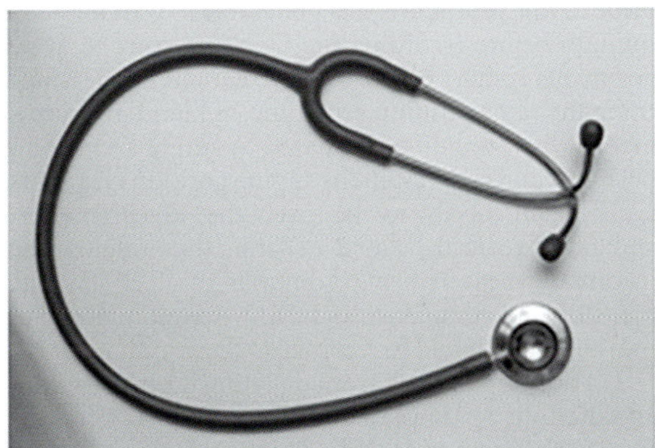

FIGURE 7.9 **Stethoscope.**

Korotkoff sounds

When assessing blood pressure with a manual sphygmomanometer, a stethoscope is used to listen to the different sounds in the artery when it is occluded and as the blood flow returns. The different sounds heard are named after Nikolai Korotkoff, the man who defined them in 1905. He defined the sounds according to five phases, reflecting different stages in the measurement of blood pressure (Table 7.7). SBP is noted when faint tapping sounds are heard initially, and these will increase in intensity as blood flow increases and changes in nature. DBP is noted when the sounds are no longer heard.

Individual variations can occur in the sequencing of these sounds. In around 5% of hypertensive people, the phase II sounds may be absent, replaced by a short period of silence—the 'auscultatory gap'. This can last through a change of 40 mmHg.

The muffling sounds of phase IV are heard when the pressure gauge is 7–10 mmHg higher than the intra-arterial diastolic pressure. This is due to a loss of transmission of pressure from the cuff to the artery. The absence of sounds associated with phase V is thought to be more closely related to the intra-arterial diastolic pressure. However, phase V sounds may be very low or absent in some adults, particularly during pregnancy.

Whether to use phase IV or phase V sounds to record blood pressure has been the subject of debate, particularly when measuring blood pressure in pregnancy. Korotkoff V is considered the most accurate phase to measure DBP (Chappell et al 2020). If Korotkoff V continues to zero, it should be documented that Korotkoff phase IV was used (e.g. phase 1 = 130, phase IV = 70, phase V = 0) (Frese et al 2011).

TABLE 7.7 BLOOD PRESSURE PHASES AND KOROTKOFF SOUNDS

Phase	Sound
I	Faint tapping sounds that increase in intensity
II	Softening, swishing sounds
III	Crisper sounds with an intense pitch, not as intense as phase I
IV	Abrupt, muffled sounds, which become soft and blowing
V	Silence—no sounds heard

Source: Johnson R, Taylor W: Skills for midwifery practice, 4th ed., Elsevier, London, 2016.

SKILL 7.1 Blood pressure estimation using a manual sphygmomanometer

1. Perform hand hygiene.
2. Confirm the woman's identity.
3. Initiate communication by introduction and obtain informed consent.
4. Encourage the woman to empty her bladder if necessary.
5. Determine the optimum site for blood pressure assessment; the right arm is preferred (Lowe et al 2015).
6. Determine previous baseline blood pressure from record if available.
7. Select appropriate cuff size (if not done, measure the arm to determine cuff size; if arm circumference is > 33 cm use a large cuff, if > 42 cm use a thigh cuff).
8. Disinfect the stethoscope.
9. If the woman has been active, allow her to rest for at least 5 minutes.
10. Position the sphygmomanometer so the base of the manometer is level with the woman's heart, whenever possible.
11. Assist the woman into a suitable position, legs uncrossed and feet flat on the ground.
12. Expose the correct upper arm, ensuring no constriction from tight clothing.
13. Support the woman's arm and ask her to turn the palm of her hand upwards.
14. Apply the cuff 2–3 cm above the site of brachial artery pulsation (in the antecubital fossa); place the cuff centrally above the artery to ensure even distribution of pressure during inflation. Ensure that there is no air in the cuff and the valve is closed.
15. If no baseline blood pressure is available systolic BP can be estimated by palpating the brachial or radial artery with the fingertips of one hand and, with the other hand, inflating the cuff rapidly by pumping the bulb until the pulse disappears. Continue to inflate the cuff 30 mmHg above this.
16. Slowly deflate the cuff by opening the valve slightly, taking note of when the pulse reappears; this gives an approximate reading of the systolic pressure and prevents confusion arising from the presence of an auscultatory gap.
17. Quickly deflate the cuff by opening the valve fully, wait for 30 seconds and then close the valve.
18. Disinfect the stethoscope, place earpieces in your ears and position the head of the stethoscope over the brachial artery.
19. Inflate the cuff to 20–30 mmHg higher than the previous blood pressure (or palpated systolic pressure).
20. Slowly deflate the cuff at 2 mmHg per second, listening for the appearance of the first clear sound (Korotkoff I).
21. Read the needle position or mercury level (systole) (at eye level) to the nearest 2 mmHg.
22. Continue to deflate the cuff slowly until the sounds are absent.
23. When the sounds are no longer audible—Korotkoff phase V (or IV if V is absent)—read the needle position or mercury level (diastole) to the nearest 2 mmHg, deflate the cuff rapidly.
24. Remove the cuff and assist with readjusting the woman's clothing, if required, and then assist her into a comfortable position.
25. Clean the bell, diaphragm and earpieces of the stethoscope with a detergent wipe.
26. Perform hand hygiene (see Chapter 1).
27. Discuss the findings with the woman.
28. Document the findings and act accordingly.

FACTORS AFFECTING ACCURACY

Care should be taken throughout to minimise the risk of inaccuracies. There are three factors that affect accuracy: technique, equipment and the operator.

The arm should be at the level of the heart (mid-sternum). If it is above this level, the blood pressure may give a false low reading, whereas placing the arm below this level can give a false high reading (BIHS 2017). Blood pressure is increased by 1 mmHg for each 2.5 cm the arm is above the level of the heart (Khan 2021). The arm should be horizontal and supported, as an unsupported, extended arm may result in the DBP rising by up to 10% (Kahn 2021).

The woman can adopt any position that is comfortable, although her legs should not be crossed at the knees as this can result in a false high recording (Lippincott et al 2015). The SBP can increase by 6.6 mmHg when the feet are not flat on the floor and legs are crossed, as noted by Edmunds and colleagues (2011). If the woman changes her position immediately prior to this procedure, it is preferable to wait for a few minutes before recording the blood pressure to avoid erroneous results. Blood pressure should be measured using the same position each time, as blood pressure is higher when standing compared to sitting and supine positions and is lowest in the supine position (Fig 7.10).

The cuff needs to be over the brachial artery and fitted correctly. Rapid deflation can result in an inaccurate measurement (Edmunds et al 2011), with the SBP underestimated and DBP overestimated. The measurement should be recorded to the nearest 2 mmHg.

Do not stop the cuff from deflating between systolic and diastolic readings or re-inflate the cuff to recheck the systolic reading as this will increase blood volume below the cuff, making the sounds softer.

If the reading is abnormal it should be repeated allowing at least 2 minutes between recordings. If

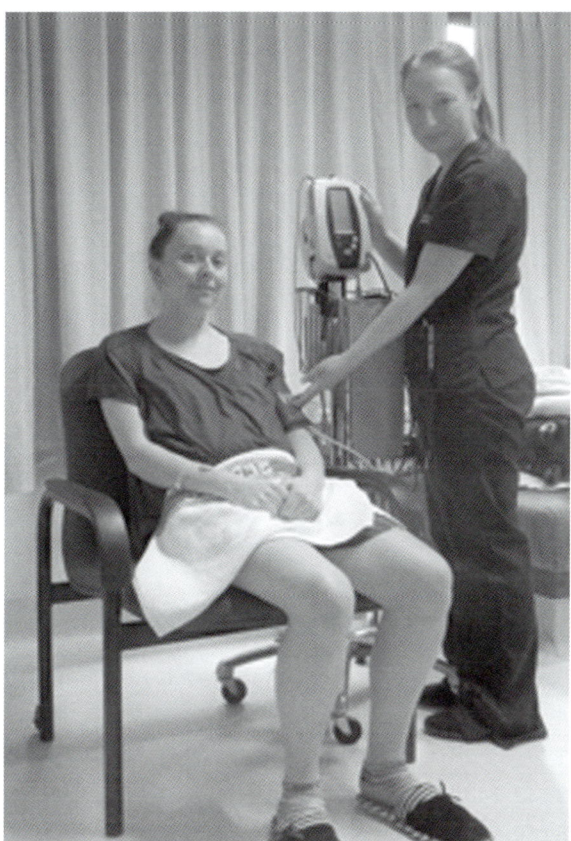

FIGURE 7.10 **Correct position for blood pressure measurement: upper arm bare, feet flat on floor, cuff at heart level, back supported.**

an abnormal blood pressure is found on the initial assessment, it should be estimated in both arms and the arm with the highest reading used for all subsequent measurements (NICE 2019). The midwife may have an unconscious bias about what they expect to hear, influenced by knowledge of earlier blood pressure measurements. Accuracy is increased if previous findings are unknown.

Manual manometers can only yield results with even numbers, rounding to the nearest five is inaccurate. End/terminal digit preference refers to the operator's preference to round the reading to the nearest end digit, usually a zero, resulting in a reading that is higher or lower than the actual measurement (Kallioinen et al 2017). Accuracy is also influenced by the individual's hearing ability. Song and colleagues (2014) found that operators with impaired hearing were more likely to underestimate the SBP and overestimate the DBP.

CENTRAL VENOUS PRESSURE

CVP is the pressure within the right atrium and reflects right ventricular end diastolic pressure (Westmead Intensive Care Unit 2016). To measure CVP a central venous catheter or peripherally inserted central catheter (Bridges 2016) is inserted into a large central vein such as the superior vena cava, femoral, brachial, subclavian or internal jugular vein and the catheter tip positioned in the right atrium or upper portion of the superior vena cava (or inferior vena cava if access is via the femoral artery).

CVP is used to estimate circulating blood volume and estimate fluid requirements (Fitzgerald, Gomersall, Ka Man et al 2015). The normal CVP range in the literature varies from 2–6 mmHg (Fitzgerald et al 2015) to 4–12 mmHg (Westmead Intensive Care Unit 2016). Trends in CVP readings and alterations related to administration of a fluid bolus are more important than a single reading (Fitzgerald et al 2015, Gomersall et al 2015). It is essential for CVP to be interpreted in the context of all clinical data (Westmead Intensive Care Unit 2016). In general, if CVP increases following a fluid bolus by 0–3 mmHg, hypovolaemia is probably present and if the CVP increases by > 3 mmHg fluid volume is probably normal or high (Gomersall et al 2015). Although traditionally CVP has been used to inform fluid management in the critically ill woman, current evidence disputes this practice (Hiroshi & Sawami 2017, Marik & Cavallazzi 2013).

Women requiring CVP monitoring are critically ill and generally managed in intensive care.

The position of the woman should always be recorded and ideally the same position used for each measurement; however, this will depend on the woman's condition. Accurate CVP measurement requires the transducer to be in line with the base of the woman's right atrium; this is the phlebostatic axis and is located at the fourth intercostal space in the mid-axillary line. An imaginary line is extended from here to the side of the chest to intersect with a second imaginary line between the front and back of the chest (Fig 7.11). This is known as the phlebostatic level and the site of intersection is marked on the side of the woman's chest to highlight the place used to obtain the reading.

CVP readings are affected by the amount of blood in the right ventricle prior to systole, the contractility of the right ventricle and the amount of resistance to blood being ejected from the right ventricle. A low CVP reading is associated with haemorrhage, hypovolaemia, dehydration, drug-induced vasodilatation and vigorous diuresis.

A high CVP reading is associated with right ventricular failure, fluid overload, fluid retention in cardiac and renal disease, pulmonary obstruction, congestion and/or embolism. Increased intrathoracic pressure results from coughing, pain (Edmunds et al 2011), decreased cardiac output, forced expiration (Valsalva) and muscle contraction (Klabunde 2012).

NEONATAL BLOOD PRESSURE

Multiple factors impact on blood pressure in the neonate including birth weight (the most significant

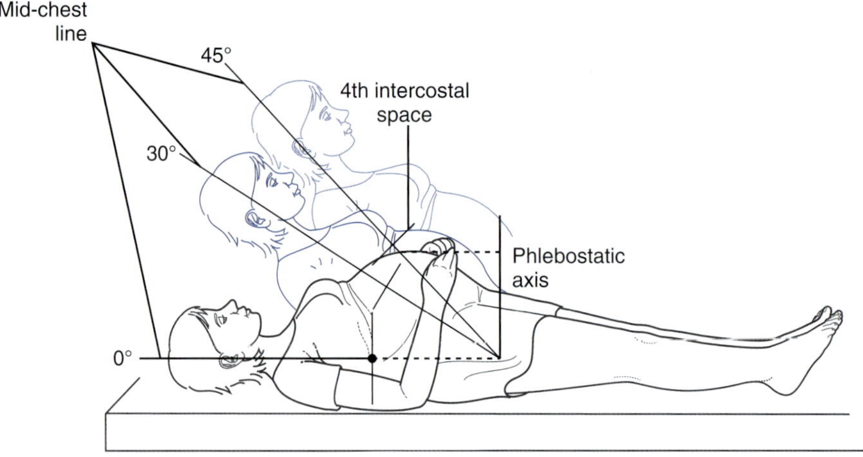

FIGURE 7.11 **Phlebostatic axis and phlebostatic level.**
Source: Johnson R, Taylor W: Skills for midwifery practice, 4th ed., Elsevier, London, 2016.

TABLE 7.8 NORMAL NEONATAL BLOOD PRESSURE, TERM INFANTS

Age	Systolic blood pressure (mmHg)	Diastolic blood pressure (mmHg)	Mean (mmHg)
1 hour	70	44	53
12 hours	66	41	50
Day 1	70±9 – 71±9	42±12 – 43±10	55±11 – 55±9
Day 3	75±11 – 77±12	48±10 – 49±10	59±9 – 63±13
Day 6	76±10 – 76±10	46±12 – 49±11	58±12 – 62±12
2 weeks	78±10	50±9	
3 weeks	79±8	49±8	
4 weeks	85±10	46±9	

Note: Measurements for Day 1, 3, 6 are from asleep to awake.
Source: Adapted from Safer Care Victoria (SCV) and the Victorian Agency for Health Information (VAHI): Neonatal eHandbook, Victorian State Government, 2016. Online 28 March 2021. Available: www.bettersafercare.vic.gov.au/clinical-guidance/neonatal.

predictor), gestational age, maternal medications, maternal hypertension and mode of birth (Sharma et al 2017). Variations in the normative blood pressure reference data for neonates and confounding factors make it difficult to determine the appropriate neonatal blood pressure range (Lalan & Warady 2015). Blood pressure increases with gestational age, birthweight and postnatal age and is lower in the preterm neonate than the term neonate (Safer Care Victoria [SCV] and the Victorian Agency for Health Information [VAHI] 2016). In the first 3 hours of life blood pressure decreases followed by an average increase of 0.2 mmHg per hour during the first 24 hours, and continues to increase gradually (Newborn Services Clinical Practice Committee 2019).

An SBP of 70 mmHg and DBP of 44 mmHg is normal during the first hour of life for term neonates. Blood pressure increases by 1–2 mmHg/day for the first 3–8 days and then increases by 1 mmHg/week for the next 5–7 weeks, stabilising around 2 months of age (Frost et al 2011). The Zubrow reference charts for neonatal blood pressure were published in 1995 and are still used by many hospitals. While systolic and diastolic pressures can be recorded, it is more usual to record the MAP. Normal values have been developed by body weight and postnatal age (Table 7.8).

In the neonatal intensive care unit (NICU), accurate blood pressure measurement is essential for appropriate treatment. Neonates, especially preterm neonates, have a poor tolerance for fluctuations in blood pressure, which can predispose them to intracranial haemorrhage and periventricular leukomalacia. Intra-arterial blood monitoring is generally considered to be the gold standard for

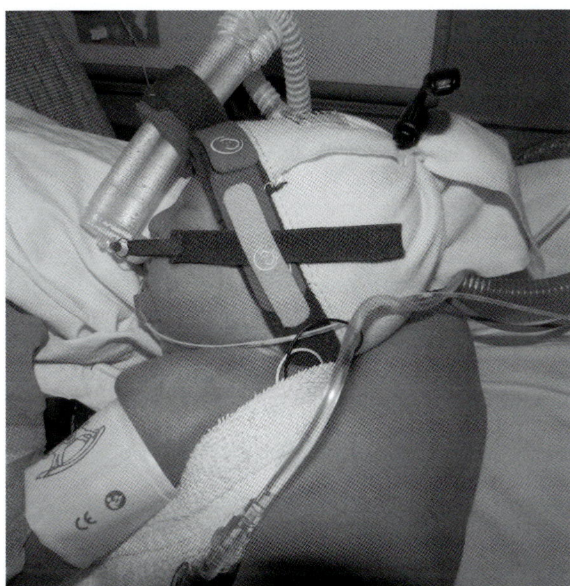

FIGURE 7.12 **Non-invasive blood pressure monitoring of neonate.**

neonatal blood pressure with the umbilical, radial and posterior tibial artery most commonly used (Sharma et al 2017). Hypertension in the neonate has a prevalence of 0.2–3% and is defined as a systolic BP > 95% for neonates of similar weight, gestation and postnatal age (Nickavar & Assadi 2014).

Blood pressure in the neonate can be non-invasive (oscillometric measurement; Fig 7.12) or invasive (intra-arterial measurement), performed via an umbilical artery catheter (UAC) or peripheral arterial catheters (Lalan & Blowey 2014). However, oscillatory blood pressure monitoring is used for the majority of neonates, with intra-arterial monitoring reserved for critically ill and unstable neonates (Dionne et al 2020). Intra-arterial BP measurement is recommended when the measurement accuracy determines treatment (Shimokaze et al 2015).

Blood pressure can be read intermittently with a manometer system (using either auscultatory or oscillatory manometers) or continuously (using a transducer attached to an arterial line, connected to an oscilloscope). Oscillometric blood pressure measurement was found to overestimate systolic BP and diastolic BP in unwell neonates (Lalan & Blowey 2014).

If the cuff is left on between measurements, it should be repositioned every 4–6 hours to reduce the risk of skin damage, nerve palsy or limb ischaemia. It is important to use the correct neonatal cuff size to obtain an accurate measurement.

SKILL 7.2 Non-invasive neonatal blood pressure measurement

An oscillometric device is used. Blood pressure is recorded as for the adult.

- Place the cuff on the selected site; the right upper arm is preferred (Dionne et al 2020).
- The correct cuff-to-arm ratio is marked on the cuff and is important to ensure correct size. The width of the cuff bladder should be appropriately 50% of the neonate's mid-arm circumference (Dionne et al 2020).
- Obtain BP measurement while neonate is asleep or quiet.
- Obtain two to three measurements if making treatment decisions.
- Compare MAP to normative values as this is the most accurate value when using oscillometric devices (Dionne et al 2020).
- Non-invasive BP may overestimate measurements when BP is low of infant is very low birthweight.
- Use oscillometric devices with caution if MAP is < 30 mmHg as they have reduced accuracy in this situation (Dionne et al 2020).

FACTORS INFLUENCING NEONATAL BLOOD PRESSURE

- Gestational age
- Postnatal age
- Birth weight
- Body weight
- Cuff size: smaller cuffs give high readings; the cuff length should be ≥ 80% of upper limb length (measured from tip of shoulder); the cuff bladder needs to be ≥ 50% of the upper arm circumference (Dionne et al 2020)
- Gender
- A state of alertness: BP is lowest in neonates who are sleeping, and increases during periods of wakefulness, agitation, crying and feeding (Nickavar & Assadi 2014)
- Maternal hypertension or pre-eclampsia
- Maternal medications, particularly antenatal steroids (Kent & Chaudhari 2013)

Role and responsibilities of the midwife

These can be summarised as:

- identifying the need to undertake blood pressure measurement
- completing the procedure correctly and accurately

- recognising and acting on any deviations from normal
- documenting the findings and acting on them accordingly
- ensuring all equipment used is properly serviced and maintained.

SUMMARY

- Various sphygmomanometers are available for use.
- Aneroid manometers are lightweight and portable; however, there is a tendency to error due to expansion and contraction of the metal parts with temperature changes.
- The mercury column manometer (the gold standard for non-invasive BP measurement) is being phased out and may be replaced with a hybrid auscultatory manometer.
- Automated manometers reduce errors such as end/terminal digit preference and threshold avoidance and can be used by people with hearing difficulties.
- All manometers should be validated, properly maintained and serviced.
- Korotkoff sounds are used to determine blood pressure: Korotkoff I, when the sounds are first heard, represents the systolic blood pressure, and Korotkoff V, when the sounds become absent, represents the diastolic blood pressure.
- Many factors can influence blood pressure accuracy, so it is important to undertake the procedure correctly and ensure equipment is properly maintained.
- Central venous pressure measurement is an advanced skill utilised for the critically ill woman.

Self-assessment exercises

The answers to the following questions may be found in the text.

1. What is the difference between systolic and diastolic blood pressures?
2. If a woman has a blood pressure of 130/70 mmHg, what are her mean arterial pressure and pulse pressure?
3. Why should blood pressure be recorded between contractions in labour?
4. What cuff size is required for a woman with a mid-arm circumference of 32 cm?
5. If using an oscillatory manometer, how often should it be calibrated?
6. What is the normal blood pressure and how is this altered during:
   a. pregnancy
   b. labour
   c. the postnatal period?
7. Identify five factors that can influence blood pressure and discuss why they occur.
8. Discuss five factors that influence the accuracy of the measurement and how the midwife can minimise this.
9. What is the central venous pressure and how can it be measured?

Resources

Best Practice Advocacy Centre New Zealand (bpac^{nz}): Better medicine, 2021. Available: www.bpac.org.nz.

British and Irish Hypertension Society (BIHS): How to measure blood pressure, 2017. Online 27 March 2021. Available: bihsoc.org/resources/bp-measurement/measure-blood-pressure.

Royal Australian College of General Practitioners: Home blood pressure diary. Excel spreadsheet, 2016. Available: www.racgp.org.au/download/Documents/AFP/2016/January/February/Fig2_Home_BP_diary.pdf

References

Agrawal A, Wenger NK: Hypertension during pregnancy, Current Hypertension Reports 22(9):64–64, 2020. Available: https://doi.org/10.1007/s11906-020-01070-0.

Alexis O: Providing best practice in manual blood pressure measurement, British Journal of Nursing 18(7):410–415, 2009.

Alpert BS, Quinn D, Gallick D: Oscillometric blood pressure: a review for clinicians, Journal of the American Society of Hypertension 8(12):930–938, 2014.

Andreas M, Kuessel L, Kastl SP, et al: Bioimpedance cardiography in pregnancy: a longitudinal cohort study on hemodynamic pattern and outcome, BMC Pregnancy and Childbirth 16:1–9, 2016.

Australian Institute of Health and Welfare (AIHW): High blood pressure, Cat. no. PHE 250, AIHW, Canberra, 2019. Online 27 March 2021. Available: www.aihw.gov.au/reports/risk-factors/high-blood-pressure/contents/high-blood-pressure

Australian Institute of Health and Welfare (AIHW): Maternal deaths in Australia, Cat. no. PER 99, AIHW, Canberra, 2020. Online 14 March 2021. Available: www.aihw.gov.au/reports/mothers-babies/maternal-deaths-in-australia

Ayres-de-Campos D: Obstetric emergencies: a practical guide, Springer, University of Porto, Portugal, 2016.

Bello N, Woolley J, Cleary K et al: Accuracy of blood pressure measurement devices in pregnancy: a systematic review of validation studies, Hypertension, 71(2):326–335, 2018.

Bishop DG, Cairns C, Grobbelaar M, et al: Heart rate variability as a predictor of hypotension following spinal for elective caesarean section: a prospective observational study, Anaesthesia 72:603–608, 2017.

Blackburn ST: Maternal, fetal and neonatal physiology: a clinical perspective, 4th ed., Elsevier Saunders, Maryland Heights, 2018.

Boardman H, Ormerod O, Leeson P: Haemodynamic changes in pregnancy: what can we learn from combined datasets? BMJ Publishing Group, London, 2016.

Bowyer L, Robinson HL, Barrett H, et al: SOMANZ guidelines for the investigation and management sepsis in pregnancy, Australian and New Zealand Journal of Obstetrics and Gynaecology 57:540–551, 2017.

Bridges E: Pulmonary artery/central venous pressure monitoring in adults, Critical Care Nurse 36:e12–e18, 2016.

British and Irish Hypertension Society (BIHS): How to measure blood pressure, 2017. Online 27 March 2021. Available: bihsoc.org/resources/bp-measurement/measure-blood-pressure/.

Brown MA: Is there a role for ambulatory blood pressure monitoring in pregnancy? Clinical & Experimental Pharmacology & Physiology 41:16–21, 2014.

Campos-Murguia A, Leon-Lara X, Munoz J, et al: Stethoscopes as potential intrahospital carriers of pathogenic microorganism, American Journal of Infection Control 42(1):82–83, 2014.

Chappell LC, Ashworth DC, Maule SP, et al: Setting and techniques for monitoring blood pressure during pregnancy, Cochrane Library 8, CD012739–CD012739, 2020. Available: https://doi.org/10.1002/14651858.CD012739.pub2

Chengyu L, Griffiths C, Murray A, et al: Comparison of stethoscope bell and diaphragm, and of stethoscope tube length, for clinical blood pressure measurement, Blood Pressure Monitoring 21:178–183, 2016.

Chestnut DH, Wong CA, Tsen LC, et al: Chestnut's obstetric anesthesia principles and practice, 5th ed., Elsevier Saunders, Philadelphia, 2014.

Davis GK, Roberts LM, Mangos GJ, et al: Comparisons of auscultatory hybrid and automated sphygmomanometer with mercury sphygmomanometer in hypertensive and normotensive pregnant women: parallel validation studies, Journal of Hypertension 33:499–506, 2015.

DeMers D, Wachs D. Physiology, mean arterial pressure, updated 22 August 2020. In: StatPearls (Internet), StatPearls Publishing, Treasure Island (FL), January 2021. Available from: www.ncbi.nlm.nih.gov/books/NBK538226/

Department of Agriculture, Water and the Environment: Ratification of the Minamata Convention on Mercury: final regulation impact statement, Australian Government, 2020.

Department of Health: Clinical practice guidelines: pregnancy care, Australian Government, Canberra, 2020.

Dionne JM, Bremner SA, Baygani SK, et al: Method of blood pressure measurement in neonates and infants: A systematic review and analysis, The Journal of Pediatrics 221:23–31.e5, 2020. Available: https://doi.org/10.1016/j.jpeds.2020.02.072.

Dorogova IV, Panina ES: Comparison of the BPLab sphygmomanometer for ambulatory blood pressure monitoring with mercury sphygmomanometry in pregnant women: validation study according to the British Hypertension Society protocol, Vascular Health & Risk Management 11:245–249, 2015.

Duffy D, McDonald S, Hayhurst B, et al: Familial aggregation of albuminuria and arterial hypertension in an Aboriginal Australian community and the contribution of variants in *ACE* and *TP53*, BMC Nephrology 17(183):431–445, 2016.

Edmunds S, Hollis V, Lamb J, et al: Observations. In Dougherty L, Lister S, editors: The Royal Marsden Hospital manual of clinical nursing procedures, 8th ed., Wiley-Blackwell, Oxford, 2011, pp. 762–776.

El Ayadi AM, Nathan HL, Seed PT, et al: Vital sign prediction of adverse maternal outcomes in women with hypovolemic shock: the role of shock index, PLoS ONE 11:1–12, 2016.

Eley V, Christensen R, Kumar S, Callaway L: A review of blood pressure measurement in obese pregnant women, International Journal of Obstetric Anesthesia 35:64–74, 2018. Available: https://doi.org/10.1016/j.ijoa.2018.04.004

Fallon N: The challenge of measuring blood pressure accurately, British Journal of Cardiac Nursing 10: 132–139, 2015.

Fitzgerald E, Gomersall C, Ka Man H, et al: Basic for nurses, Department of Anaesthesia & Intensive Care, The Chinese University of Hong Kong, Shatin, 2015.

Frese EM, Fick AH, Sadowsky S: Blood pressure measurement guidelines for physical therapists, Cardiopulmonary Physical Therapy 22(2):5–12, 2011.

Frost MS, Farshaw L, Hernandez J, et al: Neonatal nephrology. In Gardner SL, Carter BS, Enzman-Hines M, et al, editors: Merenstein & Gardner's handbook of neonatal intensive care, 7th ed., Mosby, St Louis, 2011, pp. 717–747.

Gabb GM, Mangoni AA, Anderson CS, et al: Guideline for the diagnosis and management of hypertension in adults—2016, Medical Journal of Australia 205:85–89, 2016.

Ghossein-Doha C, Khalil A, Lees C: Maternal hemodynamics: a 2017 update, Ultrasound in Obstetrics & Gynecology 49(1):10–14, 2017.

Gomersall C, Joynt G, Cheng C, et al: Basic assessment & support in intensive care, University of Hong Kong, Hong Kong, 2015.

Gomez YH, Hudda Z, Mahdi N, et al: Pulse pressure amplification and arterial stiffness in low-risk, uncomplicated pregnancies, Angiology 67(4):375–383, 2016.

Guy GP, Ling HZ, Garcia P, et al: Maternal cardiovascular function at 35–37 weeks' gestation: relation to maternal characteristics, Ultrasound in Obstetrics & Gynecology 49:39–45, 2017.

Hale S, Choate M, Schonberg A, et al: Pulse pressure and arterial compliance prior to pregnancy and the development of complicated hypertension during pregnancy, Reproductive Sciences 17:871–877, 2010.

Hay A, Ayis S, Nzelu D, et al: Validation of the Withings BP-800 in pregnancy and impact of maternal characteristics on the accuracy of blood pressure measurement, Pregnancy Hypertension Journal 6:406–412, 2016.

Head GA, McGrath BP, Mihailidou AS, et al: Ambulatory blood pressure monitoring in Australia: 2011 consensus position statement, Journal of Hypertension 30(2): 253–256, 2012.

Health Navigator New Zealand: High blood pressure, Best Practice Journal 54, 2015. Online 28 March 2021. Available: www.healthnavigator.org.nz/health-a-z/b/blood-pressure-high.

Helou A, Walker S, Stewart K, et al: Management of pregnancies complicated by hypertensive disorders of pregnancy: could we do better? Australian & New Zealand Journal of Obstetrics & Gynaecology 57: 253–259, 2017.

Hiroshi U, Sawami K: Predicting the need for fluid therapy. Does fluid responsiveness work?, Journal of Intensive Care 5:1–6, 2017.

Hogan J, Maguire P, Farah N, et al: Body mass index and blood pressure measurement during pregnancy, Hypertension in Pregnancy 30:396–400, 2011.

Iacobaeus C, Andolf E, Thorsell M, et al: Longitudinal study of vascular structure and function during normal pregnancy, Ultrasound in Obstetrics & Gynecology 49:46–53, 2017.

Kallioinen N, Hill A, Horswill MS, et al: Sources of inaccuracy in the measurement of adult patients' resting blood pressure in clinical settings: a systematic review, Journal of Hypertension 35:421–441, 2017.

Kario K, Thijs L, Staessen JA: Blood pressure measurement and treatment decisions masked and white-coat hypertension, Circulation Research 124(7):990–1008, 2019.

Kent A, Chaudhari T: Determinants of neonatal blood pressure, Current Hypertension Reports 15(5): 426–432, 2013.

Khan R: Vital signs. In Koutoukidis G, Stainton K, editors: Tabbner's nursing care, 8th ed., Elsevier, Sydney, 2021, Chapter 20: Vital sign assessment.

Klabunde RE: Cardiovascular physiology concepts, 2nd ed., Lippincott Williams & Wilkins, Philadelphia, 2012.

Kuhn JC, Falk RS, Langesæter E: Haemodynamic changes during labour: continuous minimally invasive monitoring in 20 healthy parturients, International Journal of Obstetric Anesthesia 31:74–83, 2017.

Lalan S, Blowey D: Comparison between oscillometric and intra-arterial blood pressure measurements in ill preterm and full-term neonates, Journal of the American Society of Hypertension 8(1):36–44, 2014.

Lalan SP, Warady BA: Discrepancies in the normative neonatal blood pressure reference ranges, Blood Pressure Monitoring 20:171–177, 2015.

Levy J, Gerber LM, Wu X, et al: Nonadherence to recommended guidelines for blood pressure measurement, Journal of Clinical Hypertension 18: 1157–1161, 2016.

Lippincott, Williams, Wilkins: Lippincott's nursing procedures, 7th ed., Wolters Kluwer, Philadelphia, 2015.

Loubert C, Gagnon P-O, Fernando R: Minimum effective fluid volume of colloid to prevent hypotension during caesarean section under spinal anesthesia using a prophylactic phenylephrine infusion: an up-down sequential allocation study, Journal of Clinical Anesthesia 36:194–200, 2017.

Lowe SA, Bowyer L, Lust K et al: The SOMANZ guideline for the management of hypertensive disorders of pregnancy, Australian and New Zealand Journal of Obstetrics and Gynaecology 55(1):11–16, 2015.

Marik P, Cavallazzi R: Does the central venous pressure predict fluid responsiveness? An updated meta-analysis and a plea for some common sense, Critical Care Medicine 41(7):1774–1781, 2013.

McLaughlin K, Wright S, Kingdom J, et al: Clinical validation of non-invasive cardiac output monitoring in healthy pregnant women, Journal of Obstetrics and Gynaecology Canada 39(11):1008–1014, 2017.

Meah VL, Cockcroft JR, Backx K, et al: Cardiac output and related haemodynamics during pregnancy: a series of meta-analyses, Heart (British Cardiac Society) 102: 518–526, 2016.

Melchiorre K, Sharma R, Khalil A, et al: Maternal cardiovascular function in normal pregnancy, Hypertension 67:754–762, 2016.

Ministry of Health Manatū Hauora: Observation of mother and baby in the immediate postnatal period: consensus statements guiding practice, 2012. Online 28 March 2021. Available: www.health.govt.nz/publication/observation-mother-and-baby-immediate-postnatal-period-consensus-statements-guiding-practice.

Morgan JL, Nelson DB, Roberts SW, et al: Blood pressure profiles across pregnancy in women with chronic hypertension, American Journal of Perinatology 33:1128–1132, 2016.

Morris E, McBride CA, Badger GJ, et al: 490: pregnancy induces increased arterial compliance that persists for years, American Journal of Obstetrics and Gynecology 216:S289, 2017.

Murray I, Hassell J: Change and adaptation in pregnancy. In Marshall J, Raynor M, editors: Myles textbook for midwives, 16th ed., Churchill Livingstone, Edinburgh, 2014, pp. 143–178.

Nathan HL, Cottam K, Hezelgrave NL, et al: Determination of normal ranges of shock index and other haemodynamic variables in the immediate postpartum period: a cohort study, PLoS ONE 11:1–10, 2016.

Nathan HL, de Greef A, Hezelgrave NL, et al: Accuracy validation of the Microlife 3AS1-2 blood pressure device in a pregnant population with low blood pressure, Blood Pressure Monitoring 20:299–302, 2015.

Nathan H, El Ayadi A, Hezelgrave N, et al: Shock index: an effective predictor of outcome in postpartum haemorrhage? BJOG: An International Journal of Obstetrics & Gynaecology 122:268–275, 2015.

National Heart Foundation of Australia: Guideline for the diagnosis and management of hypertension in adults, 2016. Melbourne. Accessed 20 October 2017. Online 5 July 2021. Available: https://www.heartfoundation.org.au/conditions/hypertension.

National Institute for Health and Care Excellence (NICE): Caesarean section, 2021. Online 17 August 2021. Available: www.nice.org.uk/guidance/ng192.

National Institute for Health and Clinical Excellence (NICE): Hypertension in pregnancy, 2019. Online 28 March 2021. Available: www.nice.org.uk/guidance/ng133.

National Institute for Health and Care Excellence (NICE): Intrapartum care of healthy women and their babies, 2014 updated 2017. Online 28 March 2021. Available: www.nice.org.uk/guidance/cg190.

Nelson DB, Stewart RD, Matulevicius SA, et al: The effects of maternal position and habitus on maternal cardiovascular parameters as measured by cardiac magnetic resonance, American Journal of Perinatology 32:1318–1323, 2015.

Newborn Services Clinical Practice Committee: Blood pressure—hypertension in neonates, 2019. Online 15 August 2021. Available: starship.org.nz/guidelines/blood-pressure-hypertension-in-neonates.

Nickavar A, Assadi F: Managing hypertension in the newborn infants, International Journal of Preventive Medicine 5(Suppl 1):S39–S43, 2014.

Nikolic SB, Abhayaratna WP, Leano R, et al: Waiting a few extra minutes before measuring blood pressure has potentially important clinical and research ramifications, Journal of Human Hypertension 28:56–61, 2014.

Oetzel J, Scott N, Hudson M, et al: Implementation framework for chronic disease intervention effectiveness in Māori and other indigenous communities, Globalization & Health 13:1–13, 2017.

Panaitescu AM, Baschat AA, Akolekar R, et al: Association of chronic hypertension with birth of small-for-gestational-age neonate, Ultrasound in Obstetrics & Gynecology 50:361–366, 2017.

Patel RS, Masi S, Taddei S: Understanding the role of genetics in hypertension, European Heart Journal 38(29):2309–2312, 2017.

Perinatal and Maternal Mortality Review Committee (PMMRC): Twelfth annual report of the Perinatal and Maternal Mortality Review Committee: reporting mortality 2016. Health Quality and Safety Commission, Wellington, 2018.

Pinar R, Ataalkin S, Watson R: The effect of clothes on sphygmometric blood pressure measurement in hypertensive patients, Journal of Clinical Nursing 19:1861–1864, 2010.

Priestley EM, Inaba K, Byerly S et al: Pulse pressure as an early warning of hemorrhage in trauma patients, Journal of the American College of Surgeons August, 229(2): 184–191, 2019.

Ringrose JS, McLean D, Ao P, et al: Effect of cuff design on auscultatory and oscillometric blood pressure measurements, American Journal of Hypertension 20(9):1063–1069, 2016.

Russell JA: Is there a good MAP for septic shock? New England Journal of Medicine 370(17):1649–1651, 2014.

Ruzicka M, Akbari A, Bruketa E, et al: How accurate are home blood pressure devices in use? A cross-sectional study, PLoS ONE 11:1–11, 2016.

Safer Care Victoria (SCV) and the Victorian Agency for Health Information (VAHI): Normal blood neonatal blood pressure values, 2016. Online 28 March 2021. Victorian State Government. Available: www.bettersafercare.vic.gov.au/clinical-guidance/neonatal/blood-pressure-disorders

SafeWork Australia: Preparation of safety data sheets for hazardous chemicals: Code of practice, 2016. Online 27 March 2021. Available: www.safeworkaustralia.gov.au/system/files/documents/1705/mcop-preparation-of-safety-data-sheets-for-hazardous-chemicals-v2.pdf.

Schwartz CL, Clark C, Koshiaris C, et al: Interarm difference in systolic blood pressure in different ethnic groups and relationship to the 'white coat effect': a cross-sectional study, American Journal of Hypertension 30(9):884–891, 2017.

Shahbabu B, Dasgupta A, Sarkar K, et al: Which is more accurate in measuring the blood pressure? A digital or an aneroid sphygmomanometer? Journal of Clinical & Diagnostic Research 10:11–14, 2016.

Sharma B, Ramawat P: Prevalence of inter-arm blood pressure difference among clinical out-patients, International Journal of Health Sciences 10(2):229–237, 2016.

Sharma D, Farahbakhsh N, Shastri S, et al: Neonatal hypertension, The Journal of Maternal-Fetal & Neonatal Medicine 30(5):540–550, 2017.

Sharma KJ, Rodriguez M, Kilpatrick SJ, et al: Risks of parenteral antihypertensive therapy for the treatment of severe maternal hypertension are low, Hypertension in Pregnancy 35:123–128, 2016.

Sharman J, Howes F, Head G, et al: Home blood pressure monitoring: Australian expert consensus statement, Journal of Hypertension 33(9):1721–1728, 2015.

Sharman JE, Howes FS, Head GA, et al: How to measure home blood pressure: recommendations for healthcare professionals and patients, Australian Family Physician 45:31–34, 2016.

Shimokaze T, Akaba K, Saito E: Oscillometric and intra-arterial blood pressure in preterm and term infants: extent of discrepancy and factors associated with inaccuracy, American Journal of Perinatology 32(03):277–282, 2015.

Silveira Rocha R, Gurgel Alves JA, Maia e Holanda Moura SB, et al: Simple approach based on maternal characteristics and mean arterial pressure for the prediction of preeclampsia in the first trimester of pregnancy, Journal of Perinatal Medicine 45:843–849, 2017.

Soma-Pillay P, Catherine N-P, Tolppanen H, et al: Physiological changes in pregnancy, Cardiovascular Journal of Africa 27(2):89–94, 2016.

Song S, Lee J, Chee Y, et al: Does the accuracy of blood pressure measurement correlate with hearing loss of the observer?, Blood Pressure Monitor 19(1):14–18, 2014.

Stott D, Nzellu O, Nicolaides KH, et al: Maternal haemodynamics in normal pregnancies and in pregnancies affected by preeclampsia, Ultrasound in Obstetrics and Gynecology 2017.

Tranquilli AL, Dekker G, Magee L, et al: The classification, diagnosis and management of the hypertensive disorders of pregnancy: a revised statement from the ISSHP, Pregnancy Hypertension 4:97–104, 2014.

Tuğrul E, Karaçam Z: Comparison of blood pressure and pulse readings measured on a bare arm, a clothed arm and on an arm with a rolled-up sleeve. International Journal of Nursing Studies 105:103506–103506, 2020.

United Nations: Minamata Convention on Mercury, 2013. Online 27 March 2021. Available: www.mercuryconvention.org/Convention/tabid/3426/language/en-US/Default.aspx.

Vestgaard M, Ásbjörnsdóttir B, Ringholm L, et al: White coat hypertension in early pregnancy in women with pre-existing diabetes: prevalence and pregnancy outcomes, Diabetologia 62(12):2188–2199, 2019.

Vinayagam D, Gutierrez J, Binder J, et al: G4. Does maternal obesity have an adverse effect on haemodynamics? The Journal of Maternal–Fetal & Neonatal Medicine 29:35, 2016.

Vonck S, Staelens AS, Bollen I, et al: Why non-invasive maternal hemodynamics assessment is clinically relevant in early pregnancy: a literature review, BMC Pregnancy and Childbirth 16:27–35, 2016.

Ward JP, Linden RWA: Physiology at a glance, 4th ed., John Wiley & Sons, Oxford, 2017.

Westmead Intensive Care Unit: Haemodynamic monitoring learning package, 2016. Online 27 March 2021. Available: www.aci.health.nsw.gov.au/__data/assets/pdf_file/0004/334921/Westmead_Haemodynamic_Monitoring_Learning_Package.pdf.

World Health Organization (WHO). Hypertension, 2021. Online 15 August 2021. Available: www.who.int/news-room/fact-sheets/detail/hypertension

World Health Organization (WHO). Maternal mortality fact sheet, 2019. Online 14 August 2021. Available: www.who.int/news-room/fact-sheets/detail/maternal-mortality

Worksafe New Zealand: Managing your hazardous substances: safety data sheets, 2017. Online 27 March 2021. Available: www.worksafe.govt.nz/worksafe/information-guidance/guidance-by-industry/hsno/hazardous-substances-regulations/safety-data-sheets.

Wright A, Wright D, Ispas CA, et al: Mean arterial pressure in the three trimesters of pregnancy: effects of maternal characteristics and medical history, Ultrasound in Obstetrics & Gynecology 45:698–706, 2015.

Zheng D, Giovanni R, Murray A: Effect of respiration, talking and small body movements on blood pressure measurement, Journal of Human Hypertension 26: 458–462, 2012.

Zubrow AB, Hulman S, Kushner H, et al: Determinants of blood pressure in infants admitted to neonatal intensive care units: a prospective multicenter study. Philadelphia Neonatal Blood Pressure Study Group, Journal of Perinatology 15:470–479, 1995.

CHAPTER 8

NEUROLOGICAL ASSESSMENT

Learning outcomes

Having read this chapter, the reader should be able to:

- describe the different components of the Glasgow Coma Scale (GCS)
- discuss how the midwife can complete the GCS
- identify the other observations that should be undertaken in conjunction with the GCS to gain a thorough neurological assessment
- describe abnormal neurological signs in the neonate
- identify tools used for neurological assessment of the neonate.

Neurological assessment may be undertaken when there are concerns about actual or possible alterations in a woman's level of consciousness (e.g. post-seizure, magnesium sulfate toxicity, meningitis, head injury). A full neurological assessment examines the central and peripheral nervous systems, including mental status, motor, cerebellar and sensory function, reflexes and cranial nerves (Maher 2016) and is often undertaken by medical staff or nurse practitioners.

The midwife must be appropriately trained to complete the Glasgow Coma Scale (GCS) and assess the level of consciousness competently and safely, as it provides invaluable information on a woman's neurological status. Midwives also need to be able to identify abnormal neurological signs in the neonate, such as a high-pitched cry or seizures, and escalate care as necessary. Part of the examination assesses the neonate's neurological system and midwives must notify the neonatologist or paediatrician if any concerns are detected. A full neurological assessment is then undertaken by a specialist.

This chapter focuses on the principles of neurological assessment and the midwife's role in relation to neurological assessment.

LEVEL OF CONSCIOUSNESS

Alterations in level of consciousness represent an early and sensitive indicator of neurological status. Impaired cerebral blood flow deprives the cerebral cortex and the reticular activating system (RAS) of oxygen (Cooper & Gosnell 2015). The RAS includes the brainstem and thalamus and is essential for wakefulness and awareness (Bullock & Hales 2018). The RAS has ascending and descending pathways which receive sensory information, such as pain, from the periphery and relay them to the cerebral cortex; motor information from the brain is relayed to the skeletal muscles and is involved in control of muscle tone (Bullock & Hales 2018). Midwives need to be aware of the causes of altered level of consciousness, which include the following:

- head injury
- haemorrhage
- increased intracranial pressure
- vasospasm of cerebral vasculature
- hypoxia
- hypertension
- profound hypotension
- systemic infection
- hepatic or renal dysfunction
- hypoglycaemia or hyperglycaemia
- electrolyte imbalance
- pH imbalance
- medications and other chemicals (Bullock & Hales 2018).

GLASGOW COMA SCALE

The **Glasgow Coma Scale (GCS)** is a tool for assessing level of consciousness and is a measure of brain function. Any loss or deterioration in consciousness demonstrates a deterioration in brain function. The

GCS was developed in 1974 and revised in 1979 to provide a quick and objective assessment of level of consciousness (Palmer & Knight 2006). The GCS is divided into three categories: eye opening (4 points), best verbal response (5 points) and best motor response (6 points). The three scores are totalled to score between 15 (fully conscious) and 3 (no response). The score should be recorded as a fraction using 15 as the denominator (e.g. 10/15).

The GCS provides a rapid assessment of the woman's condition and response to treatment. NICE (2014) states that a GCS >12 indicates a normal or minimally impaired level of consciousness. A score of 8 requires airway management and a drop of ≥ 2 points initiates a rapid response (NSW ACI 2013). A score of 7 or less is an indication of coma.

It is important to be aware that other factors, such as sedation and analgesia, can mask alterations in the level of consciousness (Braine & Cook 2017). NICE (2014) recommended neurological observations be completed every 30 minutes until the GCS is 15, when they can be recorded hourly for 4 hours, then every 2 hours, reverting to 30-minute assessments if the condition deteriorates.

Eye opening

Eye opening is the first GCS measurement of consciousness (Table 8.1). Eye opening assesses the integrity of the reticular activating system found in the brainstem (Okamura 2014). If a woman has damage to the eyes resulting in oedema, a score cannot be allocated and a 'C' is documented on the chart indicating that her eyes are closed (de Sousa & Woodward 2016). Some GCSs use the term 'not testable' or 'NT' to indicate that the response was not able to be assessed (Teasdale et al 2014).

If a woman's eyes are spontaneously open, the score is 4 (fully awake). If her eyes remain closed, the midwife speaks to the woman, which should provoke the eyes to open, giving a score of 3. If the woman's eyes remain closed, a peripheral painful stimulus is used—this may be a gentle shake, but if there is no response then a deeper stimulus is needed. Pressure is applied just below the lateral outer aspect of the second or third interphalangeal joint for 10–15 seconds (Okamura 2014). If the eyes open in response to painful stimuli, the score is 2.

If there is no response using a peripheral painful stimulus, a central painful stimulus is used. Central stimuli can be applying supraorbital pressure (Fig 8.1) (if no facial fracture or glaucoma) or squeezing the trapezium muscle (where the neck and shoulder meet) for 30 seconds, using the thumb and two fingers (Fig 8.2) (de Sousa & Woodward 2016). Sternal rubs are not to be used as they can result in bruising. It is important to use the same stimulus on each assessment. The type and site of the stimulus used should be documented. A score of 1 is given if the eyes remain closed (Waterhouse 2017).

TABLE 8.1 GLASGOW COMA SCALE—EYE OPENING

Category	Response	Score
Spontaneous	Eyes open spontaneously (fully awake)	4
Speech/ touch	Eyes open to verbal command or touch	3
To pain	Eyes open to painful stimuli	2
No response	No eye opening to painful stimuli	1
		'C'

Verbal response

Assessing the verbal response is an assessment of the integrity of the higher, cognitive and interpretive centres of the brain (Table 8.2) (Okamura 2014). The midwife should ascertain the level of verbal response by

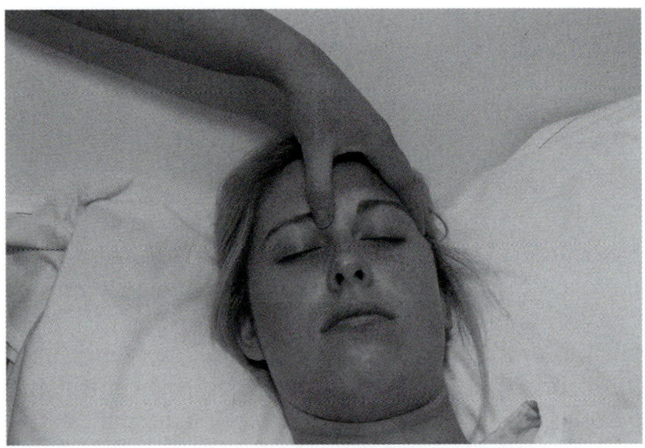

FIGURE 8.1 **Technique for pressure to the supraorbital ridge: place thumb below the eyebrow, close to the nose, and apply gradual pressure for up to 30 seconds.**

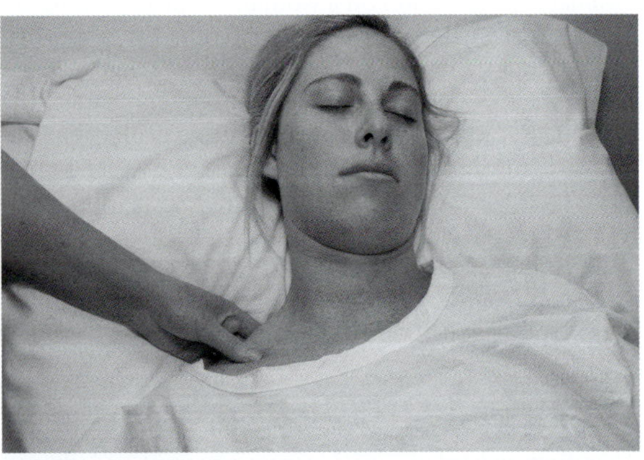

FIGURE 8.2 **Technique for squeezing trapezium muscle.**

TABLE 8.2 GLASGOW COMA SCALE—VERBAL RESPONSE

Category	Response	Score
Oriented to person, place and time	Accurate intelligible answer	5
Disoriented/talks	Speaks, but is confused regarding person, place or time	4
Inappropriate words	Words or phrases incomplete	3
Incomprehensible sounds	Moaning, groaning, grunts	2
No response	No sound in response to verbal or painful central stimuli	1

TABLE 8.3 GLASGOW COMA SCALE—MOTOR RESPONSE

Category	Response	Score
Obeys verbal commands	Able to complete movements as instructed	6
Localises to pain stimuli	Arm moves towards localised pain stimuli to try to remove it, or moves body part away from painful stimuli	5
Withdraws/flexes to pain stimuli	Movement but no localisation of pain stimuli. Withdraws from pain; e.g. arm bends at elbow without rotation of wrist	4
Abnormal flexion to pain stimuli	Abnormal flexion; e.g. wrist and forearm rotation (decorticate posture)	3
Abnormal extension to pain stimuli	Extension to pain; e.g. arm extends at elbow while wrist flexes (decerebrate posture)	2
No response to pain	No movement following central pain stimuli	1

asking questions that require answers, indicating clarity and understanding related to person, place and time.

Person questions

- Could you tell me your name?
- Could you tell me where you live?

Place questions

- Could you tell me where you are?
- Could you tell me the name of this place?

Time questions

- Could you tell me what day it is today?
- Could you tell me what month it is?
- Could you tell me what year it is?

It is important to consider the language spoken by the woman; if she does not speak English, an interpreter should be used. If a woman is intubated or has a tracheostomy and cannot speak, a score is not allocated (de Sousa & Woodward 2016). However, the NSW Adult Neurological Observation Chart indicates a score of 1 should be given and a 'T' for tracheostomy added to the chart (NSW ACI 2013).

Motor response

The motor response measures primary motor and cerebral cortex function (Table 8.3) (Okamura 2014). The woman is asked to bend, then hold out, her arms and squeeze the midwife's hands with both of her hands. The midwife can then determine if both arms can be moved and the elbows flexed; the power and release of grip from each hand can also be noted.

A score of 6 is given if the woman can complete movements as instructed. If there is no response to verbal requests, painful central stimuli is used beginning with the trapezius pinch; the next option is supraorbital pressure.

Scores of 2–5 are given according to the degree of movement and flexion occurring as a result of painful stimulus. If there is no movement of limbs following a central painful stimulus, the score is 1 (Waterhouse 2017).

PUPILLARY ASSESSMENT

While **pupillary assessment** is not part of the GCS, it is a separate and important component of the neurological assessment. The size and shape of each pupil and reaction to light are assessed. The midwife should look at the pupils to determine if they are the same shape and whether the eyes are working together. The diameter of each pupil is then measured. The average pupil is 3.5 mm under standard lighting with a normal range from 1–10 mm (Pate 2015). The pupils are usually equal in size (unequal pupils are a late sign associated with raised intracranial pressure). Some women may have pre-existing physiologic anisocoria (pupils naturally unequal).

Pupil reaction is assessed by shining a bright light from a pen torch into one eye, then the other; approach from the side rather than directly in front. The pupils should constrict briskly. A fixed pupil suggests the midbrain may be suffering from pressure as constriction and dilation of the pupils is controlled by the oculomotor nerve (cranial nerve III).

Pupils that are slow to respond or dilate suddenly and unequally can indicate cerebral oedema or traumatic brain injury (Khan et al 2017, Stocchetti et al 2017). The level of sedation administered to the woman will affect pupil reaction: pupils measuring 1–2 mm can occur when barbiturates or opiates have been used. Reactive pupils, equal in size in combination with a pinpoint pupil size, may be related to opiates or a Pontine lesion (Mayer & Marshall 2020). New onset of anisocoria (unequal pupil size) may indicate increasing intracranial pressure (ICP); a unilateral non-reactive dilated pupil indicates increasing ICP and possible brainstem compression; bilateral non-reactive dilated pupils are an ominous sign indicating midbrain damage; and midposition non-reactive pupils indicate midbrain involvement (Ryan 2019).

FINDINGS

The findings of the neurological assessment should be recorded on a neurological observation chart (Fig 8.3) in conjunction with the vital signs. While the total GCS score is recorded, it is also important to separately record the scores of the three different categories, as each one is assessing different areas of the brain. A decreasing score indicates the woman's condition is deteriorating and referral is indicated.

A severe or increasing headache, persistent vomiting, new or evolving neurological signs and symptoms (e.g. unequal pupils), a reduction to 3 or less points in eye opening or verbal responses or 2 in motor responses, agitation or abnormal behaviour should be reported promptly as they can indicate deterioration of the woman's neurological status.

Role and responsibilities of the midwife

These can be summarised as:

- ensuring appropriate training in assessing neurological observation has been undertaken prior to performing the neurological assessment
- undertaking a competent examination in which all the information is gained
- recognising deviations from normal and instigating referral
- appropriate documentation.

NEWBORN NEUROLOGICAL ASSESSMENT

Midwives complete a newborn assessment at birth and in the first few days of life a full examination of the newborn is undertaken. The examination includes neurological assessment involving observation of behaviour, posture, muscle tone, spontaneous movements, cry and reflexes. Of concern would be: a weak, irritable, high-pitched or absent cry; failure to respond to consoling actions; absent reflexes; seizures; or altered state of consciousness (Queensland Clinical Guidelines 2014). The result of the newborn examination is recorded and signed in the infant's personal health record. New Zealand has a national record; in Australia variations exist between states.

- Australian Capital Territory: *My ACT Personal Health Record* (the Blue Book)
- Northern Territory: *Health and Immunisation Record* (the Yellow Book)

SKILL 8.1 Neurological assessment

- Gather equipment and take it to the bedside:
  - pencil torch
  - observation chart
  - thermometer
  - sphygmomanometer
  - pulse oximeter.
- Perform hand hygiene.
- Inform the woman of the procedure and gain consent if conscious and responsive.
- Complete vital signs: temperature, blood pressure, pulse, respiration and arterial oxygen saturation.
- Assess level of consciousness using the GCS by assessing and scoring the following three categories:
  - eye opening (spontaneous, to verbal command, to pain or no response)
  - verbal response—ask the woman who she is, what day it is and where she is; use peripheral or central painful stimulus if no response (oriented, disoriented, inappropriate words, incomprehensible sounds or no response)
  - motor response (e.g. by asking the woman to bend and lift her arms and squeeze both your hands); if no response, use painful stimuli (verbal command, localises pain, flexes/withdraws, abnormal flexion, abnormal extension, no response).
- Assess the size and shape of the pupils and movement of the eyes.
- Assess pupillary reaction.
  - Darken the room if necessary.
  - Ask the woman to look straight ahead or hold one eyelid open, move the pen torchlight from the side of the face and briefly shine the light on the pupil.
  - Assess the degree and speed at which the pupil constricts.
  - Repeat with the other eye.
  - With both eyelids open, shine the light into one eye—the pupil in the other eye should also be observed to constrict (consensual reflex).
  - Repeat with the other eye.
- Ensure the woman is covered and comfortable.
- Document all findings on the observation chart.
- Perform hand hygiene.
- Act on findings as appropriate.

GUIDE TO ASSESSMENT OF NEUROLOGICAL OBSERVATIONS

For in-depth information please refer to the Education Package

Instructions:

1. Use of deep pain to elicit a response may be necessary
2. Central stimulus is advocated as the first choice for a painful/noxious stimulus e.g. trapezius pinch, supra-orbital pressure or sternal rub (used as a last measure)

Assessment Category	Testing Method	Possible Responses		Explanation
GLASGOW COMA SCALE				
Eyes Open (E) *Assess arousal*	Speak in a clear, strong voice. If nil response to voice progress to use of painful stimulus	Spontaneous	4	Opens eyes without stimulus
		To speech	3	Opens eyes to any verbal stimulus
		To pain	2	Opens eyes to painful stimulus
		None	1	Record as (C) if closed due to trauma or swelling
Verbal Response (V) *Assess appropriateness of speech and awareness*	Obtain the patient's attention Allow time for the patient to respond Impaired hearing may affect response	Orientated	5	Orientated to person, place and time
		Confused	4	Talks but is confused as to person, place and time. Record as "X" if Culturally and Linguistically Diverse (CALD)
		Inappropriate words	3	Uses words or phrases that make little or no sense
		Incomprehensible sounds	2	Unintelligible sounds, moaning or groaning
		None	1	No sound or speech at all Record as "T" if unable to speak due to tracheostomy or ETT
Best Motor Response (M) *Assess overall awareness and ability to respond to external stimuli* Note: if eyes are closed due to trauma and the patient is aphasic, motor response indicates the level of consciousness	Give simple command e.g. "wiggle your fingers" Allow time for the patient to respond If nil response to verbal command, progress to use of painful stimulus Record the best movement response Be careful not to misinterpret a grasp reflex	Obeys Commands	6	Follows commands, even if weakly.
		Localise to Pain	5	Moves hand towards source of pain Hand should move above nipple line
		Withdraws	4	Hand or body moves away from the source of the pain
		Flexion to Pain	3	Flexes arm (decorticate posturing)
		Extension to Pain	2	Extends elbow and internally rotates wrist (decerebrate posturing)
		None	1	Makes no response even to painful stimuli
LIMB STRENGTH Medical Research Council (MRC) Scale for Muscle Strength				
Arms and Legs *Assess limb strength* Record separately if there is a difference in results between the limbs	Instruct patient to: Move arms/legs laterally on bed; lift limb against gravity; move limb against your resistance	Normal Power	5	Active movement of body part against gravity with full resistance
		Active movement against resistance	4	Active movement of body part against gravity with some resistance
		Active movement against gravity	3	Active movement of body part against gravity
		Active movement of limb with gravity eliminated	2	Active movement of body part when effect of gravity is removed
		Flicker of movement	1	Only a trace or flicker of movement is seen or felt in the muscle
		None	0	No detectable muscle contraction
EYE SIGNS				
Pupil Size	Compare size with pupil scale	1-8mm		Record size of each pupil Record reaction to light Record as "c" if unable to open eye due to trauma or swelling. Document a lack of consensual reaction (opposite pupil fails to constrict when light is shone in eye) in health care record.
Pupil Reaction	Hold eyelid open Move small bright light toward patient from the side Shine directly into eye	Reaction Yes + No - Closed c Sluggish SL		

FIGURE 8.3 **Adult neurological observation chart.**

Source: NSW Agency for Clinical Innovation: Adult neurological observation chart—education package, 2013, p. 6. Available: https://www.aci.health.nsw.gov.au/__data/assets/pdf_file/0018/201753/AdultChartEdPackage.pdf

- New South Wales: *My Personal Health Record* (the Blue Book)
- Queensland: *Personal Health Record* (the Red Book)
- South Australia: *My Health and Development Record* (the Blue Book)
- Tasmania: *My Health Record* (the Blue Book) and My Child's eHealth Record app
- Victoria: *My Health Learning and Development Record* (the Green Book)
- Western Australia: *All About Me* (the Purple Book)
- New Zealand: *Well Child Tamariki Ora My Health Book*.

The GCS has been adapted for infants and is similar to the adult version (Table 8.4).

Disruption to blood flow and gas exchange in the neonate can result in perinatal asphyxia and neurological injury (Ahearne et al 2016). The clinical neurological examination in the neonate is performed for diagnosis, for assessment and to guide therapeutic interventions (Spittle et al 2016). In Australia and New Zealand there is a lack of consistency in the use of neurological assessments. The most common neurological assessment tool used in neonatal intensive care units is the Prechtl's General Movements Assessment and in special care nurseries the Hammersmith Neurological Examination (Allinson et al 2017). The Sarnat and Sarnat criteria (or modified Sarnat criteria) is used to assess severity of neonatal encephalopathy (Pavageau et al 2020). The Dubowitz method combines neurological and physical assessments to estimate newborn maturity (Lee et al 2017). The Dubowitz assessment has been shortened to the Ballard and New Ballard Score examination as they can be performed more rapidly (McKee-Garrett 2019).

Table 8.5 represents a summary of the areas assessed by four neonatal neurological assessment tools.

TABLE 8.4 GLASGOW COMA SCALE—INFANTS

Category	Response	Score
Eye opening	Spontaneously	4
	To speech	3
	To pain	2
	Nil	1
Best verbal response	Coos or babbles	5
	Irritable	4
	Cries to pain	3
	Moans to pain	2
	No verbal response	1
Best motor response	Spontaneously or purposeful	6
	Localises to pain	5
	Withdraws to pain	4
	Abnormal flexion to pain	3
	Abnormal extension to pain	2
	Nil	1

SUMMARY

- Neurological assessment is undertaken where there are actual or potential alterations in the level of consciousness.
- The GCS assesses the level of consciousness using response to eye opening, verbal response and motor ability.
- The midwife who has been appropriately trained can undertake the GCS and record vital signs as

TABLE 8.5 SUMMARY OF FOUR NEONATAL ASSESSMENT TOOLS

Screening tool	Screening category	Items screened
Hammersmith Neonatal Neurological Examination (HNNE) consists of 34 items in four categories	Posture and tone (motor system)	Posture, arm traction and recoil, leg traction, popliteal angle, head control, head lag, ventral suspension, flexor tone, leg extensor tone, neck extensor tone, increased extensor tone
	Reflexes	Tendon reflex, suck/gag, palmar grasp, plantar grasp, placing, Moro reflex, spontaneous movements, head raising
	Abnormal signs/patterns	Abnormal hand or toe postures, tremor, startle
	Orientation and behaviour	Eye appearances, auditory orientation, visual orientation, alertness, irritability, consolability, cry (NHS BeBop 2013)

TABLE 8.5 SUMMARY OF FOUR NEONATAL ASSESSMENT TOOLS—cont'd

Screening tool	Screening category	Items screened
Prechtl's General Movement Assessment (GMA) is a tool used to predict cerebral palsy	Birth to 8 weeks post-term Writhing	Normal Poor repertoire Cramped synchronised Chaotic
	8 to 20 weeks post-term Fidgety	Normal Absent Abnormal (Sydney Local Health District 2016)
Sarnat and Sarnat staging system is used to classify the level of encephalopathy in neonates	Level of consciousness	From stuporous to hyperalert
	Neuromuscular control	Muscle tone Posture Stretch reflexes Segmental myoclonus
	Complex reflexes	
		Suck Moro Ocular vestibular Tonic neck
	Autonomic function	Pupils Heart rate Bronchial and salivary secretions Gastrointestinal motility
	Other	Seizures Electroencephalogram findings
	Duration	From less than 24 hours to weeks (Queensland Clinical Guidelines 2017)
Dubowitz neonatal neurological examination, the Ballard and New Ballard Score identify physical and neurological maturity	Utilises neurological signs to assess neuromuscular maturity to indirectly test brain maturity	Posture, square window, arm recoil, popliteal angle, scarf sign, heel to ear are included in Ballard and Dubowitz examination; head lag and ventral suspension are included in Dubowitz

part of the woman's neurological assessment to determine any changes to her condition.

- A drop in the GCS of ≥ 2 points initiates a rapid response.

Self-assessment exercises

The answers to the following questions may be found in the text.

1. What are the three categories of the Glasgow Coma Scale?
2. What observations should the midwife undertake in conjunction with the Glasgow Coma Scale?
3. How does the midwife assess eye opening?
4. If there is no response, how is central stimuli applied?
5. How can the midwife determine the verbal response?
6. How does the midwife assess motor response?
7. What are the tools available for neonatal neurological assessment?

Resources

NSW Agency for Clinical Innovation (ACI NSW). Adult neurological observation chart—education package, 2013. Online 4 October 2021. Available: www.aci.health.nsw.gov.au/__data/assets/pdf_file/0018/201753/AdultChartEdPackage.pdf.

Hammersmith Neonatal Neurological Examination. Online 4 October 2021. Available: bebop.nhs.uk/wp-content/uploads/CDM148ScoreCards.pdf.

References

Ahearne CE, Boylan GB, Murray DM: Short and long term prognosis in perinatal asphyxia: an update, World Journal of Clinical Pediatrics 5(1):67–74, 2016.

Allinson LG, Doyle LW, Denehy L, et al: Survey of neurodevelopmental allied health teams in Australian and New Zealand neonatal nurseries: staff profile and standardised neurobehavioural/neurological assessment, Journal of Paediatrics & Child Health 53:578–584, 2017.

Braine ME, Cook N: The Glasgow Coma Scale and evidence-informed practice: a critical review of where we are and where we need to be, Journal of Clinical Nursing 26:280–293, 2017.

Bullock S, Hales M: Principles of pathophysiology, 2nd ed., Pearson Australia, Melbourne, 2018.

Cooper K, Gosnell K: Foundations and adult health nursing, 7th ed., Elsevier Mosby, St Louis, 2015.

de Sousa I, Woodward S: The Glasgow Coma Scale in adults: doing it right, Emergency Nurse 24:33–39, 2016.

Khan MN, Shallwani H, Khan MU, et al: Noninvasive monitoring intracranial pressure—a review of available modalities, Surgical Neurology International 8:51, 2017.

Lee AC, Panchal P, Folger L, et al: Diagnostic accuracy of neonatal assessment for gestational age determination: A systematic review. Pediatrics 140(6):e20171423, 2017. Available: https://doi.org/10.1542/peds.2017-1423.

Maher AB: Neurological assessment, International Journal of Orthopaedic & Trauma Nursing 22:44–53, 2016.

Mayer SA, Marshall RS: On call neurology, Elsevier, St Louis, 2020.

McKee-Garrett TM: Postnatal assessment of gestational age, UpToDate, 2019. Online 14 August 2021. Available: www.uptodate.com/contents/postnatal-assessment-of-gestational-age.

National Institute for Health and Care Excellence (NICE): CG 176 Head injury: assessment and early management, 2014. Online 10 Jan 2018. Available: www.nice.org.uk/guidance/cg176.

NHS BeBop Brainy Brain Protection: Neurological examination of the neonate, 2013. Online 10 Jan 2018. Available: bebop.nhs.uk/healthcare-professionals/neurological-examination-assessment/neurological-examination-neonate/.

NSW Agency for Clinical Innovation (ACI NSW): Adult neurological observation chart—education package, 2013. Online 10 Jan 2018. Available: www.aci.health.nsw.gov.au/__data/assets/pdf_file/0018/201753/AdultChartEdPackage.pdf.

Okamura K: Glasgow Coma Scale flow chart: a beginner's guide, British Journal of Nursing 23(20):1068–1073, 2014.

Palmer R, Knight J: Assessment of altered conscious level in clinical practice, British Journal of Nursing 15(22):1255–1259, 2006.

Pate C: The proper procedure for testing pupils: pupillary testing should be a component of every comprehensive examination, Ophthalmology Times 40(10):SS1, 2015.

Pavageau L, Sánchez PJ, Steven Brown L, Chalak LF: Inter-rater reliability of the modified Sarnat examination in preterm infants at 32–36 weeks' gestation, Pediatric Research 87(4):697–702, 2020. Available: https://doi.org/10.1038/s41390-019-0562-x.

Queensland Clinical Guidelines: Hypoxic-ischaemic encephalopathy (HIE), 2017. Online 10 Jan 2018. Available: www.health.qld.gov.au/__data/assets/pdf_file/0014/140162/g-hie.pdf.

Queensland Clinical Guidelines: Routine newborn assessment, 2014. Online 10 Jan 2018. Available: www.health.qld.gov.au/__data/assets/pdf_file/0029/141689/g-newexam.pdf.

Ryan D: Handbook of neuroscience nursing: care of the adult neurosurgical patient, Thieme, New York, 2019.

Spittle AJ, Walsh J, Olsen JE, et al: Neurobehaviour and neurological development in the first month after birth for infants born between 32–42 weeks' gestation, Early Human Development 96:7–14, 2016.

Stocchetti N, Carbonara M, Citerio G, et al: Severe traumatic brain injury: targeted management in the intensive care unit, The Lancet. Neurology 16(6):452–464, 2017.

Sydney Local Health District: Women and babies: general movements assessments (GMA) and other assessment modalities for prediction of cerebral palsy and adverse early neurodevelopment in high-risk infants, 2016. Online 10 Jan 2018. Available: www.slhd.nsw.gov.au/rpa/neonatal%5Ccontent/pdf/guidelines/GMApolicy_v4_2016.pdf.

Teasdale G, Allen D, Brennan P, et al: Forty years on: updating the Glasgow Coma Scale, Nursing Times 110(42):12–16, 2014.

Waterhouse C: Practical aspects of performing Glasgow Coma Scale observations, Nursing Standard 31: 40–46, 2017.

Wusthoff CJ: How to use: the neonatal neurological examination, Archives of Disease in Childhood—Education & Practice Edition 98:148–153, 2013.

SECTION 3

SCREENING AND TESTING

CHAPTER 9
SCREENING TESTS

Learning outcomes

Having read this chapter, the reader should be able to:

- discuss the indications for screening in the antenatal and newborn period
- recall the screening tests recommended to occur in pregnant women and newborns in Australia and New Zealand
- describe the processes for conducting and reporting the results of screening
- discuss the issue of informed consent and other ethical considerations in relation to screening
- explain the midwife's role and responsibilities in relation to each of these aspects of care.

Routine maternal health screening is offered to all pregnant women for the purpose of detecting conditions that may affect her pregnancy and/or the health of her fetus(es). Routine health screening is also offered newborns. In this chapter, the range of antenatal and newborn screening tests recommended in Australia and New Zealand at the time of writing are overviewed, and processes around screening are discussed.

ANTENATAL MATERNAL AND FETAL HEALTH SCREENING

Arguably, all care provided to a woman by a midwife or other health practitioner constitutes 'screening' by virtue of the fact that the practitioner is constantly gathering information to inform their understanding of her physiological, psychological, emotional, social, cultural, spiritual and economic condition, and to enable them to facilitate the woman's optimal wellbeing and that of her baby/babies. In this chapter, however, the term 'screening' is used to mean the range of tests offered to women in pregnancy to detect the presence of maternal or fetal physiological disease or disorder. It is recommended in Australasia that routine antenatal maternal/fetal health screening be initiated at the 'first antenatal visit, before 20 weeks' (Royal College of Pathologists of Australasia [RCPA] 2020). In New Zealand, the National Screening Unit (NSU) recommends testing begin 'as soon as possible in pregnancy' and then, as in Australia, the recommendation is that specific screening tests occur within a particular gestational age range or time point (Department of Health 2018, Ministry of Health 2017).

A key factor in screening is that the woman provides her informed consent and, in turn, the woman's capacity for providing informed consent to screening depends on her receiving objective, evidence-based information from the health professionals providing her antenatal care. There is very little research reported on the topic of midwives' conduct or their own views about their role in this regard; however, a study published in 2013 affirms that although midwives do take their responsibility for providing information about screening seriously, they have concerns about not having adequate time before screening tests must be performed (Ahmed, Bryant & Cole 2013). Etchegary and colleagues (2016) from Canada found little recollection of an informed consent process in relation to newborn screening among their study of 32 parent participants, and recognition of this issue in the United Kingdom led to the Provision of Information about Newborn Screening Antenatally (PINSA) project, which sought to determine 'how best to communicate information about newborn screening' through co-development of guidance for midwives with new parents (Ulph et al 2017, p. 370). Similarly, there is very little published research about expectant parents' understanding of antenatal screening, but it appears from what is available that it is suboptimal: in one study of 654 pregnant women, only 20% reported a good level of familiarity with the various screening methods (Nykänen et al 2017). Further consideration of how information about screening tests in pregnancy is provided to women is clearly required to ensure that everyone truly understands what they are being invited to consent to.

Indications for antenatal screening

Although antenatal screening regimens may differ from country to country, the guidance provided by the Royal Australian College of Obstetricians and Gynaecologists

(RANZCOG) is that screening tests should be offered routinely in pregnancy for the following:

- anaemia
- iron deficiency
- haemoglobin disorders
- gestational diabetes
- HIV
- hepatitis B
- hepatitis C
- varicella
- HbA1c
- syphilis
- rubella
- asymptomatic bacteriuria
- group B streptococcus
- maternal mental health
- family violence (RANZCOG 2019).

Women at higher risk of the following are also offered testing for these conditions:

- chlamydia
- gonorrhoea
- trichomoniasis
- toxoplasmosis
- cytomegalovirus
- hyperglycaemia
- asymptomatic bacterial vaginosis
- thyroid function
- vitamin D deficiency
- human papilloma virus
- cervical abnormalities (RANZCOG 2019).

Timing of first trimester screening tests and those in later pregnancy

The Royal College of Pathologists of Australasia (RCPA 2020) provides a comprehensive summary of when each recommended test should be performed. These recommendations are summarised in Table 9.1 and are further endorsed by RANZCOG (2019). Depending on the individual midwife's qualifications and/or local policy, either the midwife will be able to request screening tests for women or a medical practitioner's signature will

TABLE 9.1 TIMING OF FIRST TRIMESTER SCREENING TESTS AND THOSE IN LATER PREGNANCY

Timing	Test
First antenatal visit / before 20 weeks	**Routine** • Full blood count (including haemoglobin and platelet count); haemoglobinopathies, sickle cell and thalassaemia testing is also recommended for women from ethnic groups at high risk, including those of New Zealander Māori descent • Blood group • Antibody screen • Rubella • Hepatitis B • Hepatitis C • Human immunodeficiency virus (HIV) (HIV Ab and Ag combination) • Syphilis (treponemal pallidum particle agglutination [TPHA] or treponema pallidum particle agglutination [TPPA]) • Vitamin D • Urine microscopy, culture and sensitivity **Also consider** • Varicella-zoster antibody • Cervical cytology
After the first antenatal visit	• Obstetric ultrasound scan before 20 weeks' gestation • Screening for Down syndrome
At 26–28 weeks	• Full blood count (including haemoglobin and platelet count) • Blood group • Antibody screen • Glucose challenge test • Repeat syphilis screening in high-risk women
At 30–36 weeks	• Full blood count • Blood film • Group B streptococcus
Test any time if at high risk of infection	• Genital swab for *Chlamydia Trachomatis*, *Neisseria gonorrhoea*, HIV (Ab and Ag) • Herpes simplex virus • Cytomegalovirus • Toxoplasmosis Ab

Source: Royal College of Pathologists of Australasia: RCPA Manual: Antenatal Screening, 2020. Online 7 September 2020. Available: https://www.rcpa.edu.au/Manuals/RCPA-Manual/Clinical-Problems/A/Antenatal-screening

be required. Further, the midwife will be able to conduct some screening tests and others will need to be conducted by a pathology service. The reader is advised to investigate the policies and guidelines for their own practice context.

According to the Department of Health (2018), before testing, women should:

- be informed that having a test is their choice
- be able to provide informed consent
- have discussions about consent documented by the health professional involved
- be given the chance to ask questions about tests and treatments
- be confident their confidentiality will be maintained (unless the condition is notifiable, in which case they should be given information about the notification process)
- be given the opportunity to discuss their concerns without being coerced to reconsider if they decline to have a test
- be assured their baby will be followed up if the test is positive, and there is a process for this.

If a test result is positive, the midwife should:

- provide psychosocial support
- refer the woman for specialist care if the condition detected warrants it
- advise the woman about contract tracing if a sexually transmitted infection (STI) is identified
- offer specific support to women who are found to have a blood-borne infection as a consequence of intravenous drug use
- follow legislation if a notifiable disease has been detected.

If an STI is identified, the woman is advised to be tested for other STIs; she is also encouraged to consider contact tracing to help prevent the spread of infection (Department of Health 2018).

Contraindications

There are no physiological contraindications to any of the recommended screening tests recommended in pregnancy. Testing must not, however, be performed if the woman does not explicitly give her informed consent for it to occur.

ROUTINE NEWBORN SCREENING

In addition to maternal and fetal screening during pregnancy for harmful diseases and disorders, routine screening for all newborns to test for the likelihood of having any of a range of metabolic disorders is recommended (Box 9.1). **Newborn bloodspot screening (NBS)** uses blood taken from a heel capillary sample in the first few days of life, which is dropped onto special absorbent collection paper and transported to a screening laboratory with the micro-analytical capacity to analyse the samples accurately using tandem mass spectrometry (Arneth & Hintz 2017, Therrell et al 2015). In some countries, NBS is mandated in law and parents have no choice in the matter, and in some other countries (e.g. Canada), there is ongoing debate about whether this should be the case (Potter et al 2015). At the time of writing, parental consent is required for health professionals to conduct the NBS in both Australia and New Zealand.

In New Zealand national screening, each newborn sample is screened for 23 different conditions, and of 64,000 babies born each year, 50 will go on to be identified as having a metabolic disorder (Ministry of Health 2017). In Australia, newborn screening is undertaken by individual states and territories, with the test detecting an average of 1% of newborns as needing urgent assessment (testing) and care for one or more of the 24–30 conditions being screened.

Parents should be advised that once the newborn blood sample is received at the testing centre, it will be retained for a period of time, and in some cases, indefinitely. The reasons for this vary between jurisdictions; however, most assure parents that further testing (including DNA testing) can only be undertaken with the consent of the child's parents or the child themselves if they are old enough. In New Zealand parents either consent for the card to be returned to them or for it to be stored indefinitely; parents can request the card to be returned at any time. In some jurisdictions, parents can apply to have the card destroyed after a shorter period of time than they

SKILL 9.1 Performing a maternal screening test

- The procedure should be discussed with the woman: the conversation should include the reasons for testing as well as any harms and benefits associated with the test and any associated treatments; it should also be supported by relevant written, audio or video material (Department of Health 2018).
- Offer the woman the opportunity to ask questions and discuss any concerns she may have.
- Reassure the woman that the results of the test will remain confidential.
- Contemporaneously document the discussion in the woman's pregnancy care record, along with the woman's decision.
- Proceed to perform the test if the woman consents to it.
- Advise the woman of the process for follow-up: specifically, inform her when and how the results will be available to her, and what will happen if the test result is positive.

Box 9.1 Conditions screened for in the Newborn Screening Test: Australia and New Zealand

- Aminoacidopathies including: phenylketonuria, maple syrup urine disease, homocystinuria (tandem mass spectrometry).
- Organic acidaemias including: methylmalonic aciduria, propionic acidaemia, isovaleric acidaemia, glutaric aciduria type I (tandem mass spectrometry).
- Fatty acid oxidation defects including: carnitine transporter defect; carnitine translocase deficiency; carnitine palmitoyl transferase deficiencies; short-, medium- and very long-chain and long-chain 3-hydroxy acyl-CoA dehydrogenase deficiencies; glutaric aciduria type I (tandem mass spectrometry).
- Congenital hypothyroidism: thyroid-stimulating hormone (TSH) (immunoassay).
- Cystic fibrosis: trypsin(ogen) (immunoassay), mutation genotyping (molecular genetics: polymerase chain reaction [PCR]-based identification).
- Galactosaemia: galactose-1-phosphate, galactose (tandem mass spectrometry). (Not performed in the state of Victoria, Australia.)
- Other rare inborn errors of metabolism: may vary from state to state.

Source: Royal College of Pathologists of Australasia: RCPA manual: neonatal screen, 2020. Online 7 September 2020. Available: https://www.rcpa.edu.au/Manuals/RCPA-Manual/Pathology-Tests/N/Neonatal-screen.

would normally be kept for if they wish. The reader is advised to investigate the sample retention and destruction policy that relates to their own practice context.

Chapter 14 includes the skill for obtaining a newborn capillary sample, and information about the related considerations.

Role and responsibilities of the midwife

These are summarised as:

- knowledge and application of current evidence-based practice
- undertaking all procedures correctly
- appropriate discussion with the woman about the rationale for and implications of screening for herself and for her newborn(s)
- support of the woman, regardless of her decision
- accurate contemporaneous record keeping
- consultation, referral and advice when screening test results are positive.

SUMMARY

- Maternal antenatal screening is recommended for all pregnant women in Australia and New Zealand for the purpose of detecting conditions that may affect her pregnancy and/or the health of her fetus(es).
- Routine health screening is also offered for all Australian and New Zealander newborns.
- A key requirement in relation to screening in Australia and New Zealand is that of informed consent.
- Women who do not consent to screening must be invited to discuss their concerns, but not coerced into reconsidering their decision.
- The midwife has a responsibility to document the discussion with the woman about screening and follow-up, her consent or otherwise and the testing itself.
- For women whose screening test result is positive, the midwife should make a referral to the relevant health professional or service and assist the woman to access appropriate support.

Self-assessment exercises

The answers to the following questions may be found in the text.

1. List the screening tests recommended for pregnant women and their timing in Australia and New Zealand.
2. Discuss the pre-testing and post-testing principles underlying maternal antenatal screening.
3. Describe how to conduct an antenatal screening test.
4. List the conditions screened for in newborn bloodspot screening in Australia and New Zealand.
5. Summarise the role and responsibilities of the midwife in relation to screening.

Resources

Newborn Screening Test Information For New Zealand And Australia

Australian Government Department of Health Newborn Bloodspot Screening program information: www.health.gov.au/health-topics/pregnancy-birth-and-baby/newborn-bloodspot-screening.

Northern Territory Government website for expectant parents: nt.gov.au/wellbeing/pregnancy-birthing-and-child-health/support-new-parents.

New Zealand: Newborn metabolic screening program information: https://www.health.govt.nz/your-health/pregnancy-and-kids/first-year/first-6-weeks/health-checks-first-6-weeks/newborn-screening-tests/newborn-metabolic-screening.

Northern Territory Newborn Screening Program information: see New South Wales and Australian Capital Territory Newborn Screening Program information above.

Queensland Newborn screening test information (example from one health service): brochures.mater.org.au/brochures/mater-mothers-hospital/newborn-screening-test.

South Australia Newborn screening test information: http://www.wch.sa.gov.au/services/az/divisions/labs/geneticmed/pdfs/leaflet_01.pdf.

Victorian Clinical Genetics Services Newborn screening test information: https://www.vcgs.org.au/tests/newborn-bloodspot-screening.

Western Australia Newborn bloodspot screening information: https://pch.health.wa.gov.au/Our-services/Newborn-bloodspot-screening.

Department of Health Tasmania Newborn screening information, Screening Tests for your Baby: https://www.dhhs.tas.gov.au/pregnancy/your_baby_is_born.

References

Ahmed S, Bryant LD, Cole P: Midwives' perceptions of their role as facilitators of informed choice in antenatal screening, Midwifery 29:745–750, 2013.

Arneth B, Hintz M: Error analysis in newborn screening: can quotients support the absolute values? Analytical and Bioanalytical Chemistry 409:2247–2253, 2017.

Department of Health: Clinical practice guidelines: pregnancy care. Canberra: Australian Government, Department of Health, 2018 (updated 2019). Online 21 January 2021. Available: www.health.gov.au/resources/publications/pregnancy-care-guidelines.

Etchegary, H., Nicholls, S., Tessier, L. et al: Consent for newborn screening: parents' and health-care professionals' experiences of consent in practice. European Journal of Human Genetics 24, 1530–1534, 2016.

Ministry of Health: Pregnancy and newborn screening, 2017. Online 7 September 2020. Available: https://www.health.govt.nz/your-health/pregnancy-and-kids/first-year/first-6-weeks/health-checks-first-6-weeks/newborn-screening-tests/newborn-metabolic-screening.

Nykänen M, Vehviläinen-Julkunen K, Klemetti R: The expectations of antenatal screening and experiences of the first trimester screening scan, Midwifery 47: 15–21, 2017.

Potter BK, Etchegary H, Nicholls SG, et al: Education and parental involvement in decision making about newborn screening: understanding goals to clarify content, Journal of Genetic Counseling 24:400–408, 2015.

Royal Australian and New Zealand College of Obstetricians and Gynaecologists (RANZCOG): Routine antenatal assessment in the absence of pregnancy complications, 2019. Online 21 January 2021. Available: https://ranzcog.edu.au/RANZCOG_SITE/media/RANZCOG-MEDIA/Women%27s%20Health/Statement%20and%20guidelines/Clinical-Obstetrics/Routine-antenatal-assessment-in-the-absence-of-pregnancy-complications-(C-Obs-3b)_2.pdf?ext=.pdf.

Royal College of Pathologists of Australasia (RCPA): RCPA manual: antenatal screening, 2020. Online 21 January 2021. Available: www.rcpa.edu.au/Manuals/RCPA-Manual/Clinical-Problems/A/Antenatal-screening.

Therrell BL, Padilla CD, Loeber JG, et al: Current status of newborn screening, Seminars in Perinatology 39(3): 171–187, 2015.

Ulph F, Lavender T, Bennett R: Consent for newborn screening and storage of blood samples. British Journal of Midwifery November 2017, 25(11):730–732, 2017. Available: www.sciencedirect.com/science/article/pii/S0033350619302677.

CHAPTER 10
VENEPUNCTURE

Learning outcomes

Having read this chapter, the reader should be able to:

- discuss the indications for venepuncture
- describe how venepuncture is undertaken safely and positively using an aseptic non-touch technique
- discuss the rationale for the choice of vein and equipment used
- highlight the possible complications and how they can be avoided
- summarise the role and responsibilities of the midwife.

Venepuncture is the puncturing of a vein with a needle, usually to obtain specimens of blood for laboratory analysis, but it may also include the administration of drugs intravenously in an emergency. The ability of a midwife to undertake venepuncture facilitates individualised and holistic care for the woman from the same practitioner.

This chapter considers the indications for venepuncture, equipment preparation and skill technique.

INDICATIONS

- Antenatal screening (blood group and antibodies; full blood count; haemoglobin; Hb1Ac, HIV, hepatitis B, Rubella non-immunity, syphilis and hepatitis C).
- Assessment of full blood count and presence of Rh antibodies during pregnancy. Further repeats if Rh-negative blood group, with Kleihauer test following birth.
- Assessment of anaemia.
- Other tests may be taken if there is an existing disease (e.g. thyroid function tests, blood glucose monitoring or tolerance testing, anti-epileptic drug levels) or if other conditions are suspected (e.g. sickle cell anaemia, pre-eclampsia, thalassaemia, hepatitis B, hyperemesis gravidarum).
- Antenatal screening tests for fetal normality (e.g. alpha-fetoprotein).
- Cross-matching prior to blood transfusion or 'group and hold' prior to operative birth.

This is not an exhaustive list, but it indicates how frequently women are asked to give blood specimens. Fear of needles or of fainting can occur; midwives should be sensitive to both the physical and psychological aspects of the skill. Care and time should be taken to gain informed consent. Measures such as slow deep breaths can be used to improve the experience if the woman is very anxious. Other interventions include the **Valsalva manoeuvre** (deep inhalation and holding breath during the venepuncture), looking away and coughing gently twice without moving arms (venepuncture performed during second cough) and providing a signal to indicate the procedure is about to occur (Boerner et al 2015). An aseptic non-touch technique (ANTT) should be used (Chapter 2) to help prevent serious and debilitating bloodstream infections (Hudson Garrett 2016). Assess the need for cannulation prior to venepuncture. If a cannula is required blood can be taken during cannulation and this would avoid a woman being exposed to two procedures unnecessarily.

SUITABLE SITES

Blood is always taken from a vein, never an artery. Arterial blood is only ever sought by medical staff in specific circumstances (e.g. for blood gas analysis). The physiological additional blood volume during pregnancy and the general body warmth of the pregnant woman both create vasodilation, making venepuncture easier than it is for many other groups of people. The veins of healthy women are generally in good condition.

The midwife should be familiar with the anatomy of the arm below the elbow. For venepuncture, the most commonly used veins are those in the antecubital fossa, the median antecubital, cephalic and basilic veins (Fig 10.1). If the veins in the antecubital fossa cannot

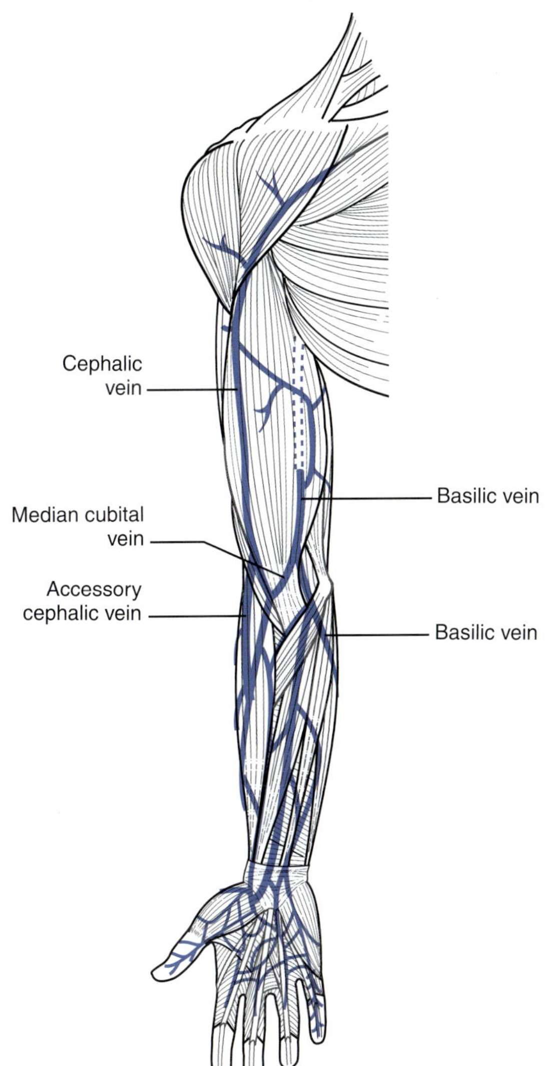

FIGURE 10.1 **Suitable veins for venepuncture.**
Source: Adapted with kind permission from Williams PL, editor: Gray's anatomy, 38th ed., Churchill Livingstone, Edinburgh, 1995.

be used, the next choice is the superficial veins on the dorsal aspect of the hand. The skin should be free from infection, inflammation and bruising.

CHOOSING A VEIN

Clearly visible veins are often nearer to the skin surface but are often smaller and harder to obtain blood samples from. Both visual inspection and palpation should be used when choosing a vein. On palpation a vein can be assessed for its size, mobility and suitability. A vein that has been repeatedly used for venous access may be thrombosed and will not feel 'bouncy' and full. The veins in the antecubital fossa are often supported by subcutaneous tissue and less likely to move or 'roll' when venepuncture is attempted.

USING A TOURNIQUET

The **tourniquet** should only obstruct venous return which allows the veins to distend and become more visible; the arterial pulse should remain palpable (Fig 10.2). The tourniquet should not be used for prolonged periods because haemoconcentration can occur after 1 minute (Higgins 2013). The longer it is applied, the more haemoconcentration occurs (Weinstein 2015). If a vein is difficult to locate, try the alternate arm or release the tourniquet for 2 minutes before reapplying it to allow the blood to return to its basal state. Blood should not be collected if a tourniquet has been in place more than 1 minute. The tourniquet should be released while the equipment is prepared and then reapplied when the midwife is ready to collect the blood. The tourniquet should be removed promptly *after* the blood has been collected (Weinstein 2015). This can be when the blood starts to flow into the collection tubes, or as soon as blood collection is completed. Haematomas may be caused if the tourniquet is not released at the appropriate time, if the arm is bent or if the needle is advanced too far and punctures the posterior wall of the vein (Scales 2008).

Clenching and unclenching the fist can cause **haemoconcentration** and repetitive muscle contraction can elevate potassium levels; therefore, this practice should be discouraged. The technique of 'tapping' the veins to increase their prominence should also be avoided because it can cause bruising and pain (Brooks 2017). Often women will know from past experience which are their 'good' veins.

SITES TO AVOID

It is important to understand the anatomy of the arm to avoid injury to the brachial artery and median nerve, which can result in pain and temporary or permanent damage. Palpating is important for making the decision

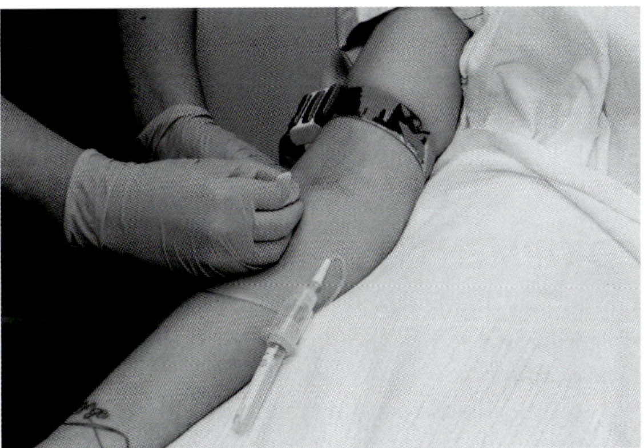

FIGURE 10.2 **Application of torniquet.**

to attempt venepuncture (Shaw 2017) and helps the midwife avoid the following structures.

- valves, which are seen as 'nodules' within the vein and make specimen collection difficult and painful if venepuncture is attempted near the valve
- arteries, which have a palpable pulse—if an artery is accidently accessed, red oxygenated blood is seen; the needle should be removed and pressure applied for at least 5 minutes with the arm in a straight position; document the error (Scales 2008)
- nerves, which often run close to arteries.

The inner aspect of the wrist should never be used for venepuncture as the radial, ulnar and median nerves are located in this area. Avoid recent puncture sites, existing bruising, areas of skin infection, arteriovenous fistula, oedema, incapacitated limbs or those with limited lymphatic drainage (e.g. mastectomy). If it is impossible to avoid an arm with an intravenous line in situ because no other options are available, the intravenous infusion should be stopped for a minimum of 5 minutes and then the venepuncture undertaken.

PAIN RELIEF

Using a calm and confident manner will help the woman feel comfortable. Ensure she is prepared and aware that discomfort or pain will usually be felt when the needle is inserted. Local anaesthetic creams may also be prescribed. If they are used, it is necessary to wait for the required time in order to obtain the full effect; this is 1–2 hours depending on which one is used.

ASEPSIS AND SKIN PREPARATION

Venepuncture can introduce microorganisms either locally into the tissues at the site or into the systemic circulation. Using an ANTT approach, the skin is the key site and should be cleansed using the locally approved skin cleanser (often a 70% alcohol-based wipe) for 30 seconds using the up-and-down, side-to-side approach (friction) and then left to air dry (for at least 30 seconds). The vein is palpated before cleaning and not touched after cleaning. Non-sterile gloves are worn and all equipment is sterile. The key parts are the needle, vacuum system and blood bottles. A disposable tourniquet is used (Brooks 2017) wherever possible. A reusable tourniquet should be cleaned after each use (Brooks 2017). The locally agreed policy should be consulted for these issues.

EQUIPMENT

Equipment should be:

- sterile, and asepsis should be maintained during the procedure
- ideally a **closed vacuum system** that also protects the midwife from contact with blood or plasma
- chosen according to the vein and the practitioner's competence.

Closed systems have a vacuum seal. This means when the needle pierces the specimen collection tube it fills with blood without any leakage and protects the midwife from contact with body fluids. Figure 10.3 shows a midwife collecting venous blood using a closed system. A 21-gauge needle should be used; this has an appropriate diameter for the viscosity of blood. Other equipment may be chosen (e.g. winged devices). The procedure is adapted according to the equipment used; midwives are advised to follow their local protocols.

Because syringes and needles increase the risk of contamination and needlestick injuries, a vacuum system should be used whenever possible. If a needle and syringe are used, they must be sterile. A needle defence system should be used and the sharps deposited safely into a sharps bin at the point of care as soon as the procedure is completed. Venepuncture using a needle and syringe requires the midwife to hold the syringe so that when the syringe plunger is drawn back; the needle is not withdrawn but remains in the vein. The specimen collection tubes should be filled in the correct order.

Poor collection techniques and mishandling of specimens increase the risk of haemolysis (breakdown of red blood cells). Haemolysis results in leakage of the components of the red cell which affects the accuracy of testing, particularly for electrolytes, possibly leading to hyperkalaemia or hypokalaemia not being detected (Makhumula-Nkhoma et al 2014).

Haemolysis can be avoided by ensuring syringes and tubes are completely dry; use gentle pressure if using a syringe as excessive pressure can collapse the vein and cause air bubbles to contaminate the specimen; avoid shaking clotted blood samples and do not use force when transferring blood to a tube (Weinstein 2015).

Specimen tubes are coded by colour and used for specific tests (Table 10.1). If in doubt of the correct specimen tube to use, contact pathology. Specimen forms must be completed correctly and the specimen transported to pathology safety and promptly.

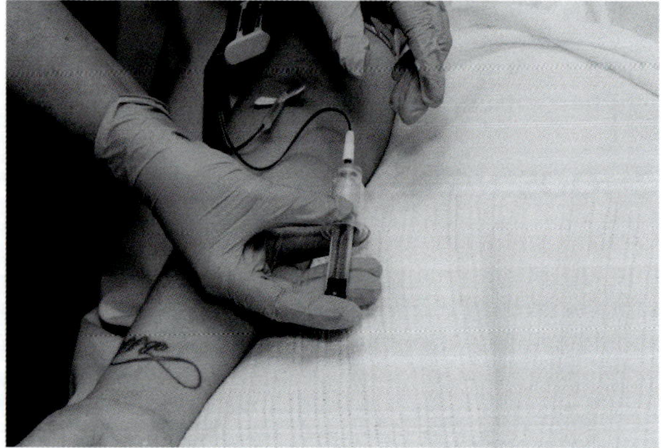

FIGURE 10.3 **Midwife collecting venous blood using a closed system.**

TABLE 10.1 BLOOD COLLECTION TUBES

Specimen tube colour	Type	Use
	EDTA (ethylenediaminetetraacetic acid) Prevents blood clotting by binding calcium and preserves structure of blood Lavender top (3–10 mL)	**Haematology** Full blood count (FBC), haemoglobin, white cell count (WCC), differential (diff), platelet count, erythrocyte sedimentation rate (ESR), red cell folate Thalassaemia screen, malaria screen Zinc proto porphyrin (ZPP) **Biochemistry** HbA1c **Molecular genetics** Genetic studies
	EDTA Pink top (4–6 mL)	**Blood bank** Cross-match (+EDTA lavender top) Group and hold (+EDTA lavender top) Group and antibody screen Direct Coombs test
	Lithium heparin gel PSTII Green top (4.5 mL)	**Biochemistry** Urea, electrolytes, creatinine, Liver function tests (LFTs), lipids, creatine kinase (CK), Troponin, glucose, iron studies, thyroid function tests (TFTs), beta hCG, C-reactive protein (CRP), calcium, magnesium phosphate, lipase, ammonia, vitamin B_{12}, folate, uric acid, PTH, amino acids, sodium valproate, digoxin, vancomycin, theophylline.
	Sodium heparin Prevents blood clots from forming by inhibiting the formation of thrombin from prothrombin Dark green top (4–6 mL)	**Biochemistry** tests requiring plasma Metabolic studies — amino acids etc. T-cell and B-cell studies Lymphocyte studies
	Sodium citrate Prevents clotting by precipitating calcium Blue top (2.7 mL)	**Coagulation tests** Prothrombin time (PT), thrombophilia tests, activated partial thromboplastin time (APTT), INR, coagulation studies (2 citrate tubes + 4 mL EDTA tube), D-dimer, fibrinogen

Continued

TABLE 10.1 BLOOD COLLECTION TUBES—cont'd

Specimen tube colour	Type	Use
	Fluoride oxalate Prevents continued metabolism of glucose by blood cells preserving blood glucose concentration (used with oxalate in tubes specifically for blood glucose measurement).	**Biochemistry** Grey top (4 mL) Lactate studies Glucose
	Serum separator tube (SST) Gold top (8.5 mL)	**Routine biochemistry** LFTs, urea, electrolytes, cholesterol, triglycerides (lipids), CK, troponin, proteins, CRP, TFTs, follicle-stimulating hormone (FSH), luteinising hormone (LH) Pregnancy test (beta-hCG), Autoantibodies Microbial, parasitic and viral serology Iron studies, vitamin B_{12}, therapeutic drug monitoring

Order of draw

1. Sterile samples such as blood cultures (aerobic then anaerobic)
2. Coagulation (blue top) sodium citrate
3. Serum separator tube (SST) (gold top)
4. Biochemistry (dark green top) sodium heparin tubes
5. Ethylenediaminetetraacetic acid (EDTA) (lavender), haematology and (pink) cross-match, group and hold, antibody screen, blood group
6. Fluoride oxalate (grey), glucose, blood alcohol

Gently invert the tube after collection.

Portable sharps boxes should be used at the point of care; a used needle should *never* be re-sheathed. Needle defence systems are increasingly available and should be used wherever possible. There is a variety of designs, but in principle the shield is moved manually or activated automatically as soon as the needle is withdrawn so the needle is covered and cannot pierce the skin again.

POSSIBLE COMPLICATIONS

- Pain increased by poor choice of site, poor technique (puncturing arteries, valves or nerves), skin cleanser that has not been left to dry and too large a needle
- Syncope; if a woman has a history of fainting, ask her to lie down
- Oedema
- Excessive bleeding
- Nerve damage
- Infection
- Bruising or haematoma
- Accidental puncture of an artery

SKILL 10.1 Maternal venepuncture

Pre-collection

Check the pathology request, the woman's identification details and the tests required.

Explain the procedure and its purpose and obtain verbal consent. (If the woman does not understand English, an interpreter should be obtained.) Ensure she has no allergies to tape or latex.

Procedure

1. Perform hand hygiene and put on non-sterile gloves.
2. Clean a plastic receiver using the locally approved wipes. Leave it to dry, remove gloves and wash and dry hands.

SKILL 10.1 Maternal venepuncture—cont'd

3. Gather equipment:
   - Vacutainer® needle and holder
   - syringe of appropriate size (depending on volume of blood required)
   - transfer device (Fig 10.4)
   - blood collection needle or safety lock, scalp vein set size 21-gauge needle (often green)
   - appropriate specimen bottles
   - approved skin cleanser, usually 70% alcohol with chlorhexidine
   - non-sterile gloves
   - antiseptic hand rub
   - sterile gauze
   - disposable tourniquet
   - adhesive plaster (if not allergic)
   - biohazard bag for transferring specimen
   - specimen request form
   - portable sharps container.
4. Explain the procedure and gain informed consent; ensure the correct specimen is being taken from the correct woman by asking her to state her name and date of birth. Check the Medical record number and check all information against the request form.
5. Identify collection site: when the woman is comfortable, support her arm in an accessible position; good light is required.
6. Apply the tourniquet approximately 5–7 cm above the antecubital fossa.
7. Identify the chosen vein by palpation, retaining the site of entry in the 'mind's eye'. Release tourniquet.
8. Perform hand hygiene and put on non-sterile gloves.
9. Cleanse the skin (key site) thoroughly using an up-and-down, left-to-right approach (> 30 seconds); wait for it to dry (> 30 seconds).
10. Assemble the needle and appropriate parts of the vacuumed system using an ANTT approach (see Chapter 2) for all key parts; reapply the tourniquet and gently unsheathe the needle.
11. Using the non-dominant hand, apply slight tension to the skin below the point of entry (this will anchor the vein).
12. Insert the needle into the vein at a 15–30° angle with the bevel (slanted edge) uppermost; be decisive but not too firm.
13. Fill the blood bottles in order and according to the system used. Gently mix those that require it.
14. If blood does not appear, the needle may be 'nudged' a little further in or withdrawn a small amount (if no blood is seen, or the woman is in acute pain, remove the needle, collect new equipment and try another site).
15. Release the tourniquet once a good flow of blood is evident or halfway through the last collection sample, withdraw the needle fully and immediately apply pressure (Brooks 2017) to the puncture site using the gauze for the next minute (the woman should be encouraged to do this, if able). Keep the woman's arm horizontal. Activate the safety device (if applicable) and place the used sharps straight into the sharps bin.
16. Apply plaster if required (check there is no allergy), once the bleeding has stopped.
17. Remove gloves and perform hand hygiene.
18. Label the specimen bottles and request form while the woman is present; send the specimen to the laboratory. Ensure the results are acted upon.
19. Dispose of other equipment correctly; clean the receiver as before.
20. Document and act accordingly.

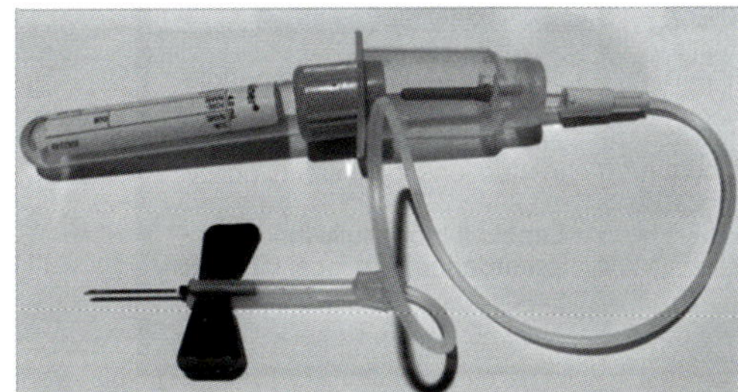

FIGURE 10.4 **Transfer device with 21-gauge butterfly needle.**

Figure 10.5 indicates the sequence for collection of venous blood using a closed system.

Brooks (2017) includes a useful practice checklist that details the significant steps in the venepuncture process.

If the midwife is unable to obtain the specimen after trying once or twice, the woman should be referred to a more experienced practitioner. Repeated attempts are inappropriate both for the woman (e.g. pain, bruising) and because usable veins should be preserved in case they are required for urgent intravenous access.

CHAPTER 11 CANNULATION

Learning outcomes

Having read this chapter, the reader should be able to:

- describe the indications for cannulation
- describe how the site is selected and the equipment chosen
- describe safe cannulation technique
- describe the correct removal of an intravenous cannula
- summarise the role and responsibilities of the midwife.

VASCULAR ACCESS

Vascular access devices are used when consistent or repeated **intravascular access** is needed for administration of medications and intravascular fluids (Marsh et al 2017). The most commonly used vascular access device is the **peripherally inserted intravenous cannula (PIVC)**. Other types of vascular access devices, such as central venous catheters (CVCs) and peripherally inserted central catheters (PICC lines), are not generally inserted by midwives. Midwives are often required to insert and care for PIVCs and, in the context of complex midwifery care, central venous access devices, such as PICC lines.

The skill of PIVC insertion and removal requires training, supervised practice and ongoing skill maintenance. The Australian Vascular Access Society (AVAS), Intravenous Nursing New Zealand (IVNNZ Inc.) and the Infusion Nurses Society (INS) provide expert information regarding vascular access (see Resources at end of chapter). Local protocols generally require cannula insertion to be undertaken by qualified staff with demonstrated competence. PIVCs are common in the clinical setting and carry a risk of localised and systemic infection (Barton et al 2017). The midwife's role and responsibility for the insertion, removal and ongoing care of PIVCs and care of **central venous access devices (CVADs)** are considered in this chapter.

CONSIDERATIONS FOR THE CHILDBEARING WOMAN

The additional blood volume in pregnancy and higher body temperature usually mean the veins are more prominent and easier to access. PIVCs should only be inserted when clinically indicated and should be removed as soon as they are no longer necessary. Complications such as poor choice of site, unsuccessful attempts and infection or occlusion increase patient discomfort, morbidity and length of hospital stay, and potentially have a financial consequence. Careful assessment should be undertaken prior to and during insertion of a PIVC to reduce the risks of complications.

INDICATIONS

There are a number of potential occasions when a PIVC may be required:

- fluid replacement or drug administration in an emergency
- administration of whole blood or blood products
- iron transfusion
- drugs requiring intravenous administration
- in preparation for a potential complication or operative birth; for example, caesarean section, multiple or breech labour or antenatal per vaginam bleed
- administration of patient-controlled analgesia
- intravenous fluid administration; for example, when nil by mouth, with epidural analgesia, postoperatively or care of a woman with hyperemesis gravidarum.

ASSESSMENT PRIOR TO PIVC INSERTION

Prior to PIVC insertion, the following should be considered:

- informed consent has been given

- any history of prior experience of PIVC insertion or similar vascular access device has been discussed; a woman may indicate she has a needle phobia or is distressed by the sight of blood
- known allergies
- current health status
- assessment of factors that may make PIVC insertion difficult or uncomfortable
- the chosen site (see below)
- the nature and duration of the medication to be administered (related to osmolality or pH) (McCallum & Higgins 2012); according to Taliaferro (pers. comm. 31 Oct 2017), this can determine which size cannula is used and may also determine the need for a different vascular access device.

Choice of site

When choosing a site for PIVC insertion, consider the following.

- Avoid:
  - the dominant arm
  - areas that are painful, phlebotic, bruised, tortuous, thrombosed, inflamed or with existing skin infection; for example, eczema, cellulitis
  - areas with compromised circulation or sensation, oedema or fracture
  - areas of flexion, such as joints, valves in the vein (seen as bulges), bony prominences, ligaments, muscle, nerves or tendons
  - areas below a previous cannulation site, as the vein may be damaged
  - a limb with an arteriovenous fistulae or shunt
  - a limb with a PICC of implanted venous access device, such as a port-a-cath
  - arteries (some are in an unexpected position).
- Select:
  - a vein (identified by its lack of pulse and the ability to empty and fill by occluding and releasing it digitally)
  - a healthy vein in good condition (feels soft and bouncy) (Cooper & Gosnell 2018) and can be palpated in the lower half of the arm; for example, dorsal venous network (back of the hand) and cephalic and basilic veins of the forearm.

Veins for cannulation can be more difficult to locate when oedema, obesity, skin pigmentation or tattoos are present (Shaw 2016). Vein location aids are becoming available and include vein imagers, ultrasound and tourniquets that cause negative pressure and increase vein visibility (Shaw 2016).

PREPARATION

Venous access is improved if the practitioner and woman are relaxed and if certain physical measures are undertaken. A tourniquet (ideally disposable) should be placed 7–8 cm above the chosen site, heat may be applied (heat pack or warm water) and gravity or gentle stroking of the vein may increase its prominence (Brooks 2017). Topical analgesia can be prescribed in some situations, particularly if the woman requests it or if a large-bore cannula is being inserted. It may take 30–60 minutes to take effect. A small amount of local anaesthetic, such as lignocaine (lidocaine), may be injected **intradermally** (see Chapter 22) at the proposed puncture site. This needs only 3–5 minutes to take effect.

ASEPSIS AND USE OF STANDARD PRECAUTIONS

Infection control measures are very important for the insertion and ongoing care of PIVCs. The aseptic non-touch technique (ANTT), in conjunction with appropriate hand hygiene practices, are recommended for cannulation (Yagnik et al 2017). A non-touch technique is used for all key parts and key sites and a general aseptic field is used with microcritical aseptic fields (ANTT 2017) (see Chapter 2). All equipment should be sterile and for single use only; a sterile dressing pack preferably designed for PIVC insertion is used, as is appropriate personal protective equipment (PPE); for example, non-sterile gloves, face shield or goggles. All sharps should be disposed of at the point of use in a sharps container.

Some local protocols indicate that a PIVC should be routinely re-sited after 72–96 hours or if clinically indicated, such as when signs of phlebitis, pain or complications are suspected. Conversely, replacement of PIVCs has been recommended by some only when clinically indicated rather than every 72–96 hours (Bolton 2015, Loveday et al 2014). A 2013 Cochrane Review did not find evidence supporting routine changing of cannulae every 72–96 hours (Webster et al 2013). A later study found that PIVC sites can remain healthy for more than 96 hours and clinical assessment is recommended for determining if an IV should be re-sited, rather than after a prescribed time limit (Helton et al 2016).

Skin cleansing of the key site should be undertaken using the locally agreed wipes/solution; ≥ 70% alcohol with 2% chlorhexidine is recommended (Gorski et al 2016). Friction is generated using the up-and-down, right-to-left approach, cleansing for at least 30 seconds. The skin should then air-dry for at least 30 seconds; the vein should not be re-palpated once the skin has been cleansed. If re-palpation is necessary, sterile gloves should be worn.

CHOICE OF EQUIPMENT

Peripheral cannulae should protect users from a sharps injury and blood spills, be easy to insert and secure (Barton et al 2017). In Australia and New Zealand, IV cannulae are colour-coded according to size (gauge), which determines the flow rate per minute. The lengths of cannulae also vary, with greater lengths required for deep veins (Fig 11.1).

The cannula chosen should suit the site and the fluid to be infused. The smallest appropriate gauge should be chosen as this improves patient comfort (Brooks 2016). A large cannula in a small vein or near a joint is more likely to irritate the vessel wall, increasing the risk of mechanical phlebitis. A larger bore cannula—16 g (grey) or 14 g (orange)—is often chosen for the childbearing woman in an emergency where high flow rates of IV fluid may be required (Table 11.1).

Cannulae may vary slightly according to the manufacturer, but generally consist of a polyurethane piece of tubing with a hub, in which there is a bevelled needle (stylet), also with a hub. Wings may be attached for ease of securing the cannula and there may or may not be a needleless injection port (Fig 11.2).

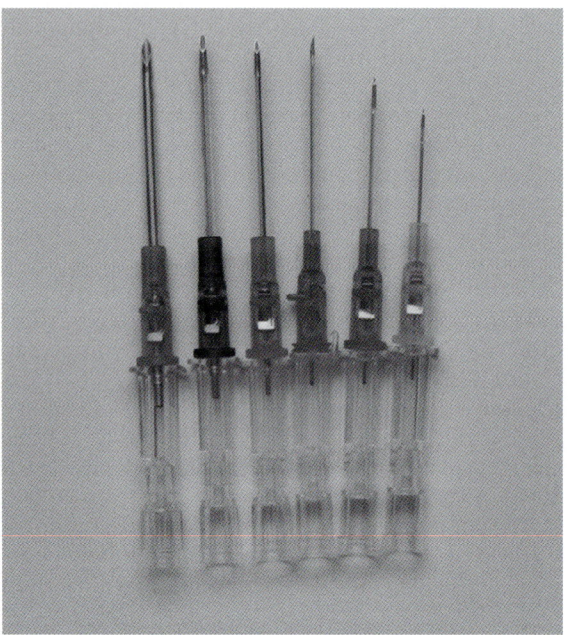

FIGURE 11.1 **IV cannulae without wings, ranging in size from small to large.**

IV cannula can form a closed system, sealed from the environment with a mechanism at the distal end of the cannula, so that blood does not leak out when the needle is withdrawn from the hub (Barton et al 2017). Safety features to prevent sharps injury include a passive safety shield and needle-free connections (Fig 11.3).

Once inserted, a closed system is maintained. Any extension tubing or needleless hubs are added and accessed using ANTT. An occlusive transparent dressing is used to help secure the cannula, allow for regular observation and permit bathing. A poorly dressed cannula increases the risks of leaking, extravasation, infection or accidental dislodgement (Marsh et al 2017). The dressing should be assessed every 6–8 hours and changed if no longer sealed or contaminated with blood or moisture (NSW Health 2013). Otherwise, the dressing may be left in place for 72 hours.

SITES FOR INTRAVENOUS CANNULATION

The most commonly used veins are the median cubital, cephalic or basilic veins of the lower arm; however, if these veins cannot be used, an alternative is the metacarpal veins on the back of the hand (Brooks 2016) (Fig 11.4).

Visual inspection and palpation of the veins will assist with identification of a vein suitable for cannulation. In cases where veins are unable to be palpated or visualised, insertion under bedside ultrasound or vein-illuminating devices is recommended (Taliaferro 2017).

DRESSING AND SECURING A PIVC

Approximately 30% of PIVCs fail prior to the completion of treatment; the risk of failure due to dislodgement, phlebitis, occlusion and infiltration is increased by a poorly secured cannula (Marsh et al 2017). Securing and stabilising a PIVC is important to reduce the risk of phlebitis and other complications (Higginson 2015). A Cochrane Systematic Review and meta-analysis found limited evidence indicating transparent dressings are more effective in prevented dislodgement, but did not find evidence indicating

TABLE 11.1 CANNULA GAUGE AND FLOW RATE

Gauge	Catheter length	Flow rate	Common use
24	14–19 mm	22–26 mL/min	Yellow: neonatal, paediatrics and elderly
22	25 mm	35 mL/min	Blue: IVABs routine IVT
20	25–45 mm	60–65 mL/min	Pink: most commonly used, IVABs, minimum size for CT scans
18	32–45 mm	105 mL/min	Green: higher flow rates, cardiac tests, ED, IVT
16	32 mm	215 mL/min	Grey: labouring women
14	32 mm	350 mL/min	Orange: emergency resuscitation

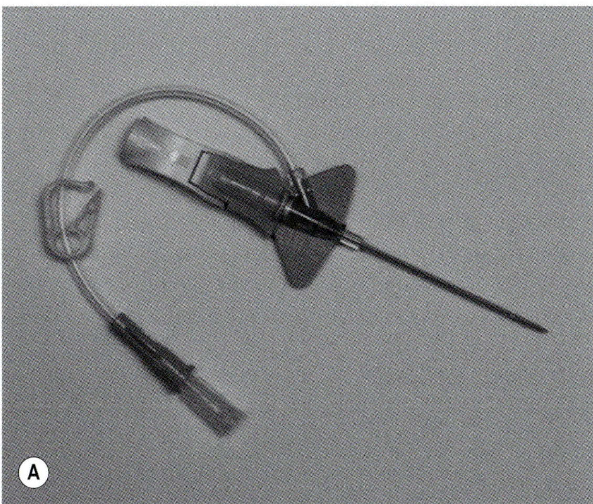

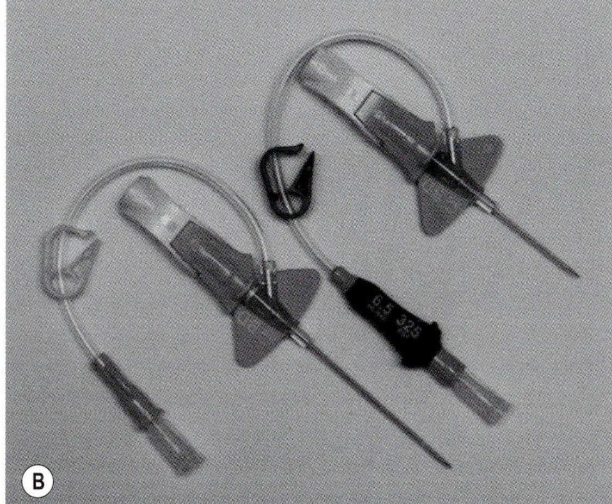

FIGURE 11.2 **IV cannula with wings.**

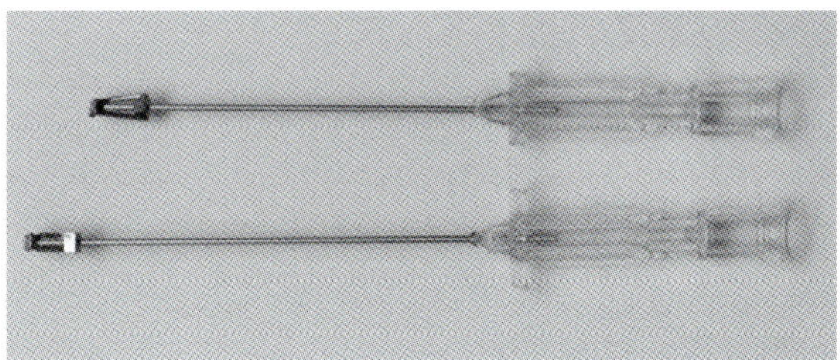

FIGURE 11.3 **IV Cannula with safety device activated.**

superiority of a transparent dressing compared to other dressings (Marsh et al 2017).

COMPLICATIONS

On insertion of the PIVC, care should be taken to stabilise the vein by applying gentle traction to the skin. The cannula can be mistakenly inserted alongside a vein, or puncture the back of the vein wall, causing pain and bruising if the angle of insertion is too great.

In the event of a failure to insert the cannula, the circumstances may dictate whether one further attempt is made or whether a more experienced colleague should be called. Many local protocols indicate inexperienced clinicians should not make more than two attempts at cannulation (NSW Health 2013). Repeated failed attempts are distressing for the woman and reduce the number of suitable veins available.

If an artery has been punctured, bright red pulsating oxygenated blood will be seen. The cannula should be removed and firm pressure applied to the puncture site for at least 5 minutes. The arm should be straight. There should be clear documentation of this incident in the notes.

The midwife needs to be alert to several possible complications from PIVC.

- **Phlebitis.** Inflammation of the vein may be caused by the presence of the cannula or its movement in the vein (mechanical phlebitis), by the drugs or fluids infused through it (chemical phlebitis) and by the presence of infection (infective phlebitis). The incidence of PIVC-related phlebitis for cannulae inserted in the emergency department (ED) is approximately 31% with a 20% incidence after 3 days and 50% after 5 days (Palese et al 2016).
- **Infiltration.** If the PIVC is dislodged, non-vesicant (non-blistering) fluids are inadvertently administered into the surrounding tissue rather than the vein. The PIVC should be removed and re-sited if still required.
- **Extravasation.** Vesicant (blistering) fluids are inadvertently administered into the surrounding tissue. Vesicant medications cause blistering and can lead to tissue necrosis, which is associated with significant morbidity (Bullock & Manias 2017). Examples include phenytoin, sodium bicarbonate, 50% dextrose, potassium and cefotaxime.

A PIVC can be assessed using scoring systems which use visual indicators. Australian research has found the inter-rater agreement of phlebitis assessment scales is poor; therefore, a particular validated phlebitis scoring system cannot be recommended (Marsh et al 2015). In the United Kingdom, the Standards for Infusion Therapy recommend use of the visual infusion phlebitis (VIP) scoring developed by Jackson in 1998 (Fig 11.5) (VIP Score 2018). Infiltration and extravasation can be avoided with optimum site choice, insertion technique and correct fixation of the cannula (Brooks 2014). The risk of phlebitis is reduced by having adequate staff with a high level of expertise (Palese et al 2016).

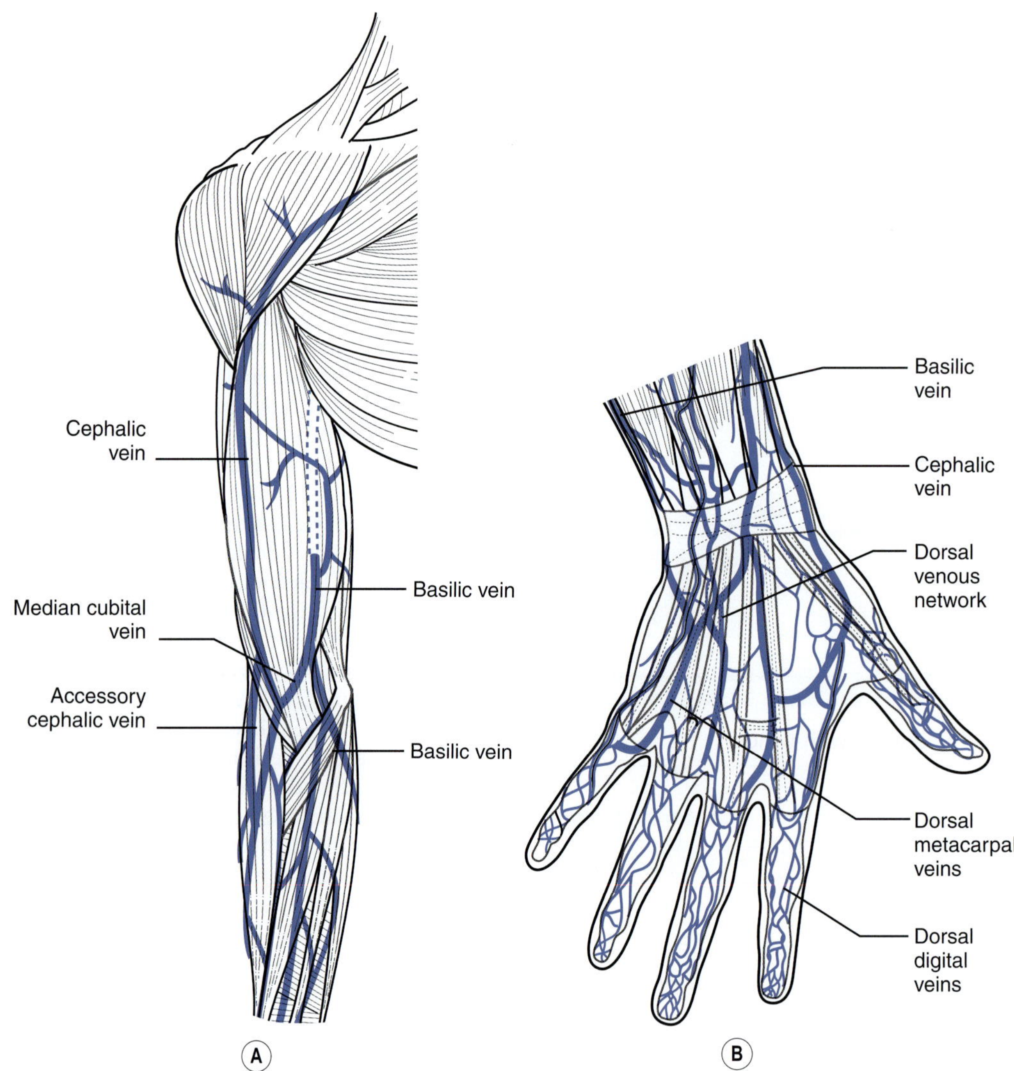

FIGURE 11.4 **Veins of the forearm and hand.**
Source: Adapted with kind permission from Williams PL, editor: Gray's anatomy, 38th ed., Churchill Livingstone, Edinburgh, 1995.

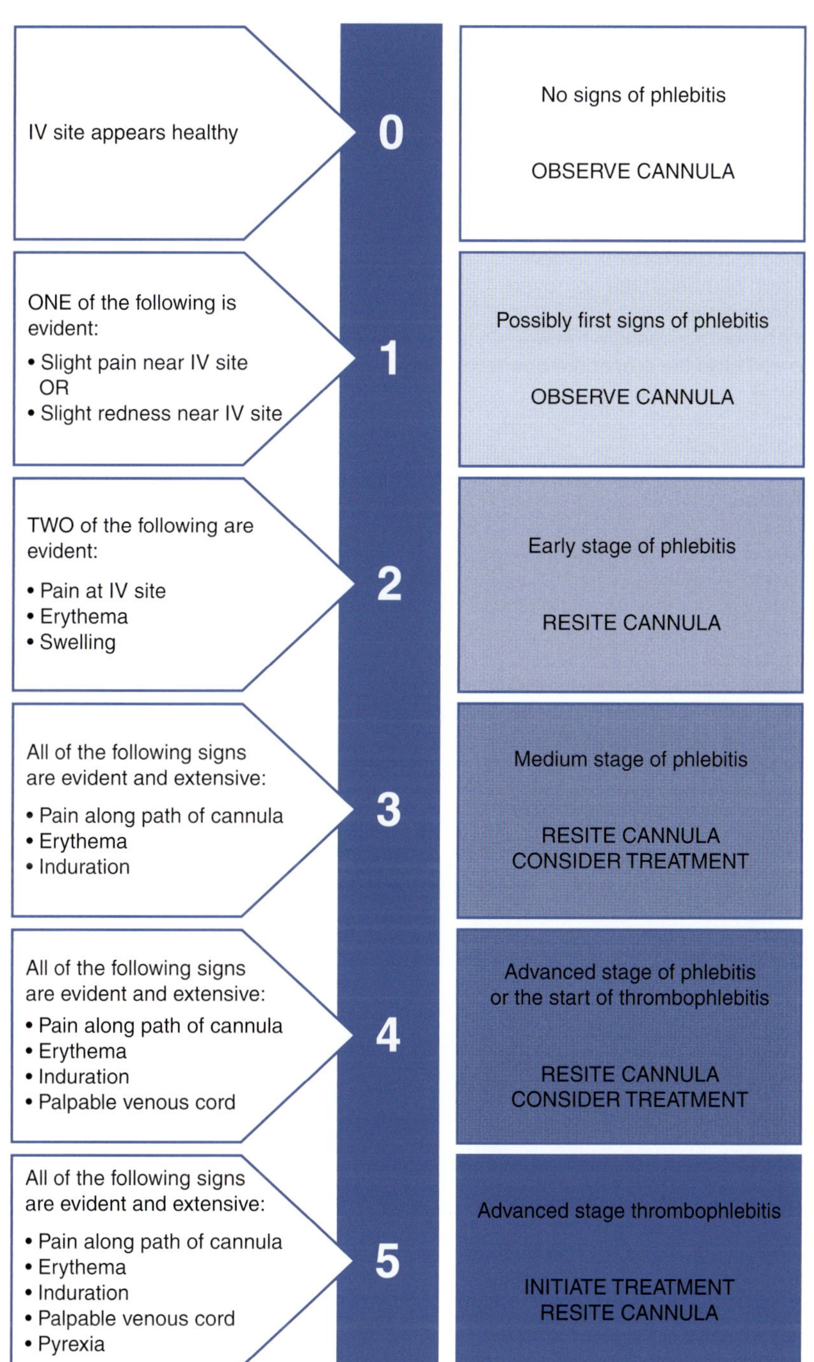

FIGURE 11.5 **Visual infusion phlebitis score.**
Source: © Andrew Jackson 1997. Reproduced with permission from Andrew Jackson, IV Nurse Consultant, The Rotherham NHS Foundation Trust UK.

SKILL 11.1 Intravenous cannulation

If topical analgesia is to be used, the vein would be selected and the cream applied and covered. The procedure would commence 30–60 minutes later (depending on which medication was applied). If using intradermal lignocaine, the prescribed amount is drawn up using ANTT as part of the preparation described below.

Preparation

1. Confirm the woman's identity by asking her to state her name and date of birth. Check her medical record number (three approved identifiers are necessary).
2. Gain informed consent and ensure the woman is aware that she can stop the procedure or ask for a rest (Shaw 2016).
3. Prepare the area; for example, good lighting, free from draughts, private.
4. Identify relevant history (e.g. anticoagulants, aspirin, needle phobia).
5. Perform hand hygiene.
6. Clean trolley or tray as per local protocol.
7. Collect equipment:
   - appropriately sized (for vein and fluid) sterile cannula and extension set
   - sterile dressing pack
   - semi-permeable occlusive dressing and hypoallergenic tape
   - approved cleansing solution/wipe (2% chlorhexidine gluconate in 70% isopropyl alcohol—if not available, chlorhexidine 0.5% in 70% alcohol; if allergic to chlorhexidine, topical povidone–iodine 10% in 70% alcohol can be used (ICCMU 2014)
   - portable sharps container
   - clean plastic tray
   - disposable tourniquet
   - two pairs of non-sterile gloves and alcohol-based hand rub
   - approved flushing solution (0.9% sodium chloride) in two preloaded 5 mL syringes
   - intradermal lignocaine with appropriate sterile needle and syringe, if using these
   - disposable sheet.

Procedure

8. Open the outer wrapper of the pack and 'drop' the dressings pack onto the tray (holding corners only).
9. Add the sterile cannula, extension set, dressing, tourniquet, skin wipe and equipment wipe (both in their packets).
10. Open the wrapper of the extension set, connect the syringe using ANTT, prime the extension set with the 0.9% sodium chloride and close clamp/s, then place it on the tray.
11. Take the trolley to the woman.
12. Perform hand hygiene.
13. Position the arm so it is supported with the disposable sheet and sterile towel (from the pack) beneath it. Assess skin and veins, avoiding areas with swelling eczema, bruising or inflammation, and identify a suitable vein.
14. Apply the tourniquet approximately 7–8 cm above the intended site so the veins can fill, but arterial flow is not obstructed.
15. Select the most likely vein by palpation (note the location), then release the tourniquet.
16. Perform hand hygiene using alcohol-based hand rub and apply gloves.
17. Cleanse the skin thoroughly with an alcohol and chlorhexidine solution/wipe for at least 30 seconds using an up-and-down, side-to-side action (crosshatching technique), creating friction. Allow it to air-dry for at least 30 seconds, then reapply the tourniquet.
18. Immobilise the vein by supporting the skin below the insertion point, with slight tension, using the non-dominant hand.
19. Insert the cannula at an angle of approximately 10–30°, bevel uppermost; as the vein is entered, a flashback of blood may be seen in the hub (this will vary according to the device used).
20. Reduce the angle of insertion almost to skin level, advance the cannula slowly a few millimetres further, pause and withdraw the needle halfway; a second flashback may be seen along the cannula.
21. Gradually advance the cannula into the vein, up to the hub, while simultaneously withdrawing the needle, remembering to remain at the same depth, following the direction of the vein. Release skin traction.
22. Release the tourniquet and withdraw the needle completely. Dispose of needle into sharps container.
23. Remove the cap off the extension set and secure it using ANTT into the cannula (usually a Luer lock).
24. Secure the cannula using the tape, usually vertically over the wings (this may vary according to the cannula type).
25. Wipe the end of the needleless port/extension set, use the four corners and the middle of the wipe, scrubbing approximately for 5 seconds each time; use another part of the wipe around the sides of the port for a further 5 seconds.
26. Open the extension line, insert the syringe and flush through using the prepared flush with a pulsation method, ending with positive pressure (see above).
27. Secure the cannula in place with a transparent dressing, ensuring that the puncture site can be visualised. Record the date and time, and attach a label to the dressing if this is the policy. Tape the extension set to the arm.

SKILL 11.1 Intravenous cannulation—cont'd

28. If required, blood specimens would be taken before connecting the extension/flushing the cannula or adding an infusion line.
29. Ensure the woman is aware of ongoing care of the cannula, asking her to report any adverse effects.
30. Dispose of equipment correctly, clean the tray, remove gloves and wash and dry hands.
31. Complete records and add a sticker to the chart (if appropriate).
32. Ensure that ongoing care of the cannula and/or infusion (see Chapter 23) is maintained (Fig 11.6).

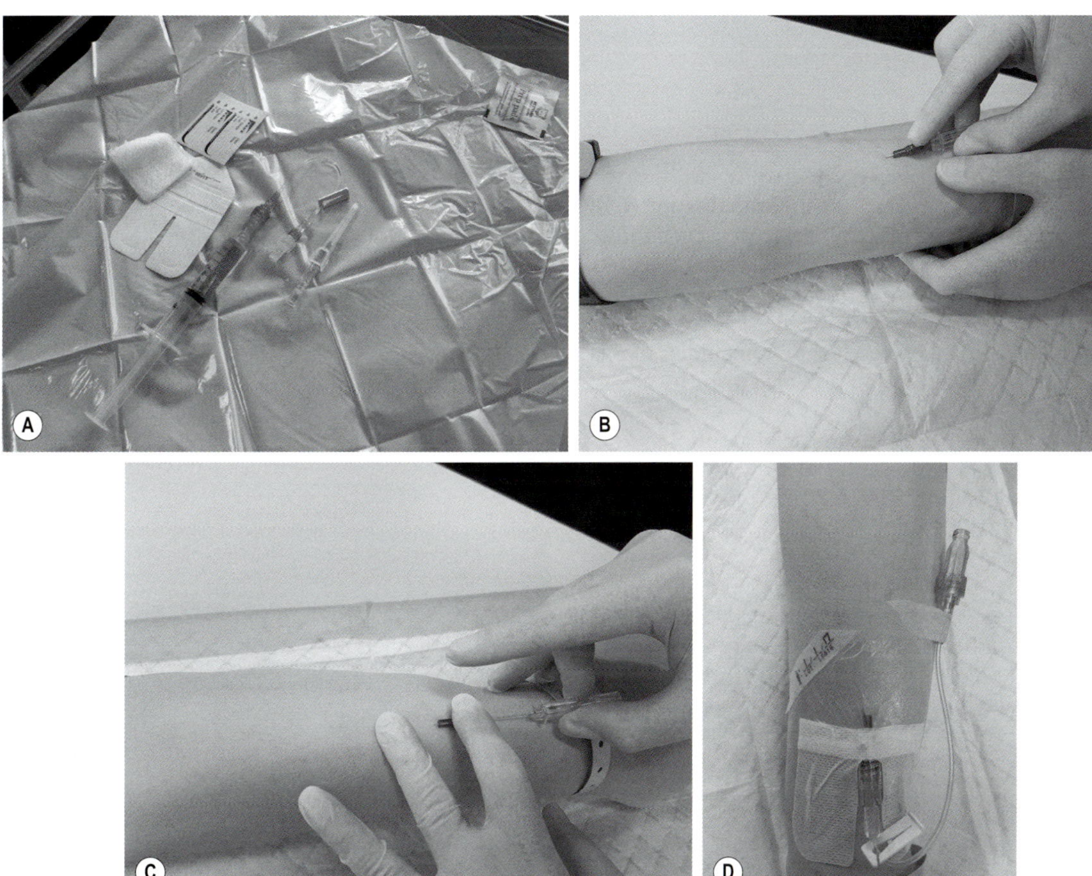

FIGURE 11.6 **Insertion of PIVC. A Setup. B, C Insertion. D Insertion complete.**

SKILL 11.2 Removal of a peripheral intravenous cannula

1. Confirm the woman's identity and gain informed consent.
2. Gather the following equipment:
    - non-sterile gloves
    - IV pressure pad or gauze
    - disposable sheet
    - portable sharps container
    - alcohol-based hand rub
3. Perform hand hygiene.
4. Position the arm so it is supported, with the disposable sheet beneath it.
5. Loosen the tape around the cannula.
6. Open the IV pressure pad/gauze, apply hand rub and then apply the gloves.
7. Begin to withdraw the cannula from the vein; prepare to place the IV pressure pad gauze

Continued

SKILL 11.2 Removal of a peripheral intravenous cannula—cont'd

immediately over the puncture site as the cannula is withdrawn.
8. Fully withdraw the cannula, then apply continuous pressure to the puncture site for 1–2 minutes.
9. Examine the cannula to confirm it is complete.
10. Dispose of the cannula correctly.
11. Once the bleeding has stopped, remove the gauze (if used) and cover the wound using a sterile adhesive dressing.
12. Ensure the woman is comfortable.
13. Dispose of remaining equipment correctly, remove gloves and perform hand hygiene.
14. Ask the woman to call if any signs of bleeding occur.
15. Complete documentation, clearly stating date and time of removal, appearance of site, whether the cannula was complete, nature of dressing applied and any further plan of care.

DOCUMENTATION

As part of the overall strategy to reduce healthcare-associated infections (HAIs), cannula care is subjected to standards of good practice principles, including documentation.

Local arrangements may include specific forms/stickers to be used alongside a detailed record of care written in the woman's notes. It should include:

- information and education provided prior to consent being granted
- details of site preparation and use of aseptic technique
- site, skin preparation, date and time of cannula insertion (NSW Health 2013)
- clinical indication
- cannula type, gauge, length and size (some local areas attach the manufacturer's printed label with the batch number to the woman's medical record)
- anything of note during the insertion procedure, including adherence to infection control protocols and the number of attempts made
- medications administered, including local anaesthetic and flushing agent
- type of dressing applied and the appearance of the insertion site afterwards
- proposed plan of care, particularly removal time
- name and signature of the midwife with date and time of documentation (Brooks 2017, Gorski et al 2016).

ONGOING CARE MONITORING

The PIVC insertion site should be observed and documented each shift (every 6–8 hours) and whenever the PIVC is accessed (Bolton 2015). The site is assessed for signs of infiltration, extravasation, inflammation, tenderness, pain, swelling, warmth and redness. If the dressing is detached, damp or soiled, it should be changed. The date and time of removal of the PIVC should be noted.

The cannula should be flushed before and after medication administration. If a continuous infusion is not in progress, the cannula should be flushed every 6–8 hours to ensure patency. The cannula is flushed with 5–10 mL 0.9% sodium chloride (normal saline) by a midwife or registered nurse who follows ANTT. Preloaded 5 and 10 mL normal saline flushes are available (Fig 11.7). The pulsation technique is used; this involves a repeated push/pause action which disturbs any adhering substances and lessens the infection risk (Goossens 2015).

Flushing the cannula serves a number of functions:

- confirms patency
- clears medications

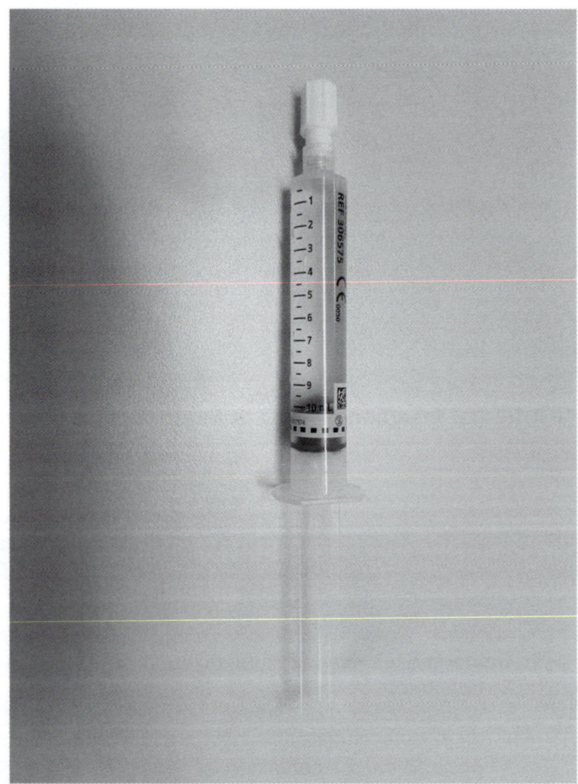

FIGURE 11.7 Preloaded normal saline flush.

- clears blood and adherents
- reduces the risk of occlusion (Goossens 2015).

If a normal saline flush is listed on the medication chart, it should be signed as for any other medication. Care of the PIVC, including visual inspection and administration of a flush, should be documented in the notes.

CARING FOR CENTRAL VENOUS ACCESS DEVICES

A Cochrane Systematic Review indicates the incidence of CVAD infections is reduced by medication-impregnated dressings (Ullman et al 2016).

Recommendations

- Prior to access, needleless connectors should be mechanically scrubbed using a 70% alcohol and chlorhexidine solution.
- Administration sets attached to an antibiotic-coated, multi-lumen CVAD should be changed at 7 days or when clinically indicated. Standard CVADs should be changed after 96 hours or when clinically indicated.
- Lumens should be cleaned with alcohol and chlorhexidine.
- IV lines attached to a CVC must be secured with no tension on catheter.
- Unused CVAD lumens/multi-flow adapters must be clamped to prevent air emboli, backflow of blood or other solutions.
- Transparent dressings should be changed at least every 7 days (earlier if not sealed, if inflamed or if blood or moisture has accumulated under the dressing).
- Only staff competent in the procedure should change CVC dressings and lines.
- The CVC insertion site should be checked every shift and any findings documented (ICCMU 2014).

Role and responsibilities of the midwife

These can be summarised as:

- making the correct selection of site and equipment
- careful insertion and removal of peripheral cannula
- undergoing appropriate training and maintenance of the skill, and assessment of competence
- educating and supporting the woman
- ongoing care and observation of the site
- correct documentation.

SUMMARY

- Peripheral intravenous cannulation is an uncomfortable, invasive procedure that may result in localised or systemic infection.
- The midwife should be appropriately trained and able to maintain the skill.
- It is an ANTT procedure, using the correct-sized cannula for the vein and nature of the fluid.
- The site is chosen with care, avoiding arteries and joints, and choosing the appropriate veins of the hand and forearm.
- Complications may arise both on insertion and in the following days. Vigilant ongoing monitoring and care is required to avoid complications.
- Documentation of insertion, monitoring and removal is thorough and contemporaneous.
- Removal is generally quick and easy; it is still an ANTT procedure.

Self-assessment exercises

The answers to the following questions may be found in the text.

1. Discuss the indications for cannula insertion.
2. Describe how to choose a suitable site for a PIVC.
3. Discuss the type of equipment selected, with a rationale for each.
4. Describe and demonstrate how a cannula is inserted correctly.
5. Discuss the complications that may arise following cannula insertion.
6. Describe how to remove a cannula correctly.
7. Summarise the role and responsibilities of the midwife when inserting and removing a PIVC.

Resources

Australian Vascular Access Society (AVAS): Online 10 October 2021. Available: avas.org.au.

Infusion Nurses Society (INS): Online 10 October 2021. Available: www.ins1.org/default.aspx.

Intravenous Nursing New Zealand (IVNNZ Inc): Online 10 October 2021. Available: www.ivnnz.co.nz.

References

ANTT: Welcome to the official home of ANTT. Online 10 October 2021. Available: www.antt.co.uk, 2017.

Barton A, Ventura R, Vavrik B: Peripheral intravenous cannulation: protecting patients and nurses, British Journal of Nursing 26:S28–S33, 2017.

Bolton D: Clinically indicated replacement of peripheral cannulas, British Journal of Nursing 24:S4–S12, 2015.

Brooks N: Chapter 3. Venipuncture and cannulation: a practical guide, M&K Publishing, Keswick, 2014.

Brooks N: Intravenous cannula site management, Nursing Standard 30:53–63, 2016.

Bullock S, Manias E: Fundamentals of pharmacology, 8th ed., Pearson, Melbourne, 2017.

Cooper K, Gosnell K: Foundations and adult health nursing, 8th ed., Mosby, St Louis, 2018.

Goossens GA: Flushing and locking of venous catheters: available evidence and evidence deficit. Nursing Research and Practice 1–12, 2015.

Gorski L, Hadaway L, Hagle M, et al: Infusion therapy standards of practice, Journal of Infusion Nursing 39(1S):1–159, 2016.

Helton J, Hines A, Best J: Peripheral IV site rotation based on clinical assessment vs. length of time since insertion, MEDSURG Nursing: Official Journal of the Academy of Medical-Surgical 25(1):44–49, 2016.

Higginson R: IV cannula securement: protecting the patient from infection, British Journal of Nursing 24:S23–S28, 2015.

Intensive Care Coordination & Monitoring Unit (ICCMU): Central venous access device post insertion management. Online 13 August 2021. Available: www.aci.health.nsw.gov.au/__data/assets/pdf_file/0010/239626/ACI14_CVAD-2-2.pdf, 2014.

Jackson A: Infection control: a battle in vein infusion phlebitis, Nursing Times 94(4):68–71, 1998.

Loveday H, Wilson J, Pratt RJ, et al: EPIVC3: national evidence-based guidelines for preventing healthcare-associated infections in NHS hospitals in England, Journal of Hospital Infection 86(Suppl 1):S1–S70, 2014.

Marsh N, Mihala G, Ray-Barruel G, et al: Inter-rater agreement on PIVC-associated phlebitis signs, symptoms and scales, Journal of Evaluation in Clinical Practice 21:893–899, 2015.

Marsh N, Webster J, Mihala G, et al: Devices and dressings to secure peripheral venous catheters: a Cochrane systematic review and meta-analysis, International Journal of Nursing Studies 67:12–19, 2017.

McCallum L, Higgins D: Care of peripheral venous cannula sites, Nursing Times 108(34/35):12, 2012.

NSW Health: Guideline: peripheral intravenous cannula (PIVC) insertion and post insertion care in adult patients. Online 16 March 2021. Available: https://www1.health.nsw.gov.au/pds/ActivePDSDocuments/PD2019_040.pdf, 2013.

Palese A, Ambrosi E, Fabris F, et al: Nursing care as a predictor of phlebitis related to insertion of a peripheral venous cannula in emergency departments: findings from a prospective study, Journal of Hospital Infection 92(3):280, 2016.

Royal College of Nursing (RCN): Standards for infusion therapy, 4th ed., RCN, London, 2016.

Shaw SJ: How to insert a peripheral cannula. RCNi, Nursing Standard 31(12):42–47, 2016.

Taliaferro K: Clinical nurse consultant of the Intravenous Access Team at Canberra Hospital and Canberra state president of AVAS, personal communication, 31 October 2017.

Ullman AJ, Cooke ML, Mitchell M, et al: Dressing and securement for central venous access devices (CVADs): a Cochrane systematic review, International Journal of Nursing Studies 59:177–196, 2016.

VIP Score: 2018. Online 13 August 2021. Available: www.vipscore.net.

Webster J, Osborne S, Rickard CM, et al: Clinically indicated replacement versus routine replacement of peripheral venous catheters, Cochrane Database of Systematic Review (4):CD007798, 2013.

Yagnik L, Graves A, Thong K: Plastic in patient study: Prospective audit of adherence to peripheral intravenous cannula monitoring and documentation guidelines, with the aim of reducing future rates of intravenous cannula-related complications, American Journal of Infection Control 45(1):34–38, 2017.

CHAPTER 12
OBTAINING SWABS

Learning outcomes

Having read this chapter, the reader should be able to:

- describe how a swab is obtained from the eye, ear, nose, throat, groin, umbilicus, vagina, wound and placenta
- discuss how to collect biochemical tests to assess for ruptured membranes and the risk of preterm labour
- discuss the role and responsibilities of the midwife in relation to obtaining swabs.

RATIONALE FOR SWAB COLLECTION

Swabs are obtained for microbiological examination to aid diagnosis and treatment of infection. It is important to identify the microorganisms causing infection so antibiotics can be matched to the specific causative organism and to reduce antibiotic resistance.

Swabs can be used to detect bacteria (culture and sensitivity), viral organisms (*Chlamydia trachomatis*), serological (antigens and antibodies, e.g. rapid antigen detection test for strep throat), mycosis (fungal, e.g. *Candida albicans*) and protozoa (malaria, trichomoniasis). Swabs have been used for large-scale testing to identify SARS-CoV-2 infections and track community transmission of COVID-19 in the context of the global pandemic.

Infection describes invasion of tissue by pathogenic microorganisms and can be endogenous (the organism is already present on the body) or exogenous (organism is transferred by other people or environmental contact) and includes hospital-acquired infections (HIAs) (Brown & Steen 2020). The majority of puerperal infections are caused by streptococcal or staphylococcal species (Brown & Steen 2020).

Early recognition and treating of infection is essential to avoid maternal sepsis. In Australia between 2015 and 2017, sepsis was responsible for 10.2% of maternal deaths and was the third most common cause of direct maternal death (AIHW 2020). In New Zealand between 2006 and 2018, pregnancy-related infection resulted in six direct maternal deaths (Health Quality & Safety Commission New Zealand 2021). Group A streptococcus (GAS) is a common microorganism involved in maternal infection, with 15% of GAS infections occurring during pregnancy and 85% occurring in the postpartum period (Stevens & Bryant 2017). Diagnostic testing for GAS may include perineal, high vaginal and endocervical swabs for culture and sensitivity (NSW Health 2016). GAS is a common cause of sore throats, particularly in children, and is often a community-acquired infection. The woman may be infected by children or others during pregnancy and the postpartum period. Women who develop GAS are more likely to have a recent history of pharyngeal or upper respiratory infection; therefore, screening for GAS (strep throat) is appropriate as the infection may be transferred to the genital tract or a caesarean section wound (Stevens & Bryant 2017). Strict adherence to hand hygiene by midwives and women, particularly before and after changing sanitary pads, may help to reduce the incidence of infection (Harper 2011).

Swabs are also taken for screening purposes and as part of infection control procedures. Screening has ethical implications because when a screen is positive women must make decisions regarding treatment. Women may be offered screening for vaginal group B streptococcus (GBS) at 35–37 weeks (Department of Health 2020). GBS can be a cause of asymptomatic bacteriuria, urinary and genital tract infection and postpartum endometritis, pneumonia and puerperal sepsis (Puopolo et al 2019). For an extensive discussion on GBS testing refer to Pairman and colleagues (2019).

Standard 3 of the Australian Commission on Safety and Quality in Health Care (ACSQHC) *National safety and quality health standards* indicates that healthcare facilities are required to have systems in place for infection prevention, control and microbiological surveillance (ACSQHC 2021). Women who have an infection must be identified rapidly to ensure they receive appropriate treatment promptly (ACSQHC 2021). Women with methicillin-resistant *Staphylococcus aureus* (MRSA) will be cared for in a single room. Local infection control policies need to be followed.

C. trachomatis is the most frequently reported notifiable diagnosis in Australia and the most commonly diagnosed sexually transmitted infection in New Zealand (New Zealand Family Planning n.d.). *C. trachomatis* screening can be discussed at the early antenatal visits and screening offered (Homer 2019). Endocervical or vaginal swabs can be used to detect *C. trachomatis.*

Swabs are also used to test for biochemical markers of ruptured membranes and assess the risk of preterm birth. Several tests have been developed for use at the point of care to detect biochemical markers present in amniotic fluid but not vaginal secretions (Ruanphoo & Phupong 2015). These include placental alpha-microglobulin-1 (PAMG-1) and insulin-like growth factor binding protein-1 (IGFBP-1). This chapter focuses on obtaining swabs from the more common sites of the eye, ear, nose, throat, groin, umbilicus, vagina, wound and placenta.

GOOD PRACTICE

Good practice for taking swabs should include the following.

- Correct identification of the woman (asking her to state her name and date of birth) and the granting of consent. Some swabs may be taken by women themselves with instructions provided. Education is important to ensure in each instance the woman understands what is being tested, and why and how the swab is obtained. It is also important to discuss the implications of a positive result and indicate when the results will be available and how they will be communicated to her.
- Clinical assessment. This helps determine if the swab is necessary and appropriate for the current clinical condition and how the result will impact on care.
- Avoiding taking unnecessary swabs. This adds to cost and can be stressful for the woman; repeat swabs should be avoided if they will not improve care.
- Collecting specimens at the right time, in the right way (avoiding contamination), using the right equipment, the right swab and transport medium, and labelled as per locally agreed policy. Failure at any of these stages wastes resources and can result in women losing confidence in the service.
- Taking swabs in a manner that protects all staff, including the midwife, transportation and laboratory services. Specimen collection should adhere to standard precautions and follow infection control protocols. Specimens should be sealed, placed in the transport bag or container and labelled 'high risk' if appropriate.
- Storing swabs correctly and ensuring that time-sensitive specimens should reach the laboratory within the recommended timeframe. Most swabs can be stored at room temperature for 24 hours and refrigerated beyond 24 hours at 2–8°C. Some specimens must not be refrigerated as refrigeration can damage some sensitive organisms.
- Documenting the collection of swabs appropriately, including time and date of collection, allows results to be located and acted on in a timely manner.

OBTAINING THE SWAB

Sterile swabs are usually made of cotton or rayon, which is attached to a shaft and placed in a transport medium immediately after collection. The swab must be sterile and within the use-by date, as expired swabs can affect results. The lid should be firmly tightened and the sample correctly labelled, including the woman's name, hospital number, date of birth, specimen taken, location from which the swab has been taken, time and date, all of which should correspond with the pathology form (this should also indicate if the woman is taking antibiotics and any signs or symptoms). The swab is then placed in a sealed biohazard bag for transport. The bag has two separate components. The sealable pouch is for the specimen so any leakage is contained and the potential for contamination is limited. The second pouch is for the laboratory request form; this avoids the specimen contaminating the form. It is taken to the laboratory as soon as possible, as some microorganisms can multiply when kept at room temperature. It is important for the midwife to be aware of how to store swabs and specimens when they cannot be transported quickly. In high-risk situations, the swab may need to be double-wrapped and labelled accordingly.

The laboratory test requested is usually 'microscopy, culture and sensitivity' (MC&S), which involves a microscopic examination for a quick initial report of the microorganism/s present, culture of the microorganism/s to identify which microorganisms are present, a microbial count to determine if they are the result of colonisation or infection and an analysis of sensitivity to antibiotics that can be administered to prevent further growth and replication.

When taking the swab, it is important the microorganisms coat the swab to increase the chances of identifying the infecting microorganism; this is best achieved by rotating the swab over the site. An aseptic non-touch technique (ANTT) (Chapter 2) should be used to avoid cross-contamination and only the affected area should be swabbed (Higgins 2013). In some situations, a sample of pus, exudate, moisture, and so on from the woman or neonate (e.g. from the umbilical stump) may need to be collected. While they can be collected via a swab stick, it may be more appropriate to use a sterile syringe to collect pus/exudate. Standard precautions, including hand hygiene, should be followed when obtaining a swab (Chapter 1). Where swabs are required from more than one site (e.g. both eyes, ears), a separate swab should be used for each site to reduce the risk of cross-infection from an infected to a non-infected area. However, usually only one swab is required from the area that appears most affected. Swabs can be self-collected if appropriate instructions are provided. Self-collection of swabs provides another option that may be more acceptable and convenient (Gaydos 2018).

There are a variety of transport mediums, as different microorganisms can thrive or die in certain mediums; thus, it is important that the correct swab and transport medium are used for the suspected microorganism. If the midwife is unsure of which swab and transport medium to use, they should ask a senior colleague or microbiologist for advice. Some colour codings for swab collection are as follows.

- Blue-top plastic shaft swab (uses Amies transport medium, a modification of Stuart transport medium which is available with or without charcoal): a bacterial swab suitable for MC&S from ear, nose, throat, eye, wounds, urogenital (for general microbiology), plus aerobes and anaerobes.
- Orange fine wire swab (Amies transport medium): suitable for MC&S from nasopharyngeal, wound sinuses, eye, ear, nose and throat.
- White-top plastic shaft swab (no transport medium): is suitable for all polymerase chain reaction (PCR) testing (except viral PCR and chlamydia/gonorrhoea).
- Green-top plastic shaft swab (viral transport medium): suitable for PCR testing (herpes simplex, herpes zoster (varicella), influenza, respiratory viruses, measles and other viruses).
- Yellow-top PCR (contains guanidine hydrochloride): suitable for cervical, vaginal or eye swab for *C. trachomatis* and or *N. gonorrhoeae*.
- Red-top collection kit for viruses: contains universal transport medium suitable for viruses such as influenza, H1N1 (swine flu), chlamydia, mycoplasma and ureaplasma specimens and rapid antigen testing (Fig 12.1).

The midwife should record in the notes which swabs have been taken and the time and date. This will ensure all staff are aware swabs have been obtained and will remind them to check the results as soon as they are ready. The woman should know why the swab(s) are undertaken and how soon she can expect to have the result.

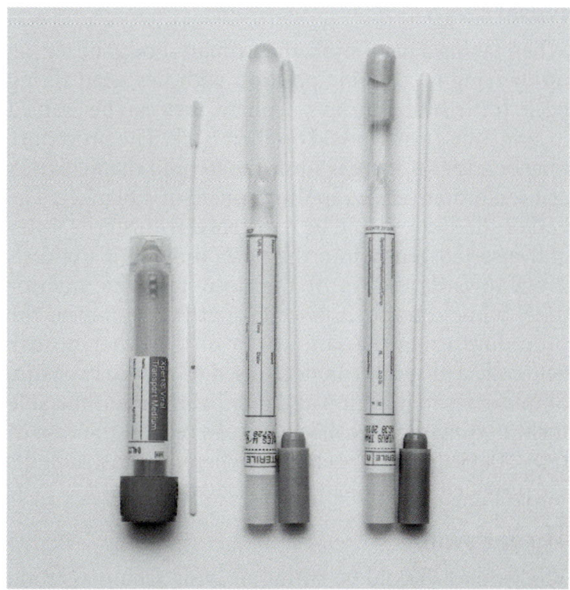

FIGURE 12.1 **The correct swab needs to be used for the desired purpose. Swabs are available for general bacterial microscopy, culture and sensitivity, PCR testing and viral testing.**

Eye swab

When obtaining an eye swab from a woman, she should be sitting upright, with her head tilted back and supported. Ask the woman to look upwards to prevent corneal damage (Dimech et al 2011). If the swab is from a neonate, they should be supported with their head held steady. The lower eyelid should be pulled down gently. The swab is held parallel to the cornea and rubbed very gently against the conjunctiva in the lower eyelid, moving from the inner canthus to the outer canthus. If *Chlamydia trachomatis* is the suspected microorganism, firmly swab the everted lower eyelid (Dimech et al 2011). It is important to avoid touching the eyelid borders or eyelashes with the swab. Usually just one swab is sufficient. If *Gonococcus* is the suspected organism, the swab should not be refrigerated as there will be no recovery of the *Gonococcus* organism and a false-negative will be reported.

Ear swab

It is important to withhold medication administered via the ears for 3 hours prior to obtaining the swab as the medication can interfere with the growth of the microorganism. To obtain a swab from the ear, the woman should sit up with her head tilting to the unaffected side. When taking a swab from a neonate, one of the parents or another midwife can hold the neonate with the head up, tilted to one side. If the neonate is too ill to be moved, lay the neonate on the unaffected side. For both the woman and the neonate, straighten the external canal by gently pulling the pinna upwards and backwards; the swab is inserted gently into and rotated around the walls of the external canal. If necessary, the external canal can be cleaned with a moistened swab to remove any debris and/or crust before inserting the swab.

Nasal swab

When taking a nasal swab, the woman should be sitting up or lying in a supine position with her head tilting back. If the swab is from a neonate, they can be cradled in someone's arms or laid on their back. The procedure may be easier if there is someone to hold the neonate's arms; alternatively, wrap the neonate in a blanket. The end of the swab should be moistened with sterile water and inserted gently into the nose, moving it upwards 2 cm towards the tip of the nose, into the anterior nares while rotating it twice (Porrit 2021). Repeat the procedure using the same swab in the other nostril. Self-collected swabs can be utilised to reduce exposure of midwives to infection and may be more comfortable for the woman. Self-collected swabs (e.g. in the case of COVID-19 testing) are effective when clear instructions are provided (Australian Government 2020).

Throat swab

The woman should be sitting or lying facing a strong light source. She should be asked to tilt her head back, open her mouth wide and say 'Ah' as she sticks out her tongue (deWit & O'Neill 2014, Porritt 2021). The tongue should be depressed using a disposable spatula and the swab inserted to the back of the throat. The swab is then rotated around the tonsillar fossa at the side of the pharynx (NSW Health 2020); this is likely to make the woman gag. When removing the swab, ensure it does not come into contact with any part of the mouth, uvula, tongue or saliva.

Groin swab

Because the skin of the groin is dry, it is important to moisten the end of the swab with sterile normal saline. The swab is then rolled along the groin, using the area of skin along the inside part of the thigh that is nearest to the genitalia.

Umbilical swab

The neonate's umbilical cord is colonised by non-pathogenic bacteria after birth (Quattrin et al 2016). An umbilical swab should be collected if signs of infection are present, including inflammation, swelling, redness or red flaring, weeping, pus, offensive odour or granuloma. The neonate should be positioned to allow easy access to the umbilicus (e.g. cradled in someone's arms or lying in a cot) and undressed to expose the umbilicus. The swab is moved gently around the umbilicus and rotated. The neonate should be re-dressed following the procedure.

Vaginal swabs

Low vaginal swabs (LVS) can be self-collected by women or collected by the midwife. If a woman is self-collecting a low vaginal swab, provide written instructions. Instruct the woman to begin by removing her undergarments, then remove the swab from the tube and avoid touching anything with the swab. In a comfortable position (lying down or standing with one leg elevated), gently part the labia and insert the swab into the vagina in a backwards direction for 2–5 cm. Rotate the swab for 10–15 seconds, remove the swab and place in the collection tube. If a vaginal–perianal swab is required, also swab across the perianal area. Local guidelines should be followed. Testing for GBS requires a low vaginal swab.

High vaginal swabs (HVS) and endocervical swabs generally require the use of a speculum to visualise the cervix (Chapter 13). The swab should be inserted through the speculum to the top of the vagina and rotated in the area required for the test (e.g. posterior fornix or cervical os). When the procedure is completed the speculum should be removed and the woman assisted into a comfortable position.

Wound swab

It is important to obtain the wound swab correctly. Wound swabs should only be collected from the affected site and avoid any contact with normal surrounding skin and tissue (Higgins 2013). Asepsis is important to minimise environmental contamination; the swab should be returned to the sterile container or transport medium immediately after collection (Higgins 2013). When obtaining a swab because of suspected uterine or perineal infection, it is best to do so before antibiotics are used. If only microorganisms from the wound surface are obtained and not those that penetrate the soft tissue, a false-positive result may ensue as the microorganisms found on the wound surface are frequently different from the microorganisms responsible for the infection (Swanson et al 2014). Prior to obtaining a wound swab, Huddleston Cross (2014) recommends using normal saline to irrigate the wound to remove surface contamination (e.g. slough, necrotic tissue, eschar) using ANNT (Chapter 2). Allow 1–2 minutes to pass before taking the swab. If the wound is dry, the swab should be moistened with sterile saline.

The swab should be rotated across a 1 cm^2 area of the wound (Levine's technique) for at least 5 seconds, using sufficient pressure to release exudate or fluid from the wound (Bainbridge 2014). The Levine technique is considered more reliable than the zigzag method of obtaining a wound swab (Ward & Holloway 2019). If there is a sinus or pocket in the wound, a separate swab should be used. Care should be taken to ensure the swab does not come into contact with the wound edge. The swab should be kept at room temperature and taken to the laboratory as soon as possible (Rebeiro et al 2020).

Placental swab

Acute **chorioamnionitis** results in gross and microscopic alterations, indicating inflammation (Gundogan & De Paepe 2013). If chorioamnionitis is suspected, swabs of the placenta for bacterial culture may be requested. It is important the midwife understands which surfaces require swabbing: the fetal surface, the maternal surface or between the membranes. If a swab of the fetal and/or maternal surface is required, the swab should be moved around the surface(s) in a zigzag direction. As the placenta passes through the birth canal it can be colonised with vaginal bacteria; subamniotic cultures significantly decrease contamination (Burton et al 2014). A **subamniotic swab** involves picking up the amnion and then making an incision in the amnion and inserting the swab between the amnion and chorion. Ensure the swab does not make contact with the edge of the amnion (Fig 12.2). A **subchorionic sample** can be collected when the amnion has become detached during birth; the amnion may be visible near where the umbilical cord inserts. Clean the surface of the chorion, covering the placenta with an alcohol swab at the site for the incision. Make a small superficial incision in the chorion with the scalpel and insert the swab just underneath the chorion (Fig 12.3). Care must be taken not to cross-contaminate the swab by touching the surface of the placenta or outer side of the membranes. Carefully place the swab in the microbiology tube. Specify on the pathology form

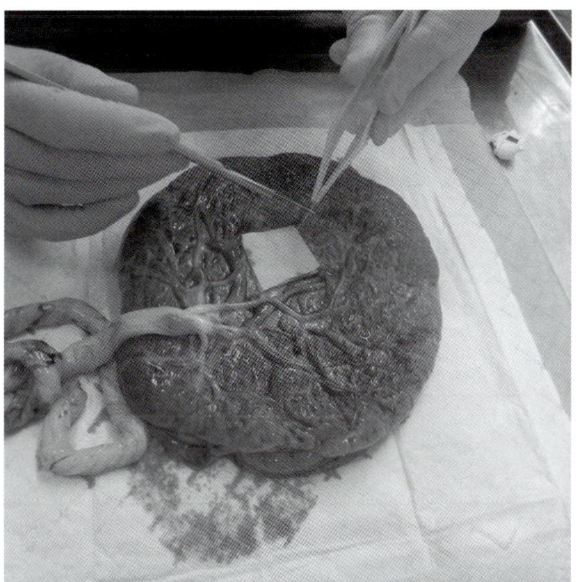

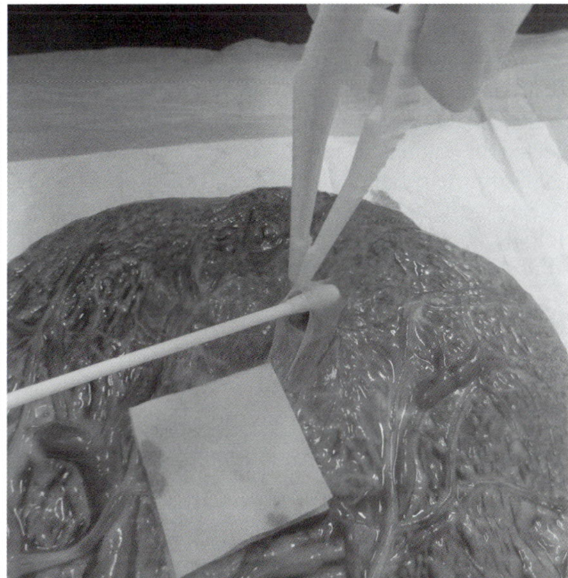

FIGURE 12.2 Collection of placental subamniotic swab.

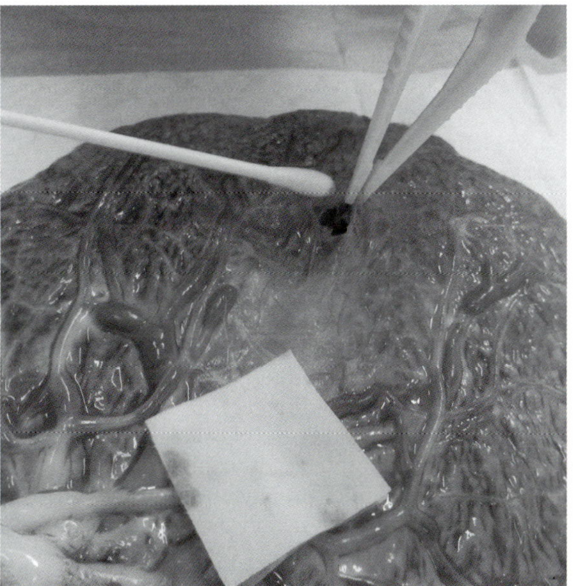

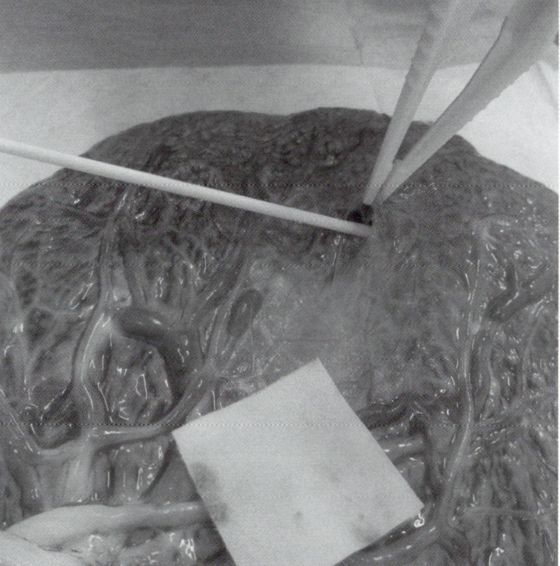

FIGURE 12.3 Collection of placental subchorionic swab.

if the swab is from a caesarean section or vaginally delivered placenta.

FETAL FIBRONECTIN TO ASSESS RISK OF PRETERM BIRTH

Fetal fibronectin (fFN) is an adhesive-like glycoprotein that bonds the developing fetal membranes to the uterus. fFN is produced between the amnion and the decidua, at the uteroplacental (or choriodecidual) junction. Fetal fibronectin is mainly confined to this junction and appears to help maintain its integrity (Fig 12.4).

Normally no fFN is present in cervicovaginal fluids between 22 and 35 weeks gestation. If the choriodecidual interface becomes disrupted by inflammation or injury, fFN is released, and this is associated with spontaneous preterm birth (Foster & Shennan 2014). fFN can be detected in vaginal secretions in early pregnancy as the glycoprotein bonds develop, and then again after 35 weeks as the bonds diminish in preparation for birth (Hologic 2020). fFN is approved for use between 22 and 35 weeks of pregnancy. An elevated fFN between 22 and 35 weeks gestation is associated with an increased risk of preterm birth. A quantitative fFN gives results in nanogram/mL. Increased levels are equated with higher risk of preterm birth in a linear fashion, as shown in Table 12.1. An fFN concentration of 50 ng/mL or less is considered negative (NICE 2015). According to Kuhrt and colleagues (2016), spontaneous preterm birth can be predicted accurately with a combination of qualitative fFN and cervical length (Kuhrt et al 2016). However, a study on nulliparous women (with a singleton pregnancy) found quantitative vaginal fFN was not supported for routine screening as it failed to predict spontaneous preterm birth (Esplin et al 2017). An fFN is collected from the posterior fornix during a speculum examination (Fig 12.5).

Another test used to predict preterm labour in women at risk of preterm labour is Actim® Partus, which tests for the presence of phosphorylated insulin-like growth factor binding protein-1 (phIGBP1-P), which is produced by the decidua and leaks into the cervix when the decidua and chorion detach. A positive test indicates the presence of tissue damage; a negative test means no significant alterations have occurred in the choriodecidual layer and birth is unlikely within the next 1–2 weeks.

Specimens for biochemical tests to predict preterm labour are collected prior to any other specimens or examination of the cervix, or transvaginal ultrasound.

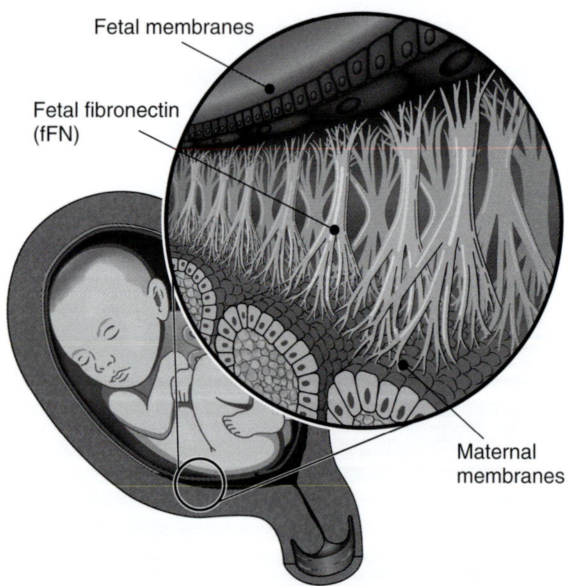

FIGURE 12.4 **Fetal fibronectin: a glue-like protein.**
Source: Hologic: What is fetal fibronectin? Online 13 August 2021. Available: https://ffntest.com/ffn/. Courtesy of Hologic, Inc. and affiliates.

TABLE 12.1 COMMERCIAL BIOMARKER TESTS FOR RUPTURED MEMBRANES

Commercially available test	Biochemical markers used	Sensitivity and specificity %
Amnioquick Duo+	IGFBP-1 and AFP	Sensitivity 96.4 Specificity 87.5
Amnisure®	PAMG-1	Sensitivity 94.4–98.9 Specificity 87.5–100
ROMplus®	IGFBP-1 and AFP	Sensitivity 99 Specificity 75
Actim® PROM	IGFBP-1	Sensitivity 95–100 Specificity 93–98

Specimen collection procedure

Step 1 Collect specimen prior to digital examination or manipulation of the cervix to avoid sample contamination.

Step 2 During speculum exam, lightly rotate swab across posterior fornix of the vagina for 10 seconds to absorb cervicovaginal secretions.

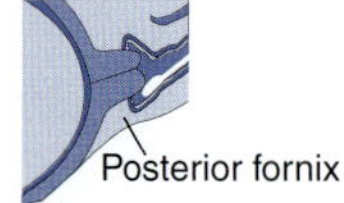

Step 3

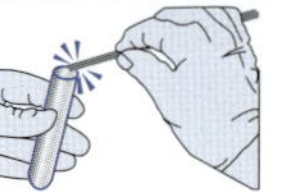

Remove swab and immerse tip in buffer. Break the shaft at the score even with the top of the tube.

Step 4 Insert the swab shaft into the hole inside the tube cap and push down lightly over the shaft, sealing the tube with a click. Ensure the shaft is inserted securely to avoid leakage. Label, and send fetal fibronectin sample to a lab near you.

FIGURE 12.5 **Collection of fFN.**
Source: Hologic: How to collect an fFN specimen. Online 13 August 2021. Available: https://ffntest.com/hcp/instructions-and-results/. Courtesy of Hologic, Inc. and affiliates.

fFN swabs should not be collected in the following circumstances:

- the presence of vaginal bleeding
- ruptured membranes
- cervical dilation > 3 cm
- before 22 weeks gestation and after 35 weeks gestation
- placenta praevia
- suspected placental abruption
- if sexual intercourse occurred in the previous 24 hours.

During collection of the sample, avoid contaminating the swab with any lubricants, cleaning agents, disinfectants or creams.

Biomarkers to assess for ruptured membranes

Ruptured membranes can be easily diagnosed when copious amounts of amniotic fluid are visible. However, it can be difficult to determine if the membranes have ruptured in many cases. Nitrazine paper can be used to test the pH of vaginal fluid, which is normally acidic ranging from 3.8 to 4.2; amniotic fluid is usually 7.0–7.3. The nitrazine paper is dipped into the suspected amniotic fluid. If a pink strip changes to blue, the membranes may be ruptured as a blue colour indicates the pH is greater than six. (Strips come in different colours, so this will not be accurate for all strips.) A false-positive or false-negative test occurs approximately 5% of the time (Duff 2020). Ferning is testing by swabbing fluid from the posterior fornix of the vagina, and placed on a glass slide. The sample is dried for 10 or more minutes and if amniotic fluid is present a ferning pattern is seen (Duff 2020).

Rapid immunoassay tests are commercially available to assist in the diagnosis of ruptured membranes (Igbinosa et al 2017). The membranes function to protect the fetus from physical damage and contaminants. The two layers of fetal membranes have a stratified structure and are able to expand during pregnancy (Palacio et al 2014). Preterm rupture of membranes may be associated with inflammatory processes triggered by endocrine or infectious events (Palacio et al 2014). When the membranes rupture, biomarkers present in higher concentrations in amniotic fluid (but not in vaginal secretions) are present in the vagina. These include placental alpha-microglobulin-1 (PAMG-1), insulin-like growth factor binding protein-1 (IGFBP-1) and alpha-fetoprotein (AFP), alone or in combination. A speculum is not required to collect a vaginal swab to assess for ruptured membranes (Fig 12.6). The manufacturer's instructions indicate that samples can be collected if urine, semen or vaginal infections are present and in the presence of trace amounts of blood. The risk of preterm birth can be estimated using a quantitative fFN (Table 12.2).

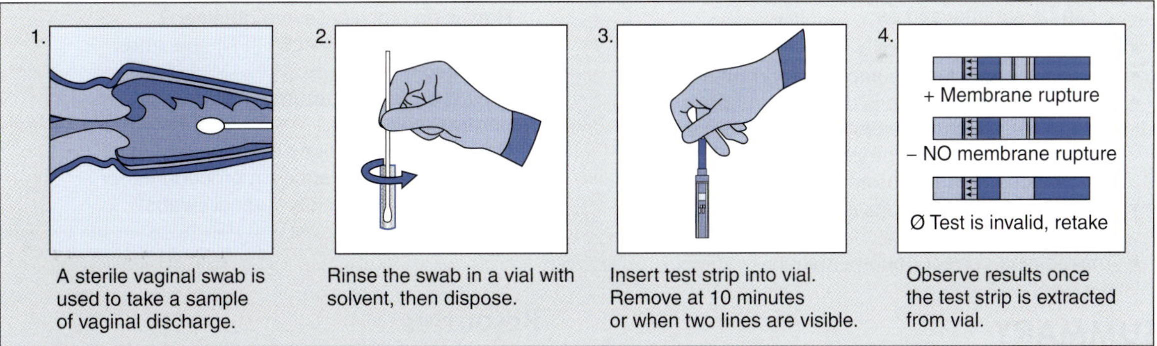

FIGURE 12.6 **Collection of swab to assess biochemical markers for ruptured membranes.**
Source: Adapted from Navamedic: AmniSure® Rapid, Reliable, Non-Invasive Test for ROM (Rupture of [fetal] Membranes), 2011. Available: www.navamedic.com/globalassets/english-master/products/amnisure/dokument/amnisure-brochure-en-110831.pdf.

TABLE 12.2 RISK OF SPONTANEOUS PRETERM BIRTH BY fFN CONCENTRATION

fFN level	Risk of birth ≤ 7 days %	Risk of birth ≤ 14 days %	Birth prior to 34 weeks %
< 10 nanogram/mL	1	1.8	1.5
11–49 nanogram/mL	0	1.6	8.2
50–199 nanogram/mL	0	7.7	11.5
200–499 nanogram/mL	14	29.0	33.0
≥ 500 nanogram/mL	38	46.0	75.0

Source: Courtesy of Hologic, Inc. and affiliates.

SKILL 12.1 Obtaining a swab

1. Discuss the procedure and gain informed consent.
2. Gather equipment:
   - non-sterile gloves and apron (if required)
   - sterile swab with transport medium
   - speculum and water-based lubricating jelly (high vaginal swab only)
   - tongue depressor (throat swab only)
   - sterile water (nasal swab only)
   - sterile normal saline (groin or wound swab).
3. Perform hand hygiene and apply apron and gloves.
4. Position the woman or neonate appropriately.
5. Ensure the area to be swabbed is exposed.
6. Open the outer packaging.
7. Remove the swab using ANTT.
8. Obtain the swab.
   - **Nasal swab**: head is tilted back to ensure the nostrils are clearly visible, moisten swab with sterile water, insert swab to the anterior nares and rotate the swab.
   - **Throat swab**: head is tilted back with mouth open and tongue protruding, depress tongue with tongue depressor and ask the woman to say 'ah', roll swab over posterior pharynx/tonsils.
   - **Skin swab**: moisten the swab with sterile saline if the area is dry, roll swab across skin or wound site.
   - Refer to the relevant section of this chapter for instructions on obtaining swabs for ear, eye, groin, vagina, umbilical cord and placenta.
9. Insert the swab into the transport medium and seal securely.
10. Label the container with the name, hospital number, date of birth of the woman or neonate, date and time the swab was obtained, nature of specimen, whether right or left (if applicable) and signature. Indicate relevant history such as current antibiotic regime. Place into transport bag.
11. Assist the woman or neonate into a comfortable position.
12. Remove and dispose of gloves and apron.
13. Perform hand hygiene.
14. Arrange transportation of the specimen to the pathology laboratory.
15. Document findings and act accordingly.

Roles and responsibilities of the midwife

These can be summarised as:

- recognising the need for a swab to be taken
- using the correct swab and transport medium
- ensuring the procedure is undertaken correctly, with minimal discomfort to the mother or neonate and with the use of appropriate standard precautions/personal protective equipment
- following up swab results and instigating referral/treatment as necessary
- maintaining correct documentation.

SUMMARY

- Obtaining a swab is a significant and simple but invasive procedure that may be undertaken on either the woman or the neonate.
- It is important to take the swab correctly and avoid contamination from adjoining structures/debris to avoid false-positive or false-negative results.

Self-assessment exercises

The answers to the following questions may be found in the text.

1. How would the midwife obtain a swab from:
   a. the ear of the neonate?
   b. the eye of a neonate?
   c. the nose of a woman?
   d. the throat of a woman?
2. How is an umbilical swab obtained?
3. How is a fetal fibronectin (fFN) specimen collected?
4. How is a test for ruptured membranes undertaken?
5. Describe how a wound swab is obtained.
6. What are the differences in procedures for obtaining high and low vaginal swabs?

Resources

Royal Children's Hospital Melbourne: COVID-19 swabbing. Online 16 March 2021. Available: https://www.rch.org.au/clinicalguide/guideline_index/COVID-19_swabbing/.

Marty FM, Chen, K, Verrill, KA (2020). How to obtain a nasopharyngeal swab specimen. New England Journal of Medicine. Videos in Clinical medicine. Online 16 March 2021. Available: https://www.nejm.org/doi/full/10.1056/nejmvcm2010260.

Australian Government (2020). Coronavirus (COVID-19) resources for health professionals, including aged care providers, pathology providers and healthcare managers. Online 16 March 2021 Available online: https://www.health.gov.au/resources/collections/coronavirus-covid-19-resources-for-health-professionals-including-aged-care-providers-pathology-providers-and-health-care-managers.

References

Australian Commission on Safety and Quality in Health Care (ACSQHC): National safety and quality health service standards. 2nd ed.—version 2. ACSQHC, Sydney, 2021. Available: www.safetyandquality.gov.au/sites/default/files/2021-05/national_safety_and_quality_health_service_nsqhs_standards_second_edition_-_updated_may_2021.pdf.

Australian Government: How to self-collect a COVID-19 swab. 2020. Online 14 March 2021. Available: https://www.health.gov.au/sites/default/files/documents/2020/06/how-to-self-collect-a-covid-19-swab.pdf.

Australian Institute of Health and Welfare: Maternal deaths in Australia. Cat. no. PER 99. Canberra, 2020, AIHW. Online 14 March 2021. Available: https://www.aihw.gov.au/reports/mothers-babies/maternal-deaths-in-australia.

Bainbridge P: How effective is wound swabbing? A clinimetric assessment of wound swabs, Wounds UK 10(4):44–49, 2014.

Brown A, Steen M: Physical health issues and complications in the postnatal. In Marshall J, Raynor M, editors: Ch 29 pp. 738–755 in Myles textbook for midwives, 17th ed., Churchill Livingstone, Elsevier, Edinburgh, 2020.

Burton GJ, Sebire NJ, Myatt L, et al: Optimising sample collection for placental research, Placenta 35:9–22, 2014.

Department of Health: Clinical practice guidelines: pregnancy care. Australian Government, Canberra, 2020.

deWit S, O'Neill P: Fundamental concepts and skills for nursing, 4th ed., Elsevier, St Louis, 2014.

Dimech J, Dougherty L, Fernandes A, et al: Interpreting diagnostic tests. In Dougherty L, Lister S, editors: The Royal Marsden Hospital manual of clinical nursing procedures, 8th ed., Wiley Blackwell, Oxford, 2011.

Duff P: Preterm prelabour rupture of membranes, 2020. UpToDate. Online 14 March 2021. Available: www.uptodate.com/contents/preterm-prelabor-rupture-of-membranes.

Esplin M, Elovitz M, Iams J, et al: Predictive accuracy of serial transvaginal cervical lengths and quantitative vaginal fetal fibronectin levels for spontaneous preterm birth among nulliparous women, The Journal of the American Medical Association 317(10):1047–1056, 2017.

Foster C, Shennan AH: Fetal fibronectin as a biomarker of preterm labor: a review of the literature and advances in its clinical use, Biomarkers in Medicine 8(4):471–484, 2014.

Gaydos, CA. Let's take a 'selfie': self-collected samples for sexually transmitted infections. Sexually transmitted diseases 45(4):278–279, 2018.

Gundogan F, De Paepe ME: Ascending infection: acute chorioamnionitis. In Baergen RN, Goldblum JR, editors: Surgical pathology clinics: placental pathology, Elsevier, Philadelphia, 2013.

Harper A: Sepsis. In: Centre for Maternal And Child Enquiries (CMACE). Saving mothers' lives: reviewing maternal deaths to make motherhood safer: 2006–08. The eighth report on confidential enquiries into maternal deaths in the United Kingdom, British Journal of Obstetrics and Gynaecology 118(Suppl 1):85–96, 2011.

Health Quality & Safety Commission New Zealand: 14th annual report of the Perinatal and Maternal Mortality Review Committee, 2021. Online 16 March 2021. Available: www.hqsc.govt.nz/our-programmes/mrc/pmmrc.

Higgins C: Understanding laboratory investigations: a guide for nurses, midwives and healthcare professionals, 3rd ed., Wiley Blackwell, Oxford, 2013.

Hologic: Information for healthcare providers: fetal fibronectin enzyme immunoassay and rapid fFN, 2020. Online 13 August 2021. Available: www.hologic.com/sites/default/files/2021-05/AW-24196-001_001_01.pdf.

Homer C: Screening and assessment. In Pairman S, Tracy S, Dahlen HG, Dixon, L: Midwifery, 4th ed., Elsevier, Sydney, 2018.

Huddleston Cross H: Obtaining a wound swab culture specimen, Nursing 44(7):68–69, 2014.

Igbinosa I, Moore III FA, Johnson C, et al: Comparison of rapid immunoassays for rupture of fetal membranes, BMC Pregnancy and Childbirth 17:1–5, 2017.

Kuhrt K, Hezelgrave N, Foster C, et al: Development and validation of a predictive tool for spontaneous preterm birth incorporating cervical length and quantitative fetal fibronectin in asymptomatic high-risk women, Ultrasound in Obstetrics & Gynecology 47(2):210–216, 2016.

National Institute for Health and Care Excellence (NICE): Preterm labour and birth, 2015: updated 2019. Online 16 March 2021. Available: https://www.nice.org.uk/guidance/ng25.

New Zealand Family Planning: Chlamydia, nd. Online 16 March 2021. Available: www.familyplanning.org.nz/advice/sexually-transmissible-infections/chlamydia.

NSW Health: Collection of nasal and throat swabs for respiratory virus testing, 2020. Online 16 March 2021. Available: https://www.health.nsw.gov.au/Infectious/Influenza/Documents/nasal-throat-swabs.pdf.

NSW Health: Maternal sepsis (puerperal fever) due to Group A Streptococcus—Information for clinician's fact sheet, 2016. Online 16 March 2021. Available: www.health.nsw.gov.au/Infectious/factsheets/Pages/maternal-sepsis-info-for-HCW.aspx.

Pairman S, Pincome J, Thorogood C, et al, editors: Midwifery preparation for practice, 4th ed., Churchill Livingstone, Elsevier, Sydney, 2019.

Palacio M, Kühnert M, Berger R, et al: Meta-analysis of studies on biochemical marker tests for the diagnosis of premature rupture of membranes: comparison of performance indexes, BMC Pregnancy and Childbirth 14:1–25, 2014.

Porritt, K: In Koutoukidis G, Stainton K, editors: Tabbner's nursing care, 8th ed., Chatswood, 2021, Elsevier Australia, Chapter 25: Nursing care of an individual: Cardiovascular and respiratory.

Puopolo KM, Madoff LC, Baker CJ: Group B streptococcal infection in pregnant women, 2019. UpToDate. Online 16 March 2021. Available: https://www.uptodate.com/contents/group-b-streptococcal-infection-in-pregnant-women.

Quattrin R, Iacobucci K, De Tina AL, et al: 70% alcohol versus dry cord care in the umbilical cord care: a case–control study in Italy, Medicine 95(14):e3207, 2016.

Rebeiro G, Wilson D, Fuller, S: Fundamentals of nursing: clinical skills workbook. Elsevier, Sydney, 2020.

Ruanphoo P, Phupong V: Evaluation of the performance of the insulin-like growth factor-binding protein-1/alpha-fetoprotein test in diagnosing ruptured fetal membranes in pregnant women, Journal of Perinatology 35:558–560, 2015.

Stevens DL, Bryant A: Pregnancy-related group A streptococcal infection, 2020. UptoDate. Online 16 March 2021. Available: www.uptodate.com/contents/pregnancy-related-group-a-streptococcal-infection.

Swanson T, Grothier L, Schultz G: Wound infection made easy. Wounds International, 2014. Online 16 March 2021. Available: www.woundsinternational.com.

Ward D, Holloway S: (2019). Validity and reliability of semi-quantitative wound swabs. British Journal of Community Nursing 24(Sup12):S6–S11, 2019.

CHAPTER 13
USE OF SPECULUM

Learning outcomes

Having read this chapter, the reader should be able to:

- discuss the indications for using a speculum
- describe how to insert and remove a speculum
- discuss what to do if the cervix cannot be visualised
- discuss the role and responsibilities of the midwife in relation to speculum use.

INDICATIONS

The midwife may need to use a speculum to:

- assess cervical dilatation during suspected preterm labour
- examine the top of the vagina and cervix for the presence of amniotic fluid when pre-labour rupture of membranes is suspected
- assess for the source of bleeding following bleeding per vaginam
- obtain a high vaginal swab
- obtain a cervical screening test.

In December 2017 Australia commenced a new National Cervical Screening Program to replace the Papanicolaou (Pap) smear (Hawkes 2018). The Pap smear tests for abnormal cells, while the new cervical screening test detects human papilloma virus (HPV), the virus responsible for 99% of cervical cancer. A cervical screening test may be offered to pregnant women who have not had such screening within the past 5 years or who have a history of abnormal symptoms, abnormal cytology or untreated cervical abnormalities (Cancer Council 2021, Department of Health 2020). The cervical screening test is not recommended in the first 6 weeks after birth. It is preferable to wait three months as early test results are often unsatisfactory due to inflammation or an insufficient sample (Cancer Council 2021). Water-based lubricants are not recommended as residual lubricant can hinder sample collection and inhibit some molecular-based tests; however, if required for comfort, a small amount of water-soluble lubricant may be used (NSW Health Pathology 2017). Collection of fetal fibronectin, high vaginal swab and biochemical tests for ruptured membranes are discussed in Chapter 12. A speculum examination is avoided in women with placenta praevia, cervical suture, previous cervical insufficiency or abruptio placentae.

TYPES OF SPECULUM

Vaginal specula come in a variety of sizes and types. They can be made of metal (reusable) or plastic (single-use, disposable). Plastic specula have a smaller range of sizes than metal specula. Metal specula should be prewarmed by running them under warm water or placing on a heating pad (Wysocki 2015).

The **Cusco speculum** is made of metal (reusable) or plastic (single-use, disposable) and usually comes in three sizes: small, medium and large (Fig 13.1). It has two short, hinged blades that are curved across their width. The blades are close together when the speculum is closed, but when open they separate and press against the vaginal walls. There is a circular opening at one end, through which the vagina and cervix can be visualised and swabs inserted when required. Attached to this are the handles that open and close the speculum using a screw mechanism. When the handles are apart the blades are closer together, and as the handles are brought closer together the blades open. Practise using the speculum to ensure familiarity with the mechanism.

The Graves and Pederson speculum work in a similar way to the Cusco speculum. The **Graves speculum** is a bivalve speculum with wide, curved, arched blades (Fig 13.2). The anterior blade is shorter than the posterior blade to enable the longer posterior blade to be positioned in the posterior fornix of the vagina. The Graves speculum comes in multiple sizes, including paediatric. The curved blades are able to separate the vaginal wall effectively and are suitable for sexually active and multiparous women.

The **Pederson speculum** is similar to the Graves speculum but has narrower blades and is designed for women with a narrow vaginal canal. This speculum is suitable for women who have never had intercourse

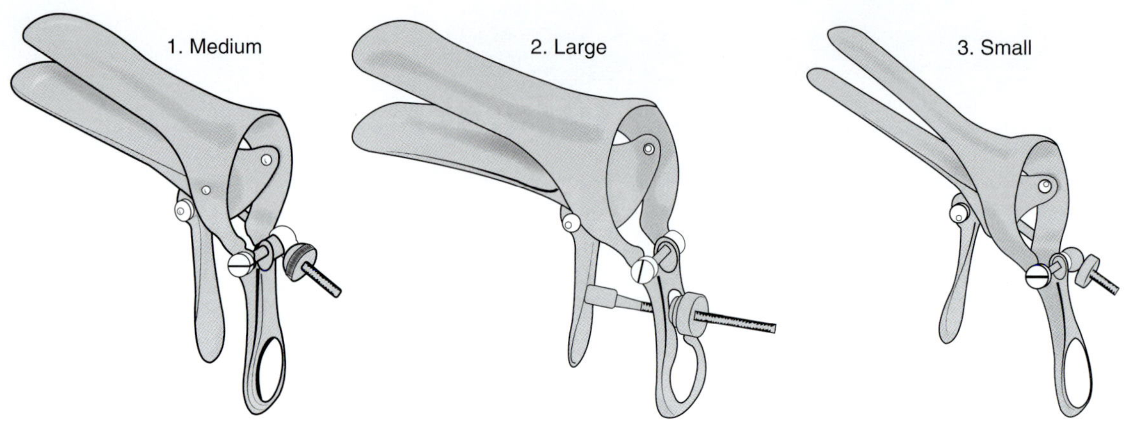

FIGURE 13.1 **Cusco speculum.**

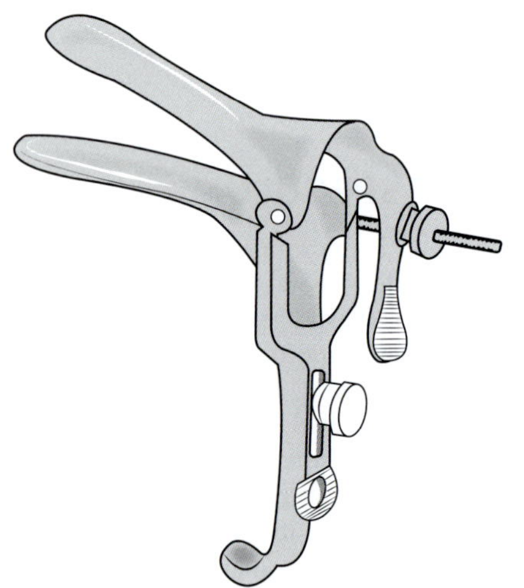

FIGURE 13.2 **Graves speculum.**

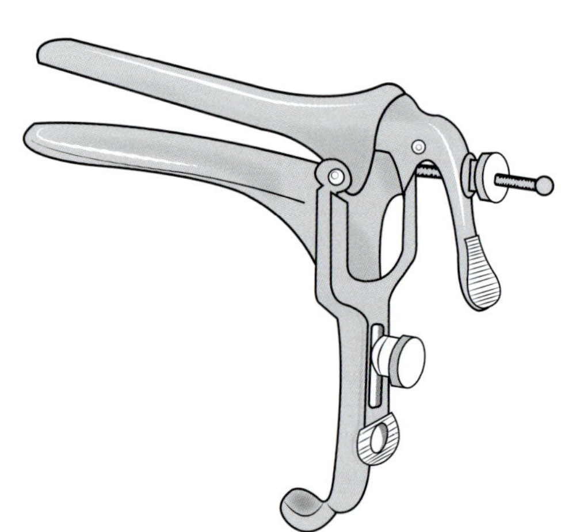

FIGURE 13.3 **Pederson speculum.**

or have scar tissue or an injury. The smaller blades may decrease the discomfort of the examination (Fig 13.3).

The **vaginal speculum** is a double-bladed speculum, where only one blade is used at a time. It holds back the posterior vaginal wall exposing the anterior vaginal wall and cervix (Fig 13.4). This speculum is often used in surgery; the groove in the middle allows secretions and blood to flow outside. An anterior wall retractor is often used in combination with the vaginal speculum to visualise the cervix.

Plastic disposable specula are commonly used. Plastic specula may include built-in lighting. Some plastic specula have a ratchet which can cause a loud clicking sound when the blades are opened and it is helpful to warn women about this sound. The sound may be minimised by lifting the adjustment tap when opening the blades (Fig 13.5).

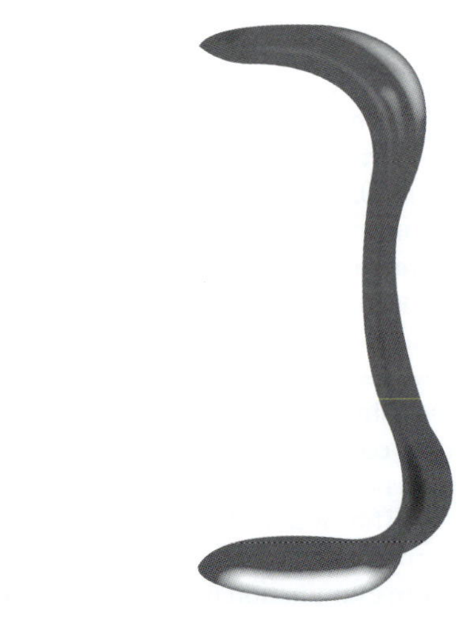

FIGURE 13.4 **Vaginal speculum.**

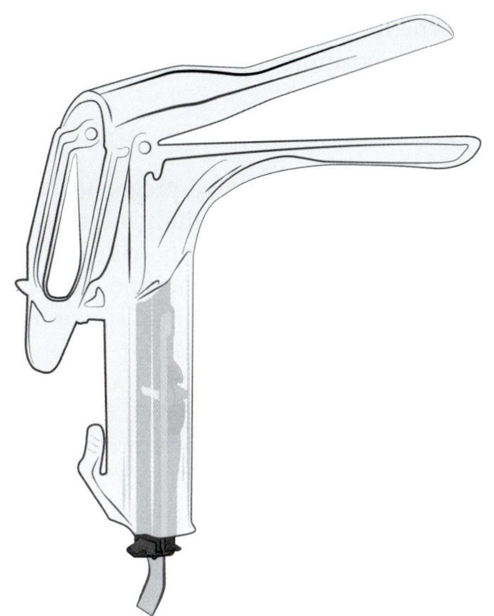

FIGURE 13.5 **Plastic speculum.**

INSERTION OF THE SPECULUM

Insertion of a speculum is an intrusive procedure and requires skilful communication and sensitivity to culture, disability, sexual minorities and personal history, as well as correct technique. It requires the concept of a shared mind, where the midwife is 'attuned' to the woman through listening and attending to her needs in a respectful and thoughtful manner (Cook & Brunton 2014). Women with a history of trauma, sexual assault or sexual abuse may be uncomfortable and anxious because they have experienced a violation of their body and their privacy (Bates et al 2011, Harris n.d.).

The procedure is not usually painful, but it can be embarrassing (Carugno et al 2020, Nagendiram et al 2020) and uncomfortable, particularly if there is a vaginal infection, lacerations or female genital mutilation. Using a cold speculum can make this discomfort worse. Women with disabilities may need to use alternative positions to assist with their comfort. Attention should be paid to the type and size of the speculum required. In general, the wider the speculum the more potential there is for discomfort; therefore, the smallest speculum that enables good visualisation should be chosen.

Women desire information so they know what to expect; they appreciate respectful sensitive communication and the opportunity to ask questions (Chorley et al 2017). It is particularly important to empower sexual assault survivors by discussing what to expect and explaining each step during the examination (Harris n.d.).

Explain the procedure to the woman to ensure she understands what to expect, is comfortable, appropriately covered and able to give informed consent and maintain her autonomy. Avoid coercive language and only proceed with what has been explicitly consented to; if anything changes, recommence the consent process (Tillman 2020). Avoid words with negative connotations such as 'this will feel very uncomfortable' because the warning and anticipation of discomfort can increase anxiety and result in higher pain scores, whereas an objective description such as 'I am now going to introduce the speculum' has been shown to decrease pain scores (Carugno et al 2020). Education involves asking the woman if she has had any issues with previous pelvic examinations and answering any questions she might have. The woman may wish to be shown how the speculum works and to observe the procedure with a mirror. Let her know she is in control and can stop the examination at any time. Women may also choose the option of guided self-insertion of the speculum (Bates et al 2011).

A water-based lubricant is applied to the speculum prior to insertion to reduce friction between the blades and the vaginal wall. Hill and Lamvu (2012) found the use of 0.3 mL of lubricant reduced the degree of pain experienced during insertion compared with using water for lubrication. If a water-based lubricant is used, a minimal amount should be applied to the outer aspect of the speculum blades. If a pathology test is being collected, review the collection instructions to ensure the lubricant is suitable. A lubricant should not be used for collection of a fetal fibronectin as it may contaminate cervicovaginal fluid.

Inform the woman when you are about to insert the speculum and encourage her to relax the pelvic floor. If a woman contracts her pelvic floor (anxiety can cause muscle tension), this can increase discomfort. The blades should be inserted either obliquely or in the anteroposterior diameter while applying gentle downward pressure. The speculum is rotated during insertion so that the handles are facing down.

The speculum should be fully inserted and then opened as far as necessary to visualise the cervix and collect any required swabs (Bates et al 2011). If the cervix is not visualised, it is possible the speculum has not been inserted far enough, in which case the blades should be closed slightly and the speculum inserted deeper or a larger speculum with longer blades used. The tip of the speculum may have slipped into the anterior fornix, which is more likely to occur if a downward pressure is not used during insertion. If this has occurred, the speculum should be withdrawn slightly and the hand holding the end of the speculum raised slightly to depress the speculum tip into the same axis as the cervix. If unable to visualise the cervix, it may help to elevate the hips by asking the woman to place a rolled towel underneath her hips. Avoid asking a woman to place her fists under her hips as this can feel disempowering.

If the lateral walls of the vagina bulge inwards on opening the blades, visualisation of the cervix will also be difficult. This is more likely to occur with obese women or where the woman has a vaginal prolapse.

To overcome this, a condom with a small cut at the tip can be placed over the speculum prior to insertion or a larger speculum can be used, although the latter may increase discomfort (Congress Alukura 2017).

Once in position, open the blades to visualise the cervix and upper part of the vagina. Facilitate visualisation by positioning a suitable overhead light (if not using a speculum with an attached light source). The light should be positioned so the midwife is looking just over the top of it. If undertaking the procedure to assess for ruptured membranes, it is important that the woman has been lying down for at least 30 minutes to allow the amniotic fluid to pool in the vagina.

When removing the speculum, take care to ensure the blades are not shut quickly while still in the vagina as they can pinch the walls of the vagina. It is better to close the blades completely once the speculum has been removed. The speculum can be rotated so it is removed using the same position as it was inserted.

ASEPSIS

Insertion of a speculum during pregnancy should be carried out using a sterile speculum and following the principles of asepsis to reduce the risk of ascending infection, which can lead to uterine and neonatal sepsis. The use of plastic, single-use disposable specula has increased. Plastic specula are single-use only; metal specula must be sterilised for reuse (Secor & Fantasia 2012). Sterile gloves should be worn if the membranes are ruptured, but non-sterile gloves are acceptable for obtaining a swab when the membranes are intact. A sterile vaginal examination (VE) pack and warm water should be used to clean the vulva if required.

SKILL 13.1 Using a speculum

1. Discuss the procedure with the woman and gain informed consent.
2. Encourage the woman to empty her bladder (collect urine sample if required).
3. If it is suspected the woman has ruptured membranes, she should lie down for 30+ minutes.
4. Gather equipment:
   - sterile or non-sterile gloves (depending on the reason for speculum use)
   - speculum and lubricant
   - disposable sheet
   - warm water (if indicated)
   - swab stick and medium, fetal fibronectin or biomarkers for ruptured membranes test (if indicated)
   - light source.
5. Ensure privacy.
6. Position the disposable sheet so that it will be under the woman's buttocks and thighs.
7. Ask the woman to remove her underwear and any sanitary pads, and lie down (if she is not already doing so) in an almost recumbent position (using a wedge to avoid aortocaval occlusion if necessary) and cover her lower abdomen and upper thighs with a sheet.
8. The woman should be asked to relax (flex) her legs at the knees with her ankles together, or feet placed on the bed. A side-lying position can also be used.
9. Perform hand hygiene and apply gloves.
10. Remove the cover to expose the genital area; the woman can be asked to do this if sterile gloves are used.
11. Lubricate the outer aspect of the blades of the speculum with a water-soluble lubricant (if appropriate for the test), keeping the blades closed.
12. If indicated, clean the genital area by swabbing the perineum from front to back using cottonwool balls or gauze soaked with warm water, passing the swabs from the examining (clean) hand to the non-examining hand; use each swab once and dispose of it.
13. Using the non-dominant hand, part the labia and insert the speculum into the vagina in a 45° downwards direction with the dominant hand (Figs 13.6 and 13.7).
14. During insertion, rotate the speculum to position the handles downwards. When the speculum is fully inserted, open the blades approximately 2 cm by unscrewing the handles and bringing them closer together (Fig 13.8). Keep the woman informed during the process.
15. Once the cervix is located (if required), screw the nut on the speculum handle until it locks (avoid over-tightening) or if using plastic speculum lock it into open position.
16. Inspect the vagina and cervix (Fig 13.9) using a good light source and, if indicated, obtain the high vaginal swab (see Chapter 12) and note any inflammation, discharge, bleeding or lesions.
17. Remove the speculum by undoing the screw, closing the blades slightly, taking care not to trap any maternal tissue, and rotating the speculum back to its insertion position then withdrawing the speculum.
18. Remove the disposable sheet and assist the woman to replace her sanitary pad and underwear.
19. Remove and dispose of gloves and equipment.
20. Assist the woman into a comfortable position.
21. Wash and dry hands.
22. Discuss any findings with the woman.
23. Document findings and act accordingly.

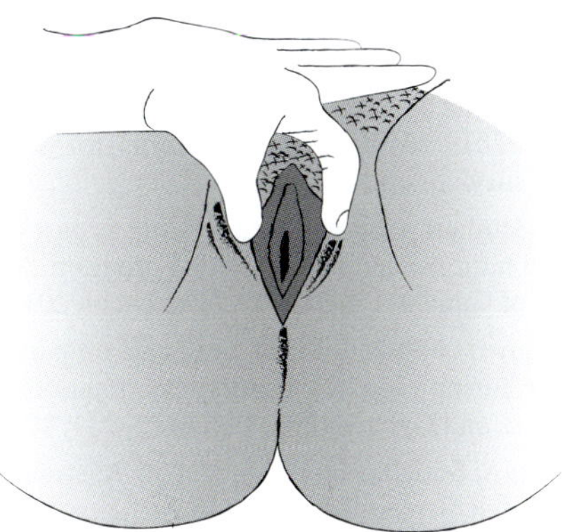

FIGURE 13.6 **Parting labia.**

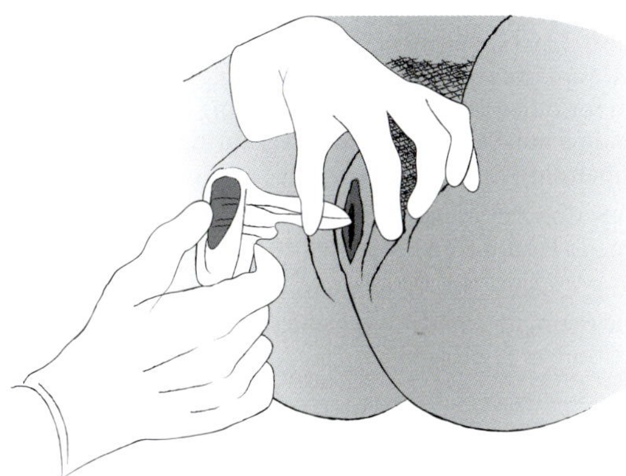

FIGURE 13.7 **Speculum insertion.**

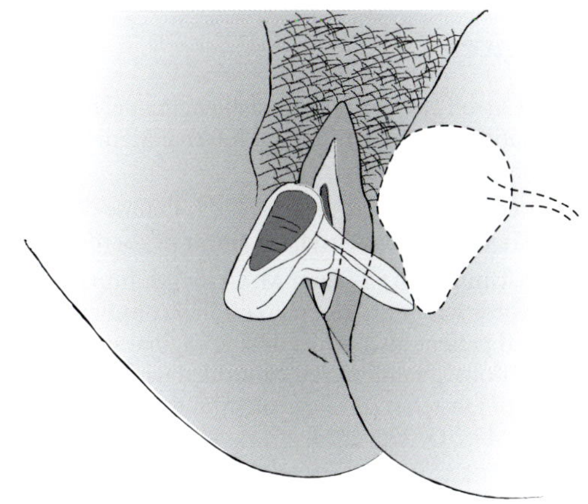

FIGURE 13.8 **Press lever to open blades.**

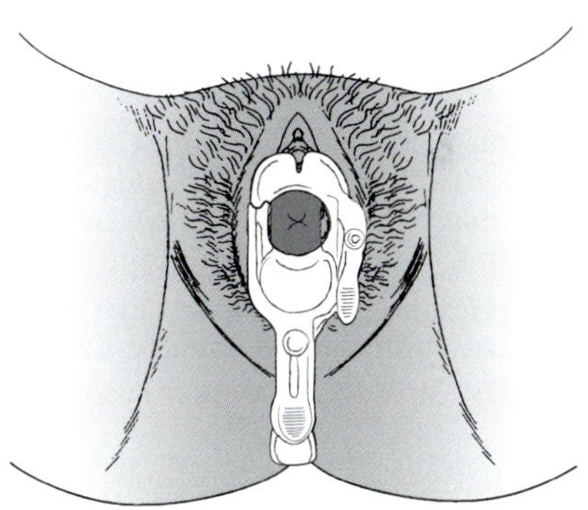

FIGURE 13.9 **Visualising cervix.**

Role and responsibilities of the midwife

These can be summarised as:

- recognising the need for using a vaginal speculum
- ensuring the procedure is undertaken correctly, with minimal discomfort
- recognising what to do if the cervix is not visualised initially
- keeping correct documentation.

SUMMARY

- The size and type of speculum should be appropriate for the clinical indication.
- Insertion of a speculum is intrusive and requires sensitivity and good communication.
- It is important to undertake the procedure correctly to reduce discomfort.
- The principles of asepsis should be followed to reduce the risk of uterine and neonatal infection.

Self-assessment exercises

The answers to the following questions may be found in the text.

1. When might a midwife need to use a speculum?
2. How may discomfort and embarrassment be reduced for the woman during this procedure?
3. Describe how the speculum should be inserted and removed.
4. What can the midwife do if the cervix is not visualised initially?

Resources

Australian Government National Cervical Screening Program: Online 20 March 2021. Available: https://www.health.gov.au/initiatives-and-programs/national-cervical-screening-program.

References

Bates CK, Carroll N, Potter J: The challenging pelvic examination, Journal of General Internal Medicine 26(6):651–657, 2011.

Cancer Council: Cervical screening, 2021. Online 27 March 2021. Available: www.cancer.org.au/cervicalscreening.

Carugno J, Timmons D, Lederer M, Grady M: Impact of using words with unpleasant emotional connotations on perceived patient discomfort during vaginal speculum examinations: a randomized controlled trial, European Journal of Obstetrics & Gynecology and Reproductive Biology 247:203–206, 2020.

Chorley A, Marlow L, Forster A, et al.: Experiences of cervical screening and barriers to participation in the context of an organised programme: a systematic review and thematic synthesis, Psycho-Oncology 26(2):161–172, 2017.

Congress Alukura: Minymaku Kutju Tjukurpa—Women's business manual, 6th ed., 2017. Online 27 March 2021. Available: https://docs.remotephcmanuals.com.au/review/g/manuals2017-manuals/d/20272.html?page=1.

Cook C, Brunton M: The influence of the Cartwright Report on gynaecological examinations and nurses' communication, Nursing Praxis in New Zealand 30:28–38, 2014.

Department of Health: Clinical practice guidelines: pregnancy care, Australian Government, Canberra, 2020

Harris N: Well woman exams for sexual assault survivors, no date. Online 20 March 2021. Available: https://www.med.unc.edu/beacon/wp-content/uploads/sites/598/2019/10/Well_woman_exams_for_sexual_assault_survivors.pdf.

Hawkes D: Human papillomavirus testing as part of the renewed national cervical screening program, Australian Journal of General Practice 47(7):412–414, 2018.

Hill DA, Lamvu G: Effect of lubricating gel on patient comfort during vaginal speculum examination, Obstetrics and Gynecology 119(2):227–231, 2012.

Nagendiram A, Bougher H, Banks J, et al.: Australian women's self-perceived barriers to participation in cervical cancer screening: a systematic review. Health Promotion Journal of Australia 31(3):343–353, 2020.

NSW Health Pathology: Changes to the National Cervical Cancer Program, 2017. Online 14 August 2021. Available: www.pathology.health.nsw.gov.au/clinical-services/changes-to-the-national-cervical-cancer-program.

Secor M, Fantasia HC: Fast facts about the gynecologic exam for nurse practitioners: conducting the GYN exam in a nutshell, New York, 2012, Springer Publishing Company.

Tillman S: Consent in pelvic care. Journal of Midwifery & Women's Health 65(6):749–758, 2020.

Wysocki S: Quality care for women's health. The internal pelvic exam, no fruits or vegetables, Journal for Nurse Practitioners 11:661–662, 2015.

CHAPTER 14

CAPILLARY SAMPLING

Learning outcomes

Having read this chapter, the reader should be able to:

- describe the procedure for obtaining a capillary blood sample
- discuss factors promoting safety and comfort for women and neonates
- describe how to take a newborn bloodspot screen
- discuss the role and responsibilities of the midwife in relation to capillary sampling.

This chapter considers capillary blood sampling for women and neonates. Capillary sampling is for tests requiring a small amount of blood. The use of finger-prick capillary samples for point-of-care testing is increasing and new devices allowing multiple tests from a single capillary sample at the point of care are being developed (Sauer-Budge et al 2017). Capillary samples collected from women are used to determine blood glucose levels and can also be used for testing haemoglobin levels. The midwife collects capillary samples from neonates as part of routine national screening in Australia and New Zealand, and also to detect or confirm deviations from normal (e.g. serum bilirubin or serum glucose).

CONSIDERATIONS WHEN TAKING CAPILLARY SAMPLES

Underpinning anatomy

The blood obtained from a capillary resembles arterial blood in oxygen content, is more likely to be contaminated with skin flora and is suitable when a small blood volume is required. The finger is used for capillary testing in women; the lateral area of the heel is the only site used in neonates and infants to approximately 6 months of age (WHO 2010). In adults the earlobe may be used in research studies.

For finger-prick and heel puncture tests blood is obtained from the capillaries contained within the skin. The arterial–venous network of the skin is located at the junction of the lower dermis and upper subcutaneous tissue. The skin should be punctured only to the depth of this junction to facilitate blood flow.

Neonatal anatomy

In neonates a deeper puncture can have serious complications. In an infant weighing 3 kg the distance from the outer skin surface to bone in the medial and lateral heel is 3.32 mm (WHO 2010). The distance from the outer skin surface to bone in the posterior heel is only 2.33 mm; therefore, this site should be avoided to reduce the chance of hitting bone. If the calcaneus (heel bone) is punctured, there is a risk of osteochondritis or osteomyelitis. The distance between the skin and bone varies depending on the weight and gestation of the neonate and the measurement site on the foot (the narrowest distance is at the posterior curve of the heel).

The plantar arteries and nerves should be avoided. Puncturing the tibial artery can cause the veins to collapse and increase the risk of introducing infection, which could lead to septicaemia. Puncturing the nerves can result in permanent damage to the nerve. Other complications include haematoma, scarring and necrosis. Skin breakdown can occur when adhesive strips are used repeatedly; it is preferable to apply pressure following the procedure.

Lancet selection

The lancet required will be slightly shorter than the estimated depth because pressure compresses the skin; hence, the depth of the puncture will be deeper than the length of the lancet (WHO 2010). Thicker lancets and deeper penetration cause more pain. Lancets are available in lengths ranging from 0.85 to 2.2 mm. For premature neonates, a length as small as 0.85 mm can be used. For a woman, the lancet is usually 2.2 mm because for a finger-prick, the depth should not be more than 2.4 mm. For a newborn heel puncture, the lancet should be < 2.0 mm (Higgins 2013). Automated lancets are used to ensure the puncture depth does not exceed the maximum permitted and also reduces sharps injury as the lancet retracts after use.

Collection order

Capillary samples are collected in the opposite order of venepuncture samples, with haematology specimens collected first, followed by chemistry then blood bank specimens in order to minimise platelet clumping effects (WHO 2010).

CAPILLARY SAMPLING FOR BLOOD GLUCOSE LEVEL—WOMEN

The incidence of diabetes is increasing and midwives will be involved in assessing blood glucose measurements in women with gestational, type 1 or type 2 diabetes mellitus to ensure good glycaemic control (Fig 14.1). Approximately 12–14% of women develop gestational diabetes around the 24th to 28th week of pregnancy (Nankervis et al 2014). Midwives may be required to provide education to ensure women can undertake self-monitoring of blood glucose levels. Many women are anxious about learning to assess their blood glucose and the impact of diabetes on themselves and their neonate (Youngwanichsetha & Phumdoung 2017). Maintaining acceptable blood glucose levels requires regular testing. Meters have a memory and data can be downloaded in various forms, including graphs and charts. Women are also encouraged to keep a diary that includes daily activities and nutritional information. Times for testing blood glucose levels include (Diabetes Australia 2021):

- before breakfast (fasting)
- after lunch/dinner
- before bed
- before rigorous exercise
- when feeling unwell.

Women with type 1 and type 2 diabetes mellitus generally require hourly blood glucose levels when they are in established labour; those with gestational diabetes who are on insulin or metformin generally require 2-hourly blood glucose levels (SA Health 2019).

The target range for blood glucose varies in Australia and New Zealand and may need to be individualised, particularly for women with preexisting diabetes (Rudland et al 2020). Consideration must be given to women with previous episodes of severe or frequent hypoglycaemia, and impaired awareness of hypoglycaemia (Rudland et al 2020). Blood glucose is measured in millimoles per litre (mmol/L); the normal range in non-pregnant women is considered to be between 4.0 to 7.8 mmol/L (Diabetes Australia 2021). Although an optimum treatment target range has not been validated for pregnancy, the Australasian Diabetes in Pregnancy Society (ADIPS) uses target levels during pregnancy based on two standard deviations above the mean values for healthy pregnant women with no known risk factors (Nankervis et al 2014). Target blood glucose levels during pregnancy will be determined by the diabetes team caring for a woman during pregnancy. Table 14.1 lists the ADIPS targets as a guide.

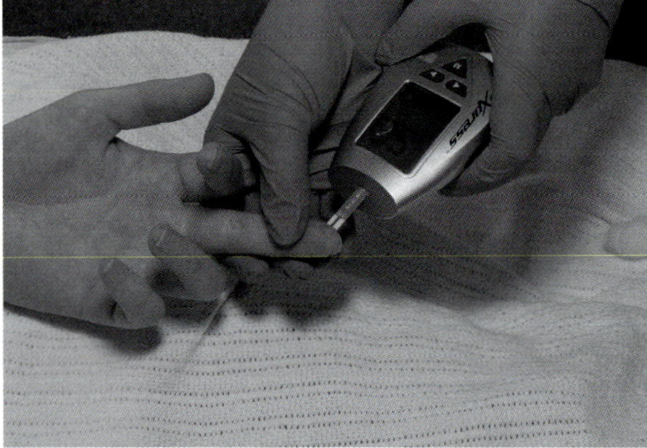

FIGURE 14.1 **Monitoring blood glucose.**

SKILL 14.1 Maternal blood glucose level

1. Gain informed consent.
2. Gather equipment:
   - lancet device and lancets
   - test strips
   - blood glucose meter (women often bring their own meter and may prefer to test their own blood glucose).
3. Perform hand hygiene.
4. Carry out accuracy check as per local protocol if required.
5. Ensure the woman's fingers are clean; washing with soap and water is satisfactory (hand sanitiser or alcohol may affect the reading and should be avoided).
6. Choose a spot on the finger; generally the side of the finger is more comfortable than the finger pad.
7. Prepare the lancet device.
8. Turn on the meter and insert the test strip (in some machines inserting the test strip turns the meter on).
9. Put on non-sterile gloves.
10. Press the lancet on the fingertip and discharge (Fig 14.1).
11. Place the test strip at the base of the drop of blood and hold the test strip until the blood is absorbed.
12. The timer will count down and the reading will appear on the screen.
13. Remove the lancet from the lancet device and place in the sharps container.
14. Perform hand hygiene.
15. Document blood glucose level and take action as required.

TABLE 14.1 BGL TARGETS FOR WOMEN WITH PRE-EXISTING DIABETES (ADIPS)

Fasting and pre-meal	4.0–5.3 mmol/L
1 hour post-meal	5.5–7.8 mmol/L
2 hour post-meal	5.0–6.7 mmol/L

Source: Rudland VL, Price SA, Hughes R, et al: ADIPS 2020 guideline for pre-existing diabetes and pregnancy, Australian & New Zealand Journal of Obstetrics & Gynaecology 60(6):E18–E52, 2020.

CAPILLARY SAMPLING—NEONATE

Repeated heel punctures can make the localised skin sore or infected and expose neonates to a painful procedure. A consistently good sampling technique reduces the risks for the neonate and limits the number of negative experiences. If repeated sampling is required, some other form of venous access (e.g. peripheral cannula) may be considered. The neonate should be kept warm, with only the foot exposed during the procedure. Holding the foot downwards encourages blood flow. Informed consent should be gained for every test and information provided indicating how and when to expect the results.

Guidelines for neonatal site selection

- Use the lateral and medial portions of the heel (plantar surface) as puncture sites.
- Draw an imaginary line from midway between the fourth and fifth toes laterally and medially from the middle of the big toe as the calcaneus rarely extends beyond these (Fig 14.2) (these points are also furthest away from the arteries and nerves).
- For each collection, select a new puncture site not previously punctured and free from bruising.

Comfort of the neonate

Many parents will find collection of capillary samples from their neonates stressful. It is helpful to explain the procedure, the neonate's expected response and strategies to reduce pain. Neonates exhibit behavioural and physiological responses to pain, including facial expressions, body movements and crying (Stevens et al 2016). Facial grimacing consisting of brow bulge, eye squeeze, nasolabial furrow is a marker of pain in neonates (Carbajal 2020, van der Vaart et al 2019, Taddio et al 2011). Physiological responses include an increased heart and respiratory rate and decreased oxygen saturation (Stevens et al 2016; Witt et al 2016), which may inhibit blood flow as the leg muscles contract and impede circulation.

Skin-to-skin contact assists with pain relief in premature infants (Olsson et al 2016). There is evidence that oral sucrose is an effective and safe method for reducing pain responses in both preterm and full-term neonates (Campbell et al 2014) (Table 14.2). Neonates breastfed during painful procedures had a shorter crying time, a smaller increase in heart rate and a smaller decrease in oxygen saturation (Singh et al 2016). Sucrose at concentrations from 20% to 30% appears to reduce pain associated with heel punctures (Matsuda 2017). Sucrose combined with interventions such as non-nutritive sucking and swaddling were the most effective (Matsuda 2017). A Cochrane Review found that sucrose reduced pain from a heel lance in term and preterm infants without serious side effects, indicating that further research is necessary to determine the minimum effective dose (Stevens et al 2016). A musical intervention where a lullaby was played for 20 minutes prior to a heel puncture and 7 minutes afterwards showed a significant reduction when sucrose and music therapy were combined (Shah et al 2017).

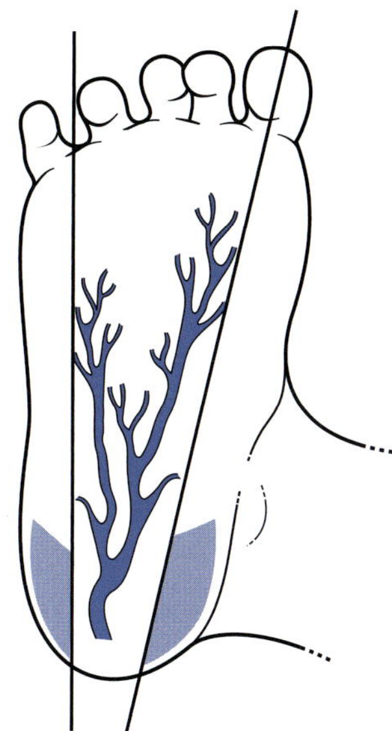

FIGURE 14.2 **The ideal sites for capillary sampling in the neonate (shaded areas).**
Source: Johnson R, Taylor W: Skills for midwifery practice, 4th ed., Elsevier, London, 2016.

TABLE 14.2 SUCROSE DOSAGE

Gestation	Dosage (24% sucrose solution)	Total dose in 24 hours
Term neonate	0.5–1.0 mL	3 mL if > 1500 g
Preterm neonate ≥ 1500 g	0.25 mL	
Preterm neonate 1000–1500 g	0.15 mL	2 mL if <1500 g
Very low birth weight (VLBW)	0.05–0.1 mL if deemed appropriate	1 mL if <1000 g

Source: Adapted from Government of Western Australia. Child and Adolescent Health Service; Pain assessment and management, 2021. Available: www.cahs.health.wa.gov.au/-/media/HSPs/CAHS/Documents/Health-Professionals/Neonatology-guidelines/Pain-Assessment-and-Management.pdf.

Sucrose results in the release of endogenous opioids (Wallace & Jones 2017). Sucrose is applied to the anterior tip of the tongue approximately 2 minutes before a painful procedure and a soother (dummy) offered with parental consent. During administration the neonates should be awake and in a feeding position to minimise the risk of aspiration. Some parents may be opposed to the idea of administering sucrose to their neonate.

Neonatal bilirubin

Midwives play an important role in the detection of **neonatal bilirubin**. Approximately 60% of neonates will develop jaundice during the first week (Pearsall & Morrow 2016). Jaundice may be haemolytic or non-haemolytic. Risk factors for haemolytic jaundice include alloimmunisation, blood group or having a sibling who was jaundiced; for non-haemolytic jaundice the risk factors are preterm birth, maternal origin from Asia, maternal obesity and having a sibling who was jaundiced (Lee et al 2016). Although rare, serious consequences may result from untreated hyperbilirubinaemia, including acute or chronic bilirubin encephalopathy and permanent brain damage known as kernicterus (Pearsall & Morrow 2016).

A capillary sample may be taken to estimate the level of unconjugated bilirubin in the blood of a jaundiced neonate. Generally an amber-coloured serum microcapillary tube is used for sample collection because bilirubin is photosensitive (Fig 14.3). Care should be taken to avoid getting air in the capillary tubes as this may result in the blood dispersing totally from the tubes during spinning, necessitating a further blood test. The appropriate amount should be collected (usually 0.5 mL) as an inadequate specimen may require the sample to be collected again.

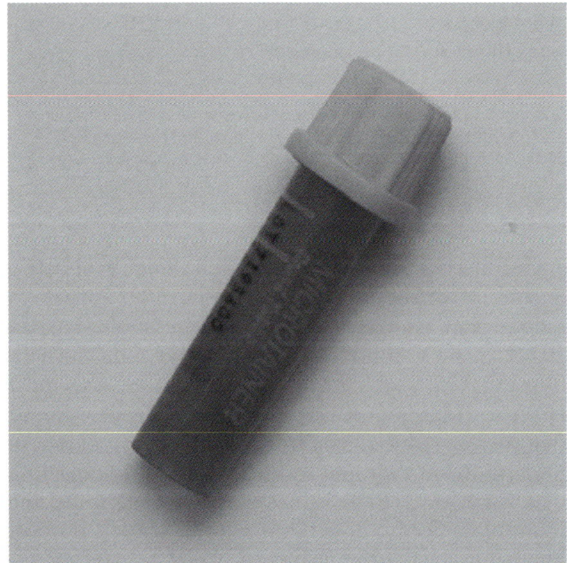

FIGURE 14.3 **Amber microcapillary tube for collecting specimen for neonatal jaundice.**

Neonatal blood glucose

A diagnostic neonatal blood glucose test is frequently taken when hypoglycaemia is suspected or as a screening test in neonates considered at risk of developing hypoglycaemia. Prior to birth the fetus receives a continuous supply of glucose. After birth the maternal glucose supply ceases and blood glucose levels fall and consequently insulin levels decrease. These changes result in the newborn commencing glucose production; however, normal concentrations of glucose are not reached for approximately 72 hours (Harding et al 2017). Hypoglycaemia is common in the hours after birth and is often transient. Defining neonatal hypoglycaemia is difficult as normal healthy neonates may have a transient, asymptomatic drop in glucose levels; in other more susceptible newborns hypoglycaemia can persist. Neonatal hypoglycaemia has been defined as < 2.6 mmol/L (Harding et al 2017) and by age and gestation (NSW Health 2016). Neonatal hypoglycaemia affects up to 15% of newborns (Hegarty et al 2016). Severe and persistent hypoglycaemia in the newborn can have serious consequences, including seizures and brain injury (Harding et al 2017).

NSW Health (2016) indicates that it is important to differentiate between an intervention threshold (where injury is not likely, but intervention is indicated) and a pathological threshold (which is likely to cause injury if left untreated). Each health district will have a policy outlining when to perform glucose screening and the interventions required if the neonate's blood sugar is low. The levels in Table 14.3 are listed as an example but may vary between health districts.

Glucose screening meters can underestimate the blood glucose level and a formal blood glucose level

TABLE 14.3 NEONATAL BLOOD GLUCOSE THRESHOLDS

Intervention threshold	
During first 24 hours in well neonates > 34 weeks	$\leq$ 2.0 mmol/L
After 24 hours in well neonates born after 34 weeks	$\leq$ 2.5 mmol/L
At any time in an unwell neonate, term or preterm	$\leq$ 2.5 mmol/L
Pathological threshold	
Urgent intervention required	$\leq$ 1.5 mmol/L (any neonate)
Symptoms of hypoglycaemia	$\leq$ 2.5 mmol/L (any neonate)

Source: NSW Health: Guideline. Women and babies: Neonatal hypoglycaemia—prevention and management, 2016. Online 31 March 2021. Available: www.slhd.nsw.gov.au/rpa/neonatal%5Ccontent/pdf/guidelines/RPAH_Hypoglycaemia_GL2016_032.pdf.

may be necessary to validate hypoglycaemia. Cleansing of the skin with alcohol-impregnated wipes affects the accuracy of the results and should be avoided. A 2016 Cochrane Review examining the efficacy of oral dextrose gel for the treatment of newborns with hypoglycaemia found treatment with 40% dextrose gel reduced separation of mothers and infants and improved the likelihood of full breastfeeding (Weston et al 2016). A randomised controlled trial in New Zealand found that a prophylactic buccal dose of 0.5 mL/kg of dextrose gel given to at-risk newborns at 1 hour of age could prevent development of hypoglycaemia (Hegarty et al 2016).

NEWBORN BLOODSPOT SCREENING

Free **newborn bloodspot screening (NBS)** is offered to all neonates born in Australia and New Zealand. Within Australia, each state has a newborn screening program funded by the state and territory governments, with services coordinated from centralised screening laboratories (New South Wales, Queensland, South Australia, Victoria and Western Australia). New South Wales has a flowchart on the screening process (Fig 14.4). In New Zealand the Ministry of Health funds a national

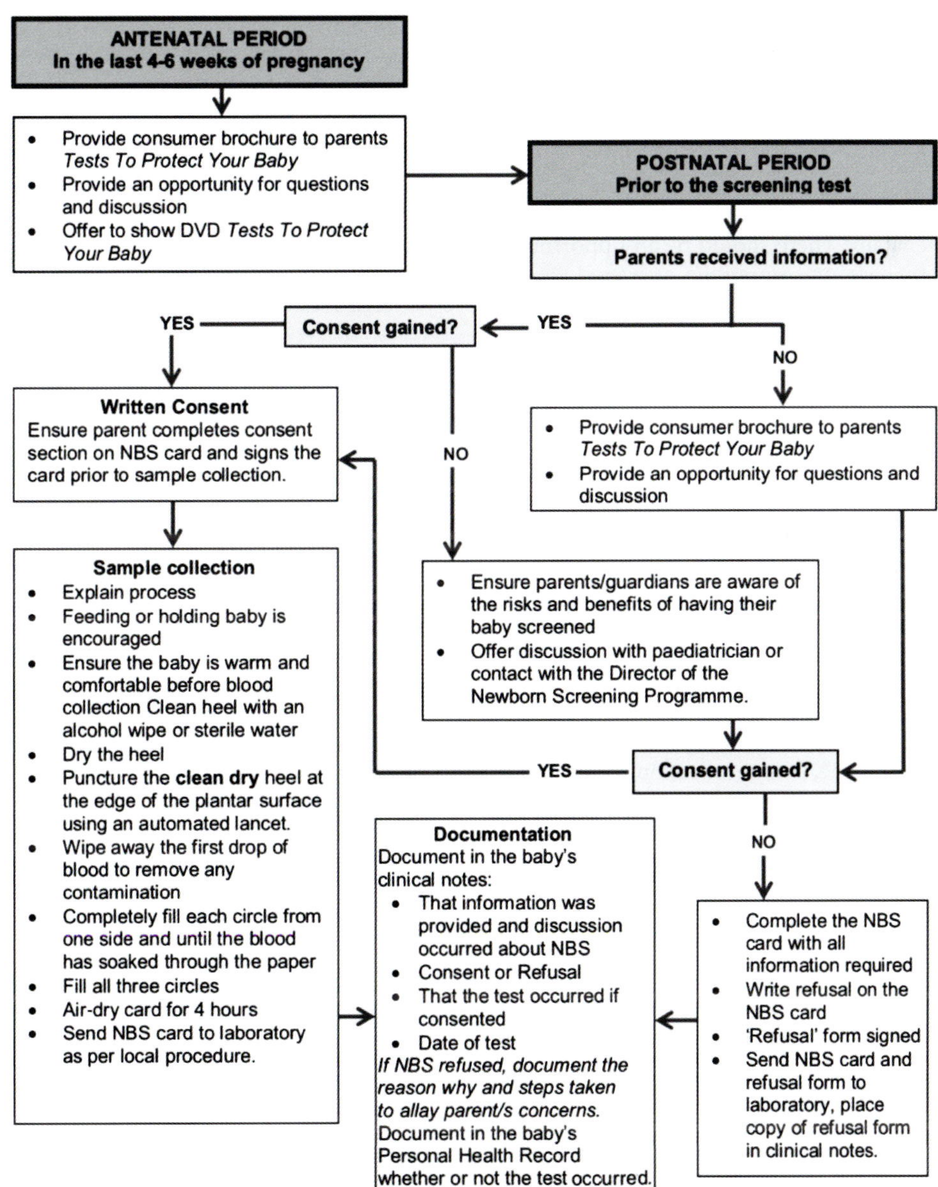

FIGURE 14.4 Newborn bloodspot screening process flowchart, New South Wales.
Source: NSW Health: Policy directive. Newborn bloodspot screening policy (PD2016_015) updated, 2021. Online 30 March 2021: Available: www.health.nsw.gov.au/policies/manuals/Documents/pmm-2.pdf.

program which has a screening flowchart for guidance (Fig 14.5). New Zealand was one of the first nations to have a national screening program. NBS has been performed in all states and territories in Australia since the 1960s (Department of Health 2017).

The national Australian NBS framework indicates that appropriate and timely information should be provided to families (Department of Health 2017). NBS detects serious disorders that can be treated following early diagnosis to prevent serious morbidity and mortality. The blood sample is collected by a heel puncture when the neonate is 48–72 hours old. Screening at this age is recommended to instigate diagnosis/treatment as early as possible and avoid serious consequences. A parent is required to sign the consent on the back of the NBS card. In order to provide informed consent, parents must understand the purpose of the test, how the sample is collected and stored, its potential future use, as well as privacy and protection processes. Australia and New Zealand have brochures available for parents; ideally these are provided antenatally. There should be an opportunity for parents to have any questions answered. For a discussion on the ethics of population screening see Pairman and colleagues (2018). The NBS program screens for around 25 medical conditions in Australia and over 20 in New Zealand, some of which are listed in Table 14.4.

Documentation

When filling in the card use a black ballpoint pen; do not use pencil, ink or felt pens. Ensure all information is legible and complete; a hospital label may be placed on the back of the card but must not cover any information or be near the bloodspots. It is essential that the name of the paediatrician, GP or midwife who will initiate follow-up of an abnormal result is written on the card.

The card should be completed fully and contemporaneously. The neonate's identification number, mother's name, date of collection, location and any relevant information is included. The information shown in Fig 14.6 is entered in the notes; some health services have a stamp available. Completion of NBS must also be documented in the neonate's personal health record.

If the neonate's parents or guardian refuse the NBS they can be provided with an opportunity to outline their concerns with the paediatrician and given a telephone number for the newborn screening program. Parents are advised to notify their healthcare worker to indicate that the infant has not been screened. Refusal, including the reason, should be documented in the newborn's clinical notes and personal health record. All the information should be completed on the newborn screening card, with the addition of refusal written on the card. The card should be sent to the newborn screening program as usual. In the event of refusal, parents may be required to sign a disclaimer form.

Collecting the newborn bloodspot screen

The bloodspot sample is obtained by a heel puncture, ideally when the neonate is 48–72 hours old. A dedicated, preprinted filter paper card is supplied. The card allows the blood to soak through to the depth required for accurate testing. Cards contain three or four circles and should be filled completely; in some cases three circles will be sufficient on a four-circle card. The card should not be used if it is damaged and the sample area should not be touched. If the sample is unable to be obtained by a heel puncture, blood from venepuncture can be used, but care must be taken to ensure the blood is not contaminated by preservatives or any other solutions. Lithium heparin or EDTA solutions may interfere with results. During collection, comfort measures such as breastfeeding are encouraged.

Storage of newborn bloodspot screen

In Australia cards must be kept for at least 2 years and are generally retained for 18 years. In Queensland the sample is kept for 28 years unless a request to destroy the card is received and then it will be destroyed after 2 years. In Western Australia the card is destroyed after 2 years. In New Zealand parents either consent for the card to be returned to them or for it to be stored indefinitely; parents can request the card to be returned at any time. The test results are normally available 1–2 working days after receipt of the sample. For normal results an individual report is not provided; however, a summary report is provided to the hospital, birth centre or homebirth midwife.

Inaccurate results may be obtained if the blood:

- is multilayered
- is multi-spotted (several smaller drops fill the circle)
- has been forced out of the heel by squeezing
- is contaminated (faeces, adult blood, alcohol, heparin or any other substance in close proximity) or compressed
- has not soaked through.

The newborn bloodspot should be collected prior to any blood transfusion. If blood was not collected prior to the blood transfusion, a repeat sample may be taken 48 hours after the blood transfusion and a repeat sample collected 2 weeks post transfusion (Sydney Children's Health Network [SCHN] 2015). The date and time of the blood transfusion should be documented on the newborn screening card under the relevant clinical information section.

Metabolic disorders, particularly congenital hypothyroidism, may be missed in neonates whose birth weight is ≤ 1500 grams. A repeat sample should be collected when the infant is more mature; this is usually between 2 to 4 weeks. Infants who were born overseas and did not receive a newborn screening test in their country of birth can be offered the newborn screening test up to 1 year of age.

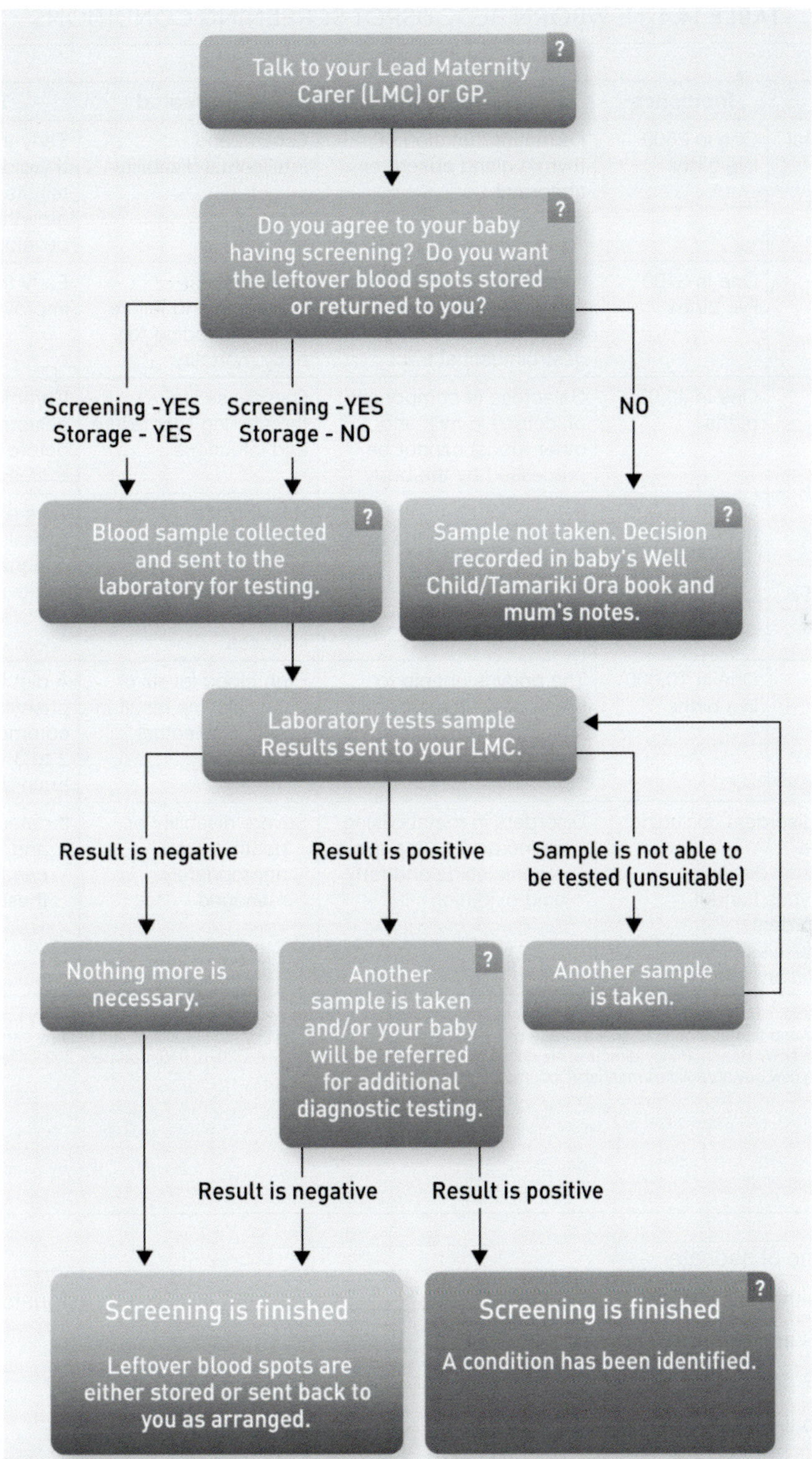

FIGURE 14.5 **Newborn metabolic screening program flowchart, New Zealand.**
Source: National Screening Unit: Newborn metabolic screening program—heel prick test: how the process works, 2014. Online 30 March 2021. Available: www.nsu.govt.nz/pregnancy-newborn-screening/newborn-metabolic-screening-programme-heel-prick-test.

TABLE 14.4 NEWBORN BLOODSPOT SCREENING CONDITIONS

Conditions screened for				
Condition	**Incidence**	**Effects of condition**	**If untreated**	**Treatment**
Primary congenital hypothyroidism	One in 2600 live births	Formation/function of thyroid gland absent or abnormal	Growth and intellectual disability	Early treatment with thyroid hormone results in normal growth and development
Cystic fibrosis*	One in 3700 live births	A genetic disorder which results in thick mucus, especially in the lungs and gastrointestinal tract	Severe chest infections and failure to thrive leading to early mortality	Early treatment improves health
Galactosaemia	One in 40,000 births	Galactose (a component of lactose in milk and other foods) cannot be processed by the body	Can cause life-threatening liver failure and infections	Commening a galactose-free diet before 2 weeks of age is lifesaving
Medium-chain acyl-coenzyme A dehydrogenase (MCAD) deficiency	One in 15,000 births	Fat cannot be completely broken down by the body	Possibly life-threatening or may result in severe disability following common childhood illnesses	Take extra precautions to make sure there is adequate energy intake during illness
Phenylketonuria	One in 10,000 live births	The body is unable to break down the essential amino acid phenylalanine	High blood levels of phenylalanine result in severe intellectual disability	A diet low in phenylalanine commenced in the first 2 to 3 weeks prevents brain damage
Rare metabolic disorders, including: • homocystinuria • maple syrup urine disease • tyrosinaemia types I and II • urea cycle disorders • organic acidopathies • fatty acid oxidation defects		Disorders in metabolising amino acids, urea cycle, organic acids and fatty acid oxidation	Severe disability or death if not appropriately managed	If detected early, diet and medications can treat most of these disorders

*Note: For cystic fibrosis, NBS detects approximately 95% of cases in neonates. Some neonates who are healthy carriers may also test positive; however, a sweat test at around 6 weeks of age will determine if the neonate has cystic fibrosis or is a healthy carrier.
Source: Adapted from NSW Health: Policy directive. Newborn bloodspot screening policy (PD2016_015) updated, 2021. Online 30 March 2021: Available: www.health.nsw.gov.au/policies/manuals/Documents/pmm-2.pdf.

Name of neonate ______________________________

Health professional ______________________________(signature)

NBS information discussed ____________________ Date __________

NBS pamphlet given to parents ____________________ Date __________

Verbal/written consent obtained ____________________ Date __________

Sample collection completed ____________________ Date __________

FIGURE 14.6 **Documentation stamp example.**
Source: Adapted from NSW Health: Policy directive. Newborn bloodspot screening policy (PD2016_015) updated, 2021. Online 30 March 2021: Available: www.health.nsw.gov.au/policies/manuals/Documents/pmm-2.pdf.

Repeat tests are requested if:

- a specific condition, such as cystic fibrosis, requires a repeat test
- the test was taken before 48 hours of age
- the specimen card has errors or omissions
- the test was taken less than 72 hours after transfusion of a blood product
- the sample is insufficient or contaminated
- there was a delay in the sample reaching the laboratory
- results were slightly abnormal.

Role and responsibilities of the midwife

These can be summarised as:

- recognising the need for capillary blood sampling
- undertaking the procedure correctly and safely
- ensuring comfort measures for the neonate
- educating and supporting the parents
- understanding blood glucose monitoring
- contemporaneous record keeping
- actioning the results, where appropriate.

SKILL 14.2 Collecting a newborn bloodspot screen or capillary sample

1. Gain informed consent from the parents; determine if they will be present and who will hold the neonate.
2. Gather equipment:
   - non-sterile gloves
   - automated fully retractable sterile lancet, blade length < 2.0 mm
   - newborn screening card or correct specimen tube/s
   - cottonwool balls or gauze swabs
   - sterile water or warm water (according to local protocol)
   - sharps container.
3. Perform hand hygiene and apply non-sterile gloves.
4. Ask the parent to hold/cuddle/comfort/breastfeed the neonate according to the chosen method of comfort; encourage a calm and relaxed atmosphere; sucrose and non-nutritive sucking may also be used.
5. Inspect the foot to select the best site (free from previous punctures or bruising), avoiding underlying nerves and bone (see Fig 14.2, p. 143).
6. Warm the newborn's foot using booties or hands; do not use cloths which have been placed in hot water (may result in scalds).
7. Ensure the neonate's leg is below the rest of the body.
8. Clean the neonate's heel with water and gauze or cottonwool and dry with gauze or cottonwool before puncturing (avoid applying alcohol, vaseline or paraffin to the heel as these substances can interfere with results).
9. Hold the ankle with the foot flexed.
10. Using a retractable sterile lancet (point depth < 2.0 mm) puncture the heel on the inner or outer border, using a quick and firm action.
11. Wipe away the first drop of blood using a sterile cottonwool swab to ensure the sample is not contaminated with fluid or debris.
12. Gently massage above the puncture site to encourage blood flow and drop blood onto one side of the filter paper (avoid squeezing as this can dilute the sample with plasma and increases the chance of haemolysis).
13. For the bloodspot screen, complete each circle ensuring blood soaks through the card to the other side. Avoid rubbing the heel on the card. For capillary sample, fill the collection tube to required level.
14. If blood does not flow, consider a second puncture using a different site on the same foot or the other foot.
15. When completed, use a cottonwool ball or gauze swab to apply gentle pressure to the site until bleeding stops; do not apply plaster or tape.
16. Place lancet in sharps container, dispose of equipment correctly.
17. Perform hand hygiene.
18. Ensure all information on the card is completed.
19. Document specimen collection and relevant results and act accordingly. The newborn bloodspot screen will need to be documented in the newborn's personal health record. A stamp may be available to document collection in the chart notes.
20. Cards should remain horizontal until completely dry, preferably using a drying rack (drying takes 4 hours). The card should be at room temperature and not exposed to artificial heat or sunlight. When stacking the cards, alternate the direction so the bloodspots cannot touch each other.
21. Dispatch samples promptly; samples should not be placed in a plastic bag, as this promotes bacterial growth and may invalidate the test results.

Source: World Health Organization (WHO): WHO guidelines on drawing blood: best practices in phlebotomy, 2010. Online 30 March 2021. Available: www.ncbi.nlm.nih.gov/books/NBK138650/pdf/Bookshelf_NBK138650.pdf.

SUMMARY

- Obtaining a capillary blood sample from the neonate should be undertaken only when required, as there are risk factors associated with this procedure. Informed consent should be gained from the parents.
- The reliability of the results partly depends upon the accuracy of the procedure. When undertaking NBS, care should be taken not to contaminate the specimen, to fill each circle with blood, to fully complete the request card and to ensure its prompt dispatch.
- The midwife should be aware of measures to minimise pain and distress for parents and neonates.

Self-assessment exercises

The answers to the following questions may be found in the text.

1. List the indications for undertaking capillary blood sampling.
2. Discuss how to avoid the risk of damage to the underlying nerves and bone when obtaining a capillary blood sample from the heel of a neonate.
3. Describe how blood flow can be encouraged during a neonatal heel puncture.
4. List the possible factors resulting in a repeat NBS being required.
5. List strategies to minimise the amount of pain felt by the neonate.
6. Discuss the role and responsibilities of the midwife in relation to capillary sampling.

Resources

Government of Western Australia. Department of Health: Your newborn baby's bloodspot screening test. https://healthywa.wa.gov.au/Articles/U_Z/Your-newborn-babys-screening-test.

International Society for Neonatal Screening (ISNS): www.isns-neoscreening.org.

National Diabetes Services Scheme and Diabetes Australia: Having a healthy baby: a guide to planning and managing pregnancy for women with type 1 diabetes. www.ndss.com.au/about-diabetes/resources/find-a-resource/having-a-healthy-baby-guide-for-women-with-type-1-diabetes/.

National Screening Unit (New Zealand): www.nsu.govt.nz/pregnancy-newborn-screening/newborn-metabolic-screening-programme-heel-prick-test.

Newborn Bloodspot Screening brochure (in English) can be downloaded from: www.schn.health.nsw.gov.au/files/attachments/newborn_screening_guidlines_2015.pdf. Also available from the Office of Kids and Families website in Arabic, Traditional Chinese, Indonesian, Japanese, Khmer, Korean, Serbian, Turkish and Vietnamese, Thai, Bengali, Nepali, Tamil and Hindi: www.health.nsw.gov.au/kidsfamilies/MCFhealth/Pages/tests-newborn-bloodspot.aspx.

Newborn Metabolic Screening Programme monitoring indicators New Zealand. Online 30 March 2021: www.nsu.govt.nz/system/files/page/newborn-metabolic-screening-programme-monitoring-indicators-feb18.pdf.

NSW & ACT Newborn Screening Tests Education Video for Parents: www.youtube.com/watch?v=KVmLpVcnI1w.

Starship Child Health New Zealand: Hypoglycaemia in the newborn. www.starship.org.nz/guidelines/hypoglycaemia-in-the-neonate/.

The Sydney Children's Hospital Network: NSW Newborn Screening Program. www.schn.health.nsw.gov.au/find-a-service/laboratory-services/newborn-screening.

References

Campbell N, Cleaver K, Davies N: Oral sucrose as analgesia for neonates: how effective and safe is the sweet solution? A review of the literature, Journal of Neonatal Nursing 20:274–282, 2014.

Carbajal R: Neonatal pain. In Emerging topics and controversies in neonatology, Springer International Publishing, 2020, pp. 485–501.

Department of Health: Newborn bloodspot screening national policy framework, 2017. Online 30 March 2021. Available: www.health.gov.au/resources/publications/newborn-bloodspot-screening-national-policy-framework.

Diabetes Australia: Blood glucose monitoring, 2021. Online 30 March 2021. Available: www.diabetesaustralia.com.au/blood-glucose-monitoring.

Harding JE, Harris DL, Hegarty JE, et al: An emerging evidence base for the management of neonatal hypoglycaemia, Early Human Development, 104:51–56, 2017.

Hegarty JE, Harding JE, Gamble GD, et al: prophylactic oral dextrose gel for newborn babies at risk of neonatal hypoglycaemia: a randomised controlled dose-finding trial (the Pre-hPOD Study), PLoS Medicine 13:1–19, 2016.

Higgins C: Understanding laboratory investigations a guide for nurses, midwives and healthcare professionals, 3rd ed., Wiley-Blackwell, Oxford, 2013.

Lee BK, Le Ray I, Sun JY, et al: Haemolytic and nonhaemolytic neonatal jaundice have different risk factor profiles, Acta Paediatrica 105:1444–1450, 2016.

Matsuda E: Sucrose for analgesia in newborn infants undergoing painful procedures, Nursing Standard 31:61–63, 2017.

Nankervis A, McIntyre HD, Moses R, et al; for the Australasian Diabetes in Pregnancy Society: ADIPS Consensus Guidelines for the Testing and Diagnosis of Gestational Diabetes Mellitus in Australia and New Zealand, 2014.

NSW Health: Guideline. Women and babies: Neonatal hypoglycaemia—prevention and management, 2016. Online 31 March 2021. Available: www.slhd.nsw.gov.au/rpa/neonatal%5Ccontent/pdf/guidelines/RPAH_Hypoglycaemia_GL2016_032.pdf.

Olsson E, Ahlsén G, Eriksson M: Skin-to-skin contact reduces near-infrared spectroscopy pain responses in premature infants during blood sampling, Acta Paediatrica 105:376–380, 2016.

Pairman S, Tracy K, Dahlen, HG, Dixon L: Midwifery, 4th ed., Elsevier, Sydney, 2018.

Pearsall R, Morrow G: Jaundice in newborns, World of Irish Nursing & Midwifery 24:51–53, 2016.

Rudland VL, Price SA, Hughes R, et al: ADIPS 2020 guideline for pre-existing diabetes and pregnancy, Australian & New Zealand Journal of Obstetrics & Gynaecology 60(6):E18–E52, 2020.

SA Health: Perinatal practice guideline: diabetes mellitus and gestational diabetes, 2019. Online 30 March 2021. Available: www.sahealth.sa.gov.au/wps/wcm/connect/public+content/sa+health+internet/clinical+resources/clinical+programs+and+practice+guidelines/womens+and+babies+health/perinatal/perinatal+practice+guidelines/perinatal+practice+guidelines?az=az-d.

Sauer-Budge AF, Brookfield SJ, Janzen R, et al: A novel device for collecting and dispensing fingerstick blood for point of care testing, PLoS ONE 12:1–13, 2017.

Shah WR, Kadage S, Sinn J: Trial of music, sucrose, and combination therapy for pain relief during heel prick procedures in neonates, Journal of Pediatrics 190: 153–158, 2017.

Singh RK, Simalti AK, Singh D: Breast feeding as analgesia in neonates: a randomized controlled trial, Journal of Nepal Paediatric Society 36:238–242, 2016.

Stevens B, Yamada J, Ohlsson A, et al: Sucrose for analgesia in newborn infants undergoing painful procedures, Cochrane Database of Systematic Reviews (7): CD001069, 2016.

Sydney Children's Health Network (SCHN): NSW and ACT newborn screening programme—sampling information and guidelines, 2015. Online 30 March 2021. Available: www.schn.health.nsw.gov.au/files/attachments/newborn_screening_guidlines_2015.pdf.

Taddio A, Shah V, Stephens D, et al: Effect of liposomal lidocaine and sucrose alone and in combination for venipuncture pain in newborns, Pediatrics 127(4): e940–947, 2011.

Van der Vaart M, Duff E, Raafat N, et al.: Multimodal pain assessment improves discrimination between noxious and non-noxious stimuli in infants. Paediatric and Neonatal Pain 1(1):21–30, 2019.

Wallace H, Jones T: Managing procedural pain on the neonatal unit: Do inconsistencies still exist in practice? Journal of Neonatal Nursing 23:119–126, 2017.

Weston PJ, Harris DL, Battin M, et al: Oral dextrose gel for the treatment of hypoglycaemia in newborn infants, Cochrane Database of Systematic Reviews (5):CD011027, 2016.

Witt N, Coynor S, Edwards C, Bradshaw H: A guide to pain assessment and management in the neonate. Current Emergency and Hospital Medicine Reports 4(1):1–10, 2016.

Youngwanichsetha S, Phumdoung S: Lived experience of blood glucose self-monitoring among pregnant women with gestational diabetes mellitus: a phenomenological research, Journal of Clinical Nursing 26:2915–2921, 2017.

SECTION 4

PRINCIPLES OF ELIMINATION MANAGEMENT

CHAPTER 15

MICTURITION AND CATHETERISATION

Learning outcomes

Having read this chapter, the reader should be able to:

- define micturition, describing normal adult urine volumes
- discuss the changes to the urinary tract related to childbearing
- describe how to facilitate normal micturition
- describe the basic anatomy and physiology of the urinary system
- describe how to insert and remove a urethral catheter.

The care and protection of the urinary tract throughout the childbirth continuum is an important component of midwifery care. Midwives are required to support normal micturition, monitor bladder health, detect infection and protect continence. Insertion, monitoring and removal of indwelling urinary catheters is a necessary skill for midwives. This chapter reviews the factors influencing micturition and the direct effects of childbearing on the urinary tract. Clinical skills related to the safe use of bedpans, urinary catheterisation and indwelling catheter care are outlined.

PHYSIOLOGY

Daily metabolism of nutrients provides the body with energy and produces waste products such as urea, ammonia and creatinine. The waste products, including excess water and electrolytes, are removed from the blood and concentrated into urine by the kidneys and then excreted via the urinary tract (Cooper & Gosnell 2018). The kidneys play a vital role in homeostasis by regulating fluid, electrolytes and acid–base balance (pH) and secreting erythropoietin (Cooper & Gosnell 2018). The renal system helps maintain the amount and composition of extracellular fluid in the body (Bullock & Hales 2018).

The kidneys are approximately 10 cm long, 5 cm wide and 5.5 cm thick (Moore et al 2018). They contain nephrons which process urine, maintain fluid balance and remove toxic waste (Cooper & Gosnell 2018). After urine is formed it passes into the two ureters, each 25–30 cm long; the ureters join the bladder at the ureterovesical junction. Urine is stored in the bladder, a collapsible muscle located behind the symphysis pubis. The bladder is within the pelvis; however, as the bladder fills with urine, it rises into the abdomen and becomes palpable.

Micturition (urination) is the act of voiding (emptying) urine from the bladder via the urethra. It requires a functioning renal system with coordination between the brain and nervous system. The bladder fills at approximately 0.5 mL/kg/hr and the sensation of needing to empty the bladder occurs in adults at a 200–400 mL volume. A full bladder activates stretch receptors which send a message to the spinal cord indicating the bladder is full. Release of urine from the bladder is controlled by two sphincters. The internal sphincter is made of involuntary muscle which contracts when the stretch receptors are activated and pushes urine past the internal sphincter where it presses on the external sphincter. The external sphincter is under voluntary control, so urine may be held until an appropriate time. The urethra carries urine from the bladder by peristalsis and terminates at the urinary meatus. A woman's urethra is approximately 4 cm long and 6 mm in diameter; the male urethra is 18–22 cm long (Moore et al 2018). The amount of urine produced varies depending on factors such as the amount of liquid consumed and the rate of fluid loss; the normal amount is 750–2000 mL per day.

A functioning renal system is essential for life. Midwives play an important role in supporting and promoting healthy micturition and preventing bladder compromise. Various factors influence micturition; these include:

- anxiety/stress
- personal habits—distraction (e.g. reading), privacy, time, etc.
- poor muscle tone due to damage or increasing age
- pain
- position
- disease
- urinary infection
- obstruction (e.g. compression from the enlarging uterus, presenting part, faecal impaction)
- damage to the nervous pathway due to trauma, disease or age
- surgery
- stress incontinence
- drugs—anticholinergics (e.g. atropine), antihypertensives (e.g. methyldopa), antihistamines (e.g. pseudoephedrine), beta-adrenergic blockers (e.g. propranolol), uterotonics (e.g. oxytocin).

Pregnancy-related physiology

Hormonal changes during pregnancy initiate major alterations in the structure and function of the renal system. Increased blood volume, cardiac output and vasodilation result in increased renal blood flow (Conrad & Davison 2014). The higher blood flow to the kidneys increases urine production. By the fourth week of pregnancy, the **glomerular filtration rate (GFR)** has increased by 20% and at term is 40% higher than in non-pregnancy (Hussein & Lafayette 2014). The increased glomerular filtration rate improves the ability of the kidneys to remove the products of metabolism from the circulation (Hussein & Lafayette 2014).

At about 10 weeks gestation, the renal calyces, renal pelvis and ureters begin to enlarge (particularly on the right side) and dilation continues to increase throughout pregnancy (Platte 2019). The kidney increases in size by approximately 30% (Hussein & Lafayette 2014). Progesterone-induced smooth muscle relaxation and compression of the ureters by the growing fetus leads to dilation of the urinary collecting system and physiological hydronephrosis (Smyth et al 2013). During the last trimester, the enlarging uterus displaces the ureters laterally; they elongate, becoming more tortuous. A dramatic rise in ureteric volume means up to 300 mL of urine can be held in the ureters with a resultant increase in urine stasis and the risk of **urinary tract infection** (UTI) (Blackburn 2018).

Progesterone relaxes the smooth muscle of the bladder and ureters, resulting in decreased tone and possible stasis of urine. Compromising of the vesicoureteral valve can allow reflux of urine. Bladder capacity doubles by term, with the bladder holding up to 1000 mL (Blackburn 2018). The bladder mucosa becomes more oedematous, predisposing it to trauma or infection. Asymptomatic bacteriuria (bacterial urine infection without typical symptoms) occurs in 2–15% of pregnancies (Smaill & Vazquez 2019). Treatment with antibiotics appears to reduce the risk of pyelonephritis, preterm birth and low birth weight (Smaill & Vazquez 2019). If untreated, up to 30% of pregnant women with asymptomatic bacteriuria develop pyelonephritis (McGarry & Tong 2015, Smaill & Vazquez 2019). The incidence of pyelonephritis increases as gestation advances.

UTIs are the most common bacterial infection in both pregnant and non-pregnant women, with an incidence of 17–20% during pregnancy (McGarry & Tong 2015). The Australian antenatal guidelines recommend testing for asymptomatic bacteriuria in early pregnancy with a urine culture. UTI during pregnancy is associated with adverse outcomes, including low birth weight and preterm labour (Platte 2019). The signs of a lower UTI (cystitis) are dysuria, urgency, frequency, haematuria, suprapubic pain and preterm labour. The signs of an upper UTI (pyelonephritis) include abrupt onset of fever/chills, nausea/vomiting, unilateral or bilateral flank pain and preterm labour (McGarry & Tong 2015). The incidence of UTI in pregnant women is 2.4 times higher in Indigenous women than non-Indigenous women; in New Zealand, Māori peoples have double the rate of hospitalisation for UTIs (Bullock & Hales 2018). The incidence of pyelonephritis during pregnancy is 0.5–2% (Platte 2019).

The enlarging uterus in the first trimester compresses the bladder, increasing the desire to micturate, resulting in **urinary frequency**. During the second trimester, the bladder is displaced upwards, allowing bladder capacity to return to normal. However, during the third trimester, pressure from the presenting part, particularly following engagement, can once again result in urinary frequency or **stress incontinence**. As the bladder is displaced into the abdomen, the urethra is elongated and bladder emptying is affected. **Nocturia** may also occur during pregnancy due to increased excretion of sodium and water occurring when the woman lies down (Blackburn 2018). The growing uterine volume places increased pressure on the pelvic floor and bladder, and may decrease the urethrovesical angle and support of the bladder neck and urethra (Bartling & Zito 2016). Pelvic floor muscle training can be effective in preventing and reducing the incidence of urinary incontinence during pregnancy and in the postnatal period (Bartling & Zito 2016). Midwives can assist women to maintain continence by teaching pelvic floor muscle exercises, providing preventative advice, early intervention symptom management and referral (O'Toole 2016).

Labour

During labour, pressure from the presenting part is exerted on the bladder, urethra and sacral plexus during descent through the pelvis. This may result in increased frequency, inhibition of the impulse to void and retention of urine, particularly if the fetus in an **occipitoposterior** position. **Urinary retention** is the inability to pass urine when the urge is present.

Lack of privacy and poor posture also contribute to retention of urine. A full or distended bladder may result in delayed descent and rotation of the presenting part, less efficient uterine contractions and increased pain (Simkin & Ancheta 2017). The bladder is displaced upwards in labour, making it physiologically an abdominal organ and decreasing the risk of bladder injury during descent of the presenting part (Marshall & Raynor 2020). Therefore, women should be encouraged to void urine at least 4-hourly during labour, and at the onset of second stage to minimise these risks (Marshall & Raynor 2020). Palpation of the bladder is an unreliable sign of the presence of urine (Doyle & Birch 2011). Decreased awareness of the need to void urine occurs if regional anaesthesia is used (e.g. epidural or pudendal block), as the drugs temporarily block the nerves supplying the bladder.

During labour, urine output should be documented for all women (Velinor 2015).

Postnatal period

Women should pass urine within 6 hours of giving birth (Blackburn 2018). However, some women may experience a delayed sensation to void due to perineal pain and swelling, particularly after an instrumental birth or perineal trauma. Following epidural anaesthesia, it may take up to 12 hours for bladder sensation to return (Marshall & Raynor 2020).

The risk of partial or incomplete ability to void is increased by:

- nulliparity (Avondstondt et al 2020, Barba et al 2021)
- trauma to the bladder or urethra (oedema, sphincter spasm)
- bladder distention in labour (Avondstondt et al 2020, Beaumont et al 2019, Lamb & Sanders 2016)
- regional anaesthesia (Avondstondt et al 2020, Perú Biurrun et al 2020)
- catheterisation during labour (Avondstondt et al 2020)
- instrumental birth (Avondstondt et al 2020, Perú Biurrun et al., 2020)
- perineal laceration (Beaumont et al 2019)
- episiotomy (Avondstondt et al 2020)
- induction or augmentation with oxytocin (Avondstondt et al 2020)
- genital tract haematoma (Lamblin et al 2019)
- prolonged second stage (Beaumont et al 2019)
- newborn macrosomia (Beaumont 2019, Perú Biurrun et al 2020)
- levator ani muscle avulsion (Gonzalez-Díaz & Perú Biurrun 2020)
- body mass index (BMI) > 39 kg/m^2 at end of pregnancy (Barba et al 2020)
- previous caesarean section (Perú Biurrun et al 2020).

Bladder overdistension can damage bladder nerves and can cause detrusor atony and voiding dysfunction (Avondstondt et al 2020). Incomplete emptying of the bladder and urinary stasis increases the risk of UTI. If a woman is unable to void within 6 hours of giving birth then measures to treat pain and swelling can be initiated to assist her to void. If urine has still not been passed, the bladder should be assessed. A bladder scanner can determine the amount of urine in the bladder and catheterisation can be considered if necessary. A displaced uterus is often caused by a full bladder and can prevent the uterus from contracting efficiently and worsen postpartum haemorrhage (Begley 2020).

Following a caesarean section the catheter is usually removed by 24 hours. Approximately 15% of women have urinary retention following catheter removal post caesarean section (Cavkaytar et al 2015). The risk of urinary retention increases with higher pregnancy weight gain, macrosomic newborn, induction of labour resulting in caesarean section and elevated pain perception at the time of first post catheter removal void (Cavkaytar et al 2015). Stress incontinence may also occur following birth as a result of damage to the perineal branches of the pudendal nerves (Wang & Ghoniem 2017). If this persists beyond the puerperium, medical attention should be sought.

During the early postnatal period, a marked diuresis occurs. Between the second and fifth postnatal days, up to 3000 mL of urine may be produced daily, with 500–1000 mL being voided at a time (Blackburn 2018). The structural changes of pregnancy slowly return to normal during the puerperium, although in some women this may take up to 16 weeks. The glomerular filtration rate declines to normal non-pregnant levels by 1 month post-birth (Hussein & Lafayette 2014).

An important part of the midwife's role and responsibilities is to detect any problems with micturition. Midwives need to be alert for difficulties women are experiencing, such as dysuria, incontinence and postnatal urinary retention. If not detected, postnatal urinary retention can result in recurrent UTIs, bladder and urinary tract damage and continence issues (Lamb & Sanders 2016). Even one episode of bladder over-distension can result in irreversible damage to the detrusor muscle and chronic alterations in urethra–vesical function (Richens 2016). Record keeping should indicate the time, amount of urine passed and the frequency, noting any symptoms associated with dysuria (e.g. stinging). Urinary incontinence in the postnatal period is associated with an increased risk of depression (Fritel et al 2016). Women with urinary incontinence report a lower quality of life (Adamczuk et al 2015, Van der Woude et al 2015).

NEONATAL PHYSIOLOGY

A neonate's bladder is an abdominal organ, being too large for the small pelvis to accommodate it. Consequently, a full bladder can compress the abdomen and increase pressure on the diaphragm (Blackburn 2018). For the neonate, micturition is an involuntary process with no control over when and where to void urine. Babies usually pass urine within the first 48 hours of life, 95% of them in the first 24 hours (Blackburn 2018). It is important the midwife records that the neonate has passed urine following birth and helps the parents to understand the expected urine output in the days that follow. Neonates from mothers who received magnesium sulfate are at higher risk of urinary retention. Urinary output is variable, depending on gestational age, fluid and solute intake, the ability of the kidneys to concentrate urine and perinatal events. Healthy newborns should pass urine in the first 24 hours.

FACILITATING NORMAL MICTURITION

The midwife has a responsibility to ensure good bladder care for all women. Wherever possible, the woman should be encouraged to void normally using the toilet. However, if a woman is immobile, a bedpan may be required (Fig 15.1). The midwife should facilitate normal micturition wherever possible. Normal micturition is influenced by factors such as stimulating the micturition reflex and maintaining good elimination habits.

STIMULATING THE MICTURITION REFLEX

Position

- An upright position, leaning forwards with feet flat on the floor. This aids relaxation of the thigh muscles and pelvic floor. Women may need to feel comfortable and have privacy.
- This is difficult to achieve in bed; use of a bedpan or commode by the bedside or use of the toilet should be encouraged.

Reduce anxiety and fear

- Anxiety can cause a sense of urgency and frequency, resulting in voiding small amounts of urine; the bladder may not empty completely as the abdominal and perineal muscles and external urethral sphincter do not relax. Anxiety can result from lack of privacy, embarrassment, fear of passing urine and the use of cold bedpans.
- Staying with a woman while she attempts to pass urine may inhibit micturition; if she feels unsteady, she may prefer someone with her; her needs should be ascertained. Warming the bedpan prior to use encourages relaxation.
- Use of the toilet can increase the sense of privacy.
- Allowing sufficient time to relax and pass urine is also important.
- Warm water poured over the perineum may aid relaxation (measure amount of fluid first if recording fluid balance).
- Pain, or fear of pain, can inhibit micturition. This is not unusual following birth with perineal trauma. Concentrated urine may increase pain; additional fluid intake should be encouraged.
- Strategies to minimise actual pain should be used (e.g. analgesia, cooling gel packs for perineal pain).

Use of sensory stimuli

- Thompson (2015) recommends the sound of running water, using the power of suggestion. If the woman is embarrassed by the noise made during micturition, particularly if others are close by, the sound of running water may mask the sound of her passing urine and help her feel more comfortable.
- A woman may find stroking the inner aspect of her thigh, placing a hand in warm water or having a drink may stimulate the sensory nerves to stimulate the micturition reflex (Thompson 2015).

Encourage good bladder habits

Good bladder habits are important, especially in the absence of the desire to void. Absence of the urge to void may be caused by prolonged use of an indwelling catheter, damage to the nervous pathways, weak pelvic floor muscles, surgery, constipation and medications. Good bladder habits include:

- regular pelvic floor exercises to increase musculature (Kissler et al 2016); this increases the maximum urethral closure pressure, promoting stronger reflex contractions following a rise in intra-abdominal pressure
- treating constipation resulting from opioids or diet
- supporting adoption of a comfortable position and routine
- encouraging adequate fluid intake (normal renal function requires approximately 2000 mL per day).

Women unable to walk to the toilet may need to use a bedpan. A smaller and lighter slipper bedpan can be used for women who have difficulty lifting up enough to use a normal bedpan.

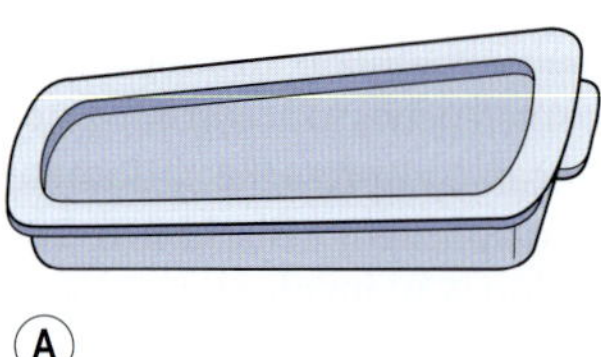

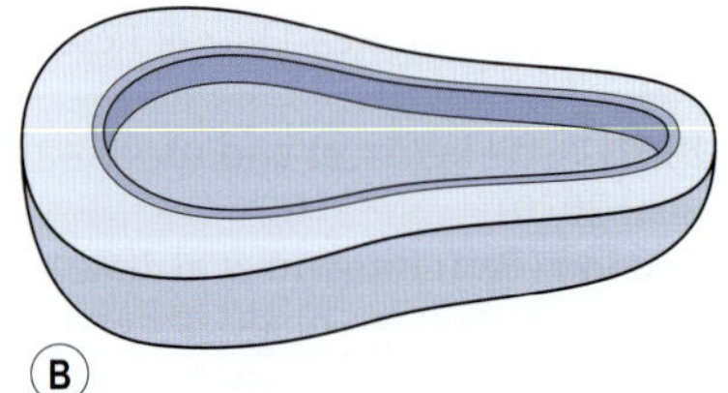

FIGURE 15.1 **Different types of bedpan. A Non-disposable slipper. B Bedpan with disposable lining.**
Source: Johnson R, Taylor W: Skills for midwifery practice, 4th ed., Elsevier, London, 2016.

SKILL 15.1 Use of a bedpan

1. Gain informed consent.
2. Prepare the environment to facilitate micturition (discussed earlier).
3. Gather equipment:
   - bedpan
   - non-sterile gloves and apron
   - liner (if used)
   - bedpan cover
   - toilet paper
   - sanitary pad, disposable bag and clean sanitary pad (if required)
   - handwashing facilities.
4. Perform hand hygiene and don non-sterile gloves.
5. Consider moving and handling issues (make sure the bed is at the correct height; assess the need for a second midwife, etc.).
6. Take the bedpan to the woman and ensure privacy.
7. Help the woman to remove her underwear and sanitary pad.
8. Place the bedpan under the woman, assisting her into a comfortable, preferably upright position. Lying on her side and then rolling back onto the bedpan may be easier for some women.
9. Stay with the woman if necessary; otherwise supply a call bell.
10. After she has voided, ensure the area is clean. If lochia is present, a damp cloth may be required prior to patting the area dry and applying a fresh sanitary pad and undergarment.
11. Remove and cover the bedpan.
12. Remove non-sterile gloves and perform hand hygiene.
13. Provide facilities for the woman to wash her hands.
14. Take the bedpan to the dirty utility room and clean as per institutional policy. Dispose of bedpan liner if used. Apply non-sterile gloves, undertake urinalysis and measure urine if required.
15. Remove non-sterile gloves and perform hand hygiene.
16. Document findings and act accordingly.

URINARY (URETHRAL) CATHETERISATION

Definition

Using aseptic technique, a sterile catheter is inserted into the bladder to drain out urine. The most common catheterisation is urethral (via the urethra). The catheter can be indwelling (left in place) or intermittent (inserted and removed) (Fig 15.2). An indwelling catheter can drain urine continually via a urine bag, or a catheter valve can be inserted into the end of the catheter allowing the bladder to be emptied periodically. Pulling on the catheter is avoided through use of a securement device (Fig 15.3). The bladder can also be catheterised through the abdominal wall using a suprapubic catheter. This is seen infrequently within the maternity setting and is generally related to bladder damage occurring with caesarean section. Bladder scanners are increasingly being used to detect the amount of urine in the bladder when a woman is unable to void (Lovell & Steen 2017). This may avoid the need for catheterisation at times.

The lining of the urethra has no natural lubrication and is sensitive and easily traumatised (Richens 2016). Efforts should be made to reduce the pain and the discomfort/trauma of catheter insertion. Usually a water-based lubricating gel is used. A pre-prepared 6 mL lignocaine (lidocaine) 2% gel can be used and takes effect after 3–5 minutes; local protocols should be followed.

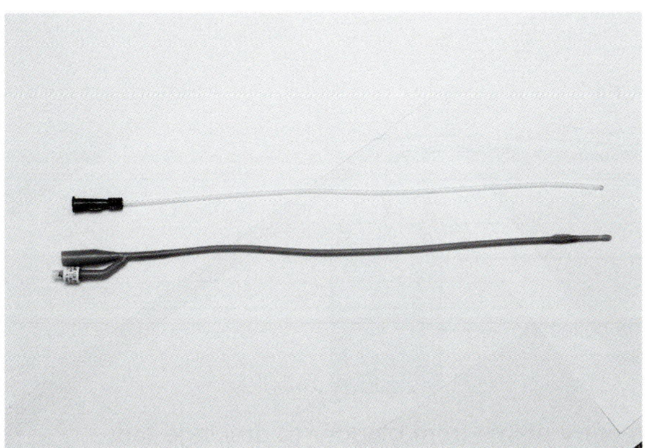

FIGURE 15.2 Indwelling and intermittent catheters.

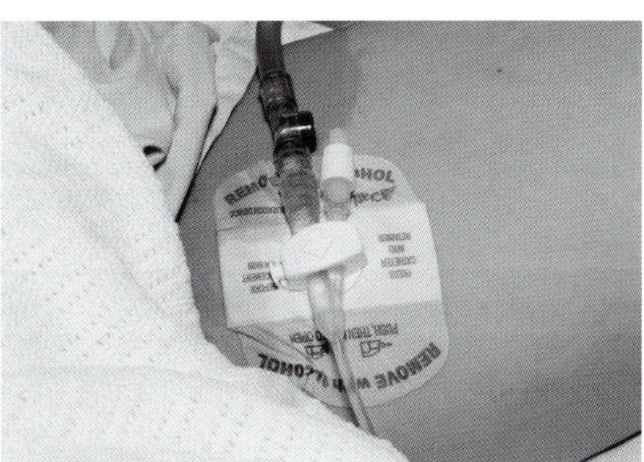

FIGURE 15.3 Securement device for catheter.

Indications

Catheterisation is an invasive procedure which can result in complications such as infection, blockage, bladder spasms, pain, urinary tract trauma and inflammation. Consequently, it should only be undertaken when clinically indicated and with full consent. Clinical indications include:

- prior to caesarean section or other abdominal surgery
- prior to instrumental birth; when the fetal head is low the angle of the catheter may need to be altered for insertion due to pressure on the urethra from the fetal head (Richens 2016)
- filling the bladder to relieve pressure on a prolapsed umbilical cord
- if a woman is unable to pass urine at any time (e.g. post-surgery or postnatal urine retention)
- epidural analgesia
- during labour when a full bladder may be impeding normal uterine activity
- during postpartum haemorrhage or for a retained placenta
- for diagnostic purposes (e.g. postnatal incontinence)
- accurate monitoring of fluid balance for acutely ill women (e.g. shock, pre-eclampsia, major haemorrhage).

On each occasion, the clinical decision is made as to whether an indwelling or intermittent catheter is the most appropriate.

Prevention of infection

An indwelling catheter carries significant risk for bacteriuria, resulting in a catheter-associated urinary tract infection (CAUTI) (Bursle et al 2015). UTIs are responsible for over 30% of HAIs, with 80% attributable to an indwelling urinary catheter (Gardner et al 2014.) The most effective way to prevent CAUTI is by removing the catheter promptly when it is no longer indicated (Bell et al 2016).

The infection risk increases according to the susceptibility of the woman, type and length of time the catheter is in situ and the quality of catheter care. Catheterisation is usually a short-term measure in maternity settings and this reduces the risk of infection. The effects of CAUTI are significant for women and result in increased costs and length of stay.

Infection-reducing measures

- Review the catheter daily and remove as soon as possible.
- Maintain comprehensive catheter care, including a sterile closed drainage system to prevent bacterial growth (Fig 15.4). Clean non-sterile gloves should be worn over decontaminated hands for every aspect of catheter care.
- Specimens should be obtained aseptically using the sampling port and care should be taken when emptying the drainage system to avoid contamination between the tap and the container.
- The drainage bag should be supported at a level lower than the bladder (maximum 30 cm) to allow free drainage and prevent backflow of the urine. A catheter holder is used to keep the bag away from the floor and reduce trauma to the urethra. Drainage bags should be changed according to manufacturer's instructions.
- The bag should be emptied when it is two-thirds full. Occluding or kinking the catheter can cause stasis of urine in the bladder and subsequent UTI.
- Ongoing catheter care includes observing the amount, colour, clarity and smell of the urine, in

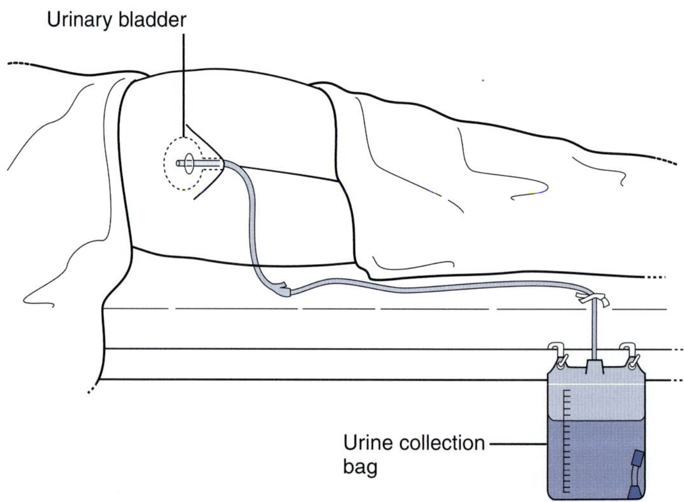

FIGURE 15.4 **Closed drainage system—no breaks or open entry points from bladder to drainage tap.**
Source: Adapted with kind permission from Jamieson EM, McCall J, Whyte L: Clinical nursing practices, 4th ed., Churchill Livingstone, Edinburgh, 2002.

conjunction with the woman's vital signs and clinical signs of illness or UTI. Information regarding all aspects of catheter care must be given to the woman.
- Maintain attendance to daily personal hygiene.
- The amount considered necessary to flush the urinary tract is 2 L of fluid per day (ACI Urology Network 2014).
- Staff should be trained and competent (adapted from Loveday et al 2014).

Choice of equipment

Catheter choice should consider reducing:
- tissue inflammation and trauma to the urethra (also improves comfort)
- mineral deposits that may cause the catheter to block
- bacterial growth.

Available catheters include sterile polytetrafluorethylene (PTFE, also known as Teflon) latex catheters and latex silicone-coated catheters. Caution must be taken to ensure women do not have a latex or Teflon allergy. If available, latex-free, hypoallergenic 100% silicone catheters are preferred. A female catheter is 20–25 cm; a standard-length catheter of 40–45 cm can be used for larger women.

The French gauge system (also known as Ch after the French inventor Joseph-Frédéric Benoît Charrière) is used to size catheters and is abbreviated as Fr. The outer circumference of the catheter determines the size. The French size equates to three times the catheter diameter in millimetres; it is based on 0.33 mm, one-third of a millimetre (Casey et al 2003). Therefore, a size 12 Fr catheter has a diameter of 4 mm.

To avoid trauma and urine leakage, the smallest lumen large enough to drain the bladder adequately, without over-distending the urethra, should be chosen. A catheter larger than 18 Fr can cause erosion of the bladder neck and urethral mucosa (Australia and New Zealand Urological Nurses Society [ANZUNS] 2013). For most women, a size 12–14 catheter is suitable.

Indwelling catheters are retained in the bladder by a balloon inflated with 5–10 mL of water (Loveday et al 2014). Catheters vary; some have a self-inflating balloon or a prefilled sterile syringe. The sterile water is squeezed from the external balloon or syringe to the internal balloon when the catheter is in the bladder. Catheters for intermittent use are short, with holes at the tip and no balloon; they are usually latex-free. All catheters are singly wrapped, sterile and include an expiry date. Catheters should be stored flat in their original packaging, away from heat and direct sunlight, and should not be bent or bundled together with elastic bands (ANZUNS 2013). Valves, drainage bags and catheter packs (containing swabs, gallipot and receivers) are also sterile and for single use only.

Documentation

Documentation of catheter insertion and management is often poor, with no information provided regarding who inserted the catheter, the indications for the catheter or ongoing management (Gardner et al 2014). As well as the clinical indication for the catheterisation, these details also need to be recorded in the woman's record:
- consent
- indication for catheterisation, date of insertion
- catheter option used (e.g. indwelling catheter [IDC], intermittent)
- type, length, size, manufacturer, batch number, expiry date and number of millilitres in balloon (sometimes a label is supplied for insertion into the woman's records)
- cleansing solution and lubricant/anaesthetic gel used
- balloon volume
- any problems encountered with the insertion
- total urine volume drained, colour of urine, sediment or abnormality (e.g. haematuria)
- plan of care, including duration/expected removal time
- specimen taken and sent (if needed)
- drainage system used
- name and signature of midwife
- follow-up action.

SKILL 15.2 Female urethral catheterisation using an indwelling catheter

This is based on the aseptic non-touch technique (ANTT) guidelines (Chapter 2), working from a suitable height and using a dressings trolley. The urethral opening and urethra are considered key sites and the sterile catheter and the connection to a sterile drainage bag are considered key parts. The procedure is adapted according to the working environment.

1. Confirm identification, explain the procedure and gain informed consent.
2. Review current medications and any known allergies.
3. Perform hand hygiene.
4. Obtain the dressings trolley, put on non-sterile gloves and clean the trolley with the locally approved wipes.
5. Gather the following equipment and place onto the lower shelf:
   - sterile urinary catheter (a second catheter should be available)
   - sterile drainage bag and holder
   - two pairs of sterile gloves
   - sterile catheter pack

Continued

SKILL 15.2 Female urethral catheterisation using an indwelling catheter—cont'd

- catheter fixation device or tape
- 1 sachet water-soluble sterile lubricating gel (anaesthetic gel if used)
- 1 sterile sachet sodium chloride 0.9% or other approved skin cleanser
- disposable waterproof sheet
- good light source
- 10 mL sterile water and sterile 10 mL syringe (not needed if catheter has a self-inflating balloon)
- batch tracking label if available.

6. Take the trolley to the woman. Ensuring privacy, position the woman (removing sanitary pad and underwear) on a disposable sheet, in a semi-recumbent position, knees bent and abducted, hips flexed and feet together.
7. Place a waterproof sheet beneath the buttocks, and replace covering so the woman is not exposed.
8. Perform hand hygiene.
9. Using ANTT, open the outer layer of the catheter pack, sliding the inner part onto the trolley. Open the inner wrapper, handling only the corners.
10. Place the sterile gloves, syringe, 0.9% sodium chloride, sterile water, catheter, drainage bag and lubricating gel onto the sterile field. Protect all key parts. Remove covering.
11. Perform hand hygiene and put on sterile gloves.
12. Using the non-dominant hand, separate the labia with gauze swabs (this minimises pressure on the labia, increases visibility and makes catheter insertion easier) (Fig 15.5); cleanse the vulva (0.9% sodium chloride or approved solution) using each swab once only, cleaning front to back, beginning with the labia majora, then to the labia minora and then centrally.
13. Remove gloves, perform hand hygiene and put on sterile gloves.
14. Establish an aseptic field by placing a fenestrated drape in position.
15. Place the receiver for urine on the sterile field between the woman's thighs, expose the tip of the catheter and apply lubrication (instil anaesthetic gel into urethra, if used); hold it using only the plastic wrapper.
16. Locate the urethra. Use the non-dominant hand to part and hold the labia with a gauze swab while the dominant hand passes the catheter gently and smoothly in an upwards and backwards direction into the urethra until urine begins to flow. Maintain asepsis by pulling back the plastic wrapper as the catheter is advanced. If the urethra is difficult to visualise, ask the woman to take a deep breath in; on expiration the urethra is easier to see (the pelvic floor relaxes).
17. Insert the catheter until urine flows and then advance it a further 2–5 cm to ensure the balloon is clear of the urethra and in the bladder. If the catheter goes into the vagina, leave it in situ and insert a new catheter into the urethra. A contaminated catheter should *never* be placed into the urethra.
18. If the woman is very uncomfortable or there is resistance at any stage, stop and seek experienced assistance.
19. Inflate the balloon by squeezing the fluid from the external balloon or syringe, then remove the syringe. The balloon must never be inflated until urine is flowing freely; if pain is felt during inflation the balloon may be in the urethra, and the catheter would need to be advanced further into the bladder before the balloon is inflated.
20. Fully remove the plastic wrapper and attach the drainage bag.
21. Clear the area, remove gloves, perform hand hygiene and apply non-sterile gloves if necessary. Assist the woman to replace her sanitary pad and underwear and to adopt a comfortable position.
22. Attach the catheter bag to the holder, securing it to the side of the bed. Additional support can be provided by taping the catheter to the leg; this reduces trauma to the urethra.
23. Discuss ongoing care (e.g. principles of infection control, sufficient mobility, oral fluids, avoiding constipation).
24. If a urine specimen is needed for culture and sensitivity, it should be taken from the catheter before the drainage bag is attached.
25. Undertake urinalysis if necessary (using the sample gained when the catheter was inserted).
26. Excessive loss of fluid from the body quickly in one episode (i.e. up to 1 L) can result in shock. The immediate drainage of urine should be observed and the flow halted with a clamp, if the volume is approaching 1 L.
27. Dispose of equipment correctly in the clinical waste bin in the room, remove gloves and perform hand hygiene. Take the trolley to the dirty utility room, clean using non-sterile gloves with approved cleanser.
28. Perform hand hygiene.
29. Document findings and act accordingly.

Intermittent catheterisation

Intermittent catheterisation is sometimes termed 'in/out' catheterisation. The procedure is exactly the same as inserting an indwelling catheter, except the catheter is a sterile single-use catheter which is removed once the urine has been drained. It is also an ANTT procedure. The container receiving the urine must be sterile and large enough to hold the expected volume.

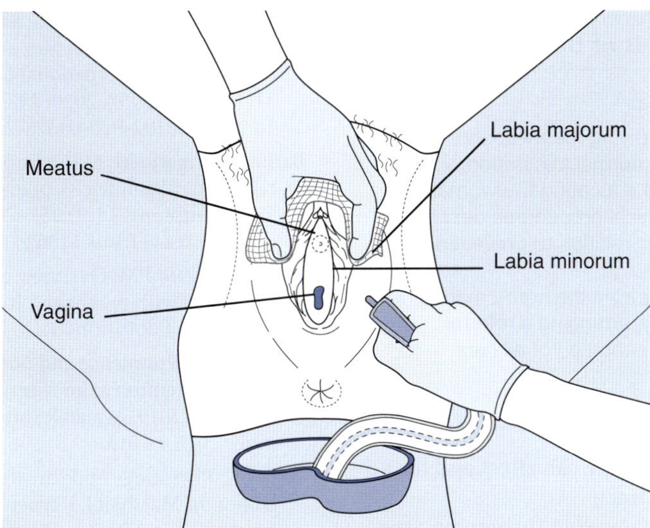

FIGURE 15.5 **Female catheterisation.**
Source: Adapted with kind permission from Nicol M, Bavin C, Bedford-Turner S, et al: Essential nursing skills, 2nd ed., Mosby, Edinburgh, 2000, p. 185.

REMOVING A URETHRAL INDWELLING CATHETER

Catheter removal should occur as soon as the woman's condition allows. Depending on local protocol, a catheter specimen of urine (CSU) may be obtained before removal to screen for infection. Traditionally, catheters are removed early in the morning. Removal of the catheter must be documented in the healthcare notes. The following information should be recorded:

- date and time of removal
- amount voided after removal
- any pain during micturition
- bladder scan results if there is a trial of void
- abnormalities noted during removal such as bleeding or pain.

SKILL 15.3 Removing a female urethral catheter

1. Gain informed consent and ensure privacy.
2. Gather equipment:
   - disposable receiver
   - 10 mL syringe (depending on catheter design) (check insertion documentation)
   - non-sterile gloves and plastic apron
   - disposable sheet
   - equipment for perineal cleansing, depending on chosen method.
3. Position the woman on the disposable sheet, as for insertion, placing the receiver between her legs; keep her covered.
4. Apply the apron, decontaminate hands and apply gloves.
5. Ask the woman to lift up the sheet covering her.
6. Deflate the balloon by removing the clamp and allowing the fluid to drain into the external balloon, or by withdrawing the water using the syringe.
7. Ask the woman to take a deep breath and then remove the catheter smoothly but quickly as she exhales, placing it into the receiver.
8. Cleanse the perineum.
9. Remove gloves and perform hand hygiene.
10. Assist the woman to replace her sanitary pad and underwear as required and to adopt a comfortable position.
11. Provide explanations regarding:
    - possible frequency and urgency of micturition due to urethral irritability, or mild haematuria due to urethral trauma
    - the need to pass urine within 6 hours, with output matching input over the next 24 hours
    - possible urinary retention
    - a fluid intake of 2 L to wash out any bladder debris.
12. Measure and record the drained urine if fluid balance is being monitored.
13. Dispose of equipment correctly and perform hand hygiene.
14. Document findings and act accordingly, ensuring the next urine output is measured and recorded.

Role and responsibilities of the midwife

These can be summarised as:

- understanding and applying the measures necessary to facilitate normal micturition, including advising and educating the woman
- undertaking all the clinical procedures described correctly, particularly in relation to preventing infection
- recognising deviations from the norm, managing them and, if necessary, arranging a referral
- keeping correct documentation of all care.

SUMMARY

- Many aspects of childbearing can affect and be affected by the urinary tract.
- Micturition can be influenced in three main ways: stimulating the micturition reflex, maintaining normal habits and ensuring adequate fluid intake.
- Catheterisation of the bladder is indicated in certain clinical circumstances. Infection is one of the greatest risks; the midwife must be aware of the care that contributes towards reducing the risk.

Self-assessment exercises

The answers to the following questions may be found in the text.

1. Which factors influence micturition?
2. Describe how childbearing affects micturition and therefore the measures the midwife can undertake to promote good urinary care.
3. Describe the advantages and disadvantages of bedpan use.
4. List the situations in which a midwife is likely to undertake catheterisation for a childbearing woman.
5. Discuss the similarities and differences between indwelling and intermittent catheterisation.
6. Which is the most likely complication to occur from catheterisation and how might this be prevented in all stages of care?

References

ACI Urology Network: Female indwelling urinary catheterisation (IUC)—adult. Clinical guideline, competencies and patient information leaflet, 2014. Online 30 March 2021. Available: www.aci.health.nsw.gov.au/__data/assets/pdf_file/0019/256132/ACI_Female_IUCv2.pdf.

Adamczuk J, Szymona-Pałkowska K, Robak JM, et al: Coping with stress and quality of life in women with stress urinary incontinence, Menopausal Review/Przeglad Menopauzalny 14:178–183, 2015.

Australia and New Zealand Urological Nurses Society (ANZUNS) 2013. Urinary catheter guidelines. Online 30 March 2021. Available: anzuns.org/guidelines/

Avondstondt AM, Hidalgo RJ, Salamon, CG: Intrapartum risk factors for postpartum urinary retention: a case-control study, International Urogynecology Journal 31(11):2395–2398, 2020. Available: https://doi.org/10.1007/s00192-020-04378-2.

Barba M, Frigerio M, Manodoro S, et al: Postpartum urinary retention: Absolute risk prediction model, Lower Urinary Tract Symptoms 13(2):257–263, 2021. Available: https://doi.org/10.1111/luts.12362.

Bartling SJ, Zito PM: Overview of pelvic floor dysfunction associated with pregnancy, International Journal of Childbirth Education 31:18–20, 2016.

Beaumont T: Prevalence and outcome of postpartum urinary retention at an Australian hospital, Midwifery 70:92–99, 2019. Available: https://doi.org/10.1016/j.midw.2018.12.013.

Begley C: Physiology and care during the third stage of labour. In Marshall J, Rayner M, editors: Myles textbook for midwives, 17th ed., Elsevier, Edinburgh, 2020.

Bell M, Alaestante G, Finch C: A multidisciplinary intervention to prevent catheter-associated urinary tract infections using education, continuum of care, and systemwide buy-in, The Ochsner Journal 16(1): 96–100, 2016.

Blackburn ST: Chapter 11. Maternal, fetal and neonatal physiology: a clinical perspective, 4th ed., Elsevier, Maryland Heights, 2018.

Bullock S, Hales M: Principles of pathophysiology, 2nd ed., Pearson Australia, Melbourne, 2018.

Bursle E, Dyer J, Looke D, et al: Risk factors for urinary catheter associated bloodstream infection, The Journal of Infection 70(6):585–591, 2015.

Casey RG, Quinlan D, Mulvin D, et al: Joseph-Frédéric-Benoît Charrière: master cutler and instrument designer, European Urology 43:320, 2003.

Cavkaytar S, Kokanalı MK, Güzel Aİ, et al: An investigation of potential risk factors for postoperative urinary retention following cesarean section, Sezaryeni Takiben Gelişen Postoperatif İdrar Retansiyonu İçin Potansiyel Risk Faktörlerinin Araştırılması 22:8–12, 2015.

Conrad KP, Davison JM: The renal circulation in normal pregnancy and preeclampsia: is there a place for relaxin?, American Journal of Physiology—Renal Physiology 306(10):F1121–F1135, 2014.

Cooper K, Gosnell K: Foundations and adult health nursing, Elsevier Mosby, St Louis, 2018.

Doyle P, Birch L: Urine elimination in pregnancy: indications for catheterisation, British Journal of Midwifery 19(9):550–556, 2011.

Fritel X, Tsegan YE, Pierre F, et al: Association of postpartum depressive symptoms and urinary incontinence. A cohort study, European Journal of Obstetrics, Gynecology and Reproductive Biology 198:62–67, 2016.

Gardner A, Mitchell B, Beckingham W, et al: A point prevalence cross-sectional study of healthcare-associated urinary tract infections in six Australian hospitals, BMJ Open 4(7):E005099, 2014.

Gonzalez-Díaz E, Perú Biurrun G: Levator ani muscle avulsion: a risk factor for persistent postpartum voiding dysfunction, International Urogynecology Journal volume 31:2327–2335, 2020. Available: https://doi.org/10.1007/s00192-020-04412-3.

Hussein W, Lafayette RA: Renal function in normal and disordered pregnancy, Current Opinion in Nephrology and Hypertension 23(1):46–53, 2014.

Kissler K, Yount SM, Rendeiro M, et al: Primary prevention of urinary incontinence: a case study of prenatal and intrapartum interventions, Journal of Midwifery & Women's Health 61:507–511, 2016.

Lamb K, Sanders R: Bladder care in the context of motherhood: ensuring holistic midwifery practice, British Journal of Midwifery 24:415–421, 2016.

Lamblin G, Chene G, Aeberli C, et al: Identification of risk factors for postpartum urinary retention following vaginal deliveries: A retrospective case-control study, European Journal of Obstetrics & Gynecology and Reproductive Biology 243:7–11, 2019. Available: https://doi.org/10.1016/j.ejogrb.2019.10.001.

Loveday H, Wilson J, Pratt R, et al: epic3: National evidence-based guidelines for preventing healthcare associated infections in NHS hospitals in England, Journal of Hospital Infection 86(Suppl 1):S1–S70, 2014.

Lovell B, Steen M: Potential to reduce urinary tract infections with the use of bladder scanners in maternity care, Australian Nursing & Midwifery Journal 24:40, 2017.

Marshall J, Raynor M: Myles textbook for midwives, 17th ed., Elsevier, London, 2020.

McGarry K, Tong IL: 5-minute consult clinical companion to women's health, Wolters Kluwer, Philadelphia, 2015.

Moore K, Agur A, Dalley A: Clinically oriented anatomy, 8th ed., Wolters Kluwer, 2018.

O'Toole J: Pelvic floor exercises for women tips and tricks, Australian Nursing & Midwifery Journal 24:44, 2016.

Platte RO: Urinary tract infections in pregnancy. Medscape, 2019. Online 30 March 2021. Available: https://emedicine.medscape.com/article/452604-overview.

Perú Biurrun G, Gonzalez-Díaz E, Fernández Fernández C, Fernández Corona, A. (2020). Post partum urinary retention and related risk factors, Urology 143:97–102, 2020. Available: https://doi.org/10.1016/j.urology.2020.03.061.

Richens Y: Urinary catheterisation: indications and complications, British Journal of Midwifery 24: 164–168, 2016.

Simkin P, Ancheta R: The labor progress handbook, 4th ed., Wiley Blackwell, Chichester, 2017.

Smaill FM, Vazquez JC: Antibiotics for asymptomatic bacteriuria in pregnancy, Cochrane Database of Systematic Reviews 2019 8:CD000490, 2019.

Smyth A, Radovic M, Garovic VD: Women, renal disease and pregnancy, Advances in Chronic Kidney Disease 20(5):402–410, 2013.

Thompson D: Urinary elimination, Chapter 34. In Potter PA, Perry AG, Stockert P, et al, editors: Essentials for nursing practice, 8th ed., Elsevier, St Louis, 2015.

Van der Woude DA, Pijnenborg JM, de Vries J: Health status and quality of life in postpartum women: a systematic review of associated factors, European Journal of Obstetrics, Gynecology & Reproductive Biology 185:45–52, 2015.

Velinor A: Urinary catheterisation in labour, British Journal of Midwifery 23:11–15, 2015.

Wang H, Ghoniem G: Postpartum stress urinary incontinence, is it related to vaginal birth? Journal of Maternal–Fetal & Neonatal Medicine 30:1552–1555, 2017.

CHAPTER 16
URINE SAMPLES

Learning outcomes

Having read this chapter, the reader should be able to:

- recognise the components of 'normal' urine and gain some understanding of the significance of the abnormal findings of urinalysis
- identify when to undertake a urinalysis and the rationale
- discuss the midwife's role and responsibilities in relation to urinalysis and the correct procedure for urinalysis.

Urinalysis is a screening tool commonly used by midwives to identify when further testing is required and should not be used in isolation when making treatment decisions. This chapter considers the components of 'normal' urine, the significance of abnormal findings and the procedure for undertaking urinalysis. Although pregnancy tests can also be undertaken using a specimen of urine, this is not discussed within this chapter.

Urine has been examined to assist in diagnosing systemic health for over 8000 years (Barasch et al 2018). Urine composition reflects the by-products generated by metabolism and the necessity to maintain the body's solute and water balance (Barasch et al 2018). The composition of urine, particularly the pH and the presence of urinary metabolites influences the bactericidal activity of urine and susceptibility to urinary tract infections and may be impacted by diet (Shields-Cutler et al 2015).

DEFINITION

Urinalysis is the testing of both the physical characteristics and the composition of freshly voided urine and is undertaken for the purposes of:

- *screening* for systemic and renal disease
- *diagnosis* of a suspected condition
- *management and planning* as a baseline and for planning and monitoring care.

In addition to assessing the physical characteristics of colour, clarity and odour of urine, urinalysis can be undertaken by laboratory testing or, more commonly and for immediate results, by using a chemical reagent strip. Urine should not be tested if it has stood for 15 or more minutes, as its characteristics may have changed (deWit & O'Neill 2014). Therefore, it is better if women provide a fresh sample at appointments. Leucocytes and erythrocytes tend to precipitate on the bottom of the container and if the sample is not mixed or is left too long the results may be inaccurate. Over time, urine samples darken in colour; odour and turbidity increase; the concentration of glucose, bilirubin and urobilinogen decreases; and the concentration of nitrite increases with pH and protein changing either way (Higgins 2013). If it is not possible to test urine soon after collection the sample should be placed in the fridge as this reduces the rate of changes.

THE PHYSICAL CHARACTERISTICS OF URINE

- Colour: Urine is yellow to amber and varies depending on urine concentration and diet. Urine voided in the morning is usually more concentrated and darker than urine voided throughout the day when fluids are consumed. Urine is coloured by urochrome (from breakdown of bile) and urobilin (from breakdown of haemoglobin) (Tortora et al 2018).
- Clarity: Freshly voided urine is usually transparent.
- Odour: Urine has a characteristically mild aromatic odour. However, if urine is left in a container the odour becomes more ammonia-like over time.

Composition of urine

Urine has a pH of 4.6–8, has a specific gravity of 1.003–1.030 and is mainly water (95%). The remaining 5% is composed of dissolved substances including electrolytes, solutes from cellular metabolism and exogenous substances such as drugs (Tortora et al 2018). The main substances in this 5% are:

- urea (from the breakdown of proteins)
- creatinine (from breakdown of creatine phosphate in muscle fibres)
- urobilinogen (from breakdown of haemoglobin)
- uric acid, sodium, potassium, phosphates, sulfates, oxalates and chlorides
- cellular components (e.g. epithelial cells, leucocytes)
- fatty acids, pigments, enzymes, hormones
- protein and glucose (present in negligible amounts, normally undetectable by routine testing).

If body metabolism or kidney function is altered, traces of substances that are not normally present in the urine may appear, or normal components may appear in abnormal amounts (Tortora 2018).

Normal occurrences during childbirth

- Pregnancy: Changes in renal tubular function make glycosuria and proteinuria more common (Blackburn 2018). Hormonal changes increase the risk of urinary tract infection and pyelonephritis.
- Labour: Ruptured membranes or contamination by a vaginal discharge or the operculum can give the appearance of proteinuria and or haematuria.
- **Ketonuria**: This may occur and, provided it is mild, is insignificant.

Indications for urinalysis

- At antenatal visits if symptoms present (follow local protocol)
- On admission to hospital for any reason, as a baseline observation
- Specific maternal disorders or treatment (e.g. hypertensive disease, diabetes mellitus, anticoagulant therapy)
- Clinical symptoms (e.g. **dysuria**, raised blood pressure)
- Altered micturition

SIGNIFICANCE OF FINDINGS

Colour

The colour of urine varies with the specific gravity: concentrated urine is dark yellow in colour whereas dilute urine can appear pale. Very dark amber or brown–green urine may contain bilirubin and this should also be suspected if urine develops a yellow foam when shaken. Haematuria also alters the colour: dark red if bleeding is within the kidneys or ureters, bright red if bleeding is from the bladder or urethra. Diet and drugs can also influence the colour. Rhubarb and beetroot change the urine to a deep red colour. Sulfasalazine can result in orange-coloured urine (Yates 2016). Vitamin B can make the urine bright yellow. *Pseudomonas* infection can give the urine a green colour (Prakesh et al 2017). Dyes such as methylene blue will also alter the colour of the urine (Puri et al 2019).

Clarity

Fresh urine is usually transparent, but when left standing may become cloudy (turbid) due to precipitation of some of the dissolved substances (e.g. uric acid). Proteinuria and bacteriuria may also cause turbidity with the most common cause a urinary tract infection (Higgins 2013). Foamy urine may be due to bilirubin or protein and infection may make the urine seem thick.

Odour

The odour of urine becomes stronger as its concentration increases. Stagnant urine smells of ammonia due to the breakdown of urea into ammonium carbonate. A sweet fruity odour may be indicative of ketones, a by-product of fat metabolism (Tortora et al 2018). Infection may cause the urine to smell offensive. The ingestion of fish, curry and other strongly flavoured food can also affect the smell of urine. Some women will have an inherited ability to form methyl mercaptan from digested asparagus, which gives urine a characteristic odour (Tortora et al 2018). Inborn errors of metabolism such as phenylketonuria cause the urine to smell musty and maple syrup urine disease is characterised by urine with a sweet odour.

Specific gravity

Specific gravity (SG) reflects the kidneys' ability to concentrate or dilute urine; a healthy adult has a specific gravity of 1.003–1.030 (Cassells 2021). Water has an SG of 1; therefore, an SG of 1.001 indicates very dilute urine and an SG of 1.035 indicates very concentrated urine (Higgins 2013). Low SG levels are associated with diuresis, over-hydration, hypercalcaemia and hypokalaemia; high levels are associated with dehydration, proteinuria and glycosuria.

pH

The pH of urine varies between 4.6 and 8 with an average of 6 (Tortora et al 2018), Urine is usually more acidic in the morning and becomes more alkaline as food is ingested. A low pH indicates the urine is more acidic and can predispose to the formation of calculi (stones) within the bladder or kidney. Diet can influence pH values, with a protein-rich diet causing the urine to be more acidic, while a high intake of vegetables increases alkalinity (Tortora et al 2018). Stale urine will have a high pH (Wilson 2005). The presence of urea-splitting organisms that convert urea into ammonia can render the urine more alkaline (Edmunds et al 2011).

Bilirubin: bilirubinuria

Bilirubin is a waste product produced by the breakdown of haemoglobin and needs to be removed from the body. The presence of bilirubin in urine is abnormal

(Martin & Martin 2019). **Bilirubinuria** means hepatic or biliary disease is present, particularly if the flow of bile into the duodenum is obstructed. A false-positive result may occur when certain drugs are taken (e.g. chlorpromazine) and a false-negative result may occur if the urine contains large amounts of ascorbic acid (Higgins 2013), particularly if the sample is exposed to sunlight, as it is unstable in light and at room temperature (Edmunds et al 2011).

Blood: haematuria

Blood in the urine is called **haematuria**. Macroscopic haematuria refers to visible blood which makes urine pink or red (Bagnall 2014), and microscopic haematuria is detected by a dipstick, but is invisible to the naked eye. Normal urine can contain very small quantities of microscopic blood; the dipstick will give a positive result if the red blood cell (RBC) count is higher than normally expected. Detectable microscopic blood occurs in up to 22% of the population and may be related to a benign cause (Higgins 2013) such as exercise-induced haematuria. Childbearing women may have contamination of urine by blood from the cervix, vagina or uterus or from haemorrhoids. Haematuria can be indicative of infection, trauma, tumours or calculi. A positive result should be confirmed by further investigation.

Glucose: glycosuria

In non-pregnant adult women glucose appears in the urine (**glycosuria**) when blood glucose levels rise (**hyperglycaemia**) above the renal threshold (approximately 10.0 mmol/L). During pregnancy, glycosuria occurs in approximately 50% of women (Lee et al 2020). Glycosuria is more common due to lowering of the renal threshold and an increased glomerular filtration rate (Murray & Hendley 2020). Glycosuria may indicate gestational diabetes or diabetes mellitus. Less common causes or glycosuria are acute pancreatitis, Cushing's syndrome, acromegaly, phaeochromocytoma and hyperthyroidism (Higgins 2013). Stress can cause the release of adrenaline, promoting break down of glycogen and release of glucose from the liver resulting in a temporary glycosuria (Tortora et al 2018). Glycosuria may also reduce the pH due to glucose metabolism by microorganisms within the urine (Edmunds et al 2011). High consumption of ascorbic acid can result in a false-negative glucose (Higgins 2013).

Ketones: ketonuria

Ketones are a by-product of fatty acid metabolism and are not commonly found in urine, as they are usually completely metabolised. In situations where there is disruption of carbohydrate metabolism, metabolic imbalances and ketone production (as a by-product of fat metabolism) can occur. This may be due to starvation, dehydration, malabsorption, the inability to metabolise carbohydrates (e.g. diabetes mellitus) or frequent vomiting and hyperemesis. Some drugs (e.g. captopril) may give a false-positive result. Ketonuria in labour is not uncommon and usually does not require treatment.

Leucocytes (white blood cells)

The enzyme leucocyte esterase is not usually detectable in urine; however, it is present in 75–85% of bacterial urinary tract infections (UTIs) (Higgins 2013). Large numbers of leucocytes in the urine are called pyuria and means that leucocytes have moved to the site of infection to destroy bacteria. False-positive results can occur if the specimen has been contaminated by leucocytes from vaginal discharge. False-negative results can occur with high levels of protein, glucose, oxalic acid and ascorbic acid and with a high specific gravity.

A urinalysis is less sensitive than microscopy and a positive test does not diagnose a UTI, although when found with nitrites it makes the diagnosis probable. If both nitrite and leucocytes are negative a UTI is unlikely.

Nitrites

Dietary nitrates are converted to nitrites in the presence of bacteria, particularly gram-negative bacteria (e.g. *Escherichia coli*). A positive nitrate indicates the presence of bacteria and is indicative of an UTI. If a dipstick is positive for nitrites a mid-stream urine (MSU) specimen should be sent for laboratory analysis. A false-negative result can occur if the bacteria have had insufficient time to convert the nitrates; for example, if the woman is experiencing frequent micturition (common with cystitis). Urine needs to be in the bladder for approximately 4 hours to allow time for bacteria to produce nitrite, making an early morning specimen preferable. High levels of ascorbic acid and urobilinogen in the urine can lead to false-negative results (Higgins 2013).

Protein: proteinuria

Protein is usually only present in very small amounts, as the molecule is too large to pass through the glomerular filtration membrane in the kidneys. However, **proteinuria** increases in pregnancy and is not concerning in the absence of signs of preeclampsia (Belzile et al 2019). Proteinuria is indicative of an increased permeability of the filtration membrane, which can occur during disease or as a result of injury, raised blood pressure or irritation of the kidney cells (Tortora et al 2018). Proteinuria may also be the result of a contaminated specimen (e.g. vaginal discharge or from increased exercise). Transient positive tests are usually insignificant; to detect larger amounts of protein an early morning specimen is required. To exclude infection an MSU specimen should be obtained, tested and sent for laboratory analysis (if necessary). A false-positive test result may occur if the urine is very alkaline or if the strip is left in the urine for too long. Significant proteinuria can indicate pre-eclampsia; therefore, a spot urine/creatine ratio or 24-hour urine is collected if the dipstick detects 1+ or more protein, particularly if blood pressure is elevated.

Urobilinogen: urobilinogenuria

Bilirubin resulting from the breakdown of haemoglobin is converted to urobilinogen by intestinal bacteria. The majority of **urobilinogen** is excreted in faeces or reabsorbed and transported back to the liver to be converted back into bile. However, the remaining urobilinogen, approximately 1% of the total, is excreted in the urine. A trace of urobilinogen is normal. Large amounts of urobilinogen may indicate liver abnormalities or excessive haemolysis. A false-negative result may occur if the sample is not fresh, has been exposed to ultraviolet light, with certain drugs (e.g. rifampicin) and with ingestion of high amounts of ascorbic acid (vitamin C). A false-positive may occur if the woman is taking phenothiazines.

Equipment for urinalysis

Urinary reagent strips or 'dipsticks' are plastic strips impregnated with chemicals that react to substances in the urine and change colour; in general, the darker the colour the higher the level (Fig 16.1). The results are given as a semi-quantitative value (e.g. trace, 1+, 2+, 3+). Dipsticks provide a quick and easy way to screen urine. A positive dipstick is not sufficient for diagnosis and should be used to inform further diagnostic steps. It is important to check the results at the correct time specified by the manufacturer—different substances will require different times to react. Use of a urine chemistry analyser reduces observer error and increases the accuracy of analysis (Correa et al 2017).

The reagent strips can degenerate with time, compounded by storage at temperature extremes or exposure to excessive humidity. Storage should be according to the manufacturer's instructions, in a cool, dry, dark area. The lid should be tight and the desiccant should not be removed from the bottle. The expiry date and condition of the reagent strip should be checked before use to ensure it is suitable to use.

SKILL 16.1 Urinalysis

1. Obtain a fresh specimen of urine for testing (if refrigerated, allow it to warm to room temperature prior to testing and invert the sample to ensure even distribution of constituents).
2. Gather equipment:
   - reagent strips (ensure they are still within their use-by date and suitable for use)
   - non-sterile gloves
   - apron (if contact with urine is likely)
   - watch with second-hand if reading manually.
3. Perform hand hygiene. Put on the apron if required and gloves.
4. Observe the colour, clarity and odour of the urine.
5. Insert the reagent strip into the urine to cover the reagent areas; remove immediately.
6. Tap the edge of the strip against the side of the urine container to remove excess urine, keeping the strip horizontal to avoid urine running down the strip and mixing the colours.
7. When reading the reagent strip manually, follow the manufacturer's instructions for timing, hold the strip close to the colour charts and read the results in good lighting (alternatively, a urine chemistry analyser may be used in accordance with the manufacturer's instructions and the results printed) (Fig 16.2).
8. Dispose of urine and equipment correctly.
9. Perform hand hygiene.

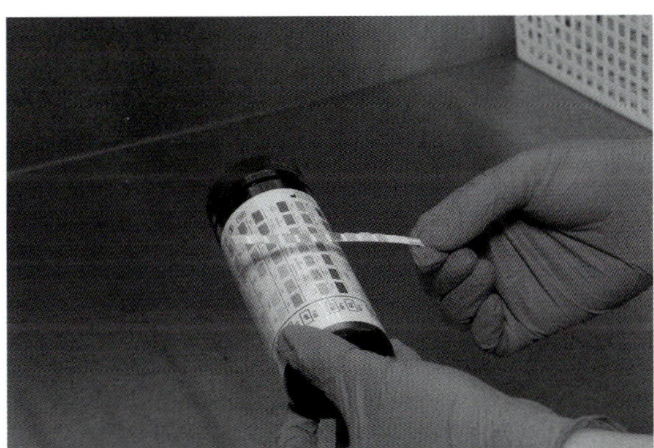

FIGURE 16.1 Manual urinalysis using reagent strip.

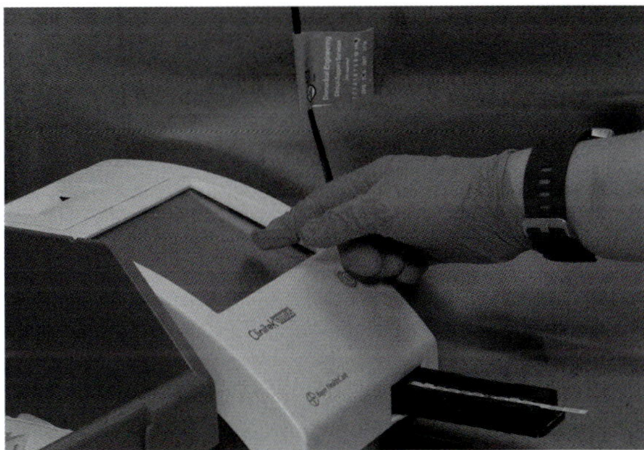

FIGURE 16.2 A reagent strip being read by a urine chemistry analyser.

Role and responsibilities of the midwife

These can be summarised as:

- undertaking the procedure correctly, using an appropriate urine specimen
- recognising deviations from normal and their significance, referring if necessary
- maintaining correct documentation.

SUMMARY

- Urinalysis may be undertaken for screening or assessment and further testing.
- Changes in pregnancy may alter urine composition with no ill effects.
- Urinalysis is quick and easy with rapid results.
- False-negative and false-positive results may occur; however, these can be minimised if the correct procedure is followed.

Self-assessment exercises

The answers to the following questions may be found in the text.

1. What are the normal constituents of urine?
2. Why might urinalysis be undertaken?
3. What observations are undertaken on urine prior to urinalysis and why?
4. List abnormal substances that may be found on urinalysis and discuss their significance.

References

Bagnall P: Haematuria: classification, causes and investigations, British Journal of Nursing 23(20): 1074–1078, 2014.

Barasch J, Bavendam T, Birder L, et al: Urine: waste product or biologically active tissue? Neurourology and Urodynamics, 37(3), 1162–1168, 2018.

Belzile M, Pouliot A, Cumyn A, Côté AM: Renal physiology and fluid and electrolyte disorders in pregnancy. Best Practice & Research Clinical Obstetrics & Gynaecology May; 57:1–14, 2019.

Blackburn S: Maternal, fetal and neonatal physiology: a clinical perspective, 5th ed., Elsevier, St Louis, 2018, pp. 351–386.

Cassells, C: Nursing care: Urinary elimination and continence. In Koutoukidis G, Stainton K, editors: Tabbner's nursing care, 8th ed., Elsevier, Sydney, 2021, Chapter 31: Nursing care: Urinary elimination and continence.

Correa ME, Côté A-M, De Silva DA, et al: Visual or automated dipstick testing for proteinuria in pregnancy? Pregnancy Hypertension 7:50–53, 2017.

deWit S, O'Neill P: Fundamental concepts and skills for nursing, 4th ed., Elsevier, St Louis, 2014.

Edmunds S, Hollis V, Lamb J, et al: Observations. In Dougherty L, Lister S, editors: The Royal Marsden Hospital manual of clinical nursing procedures, 8th ed., Wiley-Blackwell, Oxford, 2011, pp. 699–802.

Higgins C: Understanding laboratory investigations: a guide for nurses, midwives and healthcare professionals, 3rd ed., Wiley-Blackwell, Oxford, 2013.

Lee MA, McMahon G, Karhunen V, et al: Common variation at 16p11.2 is associated with glycosuria in pregnancy: findings from a genome-wide association study in European women. Human Molecular Genetics 29(12):2098–2106, 2020.

Martin C, Martin H: Urinalysis using a test strip. British Journal of Nursing 28(6):336–340, 2019.

Murray I, Hendley J: Change and adaptation in pregnancy. In Marshall J, Raynor M, editors: Myles textbook for midwives, 17th ed., Elsevier, Edinburgh, 2020.

Prakash S, Saini S, Mullick P, Pawar M. Green urine: a cause for concern? Journal of Anaesthesiology Clinical Pharmacology 33(1):128–130, 2017.

Puri S, Garg R: Intraoperative change in urine color: Be cautious for a clinical entity! AANA Journal 87(1):26–28, 2019.

Shields-Cutler R, Crowley J, Hung C, et al: Human urinary composition controls antibacterial activity of siderocalin, Journal of Biological Chemistry 290(26):15949–15960, 2015.

Thibodeau G, Patton K: Structure and function of the body, 14th ed., Elsevier, St Louis, 2012.

Tortora GJ, Derrickson B, Burkett B, et al: Principles of anatomy and physiology, 2nd Asia-Pacific Edition, Wiley, 2018.

Wilson L: Urinalysis, Nursing Standard 19(35):51–54, 2005.

Yates A: Urinalysis: how to interpret results, Nursing Times online issue 2:1–3, 2016.

CHAPTER 17

DEFECATION AND STOOL SPECIMENS

Learning outcomes

Having read this chapter, the reader should be able to:

- describe physiological changes in the gastrointestinal system during pregnancy
- discuss the factors influencing disordered intestinal mobility
- discuss the ways in which the midwife can support women with constipation
- describe how a stool specimen is collected
- summarise the midwife's role and responsibility in relation to collection of a stool specimen.

During pregnancy and the postnatal period, women experience several alterations in the gastrointestinal system which may impact on their quality of life and cause discomfort and embarrassment. Women may have difficulty discussing personal information about defecation. The midwife plays an important role in assisting women to discuss their physical symptoms, relieving discomfort and preventing complications. This chapter focuses on physiological changes, factors influencing defecation and the midwife's role in supporting women with gastrointestinal issues to ensure their wellbeing.

PHYSIOLOGY

Normal stools are semi-solid and consist of water (70%) and the end-products of digestion: residue of unabsorbed food, bile pigments, epithelial cells, mucous, bacteria, cellulose and some inorganic material. Peristalsis propels faeces through the large intestine to the sigmoid colon while up to 2 L of water is absorbed (Brown et al 2011). The longer faeces remain in the large intestine, the more water is removed and the harder the stool becomes, and vice versa. The regularity of bowel movements varies from two to three bowel movements per day to three or four bowel movements per week, depending on the individual (Tortora et al 2018).

In response to the presence of faeces the walls in the rectum expand, the brain recognises the rectum is full and the urge to defecate occurs (Bardsley 2017). The external anal sphincter is under voluntary control and can delay a bowel movement until an appropriate time (Tortora et al 2018). To inhibit defecation, an impulse is sent to the cerebral cortex. In babies and young children this ability is absent, and defecation becomes a reflex response to faeces in the rectum.

The levator ani muscle complex is composed of the iliococcygeal, pubococcygeal and puborectalis muscles, which together support the pelvic floor. The puborectalis muscle forms a supportive sling around the rectum and when contracted helps prevent leakage of faeces (Gump & Schmelzer 2016). During birth both the internal and external sphincters, along with associated nerves, can be damaged (Gump & Schmelzer 2016). Any weakness or injury to the posterior pelvic floor contributes to difficulties with defecation, including anal incontinence (Shin et al 2015).

The internal anal sphincter normally remains closed unless there is an urge to defecate. If the urge to defecate is ignored, the external anal sphincter contracts and the faeces return from the anal canal to the rectum and sigmoid colon (retroperistalsis). The stimulus then disappears until the next wave of mass peristalsis moves the faeces back into the rectum (Tortora et al 2018). If the stimulus continues to be inhibited, suppression of the reflex occurs and constipation ensues.

Once passed, faeces are usually referred to as 'stools' and can vary in appearance between individuals and even within the individual. For further descriptions of stools, refer to the Bristol stool classification (Fig 17.1).

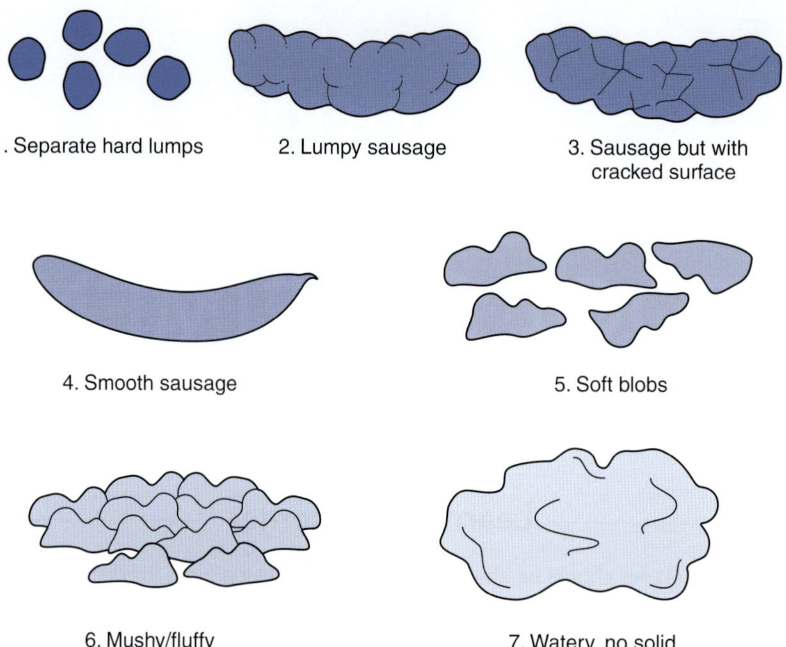

FIGURE 17.1 **Bristol stool classifications. Type 1, separate hard lumps; type 2, lumpy sausage; type 3, sausage but with cracked surface; type 4, smooth sausage; type 5, soft blobs; type 6, mushy/fluffy; type 7, watery, no solid.**
Source: Johnson R, Taylor W: Skills for midwifery practice, 4th ed., Elsevier, London, 2016.

Mental health disorders, such as anxiety and depression, appear to slow transit through the bowel increasing the risk of constipation (Lamb & Sanders 2015). A bidirectional relationship exists between high levels of stress and the microbiota–gut–brain axis (Breit et al 2018, Dinan & Cryan 2017). When a woman is under stress the gut and brain communicate via the vagus nerve resulting in decreased energy and blood flow to the gut (Enders 2014). The vagus nerve regulates smooth muscle contraction and glandular secretion in the intestine (Breit et al 2018).

Pregnancy-related physiology

During pregnancy, higher progesterone levels and the hormone relaxin decrease the mobility of intestinal smooth muscle. The peptide hormone motilin, which is responsible for stimulating motility in smooth muscles, is inhibited (Verghese et al 2015). Mechanical pressure on the rectosigmoid colon from the gravid uterus displaces the bowel, also slowing transit time (Murray & Hendley 2020). Oestrogen enlarges blood vessels and makes connective tissues softer and more pliable (Zielinski et al 2015). High levels of oestrogen and progesterone increase aldosterone, which stimulates more absorption of water and sodium from the intestines, making the stool harder (Verghese et al 2015). In combination, these factors cause bowel hypomobility and increased gastrointestinal transit time (Lamb & Sanders 2015).

During birth, the pelvic floor muscles can be damaged, particularly with forceps, fetal macrosomia, prolonged second stage and episiotomy. The levator ani muscle is part of the external anal sphincter, which is vital for control of defecation (Lamb & Sanders 2015). Labour injuries to the pelvic floor muscles and anal sphincters may result in postpartum constipation (Kuronen et al 2020). Pelvic muscle function can be improved by exercise, weight loss and biofeedback techniques (Gump & Schmelzer 2016). If problems with bowel function and continence persist, a woman should be referred for follow up.

Following birth, the bowel pattern usually returns to the normal pattern within a few days (Raynor & Catling 2017).

Constipation

Functional or primary constipation is defined as infrequent bowel movements and difficulty passing stools without underlying pathological causes (Verghese et al 2015). Secondary constipation results from medications or from underlying medical or metabolic conditions (e.g. irritable bowel syndrome and hypothyroidism) (Verghese et al 2015). The incidence of constipation is two to three times higher during pregnancy, with approximately 40% of pregnant woman affected (Kuronen et al 2020). As pregnancy continues, constipation is exacerbated by the weight of the gravid uterus and hormonal changes. Postpartum the incidence is 52% with a higher incidence of constipation after caesarean section (57%) (Johannessen & Cartwright 2020). The incidence of constipation declines rapidly to 9% by 1 month postpartum (Kuronen et al 2020). Constipation can lead to pelvic floor dysfunction, overactive bladder or pelvic organ prolapse (Kuronen et al 2020).

If faeces remain in the large intestine for longer than 5 days, more water is absorbed making the faeces hard, dry, and more difficult to pass (Thibodeau & Patton 2012). Prolonged constipation can lead to faecal impaction with a large, hardened mass which is painful to expel (Wakefield 2021), and faecal incontinence, the involuntary loss of stool and/or gas (Bezerra et al 2014). Constipation may also indirectly predispose to haemorrhoids developing. Flatus (gas) can accumulate with reduced or absent peristalsis and can lead to abdominal distension and pain (deWit & O'Neill 2014).

During pregnancy, women are at increased risk of opioid-induced constipation because opioids further reduce transit time and increase fluid absorption leading to hard stools (Li et al 2015). Iron supplements also increase the risk of constipation (Cooper & Gosnell 2018). While constipation can cause pain, discomfort and distress, the woman may experience other associated symptoms including fatigue, malaise, cramps, nausea, vomiting, confusion, restlessness, headaches and halitosis (Brown et al 2011). Constipation in pregnancy causes discomfort and may result in damage to the pudendal nerve and impair the supportive function of the pelvic floor musculature (Jefferson & Croton 2013).

Women may not wish to discuss problems such as constipation and haemorrhoids in front of their partner (Lamb & Sanders 2015). Sensitive topics can be difficult for women to bring up; therefore, it is important for midwives to provide a safe and respectful environment for women. Early recognition and treatment of constipation helps women feel more comfortable and can reduce or prevent further long-term problems such as haemorrhoids, perineal damage and anal fissures.

Straining

Straining or 'bearing down' (Valsalva manoeuvre) is best avoided as it can contribute to pelvic floor disorders including pudendal nerve damage and impaired function of the pelvic floor musculature (Kuronen et al 2020). Straining increases intra-abdominal and intrathoracic pressure, reducing blood flow to the heart, temporarily reducing cardiac output. When bearing down ends, the pressure reduces and a larger amount of blood returns to the heart which may cause a dangerous rise in blood pressure, particularly in a hypertensive individual (Dempsey et al 2014).

Straining excessively and using forceful abdominal compression over time can cause damage to the pudendal nerve and weakening of the pelvic floor (Verghese et al 2015).

Straining, particularly using the Valsalva manoeuvre of forced exhalation against a closed glottis, can result in an increase in both intrathoracic and central venous pressure. It may also result in a temporary reduction in vision with subconjunctival haemorrhage, which may occur as a result of transient subclinical retinal oedema (Connor 2010).

Haemorrhoids

Haemorrhoids are common during pregnancy and the postpartum period. It is estimated they occur in one-third of pregnancies (van der Woude et al 2014). Haemorrhoids occur when the veins in the anus swell and dilate.

During pregnancy increased intra-abdominal pressure, vascular engorgement, venous stasis, pelvic congestion, vasodilation, constipation and pushing during labour predispose women to haemorrhoids (Shin et al 2015). Haemorrhoids can be exacerbated by practices such as directed pushing, instrumental birth or episiotomy (Lamb & Sanders 2015). Other pregnancy-related factors predisposing women to haemorrhoids are the enlarging gravid uterus, which impedes venous return from the lower limbs, resulting in stagnation of blood and arteriovenous shunting within the compressed rectal veins (Murray & Hendley 2020); and relaxation of veins in the anal canal (Hall et al 2015).

Faecal incontinence

Faecal incontinence is the involuntary loss of gas, liquid or solid stool (Bezerra et al 2014) and can be related to neurological or muscular dysfunction (Raynor & Catling 2017). It affects around 10–15% of women in the general population (Turner 2017). The rate of faecal incontinence postnatally is approximately 6% at 3 months postpartum; however, many women do not disclose the problem (Shin et al 2015). Faecal incontinence may occur as overflow from constipation.

Childbirth and straining to evacuate the bowels may damage or weaken the internal and external anal sphincter. Injury or weakness in the structures of the pelvic floor increases the risk of bowel dysfunction, including faecal incontinence (Ying-Chih et al 2014). When diarrhoea is present it becomes more difficult for women with weakened muscles to contain the stool.

Constipation—predisposing factors

- Poor habits and frequently delaying defecation
- Diet (e.g. inadequate bulk; high intake of processed cheese, lean meat, eggs and pasta) (Dempsey et al 2014)
- Dehydration
- Lack of exercise or immobility (e.g. bed rest)
- Pelvic floor damage (Mayo Clinic 2015)
- Changes to normal lifestyle and routines (e.g. hospitalisation, as this causes interruption to the normal gastrocolic reflex)
- Pregnancy

- Psychological: unfavourable conditions (e.g. lack of privacy, shared toilet facilities, bedpans), fear of damaging a sutured perineum
- Pain: may be associated with haemorrhoids and fissures
- Drugs (e.g. opiates, iron supplements, antidepressants, calcium channel blockers, aluminium antacids, selective serotonin re-uptake inhibitors [SSRIs], antipsychotics, antihistamines)
- General anaesthesia
- Obstruction (e.g. faecal impaction)
- Disease (e.g. hypothyroidism, diverticular disease, neuromuscular disorders, hypercalcaemia)
- Psychiatric disorders (e.g. anorexia, depression)

Diarrhoea

Diarrhoea is an increase in the frequency, volume and fluid content of the faeces resulting from increased intestinal motility (Tortora et al 2018). In consequence, the absorption of water, nutrients and electrolytes decreases and the stool becomes semi-formed or liquid. Acute diarrhoea is common and usually self-limiting, resolving within 2 weeks; chronic diarrhoea lasts longer than 2 weeks and may be the result of an underlying disease. Diarrhoea may also lead to temporary faecal incontinence (deWit & O'Neill 2014).

Acute diarrhoea is most frequently caused by either viral or bacterial infection spread from human contact, contaminated food or water (Zielinski et al 2015).

Profuse, watery and bloody diarrhoea accompanied by fever and abdominal pain requires further investigation. Women presenting with acute diarrhoea may need to be cared for in a single room with contact and droplet precautions in place until infection is ruled out as a cause. Pregnant women with diarrhoea are at risk of dehydration and electrolyte imbalance. Fluid and electrolyte replacement is a priority and can be oral fluids, such as water, clear juice or rehydration fluid. If women are unable to tolerate fluids, intravenous fluid may be needed.

The intestinal microbiota can be disrupted when women receive antibiotics, leading to antibiotic-associated diarrhoea. The health bacteria in the gut play a role in immune function and are reduced by antibiotics allowing pathogenic organisms to multiply and cause *Clostridioides difficile*-associated diarrhoea. The use of proton pump inhibitors and H_2-receptor antagonists, particularly when combined with antibiotics, increases the risk of *C. difficile* infection (Hall et al 2015).

Diarrhoea—predisposing factors

- During the onset and early part of labour (this could result in defecation being delayed in the first 48 hours after delivery)
- Infection (e.g. helminths)
- Diet: excessive intake of certain foods (e.g. fruit, alcohol, coffee, chocolate) (Dempsey et al 2014) or food intolerance (e.g. lactose intolerance)
- Stress
- Drugs (e.g. antibiotics, iron supplements, laxatives)
- Disease (e.g. irritable bowel syndrome [IBS], Crohn's disease, ulcerative colitis, diverticulitis); with IBS, increased visceral sensitivity to rectal load occurs and is often associated with psychological comorbidity (Moulton et al 2019)
- Damage: weakened pelvic floor muscles provide little support for the anal sphincter; as the abdominal pressure rises, faeces may leak through the sphincter

PRINCIPLES: PROMOTING DEFECATION

Optimum posture

Adopting the best physiological posture aids in evacuation of the bowel. In an upright position the colon has a natural bend which helps maintain continence. Increased hip flexion occurs in a squatting position making the rectoanal canal straighter and decreasing straining during defecation (Sakakibara et al 2010). The larger rectoanal angle is believed to be due to relaxation of the puborectal and pelvic floor muscles (Sakakibara et al 2010).

Squatting or sitting forwards with the knees higher than the hips helps relax and straighten the colon, allows the weight of the torso to compress the colon and the diaphragm to move down and facilitate the action of the abdominal muscles. The abdomen should bulge out, the spine should be straight, the glottis closed, the jaw relaxed, lips open and teeth apart. The use of a footstool to raise the legs may facilitate this position (Fig 17.2). Optimal posture is difficult to achieve when sitting on a bedpan, which, accompanied by embarrassment, can inhibit evacuation of the bowel (Dempsey et al 2014).

Diet

Dietary modifications, such as a high-fibre diet and adequate fluids, should be discussed with childbearing

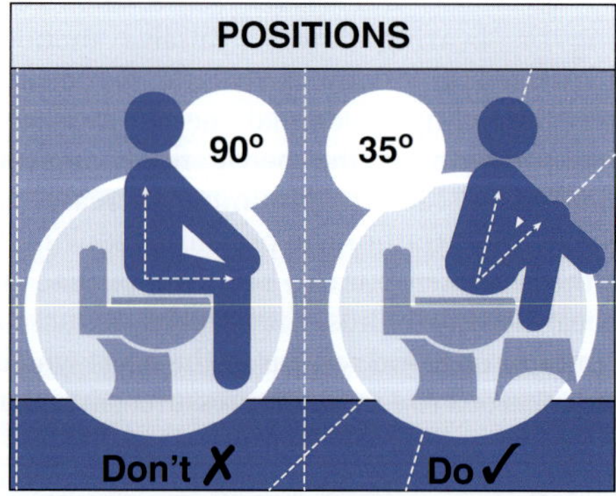

FIGURE 17.2 **Optimal position for evacuation of the bowel.**

women who are constipated (Turawa et al 2020). Dietary fibre will increase pressure on the intestinal wall, creating the stimulus for peristalsis and moving the intestinal contents more quickly so that less water is absorbed (Dempsey et al 2014). Wheat bran is a good source of fibre, iron, B vitamins, zinc and magnesium; however, it has a high capacity to absorb water (Jefferson & Croton 2013) and is associated with bloating and flatulence (Major & Spiller 2015). A high-fibre diet improves insulin sensitivity, assists with diabetes management (Mogoş et al 2017) and reduces the risk of type 2 diabetes (Ley et al 2016). The incidence of gestational diabetes may be significantly reduced by a healthy diet (Ley et al 2016) rich in fruits, vegetables and whole grains (Lowensohn et al 2016). Women with antenatal depression were found to have a poorer diet, with a higher proportion of processed foods, and those with an elevated body mass index (BMI) prior to pregnancy were at increased risk of antenatal depression in comparison with women within a healthy weight range (Molyneaux et al 2016). To prevent depression, a diet high in vegetables, fruits, legumes, wholegrains, nuts and seeds is recommended (Opie et al 2017). A low-fibre proinflammatory diet high in refined carbohydrates is associated with lower fetal growth and reduced breastfeeding (Sen et al 2016). The Nutrition Reference Values for Australia and New Zealand (National Health and Medical Research Council [NHMRC] and Ministry of Health [MoH] 2006) recommend a fibre intake of 28 g during pregnancy and 30 g for lactation, as opposed to 25 g for the non-pregnant adult female.

A healthy high-fibre diet

Increasing the amount of fibre in the diet may initially cause bloating, abdominal distention and flatulence, but this is self-limiting and the symptoms will reduce over time (Brown et al 2011). To avoid discomfort, a gradual increase in fibre is advisable. A high-fibre diet with an adequate fluid intake will prevent the stools becoming too firm to pass. Dempsey et al (2014) advise a daily fluid intake of 2–3 L when eating a high-fibre diet; although Major and Spiller (2015) indicate the evidence on drinking more water to treat constipation is lacking unless dehydration is present. Prebiotic foods pass through the stomach and small intestine undigested. Once in the large intestine they promote beneficial bacteria. Information on high-fibre and prebiotic diets is available from Monash University (see Resources at end of chapter).

Other measures include:

- conditioning; sitting on the toilet following a meal may help bowel habits be relearned, especially after breakfast—Dempsey et al (2014) suggest this is when the gastrocolic and duodenocolic reflexes cause mass propulsive movements within the large intestine
- privacy, so that the sounds and smells of defecation are not noticed; wherever possible facilitate the use of a toilet rather than a commode or bedpan
- education on care of the perineum and avoiding damage to a sutured perineum; reassurance of expected changes and return to normal bowel function following birth
- use of soft toilet paper, as this may help psychologically
- increasing mobility; constipation is associated with decreased mobility, so mild exercise will help
- easy access to clean toilet facilities; avoid using the bedpan which increases straining and oxygen consumption
- treating haemorrhoids
- using a suitable barrier cream to prevent anal excoriation
- use of oral laxatives, but these should not be the first course of action
- suppositories and micro enemas (see Chapter 21) may provide immediate but short-term relief of constipation; the cause of constipation should also be treated
- maintaining optimum posture, for example, have a stool for women to put their feet on in the toilet.

OBTAINING STOOL SPECIMENS

For childbearing women, stool specimens are likely to be screened for:

- gastrointestinal (GI) infection (e.g. infective diarrhoea)
- presence of occult blood
- parasitic infections (e.g. giardiasis, hookworm).

Stool specimens may be required to detect disease-causing pathogens (bacterial, viral or parasitic) and assist in diagnosis of gastrointestinal system disorders (Table 17.1) (Brunstein 2017). Stools can be examined for blood, mucous, infectious agents and white blood cells. The small and large intestine can be invaded by pathogenic organisms which multiply and cause infection. The most common way of contracting a gastrointestinal disorder is from ingesting contaminated food or water (Cooper & Gosnell 2018). Infectious diarrhoea is generally transmitted by the oral–faecal route via ingestion of contaminated food and water and person-to-person transmission (Kelly 2015).

Women who have travelled overseas recently may have been exposed to pathogenic bacteria and parasites. Infectious diarrhoea can cause fluid and electrolytes to be secreted into the intestinal lumen. Some bacteria produce toxic substances which can cause tissue damage. In healthcare settings, *Clostridioides difficile* infection is responsible for 20–30% of antibiotic-associated diarrhoea (Montecalvo et al 2017). Interest in the microbiome has resulted in stool specimens being collected for metabolic profiling and host-gut microbial metabolic interactions (Gratton et al 2016).

General guidelines for specimen collection should be followed. When collecting stool specimens, it is important to understand the timing and frequency of

TABLE 17.1 BACTERIAL AND PARASITIC INFECTIONS

Bacteria	Source	Diagnosis
Campylobacter species	Foodborne. Found in infected water and foods, particularly undercooked poultry and unpasteurised milk.	Stool culture (NSW Health 2017)
Salmonella species	Food- and water-borne. Found in raw eggs, raw poultry, uncooked vegetables. People may become carriers.	Stool culture Polymerase chain reaction (PCR) (SA Health 2021)
Shigella species (shigellosis)	Faecal–oral. Person-to-person. Foodborne, found in foods and water contaminated with bacteria from stool of infected person.	Stool culture (Health Direct 2020)
Escherichia coli O157:H7	Faecal–oral. Virulent toxin producing. Most strains of *E. coli* are considered normal flora and do not cause disease. *E. coli* 0157:H7 is a toxin-producing subtype which can cause serious illness. Found in raw/undercooked meats, spinach and unpasteurised milk and cider. Causes bloody diarrhoea. Can lead to haemolytic uremic syndrome.	Cultured PCR or antigen test (WHO 2018)
Clostridioides difficile, the most common cause of infectious diarrhoea in those who are hospitalised	Broad-spectrum antibiotics may lead to overgrowth. Toxin-producing strains may cause diarrhoea and other adverse outcomes. Spread by bacteria and spores in hospital environment (e.g. hands of staff).	Stool specimen (Queensland Health 2019)
Parasites		
Giardia, a protozoon (*Giardia lamblia*, *Giardia intestinalis*, *Giardia duodenalis*)	Faecal–oral. Causes giardia infection (giardiasis). Found in polluted water, raw foods, foods washed in contaminated water. Person-to-person.	Stool examination, antigen tests (Lab Tests Online Au 2020)
Cryptosporidium, a protozoon often abbreviated to 'Crypto'	Faecal–oral, person-to-person. Swimming in contaminated water. Drinking contaminated water or untreated milk.	Stool sample for microscopic identification, antigen tests (NSW Health 2018)
Threadworm/pinworm, a type of helminth known as a nematode *Enterobius vermicularis*	Faecal–oral route. Indirectly from bedding, clothing, food, overcrowding.	Stool sample, microscopic identification (Lab Tests Online Au 2020)
Tapeworm, a type of helminth with multiple varieties; the most common is *Hymenolepis* (dwarf tapeworm), known as *Taenia nana* in New Zealand	Faecal–oral transmission or ingestion of contaminated undercooked meat.	2–3 stool specimens for identification of ova and parasites (Lab Tests Online Au 2020)

the tests; some infections require repeated sampling over consecutive days. Some infective agents cannot survive for long outside the body, so the specimen must be dispatched promptly. Stool specimens should be assessed for their colour, consistency, odour and frequency, and the information recorded. The Bristol stool chart (Fig 17.1) describes the seven main types of stool classification.

Women may prefer to collect the stool specimen themselves.

SKILL 17.1 Stool specimen (adult)

1. Confirm identity, explain the procedure to the woman and gain informed consent.
2. Gather equipment:
   - clean bedpan or disposable liner
   - stool specimen container with integral scoop or spatula
   - non-sterile gloves and apron
   - biohazard bag.
3. Ask the woman to defecate into the bedpan, but not to urinate. (If incontinent, take the specimen from soiled pads, without urine contamination, if possible).
4. Wash and dry hands; apply apron and PPE.
5. Using the scoop, place the stool sample in the specimen container, filling approximately one-third of the container, and seal the lid.
6. If any parasite is visible, aim to place the entire parasite in the container.
7. Dispose of equipment and wash and dry hands.
8. Label and dispatch the specimen.
9. Document findings (including stool classification) and act accordingly.

SKILL 17.2 Stool specimen (neonate)

1. Gain parental consent.
2. Observe the neonate for signs of straining (to obtain a fresh specimen).
3. Perform hand hygiene.
4. Don non-sterile gloves and fill one-third (if possible) of the stool specimen pot with the stool taken from the neonate's nappy. Avoid contamination with urine if possible.
5. If the stool is too wet and has been absorbed, efforts should be made to catch the sample in a sterile foil bowl on the next evacuation.
6. Remove gloves and perform hand hygiene.
7. Label and dispatch the specimen (immediately for some screenings), indicating whether contamination with urine was likely.
8. Document the findings and act accordingly.

Role and responsibilities of the midwife

These can be summarised as:

- asking women about their bowel habits as part of the antenatal and postnatal examination; this should be undertaken in a respectful manner
- discussing and treating constipation as appropriate
- recording any problems, advice given and evaluating the advice in the woman's case notes
- ensuring any aperients are safe for use during pregnancy or breastfeeding
- if difficulties with defecation do not resolve, referring the woman for further investigation
- explaining the procedure and gaining consent
- ensuring correct stool specimen collection and dispatch
- understanding and applying infection control and standard precaution protocols
- correctly documenting specimen collection and acting on results.

SUMMARY

- Defecation is primarily under conscious control (in the adult).
- Inhibition of defecation can lead to constipation.
- Defecation can be promoted by a number of different factors.
- Specimens should be obtained, labelled and dispatched correctly.
- Stool specimens may be required to diagnose bacterial and parasitic infections.
- Stool specimens from the woman are obtained from a clean bedpan; from the neonate they are obtained from the nappy.

Self-assessment exercises

The answers to the following questions may be found in the text.

1. Describe the physiology of defecation.
2. Consider factors influencing the ability to evacuate the bowel.
3. Discuss how the midwife can advise women with constipation.
4. Describe three common bacterial or parasitic infections.
5. Describe how a stool specimen is obtained from a woman.
6. Describe how a stool specimen is obtained from a neonate.
7. Summarise the role and responsibilities of the midwife in relation to defecation and stool specimen collection.

Resources

Australian Clinical Labs: Faeces collection: www.clinicallabs.com.au/patient/collection-information/collection-guide/faecal-collection/faeces-collection/.

Continence Foundation of Australia: www.continence.org.au.

Lab Tests Online AU, Explaining Pathology: How samples are collected. www.labtestsonline.org.au/understanding/how-samples-are-collected.

Monash University: High fibre, high prebiotic diet for healthy individuals, 2021: www.monash.edu/medicine/ccs/gastroenterology/prebiotic.

Quest Diagnostics: For physicians and hospitals, General guidelines: www.questdiagnostics.com/home/physicians/testing-services/specialists/hospitals-lab-staff/specimen-handling/general.html.

References

Bardsley A: Assessment and treatment options for patients with constipation, British Journal of Nursing 26:312–318, 2017.

Bezerra L, Vasconcelos Neto J, Vasconcelos C, et al: Prevalence of unreported bowel symptoms in women with pelvic floor dysfunction and the impact on their quality of life, International Urogynecology Journal 25:927–933, 2014.

Breit S, Kupferberg A, Rogler G, Hasler G: Vagus nerve as modulator of the brain–gut axis in psychiatric and inflammatory disorders. Frontiers in Psychiatry, 9, 44–44, 2018.

Brown H, Crisford M, Fernandes A, et al: Elimination. In Dougherty L, Lister S, editors: The Royal Marsden Hospital manual of clinical nursing procedures, 8th ed., Wiley Blackwell, Oxford, 2011.

Brunstein J: Challenging stool sample types for MDx, Medical Laboratory Observer 49(10):56–57, 2017.

Connor A: Valsalva-related retinal venous dilation caused by defaecation, Acta Ophthalmologica 88(4):e149, 2010.

Cooper K, Gosnell K: Foundations and adult health nursing, Elsevier, Mosby, St Louis, 2018.

Dempsey J, Hillege S, Hill R: Fundamentals of nursing and midwifery a person-centred approach to care, 2nd ed., Lippincott, Williams & Wilkins Pty Ltd, Sydney, 2014.

deWit S, O'Neill P: Fundamental concepts and skills for nursing, 4th ed., Elsevier, St Louis, 2014.

Dinan TG, Cryan JF: Gut instincts: microbiota as a key regulator of brain development, aging and neurodegeneration, Journal of Physiology 595(2):489–503, 2017.

Enders G: Gut, the inside story of our body's most under-rated organ, Scribe, Melbourne, 2014.

Gratton J, Phetcharaburanin J, Mullish BH, et al: Optimized sample handling strategy for metabolic profiling of human feces, Analytical Chemistry 88:4661–4668, 2016.

Gump K, Schmelzer M: Gaining control over fecal incontinence, Medsurg Nursing 25:97–102, 96, 2016.

Hall V, Owens C, Blackwell R: Physiological and hormonal changes and GI problems experienced in pregnancy, Gastrointestinal Nursing 13:17–25, 2015.

Health Direct: *Shigella* (shigellosis), 2020. Online 3 September 2021. Available: www.healthdirect.gov.au/shigella-bowel-infection.

Jefferson A, Croton J: Using wheat bran fibre to improve bowel habits during pregnancy—a call to action, British Journal of Midwifery 21(5):331–341, 2013.

Johannessen H, Cartwright R: Constipation during and after pregnancy. BJOG: an International Journal of Obstetrics and Gynaecology May, 128(6):1065, 2020.

Kelly P: Infectious diarrhoea, Africa Health 37:22–27, 2015.

Kuronen M, Hantunen S, Alanne L, et al. Pregnancy, puerperium and perinatal constipation—an observational hybrid survey on pregnant and postpartum women and their age-matched non-pregnant controls. BJOG: an International Journal of Obstetrics and Gynaecology May, 128(6): 1057–1064, 2020.

Lab Tests Online Au: Ova, cysts and parasites, 2020. Online 2 September 2021. Available: www.labtestsonline.org.au/learning/test-index/o-and-p-or-ocp.

Lamb K, Sanders R: Constipation and haemorrhoids: a midwifery perspective for the childbearing continuum, British Journal of Midwifery 23:171–177, 2015.

Ley SH, Ardisson Korat AV, Qi S, et al: Contribution of the nurses' health studies to uncovering risk factors for type 2 diabetes: diet, lifestyle, biomarkers and genetics, American Journal of Public Health 106:1624–1630, 2016.

Li Z, Pergolizzi JV, Huttner RP, et al: Management of opioid-induced constipation in pregnancy: a concise review with emphasis on the PAMORAs, Journal of Clinical Pharmacy & Therapeutics 40:615–619, 2015.

Lowensohn RI, Stadler DD, Naze C: Current concepts of maternal nutrition, Obstetrical & Gynecological Survey 71:413–426, 2016.

Major G, Spiller R: Constipation in adults, Pulse 42–44, 2015.

Mayo Clinic: Health letter, Pelvic Muscle Dysfunction 33:4–5, 2015.

Mogoş T, Dondoi C, Iacobini AE: A review of dietary fiber in the diabetic diet, Romanian Journal of Diabetes Nutrition & Metabolic Diseases 24:161–164, 2017.

Molyneaux E, Poston L, Khondoker M, et al: Obesity, antenatal depression, diet and gestational weight gain in a population cohort study, Archives of Women's Mental Health 19:899–907, 2016.

Moulton C, Pavlidis P, Norton C, et al: Depressive symptoms in inflammatory bowel disease: an extraintestinal manifestation of inflammation? Clinical and Experimental Immunology, 197(3), 308–318, 2019.

Montecalvo M, Sisay E, McKenna D, et al: Use of a perianal swab compared with a stool sample to detect symptomatic *Clostridium difficile* infection, Infection Control & Hospital Epidemiology 38(6):658–662, 2017.

Murray I, Hendley J: Change and adaptation in pregnancy. In Marshall J, Raynor M, editors: Myles textbook for midwives, 17th ed., Elsevier, Edinburgh, 2020.

National Health and Medical Research Council (NHMRC), New Zealand Ministry of Health (MoH): Dietary fibre; extract from Nutrient Reference Values for Australia and New Zealand Including Recommended Dietary Intakes, 2006. Online 2 April 2021. Available: www.nrv.gov.au/sites/default/files/content/n35-dietaryfibre_0.pdf.

NSW Health: *Campylobacteriosis* fact sheet, 2017. Online 2 April 2021. Available: www.health.nsw.gov.au/Infectious/factsheets/Pages/Campylobacteriosis.aspx.

NSW Health: Cryptosporidiosis fact sheet, 2018. Online 3 September 2021. Available: www.health.nsw.gov.au/Infectious/factsheets/Pages/cryptosporidiosis.aspx.

Opie RS, Itsiopoulos C, Parletta N, et al: Dietary recommendations for the prevention of depression, Nutritional Neuroscience 20:161–171, 2017.

Queensland Health, 2019: CDI - Clostridium difficile infection. Online 3 September 2021. Available: www.health.qld.gov.au/clinical-practice/guidelines-procedures/diseases-infection/infection-prevention/management-advice/cdi.

Raynor M, Catling C: Myles survival guide to midwifery, 3rd ed., Elsevier, Sydney, 2017.

SA Health. Salmonella infection—including symptoms, treatment and prevention, 2021. Online 6 April 2021. Available: www.sahealth.sa.gov.au/wps/wcm/connect/public+content/sa+health+internet/conditions/infectious+diseases/salmonella+infection.

Sakakibara R, Tsunoyama K, Hosoi H, et al: Influence of body position on defecation in humans, Lower Urinary Tract Symptoms 2:16–21, 2010.

Sen S, Rifas-Shiman SL, Shivappa N, et al: Dietary inflammatory potential during pregnancy is associated with lower fetal growth and breastfeeding failure: results from project Viva, Journal of Nutrition 146:728–736, 2016.

Shin GH, Toto EL, Schey R: Pregnancy and postpartum bowel changes: constipation and fecal incontinence, American Journal of Gastroenterology 110:521–529, 2015.

Thibodeau G, Patton K: Structure and function of the body, 14th ed., Elsevier Mosby, St Louis, 2012.

Tortora GJ, Derrickson B, Burkettet, B, et al: Principles of anatomy and physiology, 2nd Asia-Pacific Edition, Wiley, 2018.

Turawa E, Musekiwa A, Rohwer A: Interventions for preventing postpartum constipation, Cochrane Library, 2020(8):CD011625–CD011625, 2020.

Turner J: Establishing a nurse-led pelvic floor and functional bowel service, British Journal of Nursing 26:640–642, 2017.

van der Woude CJ, Metselaar HJ, Danese S: Management of gastrointestinal and liver diseases during pregnancy, Gut 63(6):1014–1023, 2014.

Verghese TS, Futaba K, Latthe P: Constipation in pregnancy, Obstetrician & Gynaecologist 17:111–115, 2015.

Wakefield H: In Koutoukidis G, Stainton K, editors: Tabbner's nursing care, 8th ed., Elsevier Australia, Sydney, 2021. Chapter 32: Nursing care: Bowel elimination and continence.

World Health Organization (WHO): *E.coli* fact sheet. Online 2 April 2021. 2018. Available: www.who.int/en/news-room/fact-sheets/detail/e-coli.

Ying-Chih W, Deutscher D, Sheng-Che Y, et al: The self-report fecal incontinence and constipation questionnaire in patients with pelvic-floor dysfunction seeking outpatient rehabilitation, Physical Therapy 94:273–288, 2014.

Zielinski R, Searing K, Deibel M: Gastrointestinal distress in pregnancy, Journal of Perinatal & Neonatal Nursing 29:23–31, 2015.

SECTION 5

PRINCIPLES OF DRUG ADMINISTRATION

CHAPTER 18

MEDICATION ADMINISTRATION: LEGAL ASPECTS, PHARMACOLOGY AND ANAPHYLAXIS

Learning outcomes

Having read this chapter, the reader should be able to:

- discuss the responsibilities of the midwife in relation to medication administration
- discuss the legal aspects of autonomous administration of medicines by midwives
- identify the classifications of medications
- discuss the five 'rights' of safe medicine administration
- describe the safe administration of controlled medicines
- highlight the process for the administration of controlled medications
- understand the physiological changes influencing how medications are absorbed, distributed, metabolised and excreted for pregnant women and neonates
- describe the signs, symptoms and management of anaphylaxis.

This chapter considers the legal regulations covering medication administration by the midwife. It includes guidelines for the safe administration of medicines, and information on the management of anaphylaxis. The majority of women will take some type of medication during pregnancy and lactation. It is important to understand how the physiological changes of pregnancy affect medications. The majority of commonly used medications are relatively safe for breastfed infants as the amount of medication transferred to breastmilk is generally small. It is important for midwives to be able to provide accurate information on medication use during pregnancy and breastfeeding.

LEGAL ASPECTS OF MEDICATION ADMINISTRATION

Pharmacokinetics, pharmacodynamics and pharmacogenomics provide information on how medications work and the factors influencing their effectiveness. Medications can have positive benefits and negative effects, which must be carefully assessed. Medication use carries the risk of serious adverse reactions; therefore, medicines are regulated to protect public health and ensure they meet acceptable standards of safety, quality and efficacy.

Legislation in Australia

In Australia, Commonwealth and state and territory laws govern the quality and safety of medicines. The Commonwealth Acts affecting medicine manufacture and administration in Australia are the *Therapeutic Goods Act 1989* and the *Narcotic Drugs Act 1967*. The Therapeutic Goods Act outlines the legal requirements for the import, export, manufacture and supply of therapeutic goods in Australia and provides the basis for a uniform system to control scheduled substances.

Each state and territory has an Act and regulations for the control of medicines (Bullock & Manias 2017).

A two-tiered system regulates medicines. Higher risk medicines are *registered* and lower risk medicines are *listed* on the Australian Register of Therapeutic Goods (ARTG). All registered medicines are assessed by the Therapeutic Goods Administration (TGA) to ensure quality, safety and efficacy. All prescription medicines, most over-the-counter medicines and some complementary medicines are registered. The Pharmaceutical Benefits Scheme (PBS) details the medications subsidised by the Australian Government and helps provide timely, reliable and affordable access to medications.

Medicines are divided into schedules that classify medications according to their strength, therapeutic use, toxicity and abuse potential, safety and modes of action. Each state and territory has a slightly different schedule. The Poisons Standard is the legal title of the Standard for the Uniform Scheduling of Medicines and Poisons (SUSMP) (Table 18.1). The Poisons Standard January 2021 includes the decisions on classification of medications and poisons into schedules for inclusion in state and territory legislation.

Legislation in New Zealand

In New Zealand medicines are controlled by the *Misuse of Drugs Act 1975*, which regulates the classification of controlled drugs and establishes offences and penalties related to illicit drug use. The Act is accompanied by the Misuse of Drugs Regulations 1977, which govern the use of controlled drugs such as morphine. The regulations include midwives in their list of controlled drug prescribers (New Zealand Legislation 2021). The *Medicines Act 1981* and the Medicine Regulations 1984 govern the use of other therapeutic agents (Bullock & Manias 2017). Under the Act, drugs are classified by their potential to cause harm.

- Class A: very high risk of harm (methamphetamine, cocaine, heroin)
- Class B: high risk of harm (morphine, opium, amphetamines)
- Class C: moderate risk of harm (cannabis plant, codeine)

TABLE 18.1 STANDARD FOR THE UNIFORM SCHEDULING OF MEDICINES AND POISONS IN AUSTRALIA

Schedule	Description
Schedule 1.	The schedule intentionally left blank
Schedule 2.	**Pharmacy Medicine**—substances where the safe use may require advice from a pharmacist and are available from a pharmacy only or from a licensed person when a pharmacy service is not available.
Schedule 3.	**Pharmacist Only Medicine**—substances where the safe use requires professional advice, but which should be available to the public from a pharmacist without a prescription.
Schedule 4.	**Prescription Only Medicine** or Prescription Animal Remedy, where the use of supply should be on the order of persons permitted by state or territory legislation to prescribe and should be available from a pharmacist on prescription.
Schedule 5.	**Caution**—substances with a low potential for causing harm, the extent of which can be reduced through appropriate packaging with simple warnings and safety directions on the label
Schedule 6.	**Poison**—substances with a moderate potential for causing harm, the extent of which can be reduced by the use of distinctive packaging with strong warnings and safety directions on the label
Schedule 7.	**Dangerous Poison**—substances with a high potential for causing harm at low exposure and which require special precautions during manufacture, handling or use. These poisons should be available only to specialised or authorised users who have the skills necessary to handle them safely. Special regulations restricting their availability, possession, storage or use may apply.
Schedule 8.	**Controlled Drug**—substances which should be available for use but require restriction of manufacture, supply, distribution, possession and use to reduce abuse, misuse and physical or psychological dependence.
Schedule 9.	**Prohibited Substance**—substances which may be abused or misused, the manufacture, possession, sale or use of which should be prohibited by law except when required for medical or scientific research, or for analytical, teaching or training purposes with approval of Commonwealth and/or state or territory health authorities.
Schedule 10. (Previously Appendix C)	**Substances of such danger to health as to warrant prohibition of sale supply and use**—substances which are prohibited for the purpose or purposes listed for each poison.

Source: Federal Register of Legislation (2021). Poisons Standard June 2021. www.legislation.gov.au/Details/F2021L00650

New Zealand has three schedules for medicines, listed in Table 18.2.

Medsafe is the New Zealand medicines and medical devices safety authority, which regulates therapeutic products in New Zealand as well as administering the *Medicines Act 1981* and Medicine Regulations 1984. Medsafe ensures therapeutic products in New Zealand are used appropriately and that benefits outweigh risks.

The Pharmaceutical Management Agency (Pharmac) is the New Zealand Government's agency that determines which pharmaceutical products are publicly funded in New Zealand (see Resources section at end of chapter).

Midwives prescribing (Australia)

In Australia midwives do not receive authority to prescribe on graduation from an accredited midwifery program. To receive the authority to prescribe, midwives must complete additional accredited education (Small et al 2016) and comply with the Nursing and Midwifery Board of Australia (NMBA) Registration Standard: Endorsement for Scheduled Medicines for Midwives (Pairman et al 2019).

Midwives authorised to prescribe are identified by 'MW' in the PBS Schedule. Midwife PBS prescriptions are identifiable by colour and include the 'MW' indicator; prescriptions must include the midwife's PBS prescriber number.

The NMBA has approved the schedule 4, schedule 8 and intravenous medicines that endorsed midwives can prescribe. Endorsed midwives in Australia can prescribe medicines on the PBS schedule for midwives in accordance with state and territory legislation (see Resources section).

It is the midwife's responsibility to know and follow the prescribing accreditation for their state or territory as the medicines able to be prescribed by midwives differ between states and territories. (For a more extensive discussion of pharmacology and prescribing for midwives, see Pairman et al 2019).

TABLE 18.2 MEDICINE SCHEDULES IN NEW ZEALAND

Schedule	Description
Prescription medicines	Medicines requiring a prescription from an authorised prescriber
Restricted medicines	Medicines which can be sold by a retail outlet or supplied by a pharmacist in a pharmacy or hospital
Pharmacy-only medications	Medicines which can be sold by retail outlets or supplied only by pharmacies or hospitals, or by shops at least 10 km from the closest pharmacy which have been issued with a license

Source: New Zealand Legislation, Medicines Regulations 1984.

Midwives prescribing (New Zealand)

After graduating from an accredited midwifery program, midwives in New Zealand are able to prescribe according to their scope of practice. The Midwifery Council is required by law to prescribe the scope of practice for midwifery, which forms the legal definition of midwifery in New Zealand. Prescribing is within the midwifery scope of practice and is included under the competencies of the New Zealand Midwifery Council as Competency 2.13:

> the midwife demonstrates the ability to prescribe, supply and administer medicine, vaccines and immunoglobulin safely and appropriately within the midwife scope of practice and the relevant legislation (Midwifery Council [New Zealand] 2021).

The *Medicine Amendment Act 2013* and Misuse of Drugs Amendment Regulations 2019 allow midwives who have completed the required education to prescribe three controlled drugs (pethidine, morphine and fentanyl) during the intrapartum period.

All midwives in New Zealand must undertake a Midwifery Standards Review (MSR) at the end of their first year of practice and then every 2 years to maintain their Annual Practising Certificate (Midwifery Council [New Zealand] 2018).

Restricted substances

In Australia, the states and territories use different terms for prescribed medications. These terms include prescription drugs, prescription-only drugs, restricted substances, restricted drugs and poisons. In New Zealand the term' 'prescription medicines' is used (Bullock & Manias 2017). New Zealand midwives can prescribe up to 3 months' supply of restricted substances for women under antenatal, intrapartum and postnatal care, as well as medicines relevant to midwifery care during pregnancy until the 6-week postnatal checkup (Bullock & Manias 2017).

Controlled drugs

The supply, storage, administration, surrender and destruction of controlled drugs is tightly controlled by the legislation. Drugs should be administered in line with relevant legislation and local standard operating procedures. In Australia, the states and territories use different terms for controlled drugs, including 'drugs of dependence' and 'prohibited substances'; in New Zealand the term 'controlled drugs' is used (Bullock & Manias 2017). Controlled drugs must be stored in a locked cupboard away from other medications. A ward register for administration of controlled drugs must be maintained; the register must include:

- the name of the person the medication is being administered to

- the name of the midwife removing the medication for administration
- the prescribed medication and dose
- the name of prescriber
- the date and time of administration
- the balance of the remaining medication
- the signature of one midwife for schedule 4 medications and two midwives (or registered health professionals including registered nurses and pharmacists) for a schedule 8 medication
- any medicine from the vial not needed/wasted (ACT Parliamentary Counsel 2017).

The drug register is generally checked at the change of each shift. Any errors made in the drug register should have a line placed through them so the entry is still legible. Regulations and local protocols should be followed when medications are lost or need to be discarded or destroyed and this is done in the presence of another registered health professional such as a midwife, registered nurse or pharmacist.

Australian categories for prescribing medicines in pregnancy

To determine if a medication is safe for use during pregnancy, most prescribers and pharmacists depend on sources such as medication databases and the *Australian Medicines Handbook* (AMH) (Kennedy 2014). These sources generally consist of the Australian Drug Evaluation Committee categories for prescribing medicines in pregnancy and the manufacturer's product information (Table 18.3). In general, pregnancy and lactation are listed as requiring special precautions or contraindications. The categories are provided as a guide only; they do not provide clinical context and it is false to assume medications within the same category have a similar risk (Kennedy 2014). It is important for midwives to discuss the harms and benefits of treatments with women who are pregnant or breastfeeding. Evidence-based information on the safety of medications during pregnancy is available from the obstetric drug

TABLE 18.3 THE AUSTRALIAN CATEGORIES FOR PRESCRIBING MEDICINES IN PREGNANCY

Category A
Drugs which have been taken by a large number of pregnant women and women of childbearing age without any proven increase in the frequency of malformations or other direct or indirect harmful effects on the fetus having been observed.
Category B1
Drugs which have been taken by only a limited number of pregnant women and women of childbearing age, without an increase in the frequency of malformation or other direct or indirect harmful effects on the human fetus having been observed. Studies in animals have not shown evidence of an increased occurrence of fetal damage.
Category B2
Drugs which have been taken by only a limited number of pregnant women and women of childbearing age, without an increase in the frequency of malformation or other direct or indirect harmful effects on the human fetus having been observed. Studies in animals are inadequate or may be lacking, but available data show no evidence of an increased occurrence of fetal damage.
Category B3
Drugs which have been taken by only a limited number of pregnant women and women of childbearing age, without an increase in the frequency of malformation or other direct or indirect harmful effect on the human fetus having been observed. Studies in animals have shown evidence of increased occurrence of fetal damage, significance of which is considered uncertain in humans.
Category C
Drugs which, owing to their pharmacological effects, have caused or may be suspected of causing, harmful effects on the human fetus or neonate without causing malformations. These effects may be reversible. Accompanying text should be consulted for further details.
Category D
Drugs which have caused, are suspected to have caused or may be expected to cause, an increased incidence of human fetal malformations or irreversible damage. These drugs may also have adverse pharmacological effects. Accompanying texts should be consulted for further details.
Category X
Drugs which have such a high risk of causing permanent damage to the fetus that they should not be used in pregnancy or when there is a possibility of pregnancy.

Source: Therapeutic Goods Administration: Australian categorisation system for prescribing medicines in pregnancy, Department of Health, Australian Government, 2021. Online 28 August 2021. Available: www.tga.gov.au/prescribing-medicines-pregnancy-database.

information services located in each state and territory. Databases such as the Teratogen Information System and Reprotox are available (Kennedy 2014).

Drug information services

Any decision about taking a medication during pregnancy should involve the midwife or health professional and the woman, with all the information available on the medication and any specific circumstances considered (Department of Health 2020). In Australia, each state and territory has an obstetric drug information service (see Resources section). It is important for midwives to use current, evidence-based and reliable information sources. High-quality sources of evidence include the AMH, Therapeutic Guidelines, NPS MedicineWise, TGA, MIMS, Micromedex and BMJ Best Practice (Day & Snowden 2016). These sources provide accurate integrated evidence, expert reviews and advice (Day & Snowden 2016).

Medication safety

The Australian Commission on Safety and Quality in Health Care (ACSQHC) works to improve the safety and quality of medication use by leading and coordinating national initiatives to reduce errors and harms related to medications. In Australia a **national inpatient medication chart** (**NIMC**) has been developed (see Resources section). Medication reconciliation ensures that the medicines a woman should be prescribed match the medications they are prescribed. Whenever care is transferred, a current and accurate list of medicines should be provided because transition points are an area prone to error. The ACSQHC (2018) indicates 10–67% of medication histories contain at least one error and one-third of these errors have the potential to cause harm.

High-risk medications

High-risk medications (HRMs) have an increased risk of causing significant harm or death if misused or if errors are made. HRMs include:

- medications with a narrow therapeutic index
- medications that present a high risk when administered via the wrong route
- medications that present a high risk when system errors occur.

Electronic medication management

Electronic medication management (**EMM**) utilises digital programs to improve the accuracy, visibility and legibility of medication prescribing, thereby reducing the number of preventable adverse medication events, as well as prescribing and dispensing errors.

Quality Use of Medicines

Quality Use of Medicines (**QUM**) is a strategy aimed at improving safe and effective medicine use in Australia. Australia has responded to the World Health Organization's Global Patient Safety Challenge on medication safety by setting a goal to reduce avoidable medication errors, adverse drug events and medication-related hospital admissions by 50% by 2025 (ACSQHC 2020).

The ACSQHC provides recommendations for terminology, abbreviations and symbols used in the prescribing and administration of medications (see Resources section).

Midwives have a responsibility to be familiar with the medications they administer, including why they are given, the normal dosage, precautions, contraindications and side effects.

Midwives must follow government legislation and the policies and procedures of their workplace. Policies for checking and documenting the administration of medicines must be followed to avoid errors (Fig 18.1). Factors contributing to medication errors include:

- labelling errors
- poor communication between clinicians
- failure to verify orders or information
- disorganised medication trolleys
- inaccurate or incomplete medication prescriptions
- inadequate staffing numbers (Elliot & Liu 2010).

Medicines, when prescribed and given correctly, can make a significantly positive difference to patients. However, given incorrectly the harm caused can have far-reaching consequences, both in human and monetary terms. Accurate administration of medications requires multiple checks or 'rights'. In 2019 Australia's National Inpatient Medication Chart User Guide (Table 18.4) recommends five rights as essential to administer medications safely. However, the number of rights has been expanded in some publications (Elliot & Lui 2010).

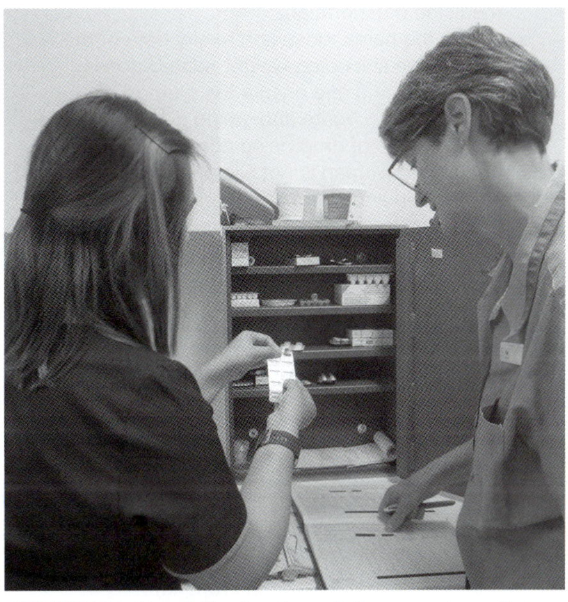

FIGURE 18.1 Carefully check and document medicines to avoid errors.

TABLE 18.4 THE ESSENTIAL FIVE RIGHTS OF MEDICATION ADMINISTRATION

1. Right medicine	Right medicine (matches the order and the person's condition). Generic names should be used when prescribing, plus approved abbreviations and clear printed handwriting. It is not the right medication if the person has an allergy.
2. Right dose	Right dose (matches the order and is safe for the person). The correct dose must be given and attention paid to decimal points to avoid large errors.
3. Right route	Right route (matches the order and is appropriate for the medicine and the person). Medications must be administered by the route prescribed. This has become more challenging as complexity increases and more options become available. Medications must be labelled correctly.
4. Right time	Right time (matches the order and its frequency and administration time directions). Medications must be administered at the correct time to ensure appropriate therapeutic serum levels; usually within 30 minutes of the prescribed time is acceptable. Medications must also be prepared at the correct time (not hours ahead) and given over the correct time (medications given too rapidly can be dangerous).
5. Right person	Right person (matches the person's identification number on the NIMC, the label on the dispensed medicine and is confirmed by the patient using three identifiers, if possible). Medication must be administered to the person it was prescribed for. Ask women to state their name and date of birth. Verify their identity using three identifiers: identification number, name and date of birth on wristband and medication chart.

Source: Adapted from Australian Commission on Safety and Quality in Health Care (ACSQHC): National Inpatient Medication Chart User Guide. ACSQHC, Sydney, 2019.

SKILL 18.1 Administration of a non-controlled medication

1. Aim to be uninterrupted.
2. Perform hand hygiene.
3. Review the signed medicine administration chart and ensure it is legible and completed correctly. Check the medicine has not already been given.
4. Obtain the right medicine from the correct storage facility. Ensure the label on the medicine dispensed is clearly written and unambiguous and check for any signs of possible tampering or medicine deterioration.
5. Check the name, dose and expiry date of the medication (including weight-related doses where relevant) and ensure the method of administration, route and timing are appropriate to the choice of drug being administered.
6. Ensure the woman is not allergic to the medication and check it is compatible with pregnancy or breastfeeding (as appropriate).
7. Prepare the medication correctly (e.g. draw up an intramuscular [IM] injection).
8. Take the medication to the woman and confirm her identity (ask her to state her name and date of birth) and confirm details on her identity band against the medicine administration chart.
9. Explain the nature and expected action of the drug, informally gaining her consent, and ensuring the drug is being given for the right reason (as expected by the woman). For a neonate, consent is given from a parent/guardian following the same discussion.
10. Observe the woman taking the medication (ensures taken at right time). If she is unable to take the medication herself, administer it by the route ordered.
11. Dispose of equipment correctly.
12. Perform hand hygiene.
13. Complete and sign the medicine administration chart and record the dose given, route, date and time of administration in other relevant documentation (e.g. partogram).
14. If any contraindications are found or a reaction develops following administration, or if the drug/route of administration is no longer suitable, contact the doctor/prescriber immediately and take appropriate action.
15. Note and document the effect of the medication (e.g. good/poor response to analgesia).

SKILL 18.2 Administration of a controlled medication

1. Obtain the signed medicine administration chart and ensure it is completed correctly.
2. Perform hand hygiene.
3. In the presence of the second practitioner, unlock the controlled drugs cupboard, check the stock of the drug in the cupboard with the drug

SKILL 18.2 Administration of a controlled medication—cont'd

register total and check tamper-proof seals are still intact.

4. Record the woman's name, amount of drug to be given, date of administration and amount remaining in the drug register.
5. Check the name, amount and expiry date.
6. Remove the drug from packaging (or draw it up) and take it to the woman.
7. Confirm her identity (ask her to state her name and date of birth) and confirm the details on her identity band against the medicine administration chart.
8. Explain the nature and expected action of the drug, informally gaining her consent, and ensuring the drug is being given for the right reason (as expected by the woman). Administer the drug and dispose of equipment safely. The second practitioner must witness the administration of the drug.
9. Sign the drug register, recording details of the time of administration.
10. Record the amount and name of the drug, route, time and date of administration in the appropriate documentation (e.g. medicine administration chart, notes, partogram). Perform hand hygiene. The second practitioner can now return to their original work.
11. Note and document the effect of the drug (e.g. good/poor response to analgesia).

PHARMACOLOGY DURING PREGNANCY AND BREASTFEEDING

For many new drugs, there is no available human pregnancy experience; if no information is available, developmental toxicity of other drugs in the same pharmacological class can be reviewed (Briggs et al 2017). It is important to know whether a drug crosses the placenta; those with a molecular weight less than 600 generally cross the placenta easily, but multiple factors can modify the amount of drug crossing the placenta (Briggs et al 2017). In the second half of pregnancy the majority of drugs (even those with high molecular weights) will cross the placenta (Briggs et al 2017).

How medications work is a product of pharmacokinetic, pharmacodynamic and pharmacogenomic properties (Patil et al 2017). **Pharmacokinetics** refers to the effect of the body on the drug and includes absorption, distribution, metabolism, transport and excretion (Zhao 2014). **Pharmacodynamics** relates to the effect of the drug on the body and the extent of observable pharmacological or therapeutic clinical responses (Zhao et al 2014). **Pharmacogenetics** refers to the genetic influences affecting drug response and inter-individual responses (Patil et al 2017). An example of pharmacogenomics occurs with codeine. Some women have the ultra-rapid metaboliser phenotype which increases the rate and extent of conversion of codeine to morphine. This results in the production of significant amounts of morphine, particularly if repeated doses are taken; the infant is exposed to morphine in the breastmilk possibly resulting in central nervous system depression and death (Hotham & Hotham 2015). Understanding how medications work helps midwives provide evidence-based information to women so they can make an informed choice regarding medications.

Changes in pregnancy

Physiological changes during pregnancy alter the pharmacokinetics and pharmacodynamics of several medications (Zhao et al 2014). Pregnancy generally increases the clearance of several drugs which has the effect of decreasing drug exposure during pregnancy (Zhao et al 2014). Unfortunately, for many medications there is no data available on pharmacokinetics during pregnancy (Zhao et al 2014). The majority of women report using at least one medication during pregnancy (Lupattelli et al 2014).

During pregnancy, the pharmacokinetics and pharmacodynamics of medications can be altered by:

- nausea and vomiting
- increased gastrointestinal transit time, which may increase the time taken to achieve optimum plasma concentration
- alterations in gastric volume and pH due to medications used to alleviate gastrointestinal disorders (e.g. proton pump inhibitors)
- alteration in drug-metabolising enzymes and transporters in the gut
- increased maternal body weight
- accumulation of body fat, which can alter the volume of distribution of some drugs
- increased extracellular and plasma volume, which increases the volume of distribution of water-soluble drugs
- lower levels of plasma albumin and alpha-1-acid glycoprotein
- the extent of drug transfer across the placenta
- alterations in the activity of hepatic drug-metabolising enzymes
- altered hepatic blood flow

- alterations in the expression of drug transporters in the liver, which can result in altered hepatic clearance of some drugs
- increased maternal renal blood flow, glomerular filtration and creatinine clearance; these can result in increased renal clearance and elimination of some medications (Zhao et al 2014).

Different doses may be required during pregnancy and their effects may be slower. It is important for pregnant women with preexisting medical conditions that require medication to have their medication requirements reviewed by their specialists/GPs on a regular basis (e.g. anti-epileptic medications).

Breastfeeding

The majority of commonly used medications are relatively safe for breastfed infants as the dose received is usually small and significantly less than the same medication given directly and safely to an infant (Hotham & Hotham 2015). Multiple factors affect the concentration of a medication in breastmilk, including maternal plasma concentration, plasma protein binding, size of the drug molecule, degree of ionisation and lipid solubility (Hotham & Hotham 2015). The risk of adverse effects on the neonate is influenced by the timing of the dose; if an infant is fed immediately before the mother takes a medication, the infant receives the lowest possible medication concentration, with the exception of medications with a long half-life; for example, diazepam (Hotham & Hotham 2015). Premature neonates have a reduced capacity for metabolism and excretion of medications, which increases the potential for toxicity (Hotham & Hotham 2015). A neonate's ability to metabolise and excrete medications is much lower than an infant at 7–8 months of age and most adverse effects have occurred in newborns less than 2 months of age (Hotham & Hotham 2015).

During breastfeeding, the following principles provide a useful guide:

- use the lowest effective dose (for potentially toxic drugs, breastmilk can be expressed and discarded in order to maintain breastfeeding)
- use routes of administration that minimise exposure
- medications with a relatively short half-life are preferred
- advise the mother to feed the infant prior to medication to reduce the concentration in breastmilk (Hotham & Hotham 2015).

The following medications are contraindicated during breastfeeding: anti-cancer drugs, lithium, oral retinoids, amiodarone and gold salts (Hotham & Hotham 2015). All midwives must know how to access evidence-based information on medication use during breastfeeding to protect the health of both mother and infant (Davanzo et al 2016). Available resources include:

- the obstetric drug information service in each state
- Drugs and Lactation Database (LactMed)
- the Australian Medicines Handbook (AMH)
- The Women's Pregnancy and Breastfeeding Medicines Guide.

Neonatal pharmacology

The neonate has significant vulnerabilities due to differences in physiology which affect drug absorption, distribution, metabolism and elimination (Ku & Smith 2015). The neonate is changing rapidly and this physiological characteristic can make the response to medications less predictable (Ku & Smith 2015). Organ systems in the neonate are less mature. The gastrointestinal tract has an increased gastric pH, lower intestinal motility and delayed gastric emptying time and lower bile acid synthesis (Ku & Smith 2015). This results in slower absorption of oral medications. Transdermal medications are more rapidly absorbed due to thinner skin and immature vasomotor control (Anderson 2017). IM absorption is affected by decreased muscle mass and less muscle perfusion, resulting in variations in absorption. Neonates have larger volumes of extracellular fluid, decreased drug protein-binding affinity and reduced concentrations of alpha-1 glycoprotein, resulting in higher free-drug concentration and a greater effect from protein-bound drugs (Anderson 2017). Increased bilirubin from neonatal jaundice can compete with some drugs for protein binding; this can lead to higher increases of free-drug concentration or increased free bilirubin (Anderson 2017). Neonates have a smaller percentage of body fat; therefore, drugs relying on redistribution to fat and muscle will have higher plasma concentration (Anderson 2017). As gestational age and body weight advance, the renal clearance of drugs increases. Neonates have immature drug targets and receptors, which may increase sensitivity to drugs and make the risk of toxicity higher (Ku & Smith 2015).

ANAPHYLAXIS

The administration of a medication is not without risk; many medications have known side effects and the midwife should be familiar with these. Known allergies should be discussed and recorded at the initial booking interview, as well as on medicine administration records and identity bands. **Anaphylaxis** is a rare but potentially fatal hypersensitivity reaction that can occur following the administration of any medication, as well as food, fluids, foreign proteins (e.g. blood transfusion, insect sting) or topical applications (e.g. plasters, latex gloves, hair dye). Reactions can take from several minutes to several hours to appear, although most severe reactions occur within several minutes.

Most reactions occur in people with no known risk factors, although it occurs more commonly with medications such as antibiotics (e.g. penicillin) and whole blood transfusions. Those with atopic disorders (e.g. asthma or eczema) are considered more vulnerable to a hypersensitivity response. Early recognition of the signs and symptoms is essential to ensure prompt management of the condition. Anaphylaxis is defined by the Australasian Society of Clinical Immunology and Allergy (ASCIA 2021) as:

- any acute-onset illness with typical skin features (such as urticarial rash or erythema/flushing and/or angioedema), plus involvement of respiratory and/or cardiovascular and/or persistent severe gastrointestinal symptoms; or
- any acute onset of hypotension or bronchospasm or upper airway obstruction where anaphylaxis is considered possible, even if typical skin features are not present.

Signs and symptoms of allergic reactions—mild or moderate

ASCIA (2021) defines these as:

- swelling of lips, face, eyes
- hives or welts
- tingling mouth
- abdominal pain, vomiting (these are signs of anaphylaxis for insect allergy).

Allergic reactions occur more slowly than anaphylaxis and symptoms tend to be less serious; it is managed by the administration of oral antihistamines with close observation for signs of improvement or deterioration and reassurance. Those who have experienced an itchy rash following the administration of a medicine should be considered sensitised and therefore at high risk of anaphylaxis should another exposure to the same medicine occur (Jordan 2010).

Signs and symptoms of allergic reactions—anaphylaxis

Anaphylaxis may present with any one of the following signs defined by ASCIA (2021):

- difficult/noisy breathing
- swelling of tongue
- swelling/tightness in throat
- difficulty speaking and/or hoarse voice
- wheeze or persistent cough
- persistent dizziness or collapse
- low blood pressure
- hives
- swelling
- pale and floppy (infants and children)
- vomiting and/or abdominal pain
- neurological symptoms (may occur; e.g. anxiety, confusion, headache)

In pregnancy, ASICA (2020) note the additional features may be present:

- persistent hypotension
- vulvar and vaginal itching
- low back pain
- uterine cramps
- fetal distress.

When anaphylaxis occurs, resuscitation may be required and the Australian and New Zealand Committee on Resuscitation (ANZCOR) guidelines should be followed (ANZCOR 2016). These guidelines are endorsed by the Australian Resuscitation Council (ARC) and the New Zealand Resuscitation Council. For life-threatening anaphylaxis, the injection of adrenaline is the first-line treatment. Adrenaline autoinjectors are safe and effective in pregnancy; adrenaline should not be withheld due to concerns with causing a decrease in placental perfusion (ASICA 2020).

Management of severe anaphylaxis

The management of severe anaphylaxis outlined below is based on the ASCIA (2020) guidelines Acute Management of Anaphylaxis in Pregnancy.

- Remove allergen trigger (in hospital, epidural infusion, intravenous [IV] infusion).
- Call for urgent medical assistance and do not leave the woman; if not in a hospital setting, call an ambulance (000 in Australia, 111 in New Zealand).
- For cardiac arrest commence resuscitation (see current ANZCOR guidelines). Peri-mortem caesarean facilitates maternal resuscitation and should be initiated by 4 minutes with baby born by 5 minutes after arrest.
- Place women who are pregnant in the left lateral position (or perform manual left uterine displacement) to prevent aortocaval occlusion. Postpartum women can be supine.
- If vomiting occurs place the woman on their side in the recovery position.
- Fatality can occur within seconds if the person stands or sits suddenly.
- Administer IM adrenaline 0.3 mg promptly (mid-anterolateral thigh) using an adrenaline autoinjector in the community setting. In hospital 0.5 mg adrenaline can be used. For women < 50 kg administer adrenaline 0.01 mg/kg IM. Doses can be repeated at 5-minute intervals if needed.
- Monitor pulse, blood pressure, respiratory rate, oxygen saturation with pulse oximetry and fetal status using continuous cardiotocography (CTG) or 5-minutely fetal heart rate if CTG is unavailable.
- Administer high flow oxygen (and airway support if required).
- Obtain IV access; if hypotensive give IV normal saline 20 mL/kg rapidly and consider additional wide-bore IV access.
- If in community transfer for medical care, let hospital staff know that an emergency caesarean section may be required.
- Caesarean section is recommended if fetal distress is present in a viable pregnancy, or management does not improve the woman's condition (e.g. hypotension persists).

Note that restoring normal maternal blood pressure does not ensure placental perfusion is adequate;

therefore, fetal monitoring is essential to guide decisions regarding timing of the birth.

Following an anaphylactic reaction, referral to an allergy clinic should be made for follow-up consultation and management (ASCIA 2021). It may be necessary for the woman to carry an adrenaline autoinjector for potential self-administration in the future. Adrenaline autoinjectors are available over the counter without a prescription at full price. In Australia they are available on PBS authority prescription; in New Zealand they are not currently reimbursed by Pharmac.

Adverse events are unintended and possibly harmful occurrences associated with medicines or vaccines (Therapeutic Goods Administration 2021). The TGA has an Advisory Committee on Medicines (ACM) where suspected adverse medication reactions can be reported by healthcare professionals, pharmaceutical companies and consumers. The TGA also has a Database of Adverse Event Notifications (DAEN), which contains information from reports of adverse events received by the TGA in relation to medicines, including vaccines. The midwife has a significant number of responsibilities in relation to the safe administration of medicines.

Role and responsibilities of the midwife

These can be summarised as:

- having a knowledge of the legal framework for the administration of medicines by midwives
- having an understanding of local protocols regarding supply, storage, record keeping and disposal of medications
- understanding pharmacokinetics during pregnancy, breastfeeding and in the neonate
- enquiring about allergies at each woman's booking interview and on each admission
- administering medications safely
- recognising and managing anaphylaxis correctly
- keeping accurate documentation.

SUMMARY

- Legislation governs the administration of medications by the midwife.
- Midwives require a good knowledge of how legislation affects the safe administration, supply, storage, surrender and destruction of medicines.
- Midwives in New Zealand may supply and administer medicines on their own autonomy. Midwives in Australia must comply with the Registration Standard: Endorsement for Scheduled Medicines for Midwives.
- Midwives should receive appropriate, thorough and ongoing training in the administration of medications; no medicine can be administered unless the midwife is familiar with its effects, possible side effects, normal dosage, precautions, contraindications, method of administration and timing.
- The correct administration of a medication should consider the five 'rights'.
- Controlled drugs and every aspect of obtaining, using and returning them is controlled by law. The midwife should be familiar with the standard operating procedures in their area of employment.
- Pharmacokinetics is the absorption, distribution, metabolism and excretion of drugs.
- Anaphylaxis is a rare but potentially fatal reaction that can result from medication administration. It is recognised by a sudden and worsening response following administration of the trigger. The woman may experience mucosal and/or skin changes, with respiratory or cardiovascular collapse. The immediate management includes the giving of IM adrenaline and action as for cardiopulmonary resuscitation.

Self-assessment exercises

The answers to the following may be found in the text.

1. What does a midwife need to know about a medicine before they can administer it?
2. List the five 'rights' of medicine administration.
3. List the steps taken to ensure all medications are correctly administered.
4. How does pregnancy affect pharmacokinetics?
5. How would the midwife recognise and manage anaphylaxis?

Resources

Australian Commission on Safety and Quality in Health care (ACSQHC) Medication charts: www.safetyandquality.gov.au/our-work/medication-safety/medication-charts/national-standard-medication-charts.

Australian Commission on Safety and Quality in Health Care (ACSQHC): Recommendations for terminology, abbreviations and symbols used in the prescribing and administration of medicines: www.safetyandquality.gov.au/publications-and-resources/resource-library/recommendations-terminology-abbreviations-and-symbols-used-medicines-documentation-0.

Australian Medicines Handbook (AMH): Available online by subscription: amhonline.amh.net.au/auth.

Department of Health, Australian Government: Quality Use of Medicines (QUM), 2020: www1.health.gov.au/internet/main/publishing.nsf/Content/nmp-quality.htm.

Department of Health, Australian Government: Therapeutic Goods Administration, 2021: Obstetric drug information services available in each Australian state and territory: www.tga.gov.au/obstetric-drug-information-services.

Department of Health and Ageing, Australian Government: 1999. National Medicines Policy 2000: www.health.gov.au/internet/main/publishing.nsf/content/B2FFBF72029EEAC8CA257BF0001BAF3F/$File/NMP2000.pdf.

Drugs and Lactation Database (LactMed): www.ncbi.nlm.nih.gov/books/NBK501922/.

European Network of Teratology Information Services (ENTIS): www.entis-org.eu.

Health Quality and Safety Commission New Zealand: Medication safety: www.hqsc.govt.nz/our-programmes/medication-safety/.

Medsafe: New Zealand Medicines and Medical Devices Safety Authority: For healthcare professionals: Information on medicines and medical devices: www.medsafe.govt.nz.

Midwifery Council (New Zealand): midwiferycouncil.health.nz.

Pharmaceutical Management Agency (Pharmac): Providing funded access to pharmaceuticals for New Zealanders, 2021: www.pharmac.govt.nz.

Poisons Standard June 2021: www.legislation.gov.au/Details/F2021L00650.

Reprotox: reprotox.org.

Teratogen Information System (TERIS): Clinical Teratology Web: a resource for clinicians: depts.washington.edu/terisdb/terisweb/index.html.

The New Zealand Formulary (NZF): Clinically validated medicines information: www.nzformulary.org.nz.

The Pharmaceutical Benefits Scheme (PBS). Midwife PBS prescribing: pbs.gov.au/browse/midwife.

The Women's Pregnancy and Breastfeeding Medicines Guide (subscription only): thewomenspbmg.org.au/subscribe.

References

ACT Parliamentary Counsel: Medicines, poisons and therapeutic goods regulation 2008, 2020. Republication no 41. Online 2 April 2021. Available: www.legislation.act.gov.au/sl/2008-42/.

Anderson BJ: Neonatal pharmacology, Anaesthesia & Intensive Care Medicine 18:68–74, 2017.

Australasian Society of Clinical Immunology and Allergy (ASCIA). Acute management of anaphylaxis in pregnancy, 2020. Online 2 April 2021: Available: www.allergy.org.au.

Australasian Society of Clinical Immunology and Allergy (ASCIA): Anaphylaxis resources, 2021. Online 2 April 2021. Available: www.allergy.org.au.

Australian and New Zealand Committee on Resuscitation: ANZCOR Guideline 9.2.7—First aid management of anaphylaxis, 2016. Online 2 April 2021. Available: resus.org.au/guidelines.

Australian Commission on Safety and Quality in Health Care (ACSQHC): Annual report 2019-20, Sydney, 2020.

Australian Commission on Safety and Quality in Health Care (ACSQHC): Medication reconciliation, 2018. Online 2 April 2021. Available: www.safetyandquality.gov.au/our-work/medication-safety/medication-reconciliation/.

Briggs GG, Freeman RK, Towers CV: Drugs in pregnancy and lactation: a reference guide to fetal and neonatal risk, 11th ed., Wolters Kluwer, Philadelphia, 2017.

Bullock S, Manias E: Fundamentals of pharmacology, 8th ed., Pearson Australia, Melbourne, 2017.

Davanzo R, Bua J, De Cunto A, et al: Advising mothers on the use of medications during breastfeeding, Journal of Human Lactation 32:15–19, 2016.

Day R, Snowden L: Where to find information about drugs, Australian Prescriber 39(3):88–95, 2016.

Department of Health: Clinical Practice Guidelines: Pregnancy care, Government Department of Health, Canberra, 2020.

Elliot E, Liu Y: The nine rights of medication administration: an overview, British Journal of Nursing 19(5):300–304, 2010.

Hotham N, Hotham E: Drugs in breastfeeding, Australian Prescriber 38:156–159, 2015.

Jordan S: Principles of pharmacology, Chapter 1. In Jordan S, editor: Pharmacology for midwives, 2nd ed., Palgrave Macmillan, Basingstoke, 2010.

Kennedy D: Classifying drugs in pregnancy, Australian Prescriber 37(2):38–40, 2014.

Ku LC, Smith PB: Dosing in neonates: special considerations in physiology and trial design, Pediatric Research 77(1–1):2–9, 2015.

Lupattelli A, Spigset O, Twigg MJ, et al: Medication use in pregnancy: a cross-sectional, multinational web-based study, BMJ Open 4(2):e004365, 2014.

Midwifery Council (New Zealand): Competencies for entry to the Register of Midwives, 2021. Online 28 August 2021. Available: www.midwiferycouncil.health.nz.

Midwifery Council (New Zealand): Practising certificates, 2018. Online 7 Feb 2018. Available: www.midwiferycouncil.health.nz/Public/06.-I-am-a-registered-midwife/2.-Practising-Certificates-.aspx.

New Zealand Legislation: Medicines Regulation Act 1984, Reprint as at 30 March 2021. Online 2 April 2021. Available: www.legislation.govt.nz.

Pairman S, Pincome J, Thorogood C, et al, eds: Midwifery preparation for practice, 4th ed., Elsevier, Sydney, 2019.

Patil A, Sheng J, Dotters-Katz S, et al: Fundamentals of clinical pharmacology with application for pregnant women. Journal of Midwifery & Women's Health 62(3):298–307, 2017.

Small K, Sidebotham M, Fenwick J, et al: Midwifery prescribing in Australia, Australian Prescriber 39(6): 215–218, 2016.

Therapeutic Goods Administration: Reporting adverse events, Department of Health, Australian Government, 2021. Online 28 August, 2021. Available: www.tga.gov.au/reporting-adverse-events.

Zhao Y, Hebert M, Venkataramanan R: Basic obstetric pharmacology, Seminars in Perinatology 38(8): 475–486, 2014.

CHAPTER 19
ORAL

Learning outcomes

Having read this chapter, the reader should be able to:

- discuss the advantages and disadvantages of the oral route, identifying what should be included in a risk assessment
- describe the different preparations available for oral use, giving an example of each
- describe the procedure for administering a drug orally to a woman and a neonate
- summarise the role and responsibilities of the midwife.

Oral medications include tablets, enteric-coated preparations, capsules, lozenges, granules, sprays, gels and liquids. Swallowed oral medications are generally absorbed in the gastrointestinal tract. Some medications are designed to be absorbed in the mouth and therefore avoid the gastrointestinal tract. This chapter considers the safe management of medication for the oral route, the preparations available and the role and responsibilities of the midwife. The procedures are described for adult and neonatal administration. It should be read in conjunction with Chapter 18.

ORAL MEDICATION

Oral administration is the most commonly used route for medication administration because of the convenience, stability and cost effectiveness (Buxton 2017). The bioavailability of oral preparations may be affected by factors influencing absorption, such as pH, gastric motility and gastric emptying time, which is influenced by the calorie content of food, metabolic state and oestrogen levels (Buxton 2017). The manufacturer's directions should be followed (e.g. before, during or after a meal) for maximum effectiveness. Medications should be administered as dispensed; crushing, dissolving, cutting or opening a tablet/capsule when this is not indicated can cause under- or overdosage. Controlled-release/extended-release medications often have an enteric coating and are designed to pass through the stomach and be absorbed slowly in the small intestine. Enteric coatings help prevent damage to the lining of the stomach. Altering these medications can cause inactivity or immediate activity, both of which can be dangerous.

Types of oral medication

Tablets disintegrate and are generally absorbed in the acidic conditions of the stomach, with the exception of buccal and sublingual tablets or wafers which are designed to dissolve in the mouth (Fig 19.1). Some tablets are chewed. *Enteric-coated* medications disintegrate only in the alkaline conditions of the intestine. *Capsules* are made of a hard gelatin (contains a solid medication) or a soft gelatin (contains a liquid medication). Sustained release medications are released slowly into the gastrointestinal tract and need to be taken less frequently. *Lozenges* are usually sucked. *Liquid* preparations are useful for women who find swallowing medications difficult. A *linctus* is a viscous syrup designed to be swallowed as a treatment for coughing. An *elixir* contains a medication insoluble in water but soluble in alcohol or other solvents, such as glycerol. *Suspensions* contain relatively insoluble solid medications which do not contain alcohol. *Emulsions* are similar, but contain a liquid medication. These preparations have a tendency to separate and need to be mixed thoroughly when prepared. They contain medications insoluble in water but have no alcohol as a solvent.

Routes for oral medication

Swallowed oral preparations such as tablets and capsules are absorbed from the gastrointestinal tract and transported into the portal circulation. They are generally swallowed whole, with a glass of water, optimally in a sitting position (Bullock & Manias 2017). If possible, the woman should remain sitting upright for a further 30 minutes. This prevents irritation to the oesophagus and other tissues. If scored, tablets/caplets may be divided in half using a tablet cutter, according to the required dosage. Wash and dry the cutter after use. Examples of tablets include analgesics, antibiotics and iron supplements.

Buccal preparations are placed between the cheek and the gum and **sublingual** preparations are placed under the tongue (Fig 19.1). Both buccal and sublingual preparations dissolve and are absorbed by the surrounding blood vessels, which drain into the superior vena cava and enter the circulation directly. Both of these routes of administration bypass the gastrointestinal tract and portal circulation (Buxton 2017). Sublingual and buccal medication are useful for women with nausea and vomiting and who may have difficulty swallowing and retaining medications. In the maternity setting, ondansetron is used to treat nausea and vomiting and can be placed on the tongue (AusDi 2021).

Lozenges are often sucked (systemic effect) or used for local effect (e.g. anaesthetic relief of sore throats, antifungal coating of the tongue). Some medications are chewed and this should be clear in the prescription.

Granules, powders and soluble tablets need to be thoroughly dissolved before administration. This is generally in water, but the manufacturer's guidelines should be followed. Examples include analgesics (e.g. paracetamol).

Elixir may be supplied prepared or require careful dilution according to the instructions. Some solutions require refrigeration. The bottle needs inverting several times to ensure thorough mixing before administration. Examples include antacids and antibiotics.

Sprays should be used according to the manufacturer's instructions. They are often sprayed into the cheek or under the tongue. Examples include glyceryl trinitrate and nicotine replacement therapy.

Some gels are used for their local action (e.g. pain relief for teething or antifungal treatment). Others such as dextrose (hypoglycaemia) or midazolam (epilepsy) are used when a rapid effect is needed.

National Inpatient Medication Chart

The National Inpatient Medication Chart (NIMC) is mandatory for all Australian public and private health services (Australian Commission on Safety and Quality in Health Care [ACSQHC] 2019). All midwives need to be familiar with the NIMC and the essential prescribing requirements including date, generic name, route, dose, frequency, administration times, indication, prescriber name and signature (ACSQHC 2019). The medication chart needs to include identification, allergies, weight, height and gestational age at birth for infants.

Approved abbreviations

A major cause of medication errors is the use of confusing abbreviations. Recommendations for terminology, abbreviations and symbols used in the prescribing and administration of medicines are available from the ACSQHC (2016). Table 19.1 lists some commonly used acceptable abbreviations.

Equipment

Medicine cups with gradations on the side are used; ideally they are disposable. As a clean transport medium, their use allows the medication to be transferred from the packet to the mouth without being touched. The gradations on the side allow liquids to be measured, as do medicine spoons. However, small or very accurate doses (e.g. paediatric doses) should be measured using an **oral/enteral syringe** (Fig 19.2). Syringes used for oral medications must not connect with intravenous ports; therefore, they are non-Luer lock so they will not

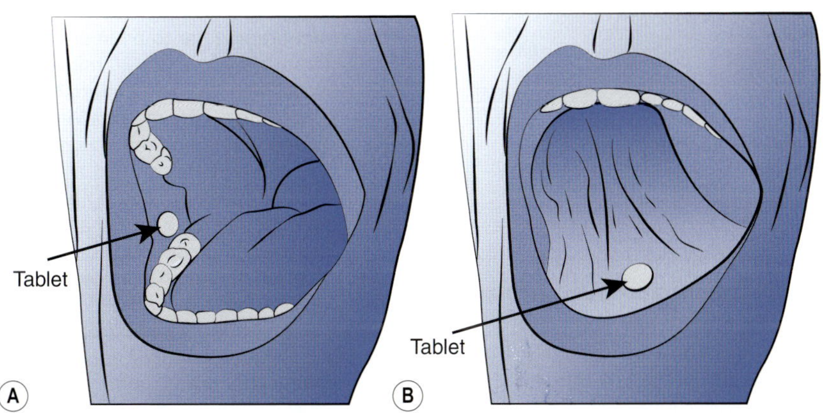

FIGURE 19.1 **Buccal and sublingual medication. A, Buccal: inside mouth, cheek area. B, Sublingual: under the tongue.**

TABLE 19.1 ACCEPTED ABBREVIATIONS

Abbreviation	Latin	Translation
bd	bis in die	twice daily
mane	mane	in the morning
tds	ter die sumendum	three times daily
qid	quarter in die	four times daily
prn	pro re nata	when required
stat	statim	immediately
tab		tablet
PO	oral	oral
subling		sublingual—under the tongue
buccal		buccal—between cheek and gum

Source: Australian Commission on Safety and Quality in Health Care, 2016.

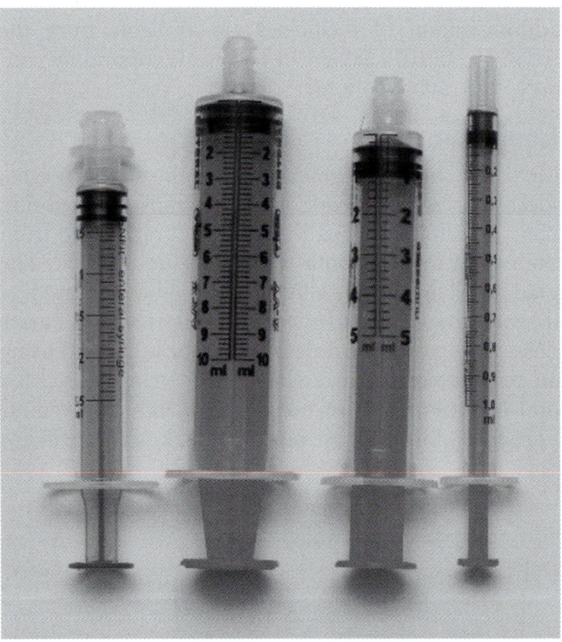

FIGURE 19.2 **Oral/enteral syringe.**

connect to intravenous tubing (this minimises risk of inadvertent parenteral administration) and are marked 'for oral use only' or 'for enteral use only'. In Australia and New Zealand, syringes and caps designed for oral medication use are generally orange or purple.

Syringes are sterile for single use only, but in some circumstances may be reused for the same client after washing. (These are then stored in a labelled plastic box.)

Education

Midwives are responsible for ensuring women are well informed about the effects, benefits, risks and possible complications of medications. Informed consent requires women to understand the expected benefits and risks of the medication. Women also need to know how to take medications correctly, and the expected effects and issues to report. Informed consent must always be gained; those with legal responsibility (e.g. parents) give consent on behalf of children. Ideally, the midwife observes the woman taking the medication administered.

SKILL 19.1 Oral medication administration

1. Ensure the woman is accessible and ready for the medication prior to dispensing it.
2. Undertake the thorough checking procedure as described in Chapter 18.
3. With clean hands, select the preparation, check the expiry date and dispense the correct dose of the drug.
   - Tablets and capsules: Tip the required number into the bottle cap, then into a medicine cup. If in foil packaging, check the strip, then push the tablets through the foil into the cup (avoid handling the medication). Return remaining medication to secure storage.
   - Elixir: Invert the bottle several times, hold the bottle with the label to the rear (to avoid obscuring the label with spilled medicine), hold the medicine cup at eye level and pour the liquid into it, ensuring the fluid is accurately on the line. Alternatively, insert an enteral syringe, invert the bottle and draw the correct number of millilitres into the syringe, also at eye level.
4. Confirm identity: Ask the woman for her full name and date of birth and check her identity band.
5. Advise the woman on how to take the medication, providing a glass of water if necessary, encouraging her to be in an upright posture and to remain so for 30 minutes. Observe her swallowing the medication. For sublingual preparations, the medication should be placed/sprayed beneath the tongue; for buccal preparations they should be placed/sprayed into the cheek or placed next to the gum; other directions to suck, chew and so on should be followed as prescribed.
6. Dispose of equipment correctly.
7. Perform hand hygiene.
8. Document the administration in the medicine administration record and any other agreed places (e.g. partogram).
9. Observe for the effects of the medication and take any necessary action.

SKILL 19.2 Oral medication administration to a neonate

1. Perform hand hygiene and undertake the thorough checking process described in Chapter 18, independently of a second colleague.
2. Confirm the identity of the neonate and reaffirm parental consent.
3. Perform hand hygiene.
4. Draw up the correct dosage accurately in an enteral syringe.
5. The neonate may be more comfortable held in the parent's arms.
6. Place the syringe into the neonate's mouth towards the cheek, squeeze a small amount (0.5–1 mL maximum) into the mouth and observe the neonate swallowing.
7. Administer the next part of the dose, observe the swallow and continue in this way until the medication is fully administered.
8. Dispose of the syringe correctly and perform hand hygiene.
9. Document administration.
10. If appropriate, observe for the effects of the medication and take any necessary action.

Precautions

- If the woman is unable to take the medication at the time of administration, it is recorded and the late administration checked before being given. A medication dispensed but not administered should be disposed of safely, never left in anticipation or returned to the bottle.
- Compliance is increased when women understand the reason for the medication, its likely effects and possible side effects. Refusal to take a drug should be recorded, with the reason and the prescribing medical officer informed.
- If a woman vomits soon after administration and only if the tablet is clearly visible, a further stat dose may be prescribed after consultation with the obstetrician. Observe the effects of the medication and take any necessary action.
- Controlled drugs may also be prescribed in an oral form; administration should be according to the local policy for controlled medication administration (Chapter 18). Tablets are counted; elixir should be measured very carefully using an enteral syringe.

ORAL ADMINISTRATION TO A NEONATE

The neonate needs to be awake and able to swallow. The parents should have given consent and should be taught the procedure if they need to repeat it themselves. The prescription is scrutinised, as per all prescriptions (Chapter 18) and local protocols adhered to (e.g. independent checking by two registered practitioners). An enteral syringe is used (as above). The majority of oral medications are in the form of elixir for neonates.

If the neonate possets, consultation with the paediatrician is necessary regarding the need for a further dose. Oral medications can be held to give with a feed as long as the feed is within 30 minutes.

Role and responsibilities of the midwife

These can be summarised as:

- practising within the standards for the safe and effective administration of medicines
- ensuring the drug is dispensed correctly, ideally in the woman's presence and given straight to her or her neonate, after thorough identity checking
- observing the effects and side effects of the administered drug
- educating the woman to aid compliance and effectiveness
- keeping correct documentation.

SUMMARY

- Oral drug administration involves thorough checking in all parts of the process, as for any other drug administration (see Chapter 18 for details).
- Oral medication may come in different forms; while the majority of oral preparations are swallowed, some are for sucking, chewing, buccal or sublingual use. Liquid preparations may be given using a medicine cup or spoon; alternatively, an enteral syringe is used.
- An assessment should be made as to whether for this woman or neonate the oral route is an appropriate one for this medication at this time.

Self-assessment exercises

The answers to the following questions may be found in the text.

1. List the advantages and disadvantages of the oral route.
2. List three steps the midwife would take before administering an oral medication.

3. Discuss the midwife's action if a medication was dispensed but the woman was not available to take it.
4. Describe how a midwife would administer a sublingual drug to a woman.
5. Describe the procedures a midwife would follow if a woman vomited her medication shortly after taking it.

Resources

Australian Commission on Safety and Quality in Healthcare (ACSQH): Standard 4 Medication Safety. Safety and quality improvement guide 2017: www.safetyandquality.gov.au/wp-content/uploads/2017/11/Medication-Safety.pdf.

Department of Health, Australian Government. National Medicines Policy (NMP): www1.health.gov.au/internet/main/publishing.nsf/Content/national-medicines-policy.

References

AusDi: Ondansetron orally disintegrating tablets full product information, 2021. Online 2 April 2021. Available: www.ausdi.com.

Australian Commission on Safety and Quality in Health Care (ACSQHC): Accepted abbreviations and symbols used in the prescribing and administration of medicines, 2016. Online 2 April 2021. Available: safetyandquality.gov.au/our-work/medication-safety/safer-naming-labelling-and-packaging-medicines/recommendations-terminology-abbreviations-and-symbols-used-medicines-documentation.

Australian Commission on Safety and Quality in Health Care (ACSQHC): National Inpatient Medication Chart User Guide. ACSQHC, Sydney, 2019.

Bullock S, Manias E: Fundamentals of pharmacology, 8th ed., Pearson, Melbourne, 2017.

Buxton ILO: Pharmacokinetics: The dynamics of drug absorption, distribution, metabolism and elimination. In Brunton LL, Hilal-Dandan R, Knollmann BC, eds: Goodman & Gilman's: The pharmacological basis of therapeutics, 13th ed., McGraw-Hill, New York, 2017.

CHAPTER 20
PER VAGINAM

Learning outcomes

Having read this chapter, the reader should be able to:

- discuss the advantages and disadvantages of the vaginal route for the administration of medicines
- describe how a medication is administered per vaginam (PV)
- discuss the role and responsibilities of the midwife before, during and after PV medication administration
- list the factors pertinent to the administration of prostaglandin PV.

The midwife is involved in the administration of medicines **per vaginam (PV)**. A range of preparations can be administered vaginally, including tablets, creams, pessaries, foams, films, rings and tape. PV medications can be used for the treatment of localised infections, contraception and for systemic use. Vaginal prostaglandins are commonly used for cervical ripening and induction of labour. In 2018, 45% of Australian women between 20 and 34 years with a singleton term baby in the vertex position had an induction of labour (AIHW 2020b). In New Zealand the induction rate was 19.4% in 2006; by 2015 this had increased to 24% (Ministry of Health 2021).

Progesterone vaginal pessaries can be used to help maintain pregnancy. New polymers are being developed for administering medications vaginally, including mucoadhesive polymers which can be manipulated to provide a local effect or a continuous release systemic effect (Misra & Shahiwala 2014). Advances in silicone elastomer vaginal ring technology are being used to combine HIV and pregnancy prevention (Murphy et al 2016). Vaginal microbicides (antiviral and antibacterial medications) are also being developed (Fernández-Romero et al 2015).

This chapter considers the midwife's role and responsibilities and the procedure for administration of PV medications, focusing largely on the administration of prostaglandin E_2 (PGE_2) and treatments for vaginal infections. This chapter should be read in conjunction with Chapters 18 and 30.

THE VAGINAL ROUTE

The vagina has a large surface area with a good blood supply and provides a favourable route of administration for local and systemic medications (Fig 20.1) (Kimball et al 2016, Machado et al 2015). Vaginal medication administration allows for lower and less frequent doses with a steady medication level unaltered by gastrointestinal factors (Krishna et al 2017).

The vaginal rugae (transverse folds) increase the surface area and the dense venous plexus covering the vagina drains into the internal iliac veins (Misra & Shahiwala 2014) allowing medications direct access to systemic circulation. The vagina and ectocervix consist of stratified squamous epithelial tissue and the endocervix consists of columnar epithelium (Fernández-Romero et al 2015). Absorption of PV medications varies with age, menstrual cycle and alterations in pH and oestrogen levels. The vaginal pH is affected by age, infection and discharge.

Vaginal medication needs to be released from the delivery system, dissolved in the vaginal fluid and penetrate the vaginal membrane. Medication is then transported across the vaginal membrane through passive diffusion (transcellular), vesicular/receptor-mediated transport or diffusion between cells (paracellular) (Misra & Shahiwala 2014).

As vaginal medications are circulated via the internal iliac veins, they bypass the liver. Vaginal medication administration can result in fewer side effects than oral medications (Pathak et al 2015). Progesterone and dinoprostone (prostaglandin E_2) are polymer-based preparations. Vaginal polymers are generally mucoadhesive and adhere to the mucous layer covering the vagina (Misra & Shahiwala 2014). The absorption varies depending on the delivery system; for example, intravaginal rings provide a controlled medication

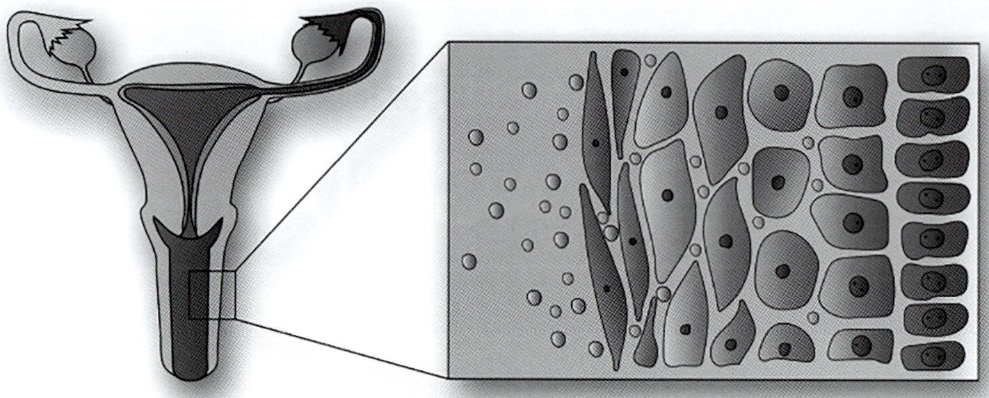

FIGURE 20.1 **Medication absorption per vaginam.**
Source: Machado RM, Palmeira-de-Oliveira A, Gaspar C, et al: Studies and methodologies on vaginal drug permeation, Advanced Drug Delivery Reviews 92:14–26, 2015.

release over time (Pathak et al 2015). Vaginal medications may cause local irritation.

When administering medications PV it is important to consider women may feel embarrassed and survivors of sexual abuse may find this method of administration traumatic. Women may prefer to self-administer the medication if this is possible.

Prostaglandins

Naturally produced **prostaglandins** increase towards term and appear to both ripen the cervix and contribute towards uterine contractions (Baddock 2018). Although vaginal gel is more rapidly absorbed than vaginal tablets or pessaries, each method of delivery of prostaglandin E_2 (PGE_2) appears equally effective (Thomas et al 2014). Synthetic prostaglandins imitate physiological ripening of the cervix and increase uterine sensitivity to oxytocin (Brown & Beckmann 2017). Prostaglandins are chemically unstable compounds and must be stored correctly. Dosages for the different compounds (e.g. gel, tablets or pessary) vary; unless otherwise prescribed, they are always placed into the posterior vaginal fornix.

The **Bishop's score** is used to determine how favourable the cervix is for birth. Bishop's scoring is undertaken prior to prescription and administration of prostaglandins and a normal cardiotocography (CTG) should be confirmed prior to PGE_2 administration and repeated when contractions begin (Laughon et al 2011). Table 20.1 shows the scores given for the five cervical features that are rated. Ongoing monitoring of fetal wellbeing should continue using intermittent auscultation or continuous monitoring as per local policy. Women who have the administration of prostaglandin as an outpatient should be given clear advice regarding when to consult/return to the maternity unit (National Institute for Health and Care Excellence [NICE] 2014).

Cervical ripening

A substantial proportion of women who are scheduled for an induction have an unfavourable cervix. Pharmacological ripening of the cervix using vaginal prostaglandins is a common procedure in Australia and New Zealand (Fig 20.2). Ripening an unfavourable cervix prior to induction of labour can improve the success rate (Baddock 2019). A low Bishop's score on admission is

TABLE 20.1 MODIFIED BISHOP'S SCORE

Cervical feature	Modified Bishop's score			
	0	1	2	3
Dilation (cm)	< 1	1–2	2–4	> 4
Length of cervix (cm)	> 4	2–4	1–2	< 1
Station (relative to ischial spines)	–3	–2	–1/0	+1/+2
Consistency	Firm	Average	Soft	–
Position	Posterior	Mid/anterior	–	–

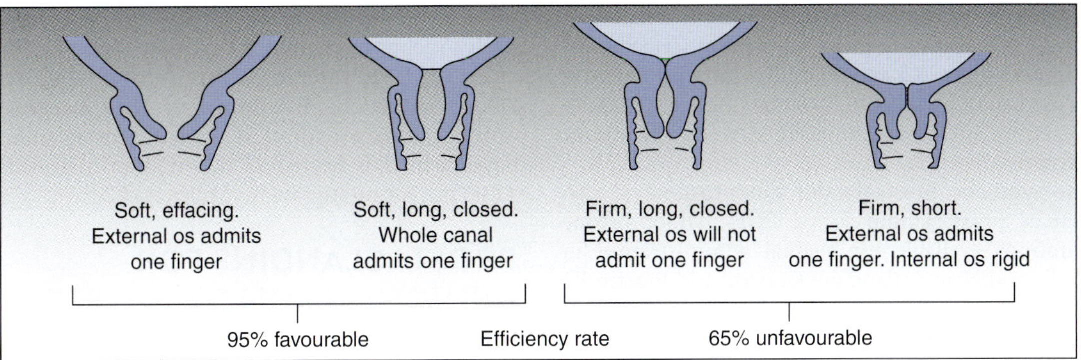

FIGURE 20.2 **Cervical ripening and induction outcome.**
Source: Oats J, Abraham S: Llewellyn-Jones Fundamentals of obstetrics and gynaecology, 10th ed., Elsevier, Sydney, 2017.

associated with a reduced likelihood of a normal vaginal birth (Raghuraman et al 2016). Prostaglandins help ripen the cervix by increasing inflammatory mediators within the cervix leading to remodelling of the cervix (Bakker et al 2017). After informed consent is given, a vaginal examination is undertaken to assess the Bishop's score. If the Bishop's score is ≥ 8 chances of a vaginal birth are favourable and the cervix is considered ripe. If the Bishop's score is ≤ 6 the chances of a vaginal birth are not favourable and the cervix is considered 'unripe'. Most women have prostaglandin administered in the hospital and then stay for observation; however, one-third of women have been shown to find outpatient cervical ripening acceptable (Sutton et al 2016). A full or modified Bishop's score may be used depending on local protocols. For women who are multiparous the Bishop's score is a poor predictor of successful induction of labour (Navve et al 2017). Parity, cervical dilatation and gestational age are factors that influence successful cervical ripening (Hiersch et al 2017). Parity, fetal station and cervical effacement are associated with successful induction (Ivars et al 2016).

PROSTAGLANDINS FOR INDUCTION

Induction of labour is offered when the perceived risk of continuing the pregnancy is greater than the risk of induction of labour (IOL). One of the common reasons for induction is postdate pregnancy, defined as ≥ 42 weeks gestation. The World Health Organization (WHO) recommends induction after 41 completed weeks of gestation. The Australian Pregnancy Care Guidelines (Department of Health 2020) recommend discussing options and preferences with women in the context of prolonged pregnancy. A 2020 Cochrane review found fewer perinatal deaths and caesarean sections with induction at or beyond 37 weeks gestation and suggested discussing options to assist women to make an informed choice (Middleton et al 2020). A Queensland study found induction of labour in nulliparous women increased the caesarean section rate significantly (Mahomed et al 2016). Care should be woman-centred, with the woman able to make a fully informed decision, being particularly aware of the risk of serious complications (NICE 2014). A plan should also be made in the event of a failed induction.

The use of prostaglandins to induce labour began in the 1960s (Thomas et al 2014). Manufactured synthetic forms of prostaglandins can be administered for the induction of labour with PV administration considered the optimum choice. A 2014 Cochrane review found PGE_2 probably results in an increased possibility of vaginal birth within 24 hours. Midwives must be familiar with the local protocol for administration of PGE_2 and carefully review a woman's history to ensure no contraindications are present. Midwives are also responsible for following drug administration procedures and checking for possible interactions. When inserting PGE_2 a water-soluble lubricant should be used as obstetric cream should not be used with PGE_2.

Most body systems can be affected by prostaglandins with side effects, including headaches and breast tenderness (Dodd et al 2019). Prostaglandins can stimulate the smooth muscle of the gastrointestinal system leading to side effects of nausea, vomiting and diarrhoea in around 5.7% of women (Bakker et al 2017). Other side effects include back pain (3.1%), a warm feeling in the vagina (1.5%) and fever (1.4%) (TGA 2020).

Some side effects are seen within 30 minutes of administration. Serious effects, such as fetal compromise, bronchospasm, uterine hypertonus, amniotic fluid embolism and uterine rupture, have been noted and care should include specific observations for these risks. Prostaglandin should be used with extreme care in grand multiparous women. Prostaglandins are bronchoconstrictors and caution should be used in women with asthma or a history of asthma (Bullock & Manais 2017).

The medication begins working within 10 minutes of administration (gel absorption is faster than pessary absorption). Women should remain in a semi-recumbent or supine position to improve absorption (usually 15–30 minutes) (Figs 20.3 and 20.4). If a retrieval device is being used, the midwife should remove the prostaglandin if any serious adverse reactions are seen (e.g. significant fetal compromise) (Fig 20.5).

The synthetic prostaglandin dinoprostone is also known as prostaglandin E_2 or PGE_2. Dinoprostone preparations available for vaginal administration in Australia and New Zealand are Cervidil and Prostin E2 vaginal gel (prostaglandin E_2) (Fig 20.4). Local protocols should be followed for administration and dosage (Table 20.2). Women induced with a dinoprostone gel gave birth vaginally in a shorter timeframe, with a similar caesarean section rate to women given a Foley catheter (Austin et al 2015). In one study 66% of women gave birth within 24 hours of administration of dinoprostone (Baloch et al 2017). A Cochrane review on prostaglandins used for labour induction found vaginal misoprostol (< 50 micrograms) was the method most likely to achieve a vaginal birth within 24 hours (Alfirevic et al 2015). However, misoprostol is not approved for labour induction in Australia or New Zealand. The optimum time for administration of prostaglandins if a daytime birth is desired is 7.00 am for primigravida and 11.00 pm for multigravida (Miller et al 2016).

PROSTAGLANDINS FOR INDUCTION FOLLOWING FETAL DEATH IN UTERO OR FOR TERMINATION OR PREGNANCY

In the event of a fetal death or a medical termination, prostaglandin E_2 (dinoprostone) OR prostaglandin E_1 analogues gemeprost (Cervagem) or misoprostol (Cytotec) may be used. The Royal Australian and New Zealand College of Obstetricians and Gynaecologists

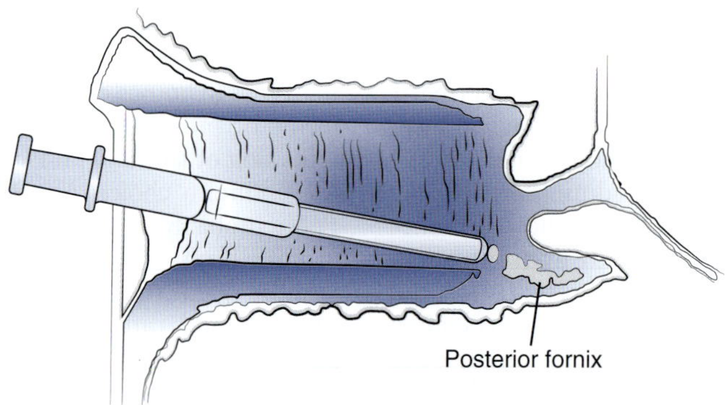

FIGURE 20.3 **Insertion of dinoprostone gel.**
Source: Adapted from Mohammed, T: Induction of labour-evidence based, Health & Medicine. 15 September, Slide 36, 2013. Online 14 May 2018. Available: www.slideshare.net/tarigms/ind-madina-26206483.

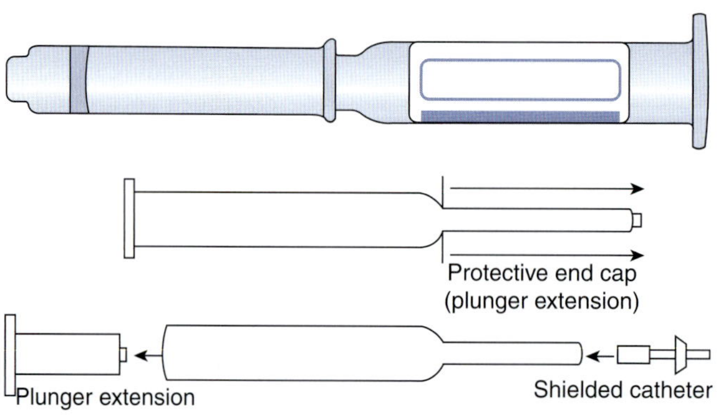

FIGURE 20.4 **Delivery system PGE_2 gel.**
Source: Adapted from Prepadil ® Gel (Generic Name Dinoprostone Cervical Gel) Concentration 0.5 mg/3.0 g. Source: www.pfizerinjectables.com/products/Prepidil.

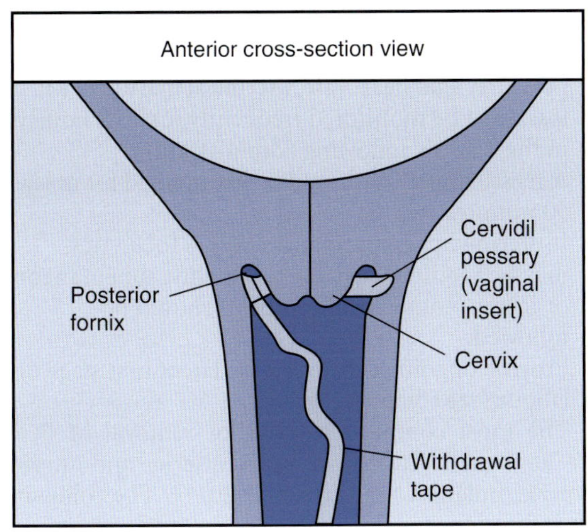

FIGURE 20.5 **Insertion of retrievable PGE_2 (Cervidil).**
Source: © Ferring Pharmaceuticals.

(RANZCOG 2016) has guidelines for the use of misoprostol on their website. Recommended dosage regimes vary considerably depending on gestational age and clinical status. The International Federation of Gynecology and Obstetrics (FIGO) has a chart with recommended doses of misoprostol (Morris et al 2017). Bronchoconstriction also occurs with PGE_1 (misoprostol) with the risk for exacerbation of asthma following PGE_1 administration < 2% (Rooney Thompson et al 2015).

Considerations prior to administration of PGE_2

Prior to administration of prostaglandins, the midwife must ensure no contraindications are present. Contraindications include:

- fetal distress, abnormal CTG
- ruptured membranes
- known hypersensitivity to prostaglandins
- unexplained vaginal bleeding during the pregnancy

TABLE 20.2 PROSTAGLANDIN ADMINISTRATION

Cervical ripening and induction of labour		
Medication	**Administration**	**Cautions**
Cervidil (10 mg dinoprostone) retrievable vaginal tape insert	Store in freezer below –18°C Keep frozen until immediately before use Use water-miscible lubricant Insert into posterior fornix Recumbent position for 30 minutes post insertion Released continuously over 24 hours	No oxytocin until > 30 minutes after removal Remove prior to amniotomy or if membranes rupture spontaneously
Prostin E2 vaginal gel (1 mg or 2 mg dinoprostone in 3 gm/2.5 mL)	Refrigerate. Remove from refrigerator at least 30 minutes prior to use and bring to room temperature Initial dosage is 1 mg Insert high into posterior fornix; avoid cervical canal Remain recumbent for ≥ 30 minutes post insertion	Further 1 or 2 mg may be given after 6 hours on basis of Bishop's score and clinical assessment Maximum dose 3 mg (or 60 microgram/kg for a 50 kg woman) over a 6-hour period
Termination of pregnancy or induction for fetal death in utero		
Prostin E2 (20 mg dinoprostone) vaginal suppository	Prostin E2: One suppository (20 mg) intravaginal (high in vagina) q3–5 hr until abortion occurs	Termination of pregnancy from 12–20 weeks gestation Evacuation of uterus following intrauterine fetal death up to 28 weeks gestation Do not exceed more than 2 days of continuous administration
Cervagem (gemeprost 1 mg vaginal pessary), a prostaglandin E analogue also known as PGE_1	Keep frozen below 10°C (do not refreeze) Warm to room temperature Destroy if not used within 12 hours Insert one pessary into posterior fornix prior to surgery	Cervical softening prior to operative procedure in first trimester, therapeutic termination of pregnancy in the second trimester
Misoprostol tablet (Cytotec 200 micrograms), a prostaglandin E_1 analogue	Store tablets at room temperature Dosage varies with gestational age and clinical indication (e.g. fetal death, incomplete or inevitable abortion) (see FIGO Misoprostol-only recommended regimens, as cited in Morris et al 2017)	Under current TGA guidelines misoprostol is not approved for induction of labour

Source: Adapted from MIMS Online, 2021, www.mimsonline.com.au.

- evidence or strong suspicion of cephalopelvic disproportion or abnormal fetal position
- women for whom oxytocic drugs are contraindicated or when prolonged contraction could be hazardous to uterine integrity (previous caesarean section or major uterine surgery)
- women already receiving intravenous oxytocin
- cases where vaginal birth is not indicated (e.g. vasa praevia)
- multiple pregnancy
- multiparous women with $\geq$ 5 term pregnancies (AusDI 2021).

Caution should be used in the following circumstances:

- asthma
- hypotension or hypertension
- anaemia, jaundice, diabetes, epilepsy
- cardiovascular or renal disease
- raised intraocular pressure or glaucoma.

Care of women following prostaglandin administration

Conscientious care following administration is important. Observations are made both for the expected action and to detect deviations from normal. These include: assessment of the contractions (strength, length and frequency); assessment of maternal and fetal wellbeing; and assessment for levels of pain.

Observation of maternal and fetal wellbeing

- Temperature, pulse, respiratory rate, blood pressure, fetal heart rate, uterine activity and PV loss must be monitored frequently (at least hourly) in the 4 hours following administration.
- A reassuring CTG should be maintained for at least 30 minutes.
- If uterine hyperstimulation occurs tocolytics may be required (usually terbutaline subcutaneous or intravenous); local protocols should be followed.
- Provide ongoing care as for the latent first stage of labour (see Chapter 30).

The most common reasons for removal of PGE_2 are abnormal fetal heart rate patterns and uterine hyperstimulation (Rugarn et al 2017). The following are indications for the removal of prostaglandins:

- prostaglandins potentiate oxytocin effects; therefore, they must be removed prior to oxytocin administration
- prior to amniotomy and if membranes rupture spontaneously
- if labour commences, uterine hyperstimulation occurs or sustained or excessive contractions are present
- following spontaneous rupture of the membranes or prior to amniotomy
- if there are indications of fetal distress.

SKILL 20.1 Administration of medicines per vaginam

1. Gain informed consent, confirm the prescription and ensure privacy.
2. Confirm gestation, review history, ascertain if membranes are ruptured or intact and assess for contraindications to medication administration. Ensure the woman has an empty bladder. Check vital signs are within normal limits.
3. Perform hand hygiene.
4. Attend abdominal palpation to confirm presentation, attitude, lie, fetal position and engagement of the presenting part.
5. Establish fetal wellbeing, fetal heart rate and normal CTG.
6. Gather equipment:
   - sterile gloves and alcohol-based hand rub
   - sterile vaginal examination pack (according to local protocol)
   - disposable sheet
   - sterile single-use water-based lubricant
   - disposable wipes
   - the PV medication.
7. Confirm the woman's identity.
8. Remove any sanitary pads or underwear, keeping the genital area covered.
9. Ask the woman to adopt an almost recumbent position (use a wedge to avoid aortocaval occlusion if necessary), with her knees bent, ankles together and knees parted, placing a disposable sheet beneath her buttocks.
10. Open the gloves, medication and suitable lubricant; place them on the sterile side of the paper (or use the vaginal examination pack).
11. Perform hand hygiene and don gloves.
12. Ask the woman to lift the covers exposing the genital area.
13. Assess Bishop's score, nature of presenting part and fetal wellbeing.
14. For PGE_2 administration, part the labia with the thumb and forefinger of the non-examining hand.
    - Lubricate the two fingers of the examining hand and gently insert into the vagina, in a downwards and backwards direction along the posterior vaginal wall to locate the cervix, ensuring the thumb does not come into contact with the woman's clitoris or anus. Slide the gel applicator between the vaginal wall and the examining hand, until it has been guided into the posterior vaginal fornix by the examining hand. The plunger is then depressed by the other hand and the gel administered. Lubricant may be applied to the tip to aid insertion.

SKILL 20.1 Administration of medicines per vaginam—cont'd

- For the application of a tablet or pessary, either insert the examining hand with the pessary secured between the fingers, guiding it into the fornix as above, or insert the examining hand into the vagina, slide the pessary in using the non-examining hand and guide it into place using the examining hand. Lubricant may be applied to the pessary to aid insertion.

15. Remove fingers and wipe the vulva with the wipes. Ensure the retrieval string is accessible (if used). Maintain the woman's dignity.
16. Remove gloves and perform hand hygiene.
17. Assist the woman to resume a comfortable semi-recumbent position.
18. Continue CTG to obtain a normal trace for at least 30 minutes.
19. Dispose of equipment correctly and wash and dry hands.
20. Document administration and findings and act accordingly.

PROGESTERONE FOR PREVENTION OF PRETERM LABOUR

Progesterone assists in maintaining pregnancy by reducing uterine contractions (Norman 2020). In 2018 in Australia, 8.7% of births were classified as preterm (birth prior to 37 completed weeks of gestation) (AIHW 2020a). In New Zealand the national average for preterm births was 7.5% between 2010 and 2014 (Filoche et al 2018). A Cochrane review found progesterone was associated with a reduction in the risk of low birthweight infants and infants born before 37 weeks (Dodd et al 2013). Women with a singleton pregnancy, no history of preterm birth and with a cervix < 25 mm prior to 24 weeks have a reduced rate of preterm birth following administration of vaginal progesterone (Campbell 2018, Skyes & Bennett 2018). In contrast, the PROGRESS trial found that vaginal progesterone after a previous spontaneous preterm birth did not reduce neonatal morbidity (Crowther et al 2017). Treatment with progesterone in women with a multiple pregnancy does not appear to reduce the likelihood of preterm birth or improve outcomes for babies (Dodd et al 2019). Approximately one-third of women using progesterone vaginal pessaries reported side effects including headaches, nausea and discomfort or pain (Crowther et al 2017). Women usually self-administer vaginal progesterone.

TREATMENT OF VAGINAL INFECTIONS

Vaginal infections are related to dysbiosis and include vulvovaginal candidiasis, bacterial vaginosis and trichomonas vaginitis (Bagga & Arora 2020). During pregnancy, increasing oestrogen levels encourage *Lactobacillus*-dominant microbiota (Krishna et al 2017, Nunn et al 2021). Lactobacillus species appear to promote vaginal homeostasis and inhibit the growth of the microorganisms responsible for vaginal infections (Ceccarani et al 2019). Vulvovaginal candidiasis is common, with approximately 20% of all women colonised with *Candida albicans*; this increases to approximately 30% during pregnancy (Aguin & Sobel 2015). The increase is possibly due to immunological changes and higher levels of vaginal glycogen (Aguin & Sobel 2015).

Women with diabetes or a recent course of antibiotics are more susceptible to *C. albicans*. Antifungal vaginal creams used to treat *C. albicans* come with an applicator which is inserted intravaginally, generally at night (e.g. clotrimazole, miconazole and nystatin). The midwife has a role in providing education on infection prevention and medication administration. Women generally self-administer the cream by sliding the applicator along the posterior vaginal wall until the medication is high in the vagina. The plunger is depressed and the applicator is removed after the medication has been ejected.

Role and responsibilities of the midwife

These can be summarised as:

- practising within evidence-based protocols
- educating and supporting the woman
- observing normality for the mother and fetus and making a referral if necessary
- keeping contemporaneous documentation.

SUMMARY

- There are both advantages and disadvantages to using the vaginal route for medication.
- For the induction of labour, prostaglandin works locally to ripen the cervix. It should be used with caution because serious, as well as less serious, side effects are possible.
- The midwife has a number of responsibilities, including all those associated with the administration of medicines and with safe and effective woman-centred care.

Self-assessment exercises

The answers to the following questions may be found in the text.

1. Describe how the midwife prepares the woman for administration of a PV medication.
2. List the possible side effects of PGE_2.
3. Describe how PGE_2 is administered PV.
4. Discuss the role and responsibilities of the midwife after the administration of PGE_2 PV.
5. Describe topical treatments available for vaginal infections.

References

Aguin T, Sobel J: Vulvovaginal candidiasis in pregnancy, Current Infectious Disease Reports 17(6):1–6, 2015.

Alfirevic Z, Keeney E, Dowswell T, et al: Labour induction with prostaglandins: a systematic review and network meta-analysis, British Medical Journal 350:h217, 2015.

AusDI: Prostin E2 Vaginal Gel product information. 2021. Online 2 April 2021. Available: www.ausdi.com.

Austin K, Chambers GM, Abreu Lourenco R, et al: Cost-effectiveness of term induction of labour using inpatient prostaglandin gel versus outpatient Foley catheter, The Australian & New Zealand Journal of Obstetrics & Gynaecology 55:440–445, 2015.

Australian Institute of Health and Welfare: Australia's mothers and babies 2018: in brief. Perinatal statistics series no. 36. Cat. no. PER 108. AIHW, Canberra, 2020a.

Australian Institute of Health and Welfare: National Core Maternity Indicators 2018: summary report. Cat. no. PER 109. AIHW, Canberra, 2020b.

Baddock S: Applied physiology for labour and birth. Chapter 22. In Pairman S, Tracy S, Dahlen HG, Dixon, L: Midwifery, 4th ed., Elsevier, Sydney, 2018.

Bagga R, Arora P: Genital micro-organisms in pregnancy, Front Public Health Jun 16;8:225, 2020.

Bakker R, Pierce S, Myers D: The role of prostaglandins E1 and E2, dinoprostone, and misoprostol in cervical ripening and the induction of labor: a mechanistic approach, Archives of Gynecology and Obstetrics 296:167–179, 2017.

Baloch R, Jabeen N, Zahiruddin S, et al: Induction of labor; efficacy and safety of intravaginal prostaglandin E2 pessary, Professional Medical Journal 24:288–292, 2017.

Brown J, Beckmann M: Induction of labour using balloon catheter and prostaglandin gel, The Australian and New Zealand Journal of Obstetrics and Gynaecology 57:68–73, 2017.

Bullock S, Manias E: Fundamentals of pharmacology, 8th ed., Pearson Education, Melbourne, 2017.

Campbell S: Prevention of spontaneous preterm birth: universal cervical length assessment and vaginal progesterone in women with a short cervix: time for action. American Journal of Obstetrics and Gynecology 218(2):151–158, 2018.

Ceccarani C, Foschi C, Parolin C, et al: Diversity of vaginal microbiome and metabolome during genital infections, Scientific Reports 9:14095, 2019.

Crowther CA, Ashwood P, McPhee AJ, et al: Vaginal progesterone pessaries for pregnant women with a previous preterm birth to prevent neonatal respiratory distress syndrome (the PROGRESS Study): a multicentre, randomised, placebo-controlled trial, PLoS Medicine 14:1–18, 2017.

Department of Health: Clinical practice guidelines: pregnancy care, Australian Government, Canberra, 2020.

Dodd JM, Grivell RM, OBrien CM, et al: Prenatal administration of progestogens for preventing spontaneous preterm birth in women with a multiple pregnancy. Cochrane Database of Systematic Reviews 1, Art. No.: CD012024, 2019.

Dodd JM, Jones L, Flenady V, et al: Prenatal administration of progesterone for preventing preterm birth in women considered to be at risk of preterm birth, Cochrane Database of Systematic Reviews (7):CD004947s, 2013.

Fernández-Romero JA, Teleshova N, et al: Preclinical assessments of vaginal microbicide candidate safety and efficacy, Advanced Drug Delivery Reviews 92: 27–38, 2015.

Filoche S, Cram F, Beard A, et al: He Tamariki Kokoti Tau-Tackling Preterm: a data-linkage methodology to explore the clinical care pathway in preterm deliveries, BMC Health Services Research May 21;18(1):374, 2018.

Hiersch L, Borovich A, Gabbay-Benziv R, et al: Can we predict successful cervical ripening with prostaglandin E2 vaginal inserts? Archives of Gynecology and Obstetrics 295:343–349, 2017.

Ivars J, Garabedian C, Devos P, et al: Simplified Bishop score including parity predicts successful induction of labor, European Journal of Obstetrics, Gynecology & Reproductive Biology 203:309–314, 2016.

Kimball AB, Javorsky E, Ron ES, et al: A novel approach to administration of peptides in women: Systemic absorption of a GnRH agonist via transvaginal ring delivery system, Journal of Controlled Release 233: 19–28, 2016.

Krishna SB, Wilson SL, Adam JK: The vaginal microbiota in women's health and disease: current understanding and future perspectives—a review, Current Trends in Biotechnology and Pharmacy 11:190–205, 2017.

Laughon SK, Zhang J, Troendle J, et al: Using a simplified Bishop score to predict vaginal delivery, Obstetrics and Gynecology 117(4):805–811, 2011.

Machado RM, Palmeira-de-Oliveira A, Gaspar C, et al: Studies and methodologies on vaginal drug permeation, Advanced Drug Delivery Reviews 92:14–26, 2015.

Mahomed K, Pungsornruk K, Gibbons K: Induction of labour for postdates in nulliparous women with uncomplicated pregnancy—is the caesarean section rate really lower? Journal of Obstetrics and Gynaecology 36:916–920, 2016.

Middleton P, Shepherd E, Morris J, et al: Induction of labour at or beyond 37 weeks' gestation. Cochrane Database of Systematic Reviews 7, Art. No.: CD004945, 2020.

Miller H, Goetzl L, Wing D, et al: Optimising daytime deliveries when inducing labour using prostaglandin vaginal inserts, The Journal of Maternal–Fetal & Neonatal Medicine 29(4):517–522, 2016.

Ministry of Health: Induction of labour in Aotearoa New Zealand: a clinical practice guideline 2019, Wellington, 2021.

Misra A, Shahiwala A: Applications of polymers in drug delivery, Smithers RAPRA, Shawbury, UK, 2014.

Morris JL, Winikoff B, Dabash R, et al: FIGO's updated recommendations for misoprostol used alone in gynecology and obstetrics, International Journal of Gynecology & Obstetrics 138:363–366, 2017. Available: https://obgyn.onlinelibrary.wiley.com/doi/10.1002/ijgo.12181.

Murphy DJ, Boyd P, McCoy CF, et al: Controlling levonorgestrel binding and release in a multi-purpose prevention technology vaginal ring device, Journal of Controlled Release 226:138–147, 2016.

National Institute for Health and Care Excellence (NICE): NICE Quality Standards (QS60) Induction of Labour April 2014. NICE, London, 2014. Available: www.nice.org.uk.

Navve D, Orenstein N, Ribak R, et al: Is the Bishop-score significant in predicting the success of labor induction in multiparous women? Journal of Perinatology 37:480–483, 2017.

Norman JE: Progesterone and preterm birth, International Journal of Gynecology and Obstetrics 150(1):24–30, 2020. Available: https://doi.org/10.1002/ijgo.13187.

Nunn KL, Witkin SS, Schneider GM, et al: Changes in the vaginal microbiome during the pregnancy to postpartum transition. Reproductive Sciences 28: 1996–2005, 2021.

Pathak M, Coombes AG, Turner MS, et al: Investigation of polycaprolactone matrices for intravaginal delivery of doxycycline, Journal of Pharmaceutical Sciences 104:4217–4222, 2015.

Raghuraman N, Stout MJ, Young OM, et al: Utility of the simplified Bishop score in spontaneous labor, American Journal of Perinatology 33:1176–1181, 2016.

Rooney Thompson M, Towers CV, Howard BC, et al: The use of prostaglandin E1 in peripartum patients with asthma, American Journal of Obstetrics and Gynecology 212:392.e1–392.e3, 2015.

Royal Australian and New Zealand College of Obstetricians and Gynaecologists (RANZCOG): The use of misoprostol in obstetrics and gynaecology, 2016. Online 2 April 2021. Available: www.ranzcog.edu.au/RANZCOG_SITE/media/RANZCOG-MEDIA/Women%27s%20Health/Statement%20and%20guidelines/Clinical-Obstetrics/The-use-of-misoprostol-in-obstetrics-(C-Obs-12)-Review-March-2016.pdf?ext=.pdf.

Rugarn O, Tipping D, Powers B, et al: Induction of labour with retrievable prostaglandin vaginal inserts: outcomes following retrieval due to an intrapartum adverse event, BJOG: An International Journal of Obstetrics and Gynaecology 124:796–803, 2017.

Sutton C, Harding J, Griffin C: Patient attitudes towards outpatient cervical ripening prior to induction of labour at an Australian tertiary hospital, Journal of Obstetrics & Gynaecology 36:921–928, 2016.

Sykes L, Bennett P: Efficacy of progesterone for prevention of preterm birth. Best practice & research. Clinical Obstetrics and Gynaecology 52:126–136, 2018.

Therapeutic Goods Administration (TGA): eBusiness Services: Product and Consumer Medicine Information. Prostin E2—Dinoprostone, 2020. Online 8 April 2021. Available: www.ebs.tga.gov.au/ebs/picmi/picmirepository.nsf/PICMI?OpenForm&t=&q=prostin%20e2&r=https://www.ebs.tga.gov.au/.

Thomas J, Fairclough A, Kavanagh J, et al: Vaginal prostaglandin (PGE2 and PGF2a) for induction of labour at term, Cochrane Database of Systematic Reviews (6):CD003101, 2014.

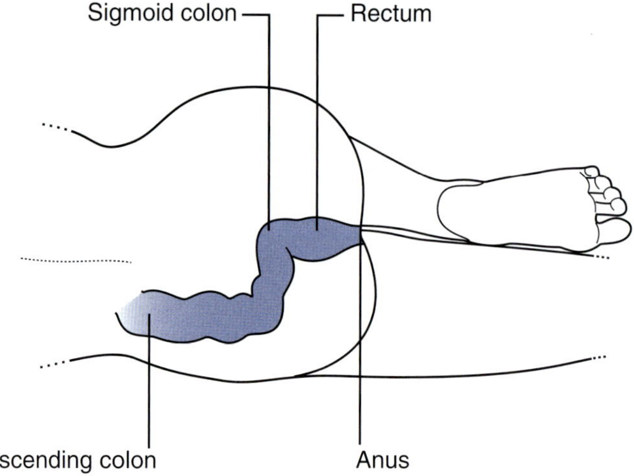

FIGURE 21.2 **Suggested positioning for insertion of PR medication.**
Source: Adapted with kind permission from Jamieson EM, McCall J, Whyte L: Clinical nursing practices, 5th ed., Churchill Livingstone, Edinburgh, 2016.

SKILL 21.1 Administration of medicines per rectum

1. The prescription is scrutinised and dispensed according to the correct procedure.
2. Confirm the woman's identity and check there are no contraindications.
3. Explain the procedure, gain informed consent and ensure privacy.
4. Perform hand hygiene.
5. If the medication is for systemic use, the woman should be encouraged to open her bowels before its administration.
6. Gather equipment:
    - suppository(ies) or (warmed) enema
    - non-sterile gloves and alcohol-based hand rub
    - disposable sheet
    - compatible lubricant, usually water-based
    - gauze swabs
    - plastic apron
    - a trolley or tray from which to work.
7. Ensure privacy and dignity and avoid unnecessary exposure. After removing underwear, the woman is asked to lie in a left lateral position with one or both of her knees flexed.
8. Place the disposable sheet beneath her buttocks and cover her with a bed sheet.
9. Put on the plastic apron, apply alcohol-based hand rub and put on gloves.
10. Ask the woman to lift the sheet.
11. Place lubricant on the gauze and lubricate the suppository or the tubing tip (if an enema). Expel the air from the enema tubing by pushing the solution through to the tip.
12. Ask the woman to take a deep breath (this relaxes the anal sphincter).
13. Lift the woman's right buttock using the left hand.

Laxative suppository

a. Insert the suppository 2–4 cm into the rectum using the right index or middle finger. Place it between the faeces and rectal wall.
b. Insert a second suppository in the same way if required.

Systemic suppository

a. Gently push the end through the anal sphincter. The finger does not need to enter the rectum.

Enema

a. Insert the enema tubing, advancing it slowly 2–5 cm. (Cease the enema if there is bleeding, complaints of pain or the woman asks you to stop.)
b. Withdraw the tubing carefully once completed, maintaining pressure on the pack to prevent the fluid flowing back into it.

14. Wipe the perineum with the gauze and re-cover the woman.
15. Remove gloves and apron.
16. Perform hand hygiene.
17. Assist the woman into a comfortable position.
18. Encourage her to retain the medication for as long as possible. Aim for laxatives to be retained for at least 10–20 minutes.
19. Ensure the call bell is accessible.
20. Assist her later, if needed, to the toilet.
21. Dispose of equipment correctly and wash and dry hands.
22. Document administration and effect and act accordingly.

Role and responsibilities of the midwife

These can be summarised as:

- appropriately checking and dispensing the drug (as for any prescription)
- understanding the action and possible side effects of the drug: the effect/side effect should always be reported and recorded; if given for laxative purposes, the quantity, colour and consistency of the stool should be recorded according to the Bristol stool classifications (Chapter 17)
- educating and supporting the woman: gaining informed consent so she has realistic expectations of the procedure and outcome
- maintaining the woman's dignity and privacy during an embarrassing procedure
- using correct administration technique, placing the medication in the correct place and upholding the infection control and personal protective equipment protocols
- avoiding potential complications
- taking appropriate care following administration: for example, assisting the woman to reach toilet facilities, if necessary (laxatives); assessing pain levels or incidence of vomiting (systemic medication)
- contemporaneous record keeping of the care given before, during and after the administration.

SUMMARY

- Administration of medicines PR may be for laxative or systemic purposes.
- The midwife should be familiar with the effect of the drug and how to administer it correctly.

Self-assessment exercises

The answers to the following questions may be found in the text.

1. Discuss the advantages and disadvantages of using the rectal route for medicine administration.
2. List the information the midwife should be familiar with before administering a laxative suppository.
3. Discuss the evidence that determines which end of a suppository should be inserted first.
4. Describe how a laxative enema is administered.
5. Summarise the role and responsibilities of the midwife when administering a medicine PR.

References

British National Formulary (BNF): BNF 66 British Medical Association, Royal Pharmaceutical Society, Pharmaceutical Press, London, 2014.

Bullock S, Manias E: Fundamentals of pharmacology, 8th ed., Pearson Australia, Melbourne, 2017.

Jordan S: Administration of medicines. In Jordan S, editor: Pharmacology for midwives, 2nd ed., Palgrave Macmillan, Basingstoke, 2010, pp. 39–61.

Lowry M: Rectal drug administration in adults: how, when, why, Nursing Times 112(8):12–14, 2016.

Peate I: How to administer an enema, Nursing Standard 30(14):34–36, 2015a.

Peate I: How to administer suppositories, Nursing Standard 30:34–36, 2015b.

- *Dorsogluteal* (gluteus maximus muscle) (maximum 4 mL): This is found on the upper outer quadrant of the buttock (Fig 22.1C). There is a risk of striking the sciatic nerve or a major blood vessel. In women with a high BMI, an injection may not reach the muscle layer.
- *Ventrogluteal* site (maximum 4 mL): This is the site of choice; the palm of the midwife's right hand is placed on the greater trochanter of the woman's left hip (or vice versa). The index finger is extended to touch the anterior superior iliac crest while the middle finger stretches as far along the iliac crest as possible. The site is in the 'V' between the index and middle fingers (Fig 22.1D).

IM injections are administered at a 90° angle to the skin (Ministry of Health 2020). Vaccine injections are generally given in the anterolateral thigh and the deltoid muscle (Department of Health 2020). The volume of solution the muscle can accommodate will vary depending on body size and age; the amounts suggested above are a guide.

The muscle should be relaxed for minimal discomfort; the site may be supported by the non-injecting hand (Shepherd 2018).

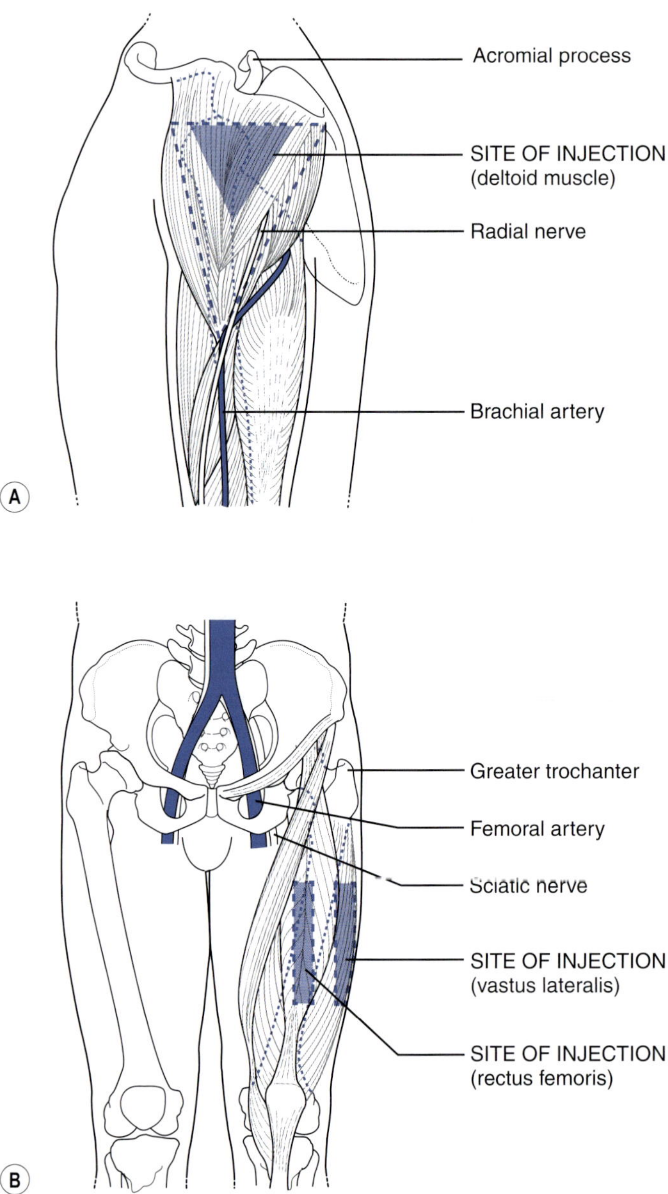

FIGURE 22.1 **Sites for adult intramuscular injection. A, Deltoid muscle. B, Rectus femoris and vastus lateralis (vastus lateralis is the one suitable site for IM injection in neonates as well).**

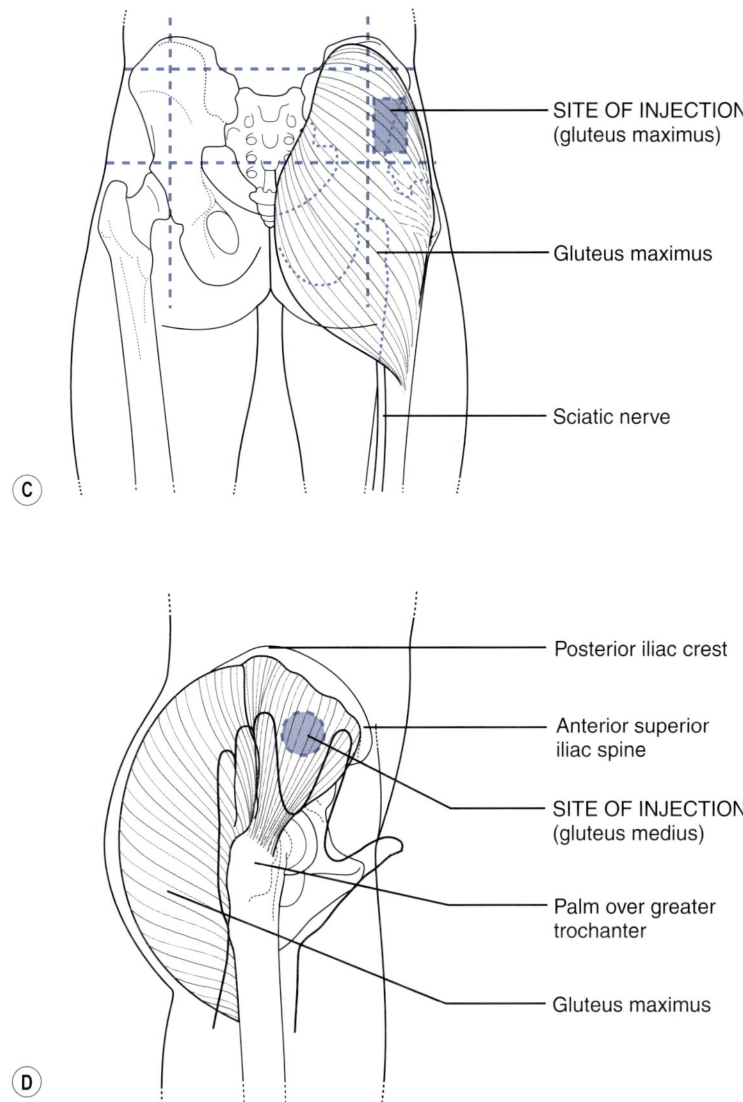

FIGURE 22.1, cont'd **C, Gluteus maximus. D, Ventrogluteal muscle.**
Source: Adapted with kind permission from Jamieson EM, McCall JM, Blythe R, et al: Clinical nursing practices, 3rd ed., Churchill Livingstone, Edinburgh, 1997.

Z-track

A **Z-track technique** (Fig 22.2) ensures the solution does not leak back to the skin and so irritate the subcutaneous tissue or stain the skin (Frotjold & Bloomfield 2021). The skin and subcutaneous tissue are moved sideways or downwards 2–3 cm and held taut, the needle is inserted and the solution is injected slowly; the needle is removed as the skin is released simultaneously to create a zigzag path (Shepherd 2018). Local protocols should be followed.

Choice of equipment

The choice of equipment depends on the site, age and body mass. A higher percentage of subcutaneous fat can mean an IM injection does not reach the muscle. Most women of normal weight would receive an IM injection with a 32 mm needle at the ventrogluteal or dorsogluteal site. At the dorsogluteal or ventrogluteal site, a 32 mm needle would result in at least 50% of women inadvertently receiving a SC injection; with a 38 mm needle 25% of obese women would still receive a SC injection instead of an IM injection (Larkin et al 2017).

In an average-sized woman, a 21-gauge (green) to 23-gauge (blue) needle is used at a 90° angle (see Fig 22.3) in any of the recommended sites. IM injections should be into muscle tissue, so too short a length of needle would make it an SC injection. The use of a filter

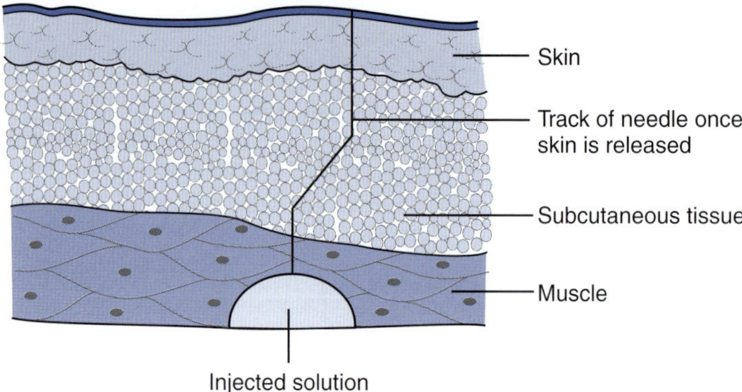

FIGURE 22.2 **Z-track injection. The skin and subcutaneous tissue are moved downwards or sideways for 2–3 cm prior to insertion of the needle and then released as the needle is removed. The solution is prevented from back tracking to the skin.**
Source: Johnson R, Taylor W: Skills for midwifery practice, 4th ed., Elsevier, London, 2016.

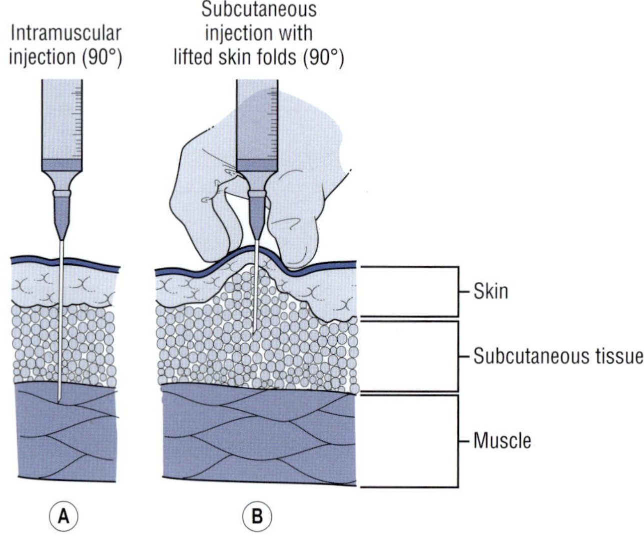

FIGURE 22.3 **A, IM injection (90°). B, SC injection with lifted skin folds, 90°.**
Source: Johnson R, Taylor W: Skills for midwifery practice, 4th ed., Elsevier, London, 2016.

needle for drawing up the solution means that a 'new' sharp sterile needle is used for injecting; this is more comfortable. The syringe is held like a dart, preventing the accidental injection of solution when injecting. Post-injection, a cottonwool ball or gauze swab is used to cover the puncture site.

Ampoules and vials

Ampoules may be glass or, increasingly, plastic, with a top that 'snaps off'. Vials tend to be glass with a rubber bung beneath the metal top. This needs cleaning with an alcohol-impregnated wipe before use to reduce the risk of cross-infection. Ampoules and vials may be completely inverted so the substance can be drawn up without any air, and so the scale on the syringe can be read correctly at eye level. Preparations may come as solutions or powder for reconstitution. In the event of needing to reconstitute a drug (e.g. penicillin), a diluent (e.g. sterile water) will be required according to the manufacturer's instructions.

IM injection for a neonate

The main anatomical site for IM injection in the infant < 12 months is the anterolateral thigh (vastus lateralis) (Fig 22.1B). In infants ≥ 12 months, the deltoid muscle is recommended. The ventrogluteal and vastus lateralis may also be used for infants ≥ 12 months (Department of Health 2020).

The maximum dose that can be injected is 1 mL. The neonate should be in a safe place (e.g. held or in a cot). A 25-gauge (orange) or 23-gauge (blue) needle is inserted at a 90° angle (Department of Health 2020).

COVID-19 vaccination

The COVID-19 vaccine is recommended for pregnant and breastfeeding women and can be given at any stage of pregnancy. The risk of serious outcomes from COVID-19 is higher for pregnant women and their fetus. Vaccination is the optimal way to reduce the risk of serious outcomes including intensive care admission and preterm birth. Vaccination does not increase the chances of complications such as preterm birth, stillbirth, small-for-gestational-age infants and birth defects (Australian Government 2021). The COVID-19 vaccination should not be given within 14 days of another vaccine (ATAGI 2021). Health professional training to administer COVID-19 vaccinations can be accessed from the Australian Government Department of Health website (see Resources at the end of this chapter).

SUBCUTANEOUS INJECTION

A **subcutaneous (SC) injection** places the medication into the connective tissue and fat beneath the skin. These tissues have a reduced blood supply in comparison to muscle, so absorption is slow and constant. Medications causing tissue irritation should not be used for SC injection as they may result in pain, necrosis and tissue sloughing (Buxton 2017). Common preparations for SC use include insulin and low-molecular-weight heparin. If heparin is inadvertently injected into muscle, IM haemorrhage and haematoma may result (Bullock & Manias 2017). Only 1–2 mL can be injected subcutaneously. SC infusions can administer medications slowly over extended time periods. Insulin pumps deliver small doses of insulin continuously by the subcutaneous route and can reduce the incidence of severe hypoglycaemia and improve glucose control.

SC injections can be inadvertently placed into muscle if the needle is injected too deeply. Needle depth and the amount of subcutaneous tissue determine whether the needle is inserted into the skin at a 45° or 90° angle. Needles greater than 6 mm are no longer recommended due to the high risk of IM injection (Australian Diabetes Educators Association [ADEA] 2017).

The lifted skin folds technique (Fig 22.4) is used to increase the distance between the skin and muscle fascia (ADEA 2017). This helps to ensure the medication is deposited in the subcutaneous tissue. The need to use a lifted skinfold takes into account factors such as the needle length (Table 22.1), injection site, body composition and age, and may be necessary when a longer needle is used. It is important to lift the skin correctly by using two fingers (thumb and first or second finger) to lift the skin upwards gently without pulling up accompanying muscle (ADEA 2017). A shorter needle (often found in pre-prepared injections or injection pens—6 mm) can be used at 90° generally without lifting the skin (Diggle 2014). The *Immunisation Handbook* (Ministry of Health 2020) indicates that when giving a SC injection in the deltoid, the needle should never be longer than 16 mm and an insertion angle of 45° should be used.

Specific considerations for insulin

The ADEA (2017) provides the following information on injecting insulin during pregnancy

- Shorter needles are preferred (pen: 4 or 5 mm length; syringe: 6 mm) for abdominal injections due to thinning of abdominal fat as a result of uterine expansion.
- In the first trimester no changes in site or technique are required.
- In the second trimester insulin can be injected over the entire abdomen as long as correctly raised skinfolds are used. The lateral aspects of

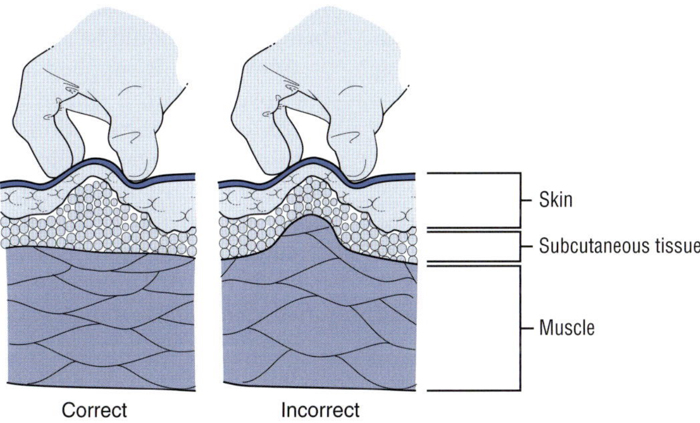

FIGURE 22.4 **Lifted skin folds—the subcutaneous tissue is lifted away from the muscle and held until the needle has been removed.**
Source: Johnson R, Taylor W: Skills for midwifery practice, 4th ed., Elsevier, London, 2016.

TABLE 22.1 GUIDE TO NEEDLE LENGTH

Guide to needle length for insulin injection SC			
	Needle size	**Angle of injection**	**Use of skin fold***
Very slender adults	4 mm	90	May
	5 mm	45 or 90	Yes
	6 mm	45 or 90	Yes
	8 mm	45	Yes
Normal weight adults	4 mm	90	No
	5 mm	90	May
	6 mm	90	Yes
	8 mm	45	Yes
Overweight/obese adults	4 mm	90	No
	5 mm	90	No
	6 mm	90	May
	8 mm	45 to 90	Yes
	12 mm	Not recommended	

*May = may be necessary; use clinical judgment.
Source: Australian Diabetes Educators Association (ADEA): Clinical guiding principles for subcutaneous injection technique, Canberra, 2017. Online 28 August 2021. Available: www.adea.com.au/wp-content/uploads/2020/07/InjectionTechniqueGuidelines_FINAL_Approved_Jan-2020-8.pdf.

the abdomen can also be used when not using a skinfold.

- In the third trimester the lateral abdomen can be used with correct skinfold technique.
- Women who do not wish to inject into their abdomen can use their thigh, upper arm or buttock instead.

Choice of site

Sites for SC injection include the buttocks, thigh and arms, although the risk of inadvertent IM injection is higher in the arms and thigh (ADEA 2017). Absorption varies with the site used; the fastest absorption is in the abdomen, followed by the arms, then thighs, with the slowest absorption in the buttock (Ogston-Tuck 2014). Site rotation decreases the risk of lipodystrophy. The ADEA (2017) recommends selecting one site and rotating within that site as absorption varies between sites.

The site should be examined prior to injection for inflammation, infection, scarring or hardness, which may all indicate poor absorption and increase the level of pain. Cleaning the skin with an alcohol swab prior to injection is not required and increases the likelihood of toughening the skin (ADEA 2017). Aspiration is not considered necessary for a SC injection (Redmond 2021).

Speed of delivery

Injections are more comfortable if injected slowly. Ogston-Tuck (2014) recommends that enoxaparin should be injected over 30 seconds. For other SC injections a specific time is not given but slow smooth injection is suggested as this reduces tissue trauma and discomfort (Redmond 2021).

Specific considerations for enoxaparin

Enoxaparin sodium (Clexane) is a low-molecular-weight heparin and is available in pre-prepared syringes at set doses. In pregnancy the dose is adjusted according to body weight and is generally administered once a day by the midwife or the woman; often the midwife needs to provide teaching, so the woman can administer enoxaparin herself. The midwife has a responsibility to teach the correct technique. Enoxaparin is administered by deep SC injection using a dart technique. Rubbing the injection site after administration may cause bruising and should be avoided (TGA 2020).

Enoxaparin is supplied in pre-filled syringes which are covered with a silicon coating. Do not wipe the needle or allow the solution to crystallise on the needle as this will damage the silicon coating (TGA 2020). The air bubble must not be expelled and should remain near the hub during administration. The air bubble remains in the syringe, ensuring the full dose has been delivered. The needle is inserted at 90° with the lifted skin folds technique (Fig 22.5A). Only when the injection is complete should the skinfold be released. Rotation of the abdominal site is necessary for long-term use. The site is rotated (e.g. right or left) and moved by at least 1 cm each day, generally in a circular pattern (Gelder 2014). A reclining position is preferable for administration. The abdomen remains a safe site during pregnancy and postnatally.

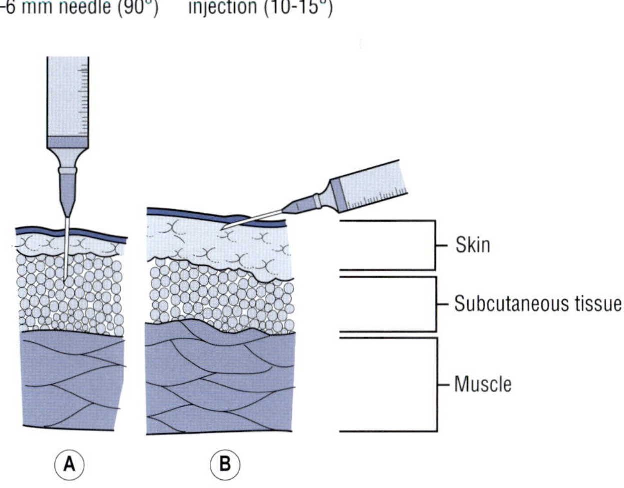

FIGURE 22.5 **A, SC injection using 4–6 mm needle length, 90°. B, ID injection (10–15°).**
Source: Johnson R, Taylor W: Skills for midwifery practice, 4th ed., Elsevier, London, 2016.

INTRADERMAL INJECTION

Intradermal administration involves injecting a small quantity of solution (up to 0.5 mL) into the dermis with a fine needle (Bullock & Manias 2017). The bevel of the needle is inserted at a 10–15° angle, with the bevel upwards so a small weal forms on the skin (Fig 22.5B). The bacille Calmette-Guérin (BCG) vaccine (tuberculosis) is given intradermally using a tuberculin or insulin syringe, usually on the upper left arm, slightly above the insertion of the deltoid muscle (Ministry of Health 2020). An **intradermal (ID) injection** can be given on the inner forearm or scapula. Midwives may inject local anaesthetic intradermally prior to cannulation (over the site of the vein to be cannulated). Local anaesthetic is also injected intradermally when infiltrating for perineal repair (Chapter 45).

SKILL 22.1 Preparing an injection

1. Review the medication order, undertake medication checking procedures (see Chapter 18).
2. Perform hand hygiene.
3. Gather equipment:
   - sterile syringe (appropriate size, not expired)
   - needle or needless access device (filter needle may be required)
   - sharps container
   - cottonwool or gauze
   - vial or ampoule
   - medicine administration chart.
4. Prepare medication.

Glass/plastic ampoule

a. Ensure all the solution is in the ampoule (not retained in the top); snap off the top (protect fingers when using a glass ampoule).
b. Draw up the medication with a syringe or needless device (or filter needle) by pulling back the plunger. Use a non-touch technique; if bubbles are aspirated, do not expel back into ampoule.
c. Invert the syringe; if any bubbles are present, tap the side gently to encourage the air to move to the top of the syringe; push the plunger to exclude the air from the syringe, ensuring none of the solution is lost and the dosage in the syringe is correct. If the syringe contains excess medication, inject the excess into the sink and recheck the medication level while holding syringe vertically.
d. Remove the drawing up needle, discard it into the sharps container and replace the needle using a non-touch technique.

Vial containing a solution

a. Remove the cap from the vial, keeping the rubber seal sterile. For a multidose vial, clean the surface of the rubber seal with an alcohol swab and allow to dry.
b. Pull back on the syringe plunger and draw an amount of air into the syringe equivalent to the volume of medication required.
c. Connect a needle or needleless access device (or vial access spike). Place the vial on

Continued

SKILL 22.1 Preparing an injection—cont'd

a flat surface, insert the access device into the rubber seal and inject air into the vial.
d. Invert the vial while holding the syringe and plunger in the dominant hand and the vial in the non-dominant hand. Ensure the tip of the needle remains below fluid level. The syringe should fill from the air pressure within the vial. It may be necessary to pull the plunger back to withdraw the correct amount.
e. Once the desired volume is in the syringe, tap the side of the barrel and dislodge any air bubbles. Draw back on the plunger and push upwards to eject any air.
f. Replace the vial access device with an appropriate-size needle.

Vial containing a powder

a. Remove the cap covering the vial containing powdered medication.
b. Draw up diluent into the syringe (the syringe normally connects directly to a sterile water ampoule).
c. Insert the needle (or needleless access device) and inject dilutant into the vial; mix the powder and dilutant by rolling between the palms (avoid shaking).
d. Draw up the required amount of reconstituted medication into the syringe.
e. Remove, drawing up the needle (or needless access device) and add the appropriate gauge and length needle.

SKILL 22.2 IM and SC injections in the adult

1. Review the medication order and consider the action, purpose, possible side effects of the medication and the patient's medical history.
2. Undertake medication checking procedures (see Chapter 18).
3. Perform hand hygiene and follow standard precautions.
4. Gather equipment:
   - sterile needle (25–26 gauge for SC, 21–24 gauge for IM); ensure the correct size for the type of injection and size and age of the client (see earlier this chapter)
   - 1 sterile syringe (appropriate size, not expired)
   - portable sharps container (if one is not in the room)
   - cottonwool or gauze
   - pre-prepared medication (may be in a preloaded syringe; e.g. enoxaparin)
   - medicine administration chart.
5. Take the prepared medicine, medication chart, sharps container and cottonwool/gauze to the woman.
6. Confirm identity by asking the woman to state her name and date of birth.
7. Ensure privacy and expose the injection site, positioning the woman accordingly (often left lateral for IM right ventrogluteal muscle).
8. Perform hand hygiene.
9. Assess site (look for bruising, muscle atrophy, amount of adipose tissue, etc.); if visibly contaminated, clean the injection site for 30 seconds, up and down, side to side, creating friction. Leave to dry for at least 30 seconds.

For SC injection

a. Identify the site, lift the skin fold if necessary (Fig 22.4) with the non-injecting hand and decisively inject at a 90° or 45° angle.
b. Inject slowly until the injection is complete, then remove the needle (release the skin folds if used).
c. Apply gentle pressure with cottonwool or gauze.
d. Activate the needle defence system.
e. Put the used sharps into the sharps container.

For IM injection

a. Using the landmarks for the chosen injection site (ventrogluteal recommended), identify the specific site for injection.
b. Using the non-dominant hand, gently stretch the skin/subcutaneous tissue 2–3 cm, then decisively inject at a 90° angle, holding the syringe like a dart.
c. Push on the plunger smoothly to inject the solution.
d. Remove the needle and release the skin at the same time.
e. Press the puncture site gently with the gauze or cottonwool; avoid massage which may cause irritation.
f. Activate the needle defence system and place the used sharps into the sharps container.

10. Assist the woman to a comfortable position.
11. Decontaminate hands.
12. Dispose of remaining equipment correctly.
13. Document administration and act accordingly; examine the site 2 hours later for any possible reactions.

Role and responsibilities of the midwife

These can be summarised as:

- correctly using equipment and choosing a site to facilitate a safe and comfortable injection technique
- knowing and applying evidence-based best practice
- educating and supporting the woman, particularly if she is anxious
- correctly disposing of sharps
- ensuring contemporaneous record keeping is correct.

SUMMARY

- Injections require the midwife to choose an appropriate length of needle and correct angle of insertion to ensure the medication is placed into the correct tissue.
- A number of factors determine which site is chosen; the ventrogluteal is the site of choice for IM injections in adults.
- Skin cleansing is not required prior to injection if the skin is clean.
- Aspiration is not necessary for SC injections or for vaccines. Aspiration may be used at times.
- Care is taken to avoid needlestick injury by using needle defence systems and sharps boxes at the point of care, and no re-sheathing of needles.

Self-assessment exercises

The answers to the following questions may be found in the text.

1. Cite examples of when injections may be necessary for a childbearing woman.
2. List the sites suitable for IM injection for both the woman and the neonate.
3. List the considerations necessary for the safe administration of SC enoxaparin.
4. Demonstrate an IM injection for a neonate.
5. Compare and contrast the similarities and differences between an IM and a SC injection in the adult, in relation to the equipment, technique and site.
6. Describe how a Z-track injection is completed.
7. Summarise the role and responsibilities of the midwife when administering an injection.

Resources

Department of Health: COVID-19 Vaccination training, 2021. Online 5 April 2021. Available: covid19vaccinationtraining.org.au/login/index.php.

References

Australian Diabetes Educators Association (ADEA): Clinical guiding principles for subcutaneous injection technique, Canberra, 2017. Online 5 April 2021. Available: www.adea.com.au/wp-content/uploads/2009/10/Injection-Technique-FINAL_170323.docx.pdf.

Australian Government: Pregnancy, breastfeeding, and COVID-19 vaccines, 2021. Online 15 November 2021. Available: www.health.gov.au/sites/default/files/documents/2021/10/covid-19-vaccination-pregnancy-breastfeeding-and-covid-19-vaccines-pregnancy-breastfeeding-and-covid-19-vaccines.pdf.

Australian Technical Advisory Group on Immunisation (ATAGI): COVID-19 vaccination—ATAGI advice on influenza and COVID-19 vaccines, 2021. Online 5 April 2021. Available: www.health.gov.au/resources/publications/covid-19-vaccination-atagi-advice-on-influenza-and-covid-19-vaccines.

Bullock S, Manias E: Fundamentals of pharmacology, 8th ed., Pearson, Melbourne, 2017.

Buxton ILO: Pharmacokinetics: The dynamics of drug absorption, distribution, metabolism and elimination. In Brunton LL, Hilal-Dandan R, Knollmann BC, eds: Goodman & Gilman's: the pharmacological basis of therapeutics, 13th ed., McGraw-Hill, New York, 2017.

Centers for Disease Control and Prevention (CDC): Advisory Committee on Immunization Practices (ACIP), ACIP vaccine recommendations and guidelines, 2021. Online 4 April 2021. Available: www.cdc.gov/vaccines/hcp/acip-recs/index.html.

Cooper K, Gosnell K: Foundations and adult health nursing, Elsevier, Mosby, St Louis, 2018.

Department of Health: The Australian immunisation handbook, Commonwealth of Australia, Canberra, 2020. Online 4 April 2021. Available: https://immunisationhandbook.health.gov.au/.

Diggle J: How to help patients achieve correct self-injection technique, Practice Nursing 25(9):451–454, 2014.

Frotjold A, Bloomfield J: Ensuring medication safety, Chapter 20. In Crisp J, Douglas C, Rebeiro G, Waters D: Potter & Perry's fundamentals of nursing, 6th ed., Australia and New Zealand edition. Elsevier, Sydney, 2021.

Gelder C: Best practice injection technique for children and young people with diabetes, Nursing Children and Young People 26(7):32–36, 2014.

Larkin TA, Ashcroft E, Elgellaie A, et al: Ventrogluteal versus dorsogluteal site selection: A cross-sectional study of muscle and subcutaneous fat thicknesses and an algorithm incorporating demographic and anthropometric data to predict injection outcome, International Journal of Nursing Studies 71:1–7, 2017.

Ministry of Health: Immunisation handbook, 3rd ed., 2020. Online 3 April 2021. Available: www.health.govt.nz/publication/immunisation-handbook-2020.

National Health and Medical Research Council (NHMRC): Australian Guidelines for the Prevention and Control of Infection in Healthcare, Canberra, 2019.

Ogston-Tuck S: Subcutaneous injection technique: an evidence-based approach, Nursing Standard 29(3): 53–58, 2014.

Palma S, Strohfus P: Are IM injections IM in obese and overweight females? A study in injection technique, Applied Nursing Research 26:e1–e4, 2013.

Redmond H: Nursing care: medication administration and monitoring, Chapter 24. In Koutoukidis, Stainton K, eds: Tabbner's nursing care, 8th ed., Elsevier, Sydney, 2021.

Shepherd E. (2018). Injection technique1: administering drugs via the intramuscular route. Nursing Times; 114: 8, 23–25.

Sisson H: Aspirating during the intramuscular injection procedure: a systematic literature review, Journal of Clinical Nursing 24:2368–2375, 2015.

Therapeutic Goods Administration (TGA): Product and consumer medicine information. Australian product information: Clexane, 2020. Online 4 April 2021. Available: www.ebs.tga.gov.au

Therapeutic Goods Administration (TGA): Product and consumer medicine information. Australian product information: Syntocinon, 2019. Online 4 April 2021. Available: www.ebs.tga.gov.au

Thomas CM, Mraz M, Rajcan L: Blood aspiration during IM injection, Clinical Nursing Research 25:549–559, 2016.

World Health Organization (WHO): WHO best practices for injections and related procedures toolkit. WHO, Geneva, 2010.

Wynaden D, Tohotoa J, Omari OA, et al: Administering intramuscular injections: How does research translate into practice over time in the mental health setting? Nurse Education Today 35:620–624, 2015.

CHAPTER 23

INTRAVENOUS MEDICATIONS AND INTRAVENOUS THERAPY

Learning outcomes

Having read this chapter, the reader should be able to:

- list indications for intravenous (IV) infusions and medications
- discuss advantages and disadvantages of the IV route
- describe the different ways in which medications can be administered intravenously
- demonstrate giving an IV drug as a bolus and by intermittent infusion
- describe the types of fluid solution commonly used for an IV infusion
- describe the formula for calculating the flow of an IV infusion
- discuss the complications associated with infusion therapy and how these are recognised and managed
- discuss how fluid balance is monitored and the significance
- discuss the role and responsibilities of the midwife when administering IV medications or IV therapy.

Midwives may be required to administer intravenous (IV) medications and IV therapy to women and neonates. This chapter examines the safe administration of IV medications and IV therapy. Antibiotics are the most common IV medication administered, although opioids, paracetamol and uterotonics are also given. IV medications can be given as a small 'bolus' or 'push', an intermittent infusion, a large-volume infusion or via a volume-controlled or patient-controlled device such as **patient-controlled analgesia (PCA)**. The skills involved in setting up, monitoring and discontinuing an IV infusion are reviewed, as well as the types of solutions used and the importance of monitoring fluid balance. Administration of IV medications and IV therapy for the neonate are not discussed.

INTRAVENOUS INFUSIONS

An IV infusion is the introduction of sterile fluid into the venous circulation through the use of pressure. Access to the circulation is usually via a **peripheral intravenous catheter (PIVC)** if IV therapy is expected to be short term. If long-term therapy is required the subclavian vein or internal jugular vein is the preferred access site, although this is rarely necessary in midwifery. Infusions can be continuous or intermittent (which may be as a secondary infusion). Errors related to IV therapy are common, despite widespread use of IV smart pumps (Blandford et al 2016). IV medication errors have a high potential to cause harm as they enter the venous blood directly and can cause rapid effects (Brindley 2020).

INDICATIONS

- Prevention of fluid and electrolyte disturbances, particularly when oral fluids/food are withheld or not tolerated (e.g. pre- and postoperatively, vomiting, diarrhoea)
- Restoring fluid and electrolyte balance (e.g. hypovolaemia, haemorrhage, shock, dehydration)
- Administration of medications (e.g. oxytocin)

EQUIPMENT

Intravenous administration set (giving set)

These are sterile pre-packed sets consisting of a long piece of air-filled tubing with a trocar at the top to insert into the bag or bottle of fluid, a drip chamber (which may contain a filter) and a cannula connection at the other end. The tubing has an adjustable roller clamp to adjust the fluid flow (Fig 23.1), which should be positioned on the upper third of the tubing. Three main types are used in midwifery: one for the administration of clear fluids, one for iron infusion (orange coloured) and one for blood transfusion (double chamber and filter). The tubing has needleless ports through which medications can be administered.

The use of a **closed system of infusion** reduces the risk of infection, with each additional connection increasing the risk of infection (Loveday et al 2014). For example, three-way taps (stopcocks) used between the cannula and infusion line are difficult to keep clean and can act as a reservoir for microorganisms that multiply in the warm, moist environment, increasing the risk of infection (Felver 2015).

Needleless connectors

A **Luer lock** is used to secure a needleless connector to an IV cannula (Fig 23.2). It is designed to eliminate the use of needles and reduce sharps injuries. Needleless connectors should be disinfected prior to use and aseptic non-touch technique (ANTT) should be used when manipulating needleless connectors.

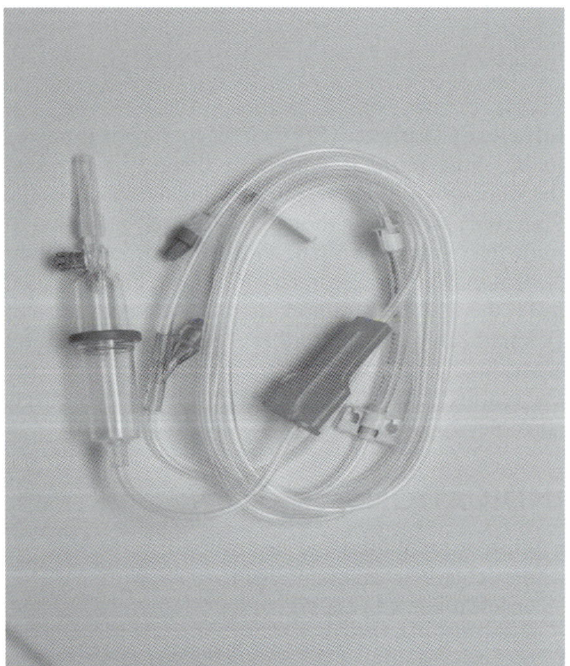

FIGURE 23.1 An intravenous administration set.

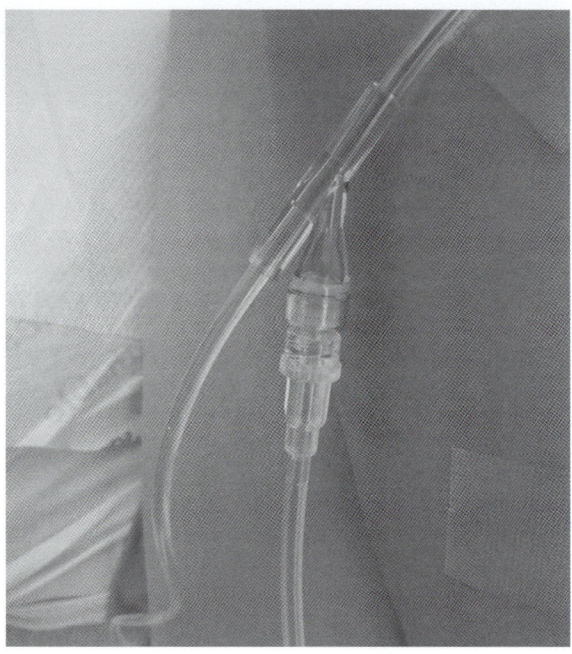

FIGURE 23.2 A needleless connector.

Many needle-free connectors have a silicon piston which allows fluid to pass through when the device is compressed and returns to its original position when compression is released (Harrold 2019). Extension sets are often added to needleless connectors because they decrease movement and manipulation of the cannula (Gorski et al 2016).

Calibrated burette sets

Calibrated burette sets (volume control devices) can be used when a medical infusion device is unavailable, to obtain greater control over the flow rate. Calibrated burette sets allow for very small amounts of fluid to be administered and are more likely to be used in the neonatal unit than the maternity unit or to administer diluted medications.

Medical infusion devices

A variety of infusion devices allow the infusion flow to be regulated electronically, administering a prescribed amount of fluid over a set time (Fig 23.3). Infusions administered using gravity are more likely to result in harm than an infusion administered with a device (Blandford et al 2019).

The midwife should know how the infusion devices work and ensure they are properly cleaned and maintained. Inappropriate cleaning products have resulted in damage to infusion pumps, which may in turn cause malfunction and disruption to infusion flow (Giuliano & Niemi 2016). Whenever possible, the pump should be connected to a power source to maintain the battery charge. Relying on

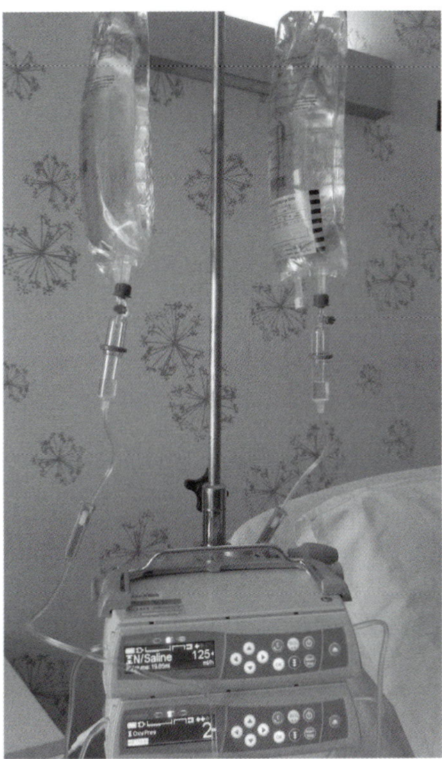

FIGURE 23.3 **A medical infusion device.**

the battery to continue the infusion for many hours is not best practice; if the battery is depleted the device can cease operation rapidly (Giuliano & Ruppel 2017). The infusion device alarm does not detect the presence of complications such as infiltration; therefore, it is important to continue to check the site and ensure the woman is aware of signs and symptoms she needs to communicate to the midwife. Pump alarms can disturb sleep, cause concern to women and limit mobility (Wheeler et al 2020).

Calculating the flow rate of the intravenous fluid when no infusion device is used

When no infusion device is available, the infusion can be administered using gravity, and the flow rate calculated and set manually. The midwife should refer to the administration set being used for details of the number of drops per millilitre (mL), referred to as the drop factor. Commonly the drop factor is 20 drops/mL for macrodrip chambers and 60 drops/mL for microdrip chambers (Raghunathan 2021). The drop factor is determined by the size of the tubing lumen; microdrips administer 60 drops per mL and are useful for the administration of small fluid volumes whereas a macrodrip is usually used for rates greater than 75 mL/hour (Bowen 2014). The following formula is used to calculate the number of drops per minute (Brindley 2020):

$$\frac{\text{volume required (mL)}}{\text{infusion duration (hour)}} \times \frac{\text{set value (drops/mL)}}{\text{minutes in 1 hour (60)}} = \text{drops rate (drops/mL)}$$

For example, if 1000 mL of normal saline solution is prescribed for manual IV infusion over an 8-hour period using an administration set with a drop factor of 20, the flow rate will be:

$$\frac{1000}{8} \times \frac{20}{60} = \frac{20{,}000}{480} = 41.6$$

Round the figure up to 42 drops per minute.

It is important to ensure the fluid is infused over the correct period of time to prevent over-or under-infusion, both of which can have serious consequences. The flow rate should be checked regularly to ensure the rate is correct; Raghunathan (2021) suggests every 15 minutes, then hourly when stable. The flow rate is influenced by a number of factors; for example, the height of the fluid in relation to the insertion site, the fluid type (the characteristics of the fluid; see Table 23.1). The woman's blood pressure, movements and position, patency of the cannula and kinks in the tubing (Bowen 2014).

If the infusion roller clamp is open allowing free flow, the volume of fluid delivered in a specific timeframe will vary. Pierce and colleagues (2013) found that 250 mL phenylephrine placed at 80 cm and running through a microdrip and an 18-gauge cannula would empty in < 10 minutes, whereas a 1000 mL bag of crystalloid at 100 cm through a 14-gauge cannula would empty in less than 30 minutes. This highlights the importance of regularly checking the flow rate.

Intravenous (IV) smart pumps

IV smart pumps (electronic infusion pumps) are programmed with medication libraries and dose error reduction software (Brindley 2020). These bypass the requirement to input the infusion rate and volume manually because when the midwife selects a medication from the IV pump library, the infusion rate is automatically calculated. Each program has predetermined limits which can be set as 'hard' (meaning they cannot be overridden) or 'soft' (meaning they can be overridden) (Blandford et al 2016). The smart pump alerts the midwife if the infusion rate is higher than usual dosing limits (Giuliano 2015). The pump will sound an alarm if the flow of fluid is obstructed; most have in-line pressure detection monitors which set off an alarm at a set pressure threshold (Gouveia 2016). Pumps should include air sensors to detect and prevent the passage of air bubbles (Gorski et al 2016). Smart pumps also have a mechanism to control free flow of fluid (Harrison 2016). The new generation of smart pumps have wireless and barcode technology linked to the hospital pharmacy (McKeag 2015). Older volumetric pumps can be programmed to deliver a set amount of fluid in a set amount of time, but do not include medication libraries.

The pump alarm is activated when:

- there is a blockage preventing the flow of fluid
- fluid volume has been delivered
- increased pressure is required (e.g. infiltration)
- the battery is low
- air is detected in the line.

When pre-programmed pumps are unavailable, the midwife should calculate the rate of infusion (mL/hour) using the manufacturer's instructions. Generally the formula used is:

$$\frac{\text{volume to be infused (mL)}}{\text{number of hours}} = \text{flow rate (mL / hour)}$$

For example, if an infusion pump is to administer 500 mL of Hartmann's solution over a 4-hour period, the rate will be:

$$\frac{500}{4} = 125 \text{ (mL / hour)}$$

INFUSION ERRORS

The use of medical infusion devices is complex and does not remove infusion errors. Possible errors include: incorrect rate; changed orders with incomplete documentation; failure to follow procedures such as labelling; incorrect start time; wrong drug, fluid or dilutant; incorrect positioning of roller clamp; incorrect use of the drug library; and allergy oversight (Lyons et al 2018). Between 2002 and 2013, Australia's Therapeutic Goods Administration (2014) received 1016 incident reports related to infusion devices; in 36 incidents the patient died; 99 incidents had the potential to be fatal without medical intervention and 153 incidents resulted in serious injury.

Intravenous fluid

A variety of solutions can be administered intravenously (Table 23.1). Solutions are classified as crystalloids or colloids depending on their ability to diffuse through a membrane. Approximately 60% of body weight consists of water, with two-thirds intracellular (inside the cells) and one-third extracellular (outside the cells) (Bullock & Hales 2018).

Crystalloid solutions

Crystalloids contain electrolytes and are classified by tonicity, which is the concentration of electrolytes in comparison with body plasma.

- **Isotonic** means equal concentration (equal tonicity): the crystalloid solution has the same composition as plasma and will be distributed equally between intracellular and extracellular fluid. Isotonic fluids will expand the extracellular fluid volume (ECV) without moving water in or out of cells.

TABLE 23.1 INTRAVENOUS INFUSION SOLUTIONS COMMONLY USED IN MIDWIFERY

Solution	Example	Indication for use
Crystalloid: isotonic solutions (same tonicity as blood)	0.9% sodium chloride Lactated Ringer's (Hartmann's) 5% dextrose in water, Plasma-Lyte	To compensate for fluid loss by expanding the circulating volume
Crystalloid: hypotonic solutions (lower particle concentration)	0.45% sodium chloride	To compensate for fluid loss by moving fluid into intracellular spaces
Crystalloid: hypertonic solutions (higher tonicity than plasma)	10% dextrose in water 20% dextrose in water 50% dextrose in water 20% albumin	To compensate for fluid loss by moving fluid from intra- to extracellular spaces
Colloids: undissolved particles (protein, starch, sugar) too large to pass through capillary walls	5% or 25% albumin	Draws fluid from interstitial and intracellular spaces. Used when crystalloids ineffective
Plasma expanders: Colloid fluids	Dextran, Gelofusine (succinylated gelatin),	To expand plasma volume by drawing fluid from interstitial spaces. Used to treat hypovolaemia
Iron solutions	Iron sucrose Iron polymaltose Ferric carboxymaltose	To treat iron deficiency anaemia
Blood and blood products	Whole blood Packed cells	To maintain circulatory volume, increase particular blood components

Source: Johnson R, Taylor W: Skills for midwifery practice, 4th ed., Elsevier, London, 2016.

- **Hypotonic** means low concentration (low tonicity): the crystalloid solution has less electrolytes than plasma and will result in fluid moving from the intravascular to the extravascular space. Water from the ECV is drawn into the cells (e.g. dextrose 5%).
- **Hypertonic** means high concentration (high tonicity): the crystalloid solution has more electrolytes than plasma and will result in fluid moving by osmosis from the extravascular spaces into the intravascular space (e.g. albumin 20%).

IV fluids are usually contained within a soft plastic bag, but may also be in a glass bottle or semirigid plastic container; these may have calibrations on the side to indicate how much fluid is in the container. However, the fluid bag graduations are inaccurate and do not represent the amount of fluid left in the bag (Nowicki 2013). The soft bags have a double plastic layer that is pulled apart or twisted off and the trocar inserted through the opening. Glass containers have a rubber bung covered with a sterile seal. Once the sterile seal is removed, the trocar is inserted through the bung, along with a sterile air inlet needle for venting to equalise pressure within the bottle and facilitate fluid flow.

Prior to use, glass containers should be checked for cracks and chips, and plastic containers squeezed to ensure there are no leaks (Raghunathan 2021). Glass or semirigid containers require venting (Gorski et al 2016). The fluid should be checked to ensure there is no discolouration, cloudiness, particles or precipitate present. If in doubt, do not use.

IV solution bags must not be respiked, as they are designed for single use only (Therapeutic Goods Administration 2017). If the giving set spike is disconnected, air may enter the bag and, when reconnected, may result in air entering the IV line with the potential to cause an air embolism. IV administration sets must always be primed correctly to ensure no air is in the line (Therapeutic Goods Administration 2017). IV pumps have a setting for priming IV administration sets and purging air from the tubing.

Checking the infusion solution prior to administration

A doctor or midwife with prescribing rights must prescribe the solution, which is checked by two registered health professionals (registered midwife, registered nurse, medical doctor) to ensure the correct infusion is given to the correct woman. The midwife should check the following:

- the woman's name, date of birth and hospital number
- the medication administration chart: type of infusion fluid, and amount to be infused, which should be accurately written up and signed; the method of administration, route and timing must be compatible with the IV fluid
- the fluid bag contains the correct solution and volume and has not expired
- the fluid does not have signs of discolouration, cloudiness or sediment, and the container does not have signs of contamination or damage
- all IV fluids and additives are compatible
- the flow rate is calculated, if an infusion device is not available
- the program is correct, if an infusion device is used
- the batch number, which for some infusions is recorded on the medicine administration chart.

SKILL 23.1 Commencing an intravenous infusion using a fluid bag

1. Use ANTT to reduce the risk of infection (see Chapter 2).
2. Confirm the identity of the woman (ask her to state her name and date of birth) and confirm details and medical record number on her identity band against the medicine administration chart and gain informed consent.
3. Ensure a patent cannula is in situ (see Chapter 11 for IV cannulation).
4. Perform hand hygiene.
5. Gather equipment:
   - IV administration set (giving set)
   - extension tubing (if required)
   - medication/fluid order sheet
   - IV infusion solution (ordered by doctor and checked as above)
   - sterile or clean receiver
   - alcohol-based hand rub plus non-sterile gloves
   - IV pole
   - infusion pump
   - label if required
   - 70% alcohol/2% chlorhexidine (or locally approved skin cleanser).
6. Perform hand hygiene.
7. Don non-sterile gloves.
8. Remove outer wrapping from infusion solution and hang on IV pole.
9. Open the administration set and close the roller clamp below the drip chamber.
10. Remove the cover from the trocar at the top end of the tubing and from the infusion bag, without touching either opening (both ANTT key parts).
11. Insert the trocar into the bag of IV solution.
12. Gently compress the drip chamber to half or two-thirds full to reduce the risk of air bubbles in the tubing.

Continued

SKILL 23.3 Ongoing care of the intravenous infusion—cont'd

in the progress notes. Transparent dressings are preferable as they allow visualisation of the site.

- If the woman's clothing needs to be changed while an infusion is in progress, avoid disconnecting the tubing but pass the bag of fluid and tubing through the clothing. This is easily achieved if the arm without the tubing is removed from the clothing first, followed by the arm with the infusion in situ. When putting on clothes, the fluid bag and tubing are passed through the sleeve (in the same direction the arm is placed through it) followed by the arm with the infusion in situ and then the unaffected arm through the other sleeve.
- If the woman is mobilising (e.g. to walk to the toilet), the infusion/medical infusion device should be placed onto a pole with wheels and the woman encouraged to hold onto the pole using the hand with the infusion in situ to push the pole while walking (Felver 2015). Avoid disconnecting IV administration sets for showering or mobilising.
- Keep the pump dry at all times.

SALINE LOCKS AND FLUSHING A CANNULA

If IV fluids are being discontinued but the IV cannula needs to remain in situ for intermittent medication administration or for IV access in case of an emergency, a saline lock is required. The cannula will need to be flushed regularly to prevent occlusion, to avoid mixing incompatible fluids or medications and to ensure the cannula remains patent. Flushing impedes attachment of fibrin, drug precipitates, biofilm and other deposits in the intraluminal catheter wall that contribute to occlusion (Goossens 2015, Keogh et al 2020). 'Flushing the cannula' is defined as manual injection of normal saline to maintain patency and push residual medication into the vein. 'Locking the cannula' also refers to the injection of a limited volume of fluid to maintain cannula patency. The terms 'flushing' and 'locking' are often used interchangeably (Goossens 2015). The risk of infection of the IV cannula is increased by contamination of the cannula hub or needle-free connector; therefore, ANTT is essential when locking or flushing a cannula. An Australian study found regular assessment of catheter and insertion site, flushing pre and post drug administration, flushing the cannula at least every 8 hours when not in use, a flush volume at least twice the length and diameter of the catheter, using manufactured pre-filled flush syringes, and a gentle, pulsatile technique, plus documentation decreased PIVC failure (Keogh et al 2020).

SKILL 23.4 Using a saline lock and flushing a cannula

Using a saline lock

1. Gather equipment (sterile 0.9% sodium chloride for injection, approved swab for cleaning).
2. Perform hand hygiene.
3. Stop the IV infusion by closing the roller clamp and/or turning off (or pausing) the infusion device.
4. Disinfect the catheter hub or needle-free connector (create friction by scrubbing in a twisting motion for 15 or more seconds) with a single-use alcohol-impregnated swab or 70% alcohol and 2% chlorhexidine swab (Harrold 2019). If an allergy is present 10% povidone-iodine can be used as an alternative. Let the hub or needle-free connector air dry completely (Harrold 2019).
5. Open the single-dose sterile 0.9% normal saline package. Loosen and remove the IV tubing from the hub and connect the sterile 0.9% sodium chloride for injection (the volume of the flush should equal twice the volume of the catheter and extension tubing).
6. Flush the cannula by slowly injecting the flush solution with a pulsatile (push-pause) motion as this appears more effective at removing debris compared to a continuous push of fluid (Gorski et al 2016).
7. After flushing the cannula, remove the syringe and discard.
8. Clamp extension tubing if present on a PIVC.

Flushing an IV cannula

- PIVCs must be flushed at least every 8 hours if a continuous infusion is not in progress (Keogh et al 2020).
- The cannula should be flushed with 0.9% normal saline before and after the administration of medications with a volume equal to double the internal volume of the cannula (and extension if used), generally 2–5 mL (Gorski et al 2016).
- The cannula should be flushed to maintain patency and to prevent mixing of incompatible medications and solutions.

SKILL 23.4 Using a saline lock and flushing a cannula—cont'd

- Sterile 0.9% sodium chloride for injection is used unless an alternate solution is recommended by the manufacturer.
- Pre-prepared saline flushes are preferred because they reduce the risk of infection (Gorski et al 2016). Sterile water should not be used to flush cannulas and force should not be used during the flush (Gorski et al 2016).
- The catheter must be flushed:
  - after cannula insertion
  - before and after each fluid infusion or injection of a medication; if more than one medication is given, the cannula should be flushed in between to avoid drug incompatibilities (Gahart et al 2016) and the flush needs to have enough volume to clear the medication from the cannula
  - prior to and after drawing blood.

SECONDARY AND CONCURRENT INFUSIONS

At times a second infusion may be connected to the primary infusion, often for the purpose of medication administration. The second administration set and all connectors must be primed to prevent the administration of a large amount of air into the circulation. A secondary infusion ('piggy-back') is connected to a needleless port in the primary IV administration line. It is important the fluids in both tubing sets are compatible (in case there is mixing of fluid) to prevent precipitates forming and obstructing the flow. A concurrent infusion refers to two infusions running through a single IV port (e.g. Y-connector), both with their own infusion device to control the rates of flow individually. Where more than one administration set is used, it is vital to label each one correctly.

COMPLICATIONS

Phlebitis

A number of complications can develop from IV infusions, including infection at the cannula site and phlebitis (inflammation of the vein). Mechanical phlebitis results from irritation of the vein wall. Chemical phlebitis results from infusion of an irritating substance (e.g. hypertonic), rapid infusion (Felver 2015) or antiseptic being pulled into the vein during insertion because the antiseptic was not given time to dry (Gorski 2018). Bacterial phlebitis can result from poor aseptic technique and can lead to a catheter-associated bloodstream infection (Gorski 2018). The area will be painful, swollen and inflamed along the vein (seen as a red streak), which may feel hard and warm to touch. A warm, moist compress applied to the affected site can reduce discomfort (deWit & O'Neill 2014). If phlebitis or infection occur the cannula should be re-sited.

Infiltration and extravasation

Infiltration is leakage of the IV solution into the tissue surrounding the cannula, causing pain and swelling. Extravasation is when the IV fluid or medication is vesicant (blister forming). Infiltration and extravasation can occur when the cannula becomes dislodged or has penetrated the vessel wall. The signs and symptoms of extravasation include cool skin temperature at the site, blanched taut skin, pain, burning, discomfort, oedema, decreased mobility of the extremity and leaking of fluid from the insertion site. The infusion rate is reduced and there is an absence of blood return or a pale pinkish blood return (Gorski 2018). The infusion should be discontinued immediately and restarted at a new site (Gorski 2018).

Haematoma

Haematoma and ecchymosis refer to a swelling comprising blood confined to subcutaneous tissue as the result of a break in a blood vessel allowing blood to leak into the surrounding tissue (Gorski 2018). This often results from trauma due to venipuncture technique or use of a large-gauge cannula. The skin may appear discoloured with swelling and discomfort present.

Thrombosis

A blood clot (**thrombus**) can form within a blood vessel and lead to an interruption in blood flow to the traumatised tissue at the cannula site. The area will appear similar to phlebitis and the infusion may stop if the clot occludes the cannula. Bowen (2014) suggests applying a warm compress and re-siting the infusion, but cautions against rubbing or massaging the affected area.

Speed shock

Speed shock occurs when a large volume of IV fluid or a medication bolus is administered too rapidly. A rapidly administration enables plasma levels to reach toxic proportions and shock the vital organs leading to serious complications including syncope, shock and cardiac arrest (Gorski 2018). The woman may develop a flushed face, pounding headache, dizziness, chest tightness tachycardia, irregular pulse and hypotension. As the reaction increases, the woman can become shocked, lose consciousness and cardiac arrest can follow. If a reaction is suspected, the infusion should be stopped immediately and urgent medical assistance sought, vital signs are monitored and symptoms treated.

Fluid/circulatory overload

This occurs when excessive amounts of isotonic fluids are given. The extracellular volume increases in proportion to the amount of fluid administered and is not drawn into the intracellular compartment. This may occur if the fluid rate is too rapid or the amount required miscalculated. The woman can develop engorged neck veins (jugular), hypertension, tachypnoea, dyspnoea, tachycardia (pulse may be bounding), elevated central venous pressure measurement and peripheral oedema. The fluid balance chart will show a high positive balance. If this develops, the infusion should be stopped or slowed, the woman sat upright, oral fluids may need to be withheld, medical assistance sought, vital signs monitored and symptoms treated.

Air embolism

Air embolism is a preventable complication. It occurs when there is direct communication between air and the vascular system with a pressure gradient supporting passage of air into the circulation (Natal 2017). It is important to prime IV lines, remove air from IV tubing, syringes, needleless connectors and extension sets as well as ensuring connections do not allow air entry (Gorski 2018). Estimations indicate 5 mL/kg of air is required for significant injury including shock and cardiac arrest; however, complications have been observed with 20 mL of air injected into an IV (Natal 2017).

Symptoms include dyspnoea, tachypnoea, tachycardia and hypotension. Treatment is to occlude the cannula to prevent any further air entering the system, call for urgent medical assistance, monitor vital signs and treat the symptoms.

Sepsis

This may occur if ANTT is not maintained during insertion of the cannula or connecting/changing fluids and equipment. Bowen (2014) suggests frequent dressing changes may be a cause of sepsis. The insertion site will appear red and be tender. The woman can develop fever, malaise, headache, nausea, vomiting, tachycardia and tachypnoea. If suspected, medical assistance is called for, the infusion site changed, blood cultures obtained and, if indicated, antibiotics administered.

Monitoring fluid balance

A fluid balance chart should be started at the beginning of the infusion and maintained throughout to ensure the woman is tolerating the amount of fluid being infused. A fluid balance chart records all fluids taken into the body through the IV and oral routes (and very rarely for the adult via a nasogastric tube) and all fluid lost from the body, mainly in urine, but includes vomit, wound drainage, diarrhoea, nasogastric drainage and blood loss. Normally fluid intake and output balance each other; however, if the amount of fluid taken in exceeds the amount excreted, circulatory overload can result. Cardiac failure can ensue, characterised initially by increasing dyspnoea and peripheral oedema, unless fluid intake is restricted. A reduction in plasma osmolarity and oedematous cells can also result in convulsions and coma if the brain cells swell. If output exceeds intake, dehydration with shrinkage of cells and tissues can occur.

It is important for the midwife to accurately measure and record all fluid intake (oral, IV) and fluid output and keep a cumulative total. Up-to-date cumulative totals enable quick assessment of the fluid balance status of the woman; any change, such as decreasing urinary output, warrants escalation. Fluid balance charts do not usually consider fluid obtained from food (although some food, such as yoghurt, may be included) or insensible fluid loss; however, Bowen (2014) suggests these two usually balance each other out. The total amount of intake and output is calculated at the end of each 24-hour period and a calculation as to whether the woman is in balance or has a positive (excess intake) or negative (excess output) balance is documented in the appropriate records and acted on accordingly. The overall balance should be carried forward to the next 24-hour period as the intake–output balance may not be achieved for 2–3 days (Bowen 2014).

IV MEDICATIONS

IV-administered medications avoid the absorption process (Bullock & Manias 2017) and travel through the bloodstream, where they are rapidly distributed into the body tissues (Lee 2014). IV medications are administered directly into a vein, usually through an IV cannula. The needleless port of the cannula is accessed using a syringe (to give a bolus) or connected to a syringe driver or a piggy-back IV mini-bag with medication additive (for intermittent infusion) or to patient-controlled analgesia (PCA) infusion. For many IV medications, tolerance is improved when they are infused slowly rather than given as a bolus (Siwale & Sani 2016). Intermittent IV infusion refers to successive IV medication infusions administered over a short period (e.g. 20–30 minutes) (Siwale & Sani 2016).

INDICATIONS FOR IV USE

- When rapid absorption and effect is required
- When constant therapeutic blood levels of a drug are required
- When drugs are contraindicated by other routes (e.g. oral, intramuscular [IM])
- Where peripheral perfusion is poor, reducing the effect of drugs administered by injection

DISADVANTAGES OF THE IV ROUTE

- Requires a patent peripheral IV cannula which may cause pain in the short term
- An invasive procedure increasing the risk of infection
- Rapid absorption of the medication increases the risk for an adverse reaction
- Increased potential for medication errors (e.g. drug and physiochemical incompatibility), particularly if multiple drug infusions are required at the same time and the drugs are allowed to mix (Westbrook et al 2012)
- Increased potential for bacterial or particulate contamination if drugs are being diluted or added to other fluids (Bertsche et al 2008)

SAFETY CONCERNS

All medications administered IV should be considered high-risk as their effect is immediate, they are irretrievable and can result in serious adverse effects (Gahart et al 2016). All high-alert IV medications should be administered using a programmable infusion pump with dose error reduction software (Gilchrist 2016).

Despite improvements in IV medication administration, particularly with advancing technology, a high risk remains for error compared with other forms of administration (Fanikos et al 2017). Around one-third of adverse drug events are related to the administration phase and include failing to follow: the prescription, preparation or administration and institutional instructions (Fanikos et al 2017). These errors account for 44–62% of errors related to injectable medications (Fanikos et al 2017). According to Westbrook and colleagues (2012), the following steps will help to avoid procedural and clinical errors when administering IV medications.

To avoid procedural failures:

- Read the medication label.
- Check identification with details on the medication chart.
- Do not store medications temporarily in an insecure environment.
- Record administration on the medication chart.
- Use ANTT.
- Check pulse or blood pressure prior to administration (when necessary).
- Check blood sugar level prior to administering insulin.
- Two registered health professionals sign the dangerous drug register.
- Two registered health professionals check preparation and witness administration of the dangerous drug.
- Two registered health professionals sign medication charts when applicable.

To avoid clinical errors:

- Ensure correct IV rates.
- Ensure correct mixture.
- Ensure correct volume.
- Check there is no drug incompatibility (incorrect diluent).
- Check medication has not already been given.
- Give medication at the right time in the right formulation to the right person.
- Check if any allergies are present.

The Institute for Safe Medication Practice (ISMP 2015) advises discarding any unattended, unlabelled syringes containing any type of solution and recommend that the syringe is always labelled once the medication is drawn up, unless this is done by the patient's bedside and administered immediately. Using pre-prepared, ready-to-administer forms of medication is recommended, wherever possible (ISMP 2015). However, midwives often need to prepare medications. The manufacturer's instructions on diluent (usually water or normal saline 0.9%) and volume should be followed; powders must be diluted. If the powder does not dissolve, it should be discarded and another dose of the medication and diluent mixed.

To promote safe medication management, the 'five rights' (see Chapter 18) should be checked in relation to the drug, the diluent and the flush by two midwives (or midwife and another registered health professional), one of whom must be the administrator of the drug. Both midwives should ensure they independently check that the medical infusion device is set to the correct program for delivery of the medication (if used).

The cannula site should be assessed for patency and signs of compromise, such as infiltration and extravasation before the medication is given (see Chapter 11). If the cannula is not patent, accidental injection of drugs into the tissues rather than the vein can occur, resulting in pain, sloughing of the tissues and abscess formation (Hall 2015).

If there is any doubt, the cannula should be flushed and, if not patent it should be removed and a new one sited elsewhere, if IV medications are still required. The IV infusion should be ceased immediately if the woman has pain, burning or stinging at the insertion site (Gorski et al 2016).

Aseptic non-touch technique (ANTT)

It is important to use an ANTT approach to reduce the risk of infection (Hugill 2017). ANTT should be used when reconstituting the medication and when handling the syringe and needleless port (key parts). The use of gloves will also protect the midwife's hands from contact with the medication constituents during drawing up.

Bolus/push administration (direct intermittent injection)

An IV bolus introduces a concentrated dose of a drug through a needleless port (often via an extension set) directly into the circulation, usually with a small amount of fluid (Hall 2015). This is useful when there is concern about fluid overload, but the high concentration can also cause a chemical phlebitis, particularly if poor administration technique (such as rapid administration) is used (Zheng 2016). The bolus is administered as a 'push' as the midwife will physically push the drug through the woman's cannula. An IV bolus is absorbed rapidly, produces high drug concentrations (Rang 2016) and there is no time to correct errors (Hall 2015) Bolus IV administration has higher rates of serious errors than IV infusions (ISMP 2015, Westbrook et al 2012). It is important the midwife is aware of the manufacturer's recommendations for administration as overly rapid administration can be a factor in adverse reactions (Paparella & Mandrack 2016). No IV drug should be administered in less than 60 seconds (deWit & O'Neill 2014), and most should be administered over 3–10 minutes, but if there are no recommendations for the rate of administration, manufacturers suggest proceeding slowly over 5–10 minutes (Ansell & Dougherty 2011). Further advice can be sought from the hospital pharmacist if any doubt exists. It is particularly helpful to give the drug slowly if there is a possibility of an anaphylactic reaction occurring, as this usually happens quickly, and it enables the midwife to stop administration immediately (see Chapter 18). When drawing up from an ampoule always use a filter needle (Gorski et al 2016).

SKILL 23.5 Intravenous bolus

1. Review the medication administration record for type of medication, dosage, route and time (see Chapter 18).
2. Check that the cannula is patent and has a needleless injection port attached (extension sets reduce manipulation of the cannula).
3. Perform hand hygiene.
4. Gather equipment:
   - medication administration record (MAR)
   - disposable gloves
   - medication in vial or ampoule
   - plastic tray
   - sterile syringe
   - needleless access device or needle (filter needle may be required)
   - antiseptic swab
   - pre-prepared sodium chloride flush in 5 or 10 mL syringe
   - sharps container
   - watch with second hand or digital display.

5A. **If a diluent is used:**
   a. Perform hand hygiene and put on non-sterile gloves.
   b. Open the diluent by snapping off the top.
   c. Insert syringe into the diluent (syringe normally connects directly to sterile water ampoule) and draw up the required amount by pulling back the plunger. Use ANTT.
   d. Remove the cap from the vial, keeping the rubber seal sterile.
   e. Insert needleless access device (or needle) and inject diluent into vial. Mix the powder and diluent by rolling the vial between the palms (avoid shaking it).
   f. Draw up the required amount of reconstituted medication into the syringe.
   g. Remove drawing up needle (or needleless access device).

5B. **If there is no diluent:**
   a. Open the medication by snapping off the top, having first ensured all the liquid is at the bottom of the ampoule/vial. If a vial is used with a rubber bung, the bung should be cleaned with the approved cleanser for 15–20 seconds, up-and-down, side-to-side, creating friction; then left to dry for at least 30 seconds.
   b. Unsheathe the needleless access device (or needle) and insert it into the ampoule/vial to withdraw the required amount of medication; if the ampoule has a rubber bung, McKenna & Lim (2014) recommend drawing air into the syringe equal to the volume of the drug required; the needle is inserted centrally and the air injected, taking care not to inject into the solution. Keep the needle in the solution to prevent air from being aspirated into the syringe.

6. When the required volume of medication is drawn up, invert the syringe and examine it for air. If necessary, tap the syringe gently to encourage the air to the top of the syringe; push the plunger to exclude the air from the syringe, ensuring no solution is lost and the dosage in the syringe is correct.
7. Remove the needleless access device (or needle) from the syringe without touching the end of the syringe and place in the sharps container.
8. Cover the end of the syringe with a sterile cap/cover without touching the key parts and place it on the plastic tray.
9. Label the syringe.
10. Place pre-prepared flush and antiseptic wipe on the plastic tray.
11. Remove gloves and perform hand hygiene.
12. Take the medicine administration chart, sharps container and tray to the woman.
13. With both midwives present, confirm the woman's identity by asking her to state her

SKILL 23.5 Intravenous bolus—cont'd

name and date of birth and checking her identity label against the medication administration chart.

14. Perform hand hygiene and don non-sterile gloves.
15. Scrub the tip of the IV port (needleless connector) with the approved cleanser for 15–20 seconds, up-and-down and side-to-side, creating friction and using different parts of the wipe. Then clean away from the tip using a non-touch technique. Leave to dry for at least 30 seconds.
16. If present, check the infusion is running correctly, then stop it.
17. If using a flush, remove the cap/cover from the syringe containing the flush.
18. Attach the syringe to the needleless port and inject the flush, observing around the cannula site for swelling, then disconnect the flush.
19. Remove the cap/cover from the syringe containing the medication.
20. Attach the syringe and inject the first 1 mL of the medication according to the manufacturer's recommendations, observing the woman's condition throughout.
    - If an infusion is present, it can be restarted; if no problems are noticed, stop the infusion and continue to administer the rest of the medication at the correct rate.
    - If the infusion fluid is incompatible with the medication, Ansell & Dougherty (2011) recommend stopping the infusion and flushing the line before and after the medication administration and then restarting the infusion.
    - If no infusion is present, continue to inject the medication according to the manufacturer's instructions.
21. If an adverse reaction develops while administering the medication, stop the administration, call the doctor and manage accordingly.
22. Repeat the flush with the remaining normal saline, using pulsation and positive pressure, as described previously. Recommence the infusion at the appropriate rate (if required).
23. Dispose of equipment correctly.
24. Remove gloves.
25. Perform hand hygiene.
26. Document administration and effects and act accordingly.

INTERMITTENT INFUSION (LARGER VOLUME)

The medication can be added to a larger volume (25–250 mL) of compatible fluid and administered as an infusion over 15 minutes to 2 hours (Ansell & Dougherty 2011). This should be in line with the manufacturer's instructions and locally approved guidelines. The infusion should be administered through a medical infusion device to ensure it runs over the correct time period. The intermittent infusion is achieved by:

- adding medications to a burette giving set of an existing infusion, with the existing infusion being stopped until the medication has been administered; or
- attaching a prepared infusion containing the medication to a giving set and connecting this to the cannula if there is no existing infusion; or
- connecting the prepared infusion of the medication (and giving set) to a needleless port, ideally the one closest to the cannula (ISMP 2015), stopping the existing infusion until the medications have been administered. If there is no infusion running, the cannula will require flushing before and after medication administration, as described earlier. Hand hygiene and ANTT are essential at each stage of the procedure to ensure microorganisms are not introduced into the closed system.

If a medication is added to a bag of IV fluid, the following are important.

- ANTT is used when drawing up and adding medication.
- The fluid and medication are compatible.
- Care is taken not to puncture the bag.
- An additive label is applied with the right medication, dose, name and medical record number of the woman, and date and time the medication was added, and signed by those involved in the checking procedure.
- The medication and fluid are thoroughly mixed (by inverting the bag gently).
- The checking procedures are the same as for bolus administration.
- The flow rate is correct.

Documentation in the woman's notes should include the amount of the medication and diluent used (if any), time and duration of administration and whether by a bolus or intermittent infusion. The woman's response should be noted and documented. If the cannula has been flushed, documentation should also include the flush used, the amount and whether it was before, after or both. The medication chart should also be signed.

SYRINGE DRIVER

A syringe driver is a small, powered (mains and/or battery) infusion pump used to gradually administer a medication (or small amounts of fluid) contained within a syringe, by driving the plunger of the syringe at an accurately controlled rate. Tubing connects the syringe to the cannula and this is primed as for any other IV tubing prior to use. The syringe contains a medication, usually pre-diluted to a specific strength (this should not be diluted further), although the initial dilution can be made up in the clinical area. A 60 mL syringe is usually the largest size that can be accommodated with these devices and most pumps use smaller syringes.

Errors in the use of syringe drivers occur in a number of areas, including incorrect medication rate, overly rapid infusion and user error (Lee 2014). The midwife should have received training on the use of syringe drivers, including how to correctly insert the syringe and to have a second person confirm the infusion rate. The device should be serviced regularly according to manufacturer's instructions.

Most new syringe drivers use mL/hr to calculate the administration rate and some can be programmed for the medication used. The safety compliance of syringe drivers is important and safety features should include the device not being able to be started if the syringe is not fitted correctly, volume-infused display, unintended bolus protection and an alarm to alert infusion is near the end (Lee 2014).

The setting up of the pump relies on several standard principles.

- Use of ANTT.
- Calculation of the amount of drug required over the given period of time with appropriate solution for dilution.
- Use of an appropriately sized sterile syringe inserted, so the plunger is secure.
- Sterile preparation and dilution of the medication (may be supplied pre-prepared).
- Sterile tubing fits the needleless port; the tubing must be primed and attached, after measurement and calculation of the rate or accessing the correct program.
- The syringe must be labelled correctly with the name, dose and volume of the drug and expiry date.
- The syringe driver should be maintained and in full working order; alarms for 'occlusion' and 'infusion complete' must be working and the midwife must make regular observations of the pump to ensure the infusion is delivering the correct amount of fluid.

PATIENT-CONTROLLED ANALGESIA (PCA)

Patient-controlled analgesia (PCA) is primarily used for postoperative analgesia. For PCA, the woman presses a button to administer a pre-set, titrated dose of analgesic medication known as the demand dose. Women using a PCA should be educated on its use. This gives the woman control over when and how she uses the PCA in response to her individual needs. A lockout interval is programmed to prevent doses being administered too quickly, prevent over-medication and provide time for the initial dose to take effect (usually 5–10 minutes). The pump can also be programmed to deliver a continuous amount (basal dose) over a set period of time, usually 1–4 hours. The maximum dose is the lockout dose; this means if the maximum amount is reached, no more doses can be given (Schumacher et al 2018). The lockout period is from when a dose has been given until the time the next dose can be given. Each device has an inbuilt tamper-proof mechanism to prevent the woman, visitors or others from changing the dose and/or frequency of the bolus. The PCA should be checked frequently to determine the number of successful demands and the number of attempts.

When a PCA is used, there is a tendency to use less medication as women can self-administer before the pain becomes difficult to manage (McKenna & Lim 2014) and women report lower pain scores (Singer et al 2021). Anxiety levels are reduced because the woman is in control of her pain medication (deWit & O'Neill 2014). According to Ismail and colleagues (2012), pain control was improved and there was less need for rescue analgesia for breakthrough pain, a lower incidence of nausea and vomiting and greater patient satisfaction when PCA pethidine was used for post-caesarean section analgesia. Similar results were found when tramadol was administered via a PCA rather than as a continuous IV infusion (Demirel et al 2014). Another advantage of PCAs is that they can maintain a reasonably constant concentration of the medication within the blood.

Side effects of the PCA are related to the medication being administered. Opioid medications are commonly used for analgesia and they function by attaching to opioid receptors (Schumacher et al 2018). Common side effects from opioid use include nausea, vomiting, pruritus, respiratory depression, drowsiness and sedation (Bounes et al 2017). Postoperative opioids are also associated with reduced gastric motility (slowed bowel function, ileus), urinary retention and shivering (Donald de Boer et al 2017).

PCAs for analgesia generally use a 50 mL syringe. A standardised medication concentration and preprinted orders are preferred (Gorski et al 2016). The PCA medication ordered is checked by two midwives (or midwife and registered nurse, pharmacist or doctor) and diluted to the correct concentration with normal saline. Any changes in settings must also be double-checked. The following medications can be administered via a PCA: fentanyl, morphine, hydromorphone, remifentanil, tramadol and ketamine.

The midwife establishing the infusion must set:

- the lockout interval
- a 1-hour or 4-hour dose limit
- a limit to the amount of medication received with each demand.

The risk of PCA-associated respiratory depression is 0.5%; this is a serious side effect and women with PCAs must be monitored frequently (Dobbins 2015). Observations should include pulse oximetry; supplemental oxygen may be required. When the PCA is taken down, any remaining medication must be discarded by two registered midwives (or appropriately registered health professionals) following local policy, including documentation in the S8 drug book.

SUMMARY

- IV drugs have a swift effect, which, while advantageous, can also be problematic if an adverse reaction occurs.
- ANTT should be used throughout the setting up and administration of an IV drug.
- IV drugs may be given in the following ways:
  - intermittent direct bolus or 'push' injection
  - intermittent infusion
  - additives to an infusion
  - syringe driver
  - patient-controlled analgesia.
- The midwife needs to be competent in the administration of medication IV and the correct use of all devices used in their clinical area of practice and maintain this competency.
- When given as a 'bolus' injection, it is important to administer the drug slowly to reduce the risk of phlebitis and adverse reactions.
- An IV infusion is a means of giving fluid or drugs directly into the venous circulation.
- Medical infusion devices are used to administer the infusion at a set rate.
- IV infusion is associated with several complications and regular monitoring of the woman is required during the procedure.
- A woman with an IV may require assistance to care for herself and her neonate.

Role and responsibilities of the midwife

These can be summarised as:

- adhering to local regimens for training and updating of skills
- using correct administration procedure and complying with local guidelines
- advising the woman of changes to medications strengths/rates of medication
- observing the woman for any unexpected or adverse responses
- maintaining competency in the setting up and monitoring of IV infusions
- minimising the risk of infection during all procedures by using ANTT
- being familiar with the medical infusion devices available and ensuring they are properly used and maintained
- identifying complications and how to treat them, referring as necessary
- recognising the significance of fluid balance and accurate fluid balance charts
- keeping contemporaneous records.

Self-assessment exercises

The answers to the following questions may be found in the text.

1. What are the advantages and disadvantages of administering drugs via the IV route?
2. Discuss the ways in which IV drugs can be administered.
3. Describe how you would administer a bolus dose of IV antibiotics.
4. How do the principles of ANTT apply to IV drug administration?
5. Discuss the advantages of patient-controlled analgesia.
6. Summarise the role and responsibilities of the midwife when administering drugs intravenously.
7. What are the indications for an IV infusion?
8. When would an isotonic solution be used rather than a hypotonic or hypertonic solution?
9. What is the formula for calculating the flow rate of an IV infusion when a medical infusion device is not used?
10. Identify four complications associated with IV infusion therapy and how you would recognise and manage these.
11. Describe how an IV infusion is set up and commenced.
12. What are the ongoing responsibilities of the midwife during the infusion?
13. How is fluid balance recorded and why is this important?

References

Ansell L, Dougherty L: Medicines management. In Dougherty L, Lister S, eds: The Royal Marsden manual of clinical nursing procedures, 8th ed., Wiley-Blackwell, Chichester, 2011.

Bakan M, Topuz U, Esen A, et al: Inadvertent venous air embolism during cesarean, Brazilian Journal of Anesthesiology 63(4):362–365, 2013.

Bertsche T, Mayer Y, Stahl R, et al: Prevention of intravenous drug incompatibilities in an intensive care unit, American Journal of Health-System Pharmacy 65(19):1834–1840, 2008.

Blandford A, Dykes P, Franklin B, et al: Intravenous infusion administration: a comparative study of practices and errors between the United States and England and their implications for patient safety, Drug Safety 42(10):1157–1165, 2019.

Blandford A, Furniss D, Lyons I, et al: Exploring the current landscape of intravenous infusion practices and errors (ECLIPSE): Protocol for a mixed-methods observational study, BMJ Open 6:e009777, 2016.

Bounes V, Charriton-Dadone B, Levraut J, et al: Predicting morphine related side effects in the ED: an international cohort study, The American Journal of Emergency Medicine 35(4):531–535, 2017.

Bowen L: Fluid, electrolyte and acid-base balance. In Dempsey J, Hillege S, Hill R, eds: Fundamentals of nursing and midwifery, 2nd ed., Lippincott, Williams & Wilkins, Sydney, 2014.

Brindley J: How to undertake intravenous infusion calculations, Nursing Standard 35(3):47–50, 2020.

Bullock S, Hales M: Principles of pathophysiology, 2nd ed., Pearson Australia, Melbourne, 2018.

Bullock S, Manias E: Fundamentals of pharmacology, 8th ed., Pearson Australia, Melbourne, 2017.

Demirel I, Ozer AB, Atilgan R, et al: Comparison of patient-controlled analgesia versus continuous infusion of tramadol in post-cesarean section pain management, Journal of Obstetrics and Gynaecology Research 40(2):392–398, 2014.

deWit SC, O'Neill P: Fundamental concepts and skills for nursing, 4th ed., Elsevier, St. Louis, 2014.

Dobbins E: Sidestep the perils of PCA in post-op patients, Nursing 45(4):64, 2015.

Donald de Boer H, Detriche O, Forget P: Opioid related side effects: postoperative ileus, urinary retention, nausea and vomiting and shivering: a review of the literature, Best Practice & Research Clinical Anaesthesiology 2017.

Fanikos J, Burger M, Canada T, et al: An assessment of currently available IV push medication delivery systems, American Journal of Health-System Pharmacy 74:e 230–e235, 2017.

Felver L: Fluid, electrolyte and acid-base balance. In Potter PA, Perry AG, Stockert PA, et al, eds: Essentials for nursing practice, 8th ed., Elsevier, St. Louis, 2015.

Frimpong A, Caguioa J, Octavo G: Promoting safe IV management in practice using H.A.N.D.S, British Journal of Nursing 24(2):138, 2015.

Gahart BL, Nazareno AR, Ortega MQ: Gahart's 2016 intravenous medications: a handbook for nurses and health professionals, 32nd ed., Elsevier Mosby, St Louis, 2016.

Gilchrist A: 5 new best practices for medication safety all hospital pharmacists should know, Pharmacy Times 82:H10, 2016.

Giuliano K: IV Smart pumps: the impact of a simplified user interface on clinical use, Horizons (Suppl):13–21, 2015.

Giuliano K, Niemi C: The urgent need for innovation in IV infusion devices, Nursing 46(4):66–68, 2016.

Giuliano KK, Ruppel H: Are smart pumps smart enough? Nursing 47(3):64–66, 2017.

Goossens GA: Flushing and locking of venous catheters: available evidence and evidence deficit, Nursing Research and Practice 985686, 2015. Available: https://doi.org/10.1155/2015/985686.

Gorski L: Phillips's manual of IV therapeutics: evidence-based practice for infusion therapy, 7th ed. F. A. Davis Company, 2018.

Gorski L, Hadaway L, Hagle ME, et al: Infusion therapy: standards of practice, Journal of Infusion Nursing (Suppl 39):1S, 2016.

Gouveia S: In-line pressure monitoring in IV infusions: benefits for patients and nurses, British Journal of Nursing 25(19):S28–S33, 2016.

Hall A: Administering medications. In Potter PA, Perry AG, Stockert PA, et al, eds: Essentials for nursing practice, 8th ed., Elsevier, St. Louis, 2015.

Harrison L: Safely managing smart pumps in the clinical setting, Nursing Management 47(6):20–21, 2016.

Harrold K: Guide to the safe use of needlefree connectors, British Journal of Nursing 28(Sup14b):1–6, 2019. Available: https://doi.org/10.12968/bjon.2019.28.Sup14b.1.

Hugill K: Preventing bloodstream infection in IV therapy, British Journal of Nursing 26(14):S4–S10, 2017.

Institute for Safe Medication Practice (ISMP) 2015. ISMP Safe practices guidelines for adult IV push medications. Online 10 April 2021. Available: www.ismp.org/sites/default/files/attachments/2017-11/ISMP97-Guidelines-071415-3.%20FINAL.pdf.

Ismail S, Afshan G, Monem A, Ahmed, A: Postoperative analgesia following caesarean section: intravenous patient controlled analgesia versus conventional continuous infusion, Open Journal of Anesthesiology 2:120–126, 2012.

Keogh S, Shelverton C, Flynn J, et al: Implementation and evaluation of short peripheral intravenous catheter flushing guidelines: a stepped wedge cluster randomised trial, BMC Medicine 18, Article no. 252, 2020. Available: https://doi.org/10.1186/s12916-020-01728-1.

Lee PT: Syringe driver safety issues: an update, International Journal of Palliative Nursing 20(3):115–119, 2014.

Loveday HP, Wilson JA, Pratt RJ, et al: epic3: National evidence-based guidelines for preventing healthcare-associated infections in NHS hospitals in England, Journal of Hospital Infection 86:S1–S70, 2014.

Lyons I, Furniss D, Blandford A, et al: Errors and discrepancies in the administration of intravenous infusions: a mixed methods multihospital observational study, BMJ Quality & Safety 27(11):892–901, 2018.

McKeag N: Infusion pumps: constantly evolving, British Journal of Nursing (Oncology Supplement) 24(10), 2015.

McKenna L, Lim AG: Medications. In Dempsey J, Hillege S, Hill R, eds: Fundamentals of nursing and midwifery, 2nd ed., Lippincott Williams & Wilkins, Sydney, 2014.

Natal BL: Venous air embolism, Medscape, 2017. Online 10 April 2021. Available: https://emedicine.medscape.com/article/761367-overview#a5.

National Institute for Health and Care Excellence (NICE): Infection prevention and control 2014. Quality standard 61 NICE. Online 10 April 2021. Available: www.nice.org.uk/guidance/qs61.

Nowicki RWA: Inaccuracy of fluid container volume markings, Anaesthesia 68:640–654, 2013.

Paparella S, Mandrack M: IV push medication administration: Making safe choices; choosing best practice, Journal of Emergency Nursing 42(1):64–67, 2016.

Pierce ET, Kumar V, Zheng H, Peterfreund, A: Medication and volume delivery by gravity-driven micro-drip intravenous infusion: potential variations during 'Wide-Open' flow, Anesthesia and Analgesia 116:614–618, 2013.

Raghunathan, K: Nursing care of an individual. In Koutoukidis G, Stainton K, eds: Tabbner's nursing care, 8th ed., Elsevier, Sydney, 2021.

Rang, H: Rang and Dale's pharmacology, 8th ed., Elsevier Churchill Livingstone, 2016.

Schumacher MA, Basbaum AI, Naidu RK: Opioid agonists and antagonists: Basic and clinical pharmacology, 14th ed., McGraw-Hill, New York, 2018.

Singer M, Grebenyuk E, Ackroyd S, Hart L: 868 Patient controlled epidural analgesia for post-caesarean pain management in women with opioid use disorder, American Journal of Obstetrics and Gynecology, 224(2):S540–S540, 2021. Available: https://doi.org/10.1016/j.ajog.2020.12.891.

Siwale RC, Sani SN: Multiple-dosage regimens. In Shargel L, Yu AC, eds: Applied biopharmaceutics and pharmacokinetics, 7th ed., McGraw-Hill, New York, 2016.

Spencer S, Gilliam P: Teaching patients about their short peripheral IV catheters, Nursing 45(2):64, 2015.

Therapeutic Goods Administration, Medical devices safety update Volume 5, Number 4, July 2017, Australian Government, Department of Health, 2017. Online 10 April 2021. Available: www.tga.gov.au/publication-issue/medical-devices-safety-update-volume-5-number-4-july-2017.

Therapeutic Goods Administration: Medical devices safety update, Volume 2, Number 4, July 2014. Australian Government, Department of Health, 2014. Online 10 April 2021. Available:. www.tga.gov.au/publication-issue/medical-devices-safety-update-volume-2-number-4-july-2014.

Tollefson J, Hillman E: Clinical psychomotor skills: assessment tools for nurses, 7th ed., Cengage Learning, 2019.

Westbrook JI, Reckmann M, Ling L, et al: Effects of two commercial electronic prescribing systems on prescribing error rates in hospital in-patients: A before and after study, PLoS Medicine 9:1–11, 2012.

Wheeler C, Furniss D, Galal-Edeen G, et al: Patients' perspectives on the quality and safety of intravenous infusions: a qualitative study, Journal of Patient Experience 7(3):380–385, 2020.

Wilkins RG, Unverdorben M: Accidental infusion of air a concise review, Journal of Infusion Nursing 35(6):404–408, 2012.

Zheng H: Intravenous infusion. In Shargel L, Yu AC, eds: Applied biopharmaceutics and pharmacokinetics, 7th ed., McGraw-Hill, New York, 2016.

CHAPTER 24
BLOOD AND IRON TRANSFUSION

Learning outcomes

Having read this chapter, the reader should be able to:

- list reasons for iron or blood transfusion in maternity care settings
- discuss why O Rh-negative blood is the universal donor and AB-positive the universal recipient
- consider the midwife's role in safe blood product transfusion practice
- discuss the midwife's role in safe iron infusion practice.

Blood transfusions can be lifesaving in the event of severe maternal haemorrhage. Midwives need to be able to administer blood products and iron safely. In the event of a critical haemorrhage, midwives need to understand the massive transfusion protocol. Women who are anaemic have less tolerance for blood loss; anaemia during pregnancy is related to adverse outcomes for mother and infant. Anaemia during pregnancy is associated with uterine atony and increased blood loss (Frass 2015). In pregnancy, anaemia is commonly caused by reduced red blood cell production resulting from depleted iron stores. Clinical outcomes can be improved by evidence-based transfusion management and careful consideration of all available therapies to correct anaemia, including iron infusion. This chapter examines the safe administration of blood and iron infusions and the midwife's role and responsibilities.

The severity of postpartum haemorrhage (PPH) is increasing (Flood et al 2017, McDonnell & Browning 2017). However, the incidence of blood transfusion is declining. In New South Wales during 2017, the percentage of women receiving a blood transfusion following vaginal birth was 0.97%, a decrease from 1.32% in 2015; following caesarean section this figure was 0.94%, a decrease from 1.25% (Centre for Epidemiology and Evidence 2018). Blood transfusion is not without risk and in response to evidence of transfusion-related adverse outcomes the National Health and Medical Research Council (NHMRC), the Australian and New Zealand Society of Blood Transfusion (ANZSBT) and the National Blood Authority (NBA) have developed patient blood management guideline modules which provide an excellent resource for midwives.

DEFINITIONS

Iron infusion: Iron is administered intravenously into the venous circulation. An iron infusion is recommended for women with:

- iron-deficiency anaemia requiring rapid restoration of haemoglobin (Hb) and iron stores
- inadequate response to oral iron
- poor tolerance or absorption of oral iron (NBA 2015).

Blood transfusion: Whole blood or components of blood are introduced into the venous circulation to decrease morbidity and mortality. A shortage of red blood cells results in hypoxia; the circulatory system needs to have sufficient blood within the vessels to sustain blood pressure, heart rate and all other circulatory functions. Blood transfusion is recommended for women with:

- hypovolaemia (e.g. after a significant haemorrhage)
- low haemoglobin
- some clotting disorders and blood diseases.

Blood can be administered in different forms: whole blood, packed red cells (plasma removed), platelet concentration, fresh frozen plasma, white blood cells and cryoprecipitate (clotting factors) (Jones

& Heyes 2014, Watson & Hearnshaw 2010). Anti-D immunoglobulin is also a human blood product.

Massive transfusion: This is defined as transfusion of five or more units within a 4-hour period. Massive transfusion necessitates resuscitation measures, including:

- commencing active warming to avoid hypothermia
- avoiding excessive crystalloids to decrease risk of dilutional coagulopathy
- low-volume resuscitation—tolerate permissive hypotension (systolic BP 80–100) to balance haemostasis and organ perfusion
- not relying on haemoglobin alone as transfusion trigger (NBA 2015).

Postpartum haemorrhage (PPH): This is ≥ 500 mL blood loss following vaginal birth and 1000 mL after caesarean birth (Collis & Guasch 2017). PPH occurs in approximately 6% of births (Kerr et al 2016).

Severe PPH: This is blood loss ≥ 1000 mL or any amount of blood loss resulting in haemodynamic compromise (shock).

Massive PPH: Also called obstetric critical bleeding, this is defined by NSW Health (2021) as any of the following:

- blood loss ≥ 2000 mL
- blood loss is life-threatening
- a massive blood transfusion may be needed.

Other definitions include blood loss of > 2500 mL, Hb drops to < 40 g/L, transfusion of ≥ 5 units of packed red blood cells (RBCs) or coagulopathy requiring treatment or need for invasive procedures (Collis & Guasch 2017). Useful clinical signs are a pulse greater than 110 and systolic blood pressure less than 90 (Hunt et al 2015). With massive haemorrhage, coagulopathy often occurs and coagulation factors such as fibrinogen and fresh frozen plasma may be required (Seto et al 2017).

Anaemia: This occurs when a decrease in the number of red blood cells reduces oxygen-carrying capacity to such an extent that the body's physiological requirements are no longer met (World Health Organization [WHO] 2011). The reason for the reduction in the number of erythrocytes is generally from altered red blood cell production, bleeding or increased destruction of red blood cells (Bullock & Hales 2018). The normal range for Hb concentration during pregnancy in Australia has not been defined; however, < 110 is often used in first trimester and < 105 in second and third trimester of pregnancy. The WHO recommendations are commonly used. Anaemia in pregnancy is defined by the WHO (2011) as < 110 g/L for pregnant women and is further categorised in Table 24.1.

Cell salvage: This is the collection of blood lost during surgery: the RBCs are washed, filtered and reinfused (Collis & Guasch 2017). A key aim is to reduce allogenic transfusion and decrease transfusion-related adverse events (NBA 2015).

TABLE 24.1 WHO ANAEMIA DEFINITIONS

Anaemia definitions	Haemoglobin in g/L
During pregnancy	< 110
	100–109 mild
	70–99 moderate
	< 70 severe
	< 40 critical
Postpartum	< 100

Source: Adapted from World Health Organization (WHO): Haemoglobin concentrations for the diagnosis of anaemia and assessment of severity, 2011. Online 29 August 2021. Available: www.who.int/vmnis/indicators/haemoglobin.pdf.

ERYTHROPOIESIS-STIMULATING AGENTS (ESAS)

The hormone erythropoietin (EPO) is synthesised by the kidney and assists the maturation of red blood cells within the bone marrow (Arnlind et al 2016). ESAs can be considered antenatally for women with an increased risk of haemorrhage and should be used in conjunction with iron therapy (NBA 2015). ESAs may be considered for treatment of Jehovah's Witnesses with acute anaemia (Dills et al 2016).

ESAs including erythropoietin have also been used to improve red cell production and reduce the need for transfusion in preterm infants (Lowe et al 2017).

CARE DURING PREGNANCY

Blood group and antibody testing are recommended for all pregnant women. Follow-up testing is beneficial for women who are RhD negative or have alloantibodies which could cause haemolytic disease of the newborn (NBA 2015). Women with alloantibodies that are clinically significant should have a blood group and antibody screen on their admission to hospital and when they are in labour, to ensure the appropriate blood is available without delay (NBA 2015).

WOMEN UNABLE TO HAVE BLOOD PRODUCTS

The administration of blood and blood products is not always an option. Some women may object to blood products due to religious beliefs and others may have complex red cell antibodies which exclude blood transfusion (Kidson-Gerber et al 2016). Women who cannot have a transfusion should be identified at the first antenatal visit, and refusal or inability to have blood products documented in the medical record. Women with complex red cell antibodies require referral to a haematologist (Kidson-Gerber et al 2016).

The religious beliefs of Jehovah's Witnesses prohibit blood transfusion of whole blood, red cells, plasma, platelets and white cells (Kidson-Gerber et al 2016). Other products including immunoglobulins, albumin, vaccines, solid organs and coagulation-factor preparations may be accepted (Kidson-Gerber et al 2016). Autologous blood transfusion is only accepted if the blood is circulating in a closed loop that remains continuous with the body (Scharman et al 2017). In Australia it is generally accepted that women who are pregnant or postpartum have the right to refuse treatment (Kidson-Gerber et al 2016).

The following management strategies are recommended.

- Maximise haemoglobin, iron, B_{12} and iron stores antenatally.
- Monitor haemoglobin and ferritin regularly.
- Use intravenous (IV) iron when oral iron therapy proves ineffective or is poorly tolerated.
- Inform senior staff of the woman's admission for labour.
- Consider IV cannula for labour (large bore).
- At birth, minimise blood loss with active management of third stage, measure blood loss accurately, observe fundal tone, record vital signs.
- Withhold antiplatelet and anticoagulant drugs prior to birth.
- Assess for risk of PPH; women at risk of major haemorrhage (e.g. placenta praevia/accreta) require a multidisciplinary plan (NBA 2015).
- Develop an advance care plan and blood management plan antenatally (discuss acceptable options, including cell salvage, cryoprecipitate, fibrinogen or prothrombin).
- In the context of haemorrhage, achieve haemostasis as quickly as possible.
- IV iron infusion is appropriate for optimising haemoglobin in postpartum women with anaemia (Kidson-Gerber et al 2016) and ESAs can also be considered (NBA 2015).

CLINICAL CONSIDERATIONS

The three pillars of blood management are defined by the NBA (2015) as:

- optimising blood volume and RBC mass
- minimising blood loss
- managing anaemia.

Discussion

Iron transfusion, cell salvage and techniques, such as autologous donation or ESAs, are developing technologies and can decrease the use of blood transfusions, which has a significant effect both in human and financial terms. The midwife has a responsibility in providing effective antenatal care and managing the third stage of labour, as well as during maternal haemorrhage. The need for transfusion should be reviewed carefully for each individual.

Patient blood management has the goal of improving clinical outcomes and avoiding unnecessary exposure to blood components (NBA 2015). Early blood transfusion restores oxygen-carrying capacity and is determined by the clinical picture. O negative blood should be used until cross-matched blood is available. NSW Health (2021) recommends considering blood transfusion in the context of active bleeding as follows.

Actively bleeding

- Bleeding is rapid or ongoing
- Signs of shock are present

OR

- Bleeding continues after 3.5 L of warmed clear fluid have been infused rapidly

Not actively bleeding

For women who are not actively bleeding, the transfusion of red blood cells is determined by Hb and assessment of clinical status (NBA 2015). Iron transfusion can be considered as an appropriate alternative in the clinical situation.

If a blood transfusion is indicated, a single unit of RBC should be transfused, followed by clinical assessment and review to determine if further transfusion is required (NBA 2015). The majority of PPH episodes are recognised early and treated before the threshold for initiating the massive transfusion protocol.

Haemoglobin levels

Evidence for the treatment of anaemia with an RBC transfusion is not available for women during pregnancy or postpartum. The NBA (2015) considers the following suggestions reasonable:

- Hb > 90 g/L, RBC not usually appropriate
- Hb 70–90 g/L, RBC is not associated with decreased mortality
- Hb < 70 g/L, RBC transfusion may be associated with decreased mortality and is possibly appropriate; consider other therapies if available (NBA 2015).

MASSIVE TRANSFUSION

In women with severe haemorrhage, initiating a massive transfusion with RBC and other blood components may be lifesaving (NBA 2015).

In women with critical bleeding, timely escalation should occur to ensure appropriate management and use of RBC and other blood components which may reduce morbidity and mortality (NBA 2015).

If major maternal haemorrhage requiring massive transfusion occurs, the NBA (2015) suggests:

- fresh frozen plasma (FFP): 15 mL/kg
- platelets: 1 adult therapeutic dose
- cryoprecipitate: 3–4 g

OR
- follow direction from haematologist/transfusion specialist.

HAEMOVIGILANCE REPORTING

Haemovigilance is important to identify and prevent adverse events related to transfusion, and includes surveillance procedures covering all aspects of transfusions. Adverse transfusion-related events are first reported internally using incident reports. The health service organisation reviews the incident. Following local or central review, the data from each state or territory department of health is aggregated and the annual *Australian Haemovigilance Report* is produced. The report aims to improve practice standards and ensure the safety of people receiving blood (NBA 2020).

The National Safety and Quality Health Service Standards (NSQHS) Standard 7 Blood and Blood Products is designed to ensure safe transfusion of blood and blood products (ACSQHC 2021). The responsibility for safe and effective transfusion rests with the multidisciplinary team, but especially with those directly administering it (e.g. the midwife). The stages of safe transfusion practice are considered in detail below.

UNDERSTANDING BLOOD GROUPS

The ABO group is the most essential pre-transfusion test and a full ABO group, RhD type and antibody screen (e.g. group and screen) should be performed. Blood groups are defined as A, B, AB or O Rh-negative or Rh-positive. The group is determined by the presence of an antigen on the red cell surface and an antibody in the serum. Individuals with group A, for example, have A antigens on their surface and B antibodies in the serum (Table 24.2). Eighty-five per cent of the population has an additional antigen on their red cells—the Rh factor. If Rh-positive blood is introduced into a Rh-negative person, antibodies form, with a haemolysing effect on the next introduction of Rh-positive blood. Blood group O is known as the universal donor (having no antigens for antibodies to fight), while group AB is known as the universal recipient (having no antibodies to fight foreign antigens). Therefore, the true universal donor is O Rh negative (Rh−) and the true universal recipient is AB Rh-positive (Rh+).

An incompatible blood donation initiates the antigen–antibody reaction, causing red blood cells to agglutinate (clump together); this is a serious transfusion reaction, potentially leading to kidney failure and death.

TABLE 24.2 ANTIBODIES/ANTIGENS OF THE BLOOD GROUPS

Group	Antigen	Antibody
A	A	B
B	B	A
AB	AB	None
O	None	AB

MATERNAL ANTIBODIES

The presence of maternal antibodies (e.g. anti-D, anti-Kell) means that cross-matching should be undertaken carefully to ensure a safe match. Maternal antibodies can have life-threatening consequences for the fetus. Blood group and Rh factor screening of maternal blood generally takes place at booking and, if the woman is Rh-negative, prophylactic anti-D (single dose, 625 IU) is offered at 28 and 34 weeks gestation (Department of Health 2020). If postnatal administration of anti-D is required, it should be administered within 72 hours. Rh-negative women who do not receive anti-D are at risk of developing anti-D antibodies, known as sensitisation. This sensitisation is known as red blood cell alloimmunisation, maternal alloimmunisation or Rh-isoimmunisation. If a woman becomes sensitised, her anti-D antibodies are able to cross the placenta and destroy fetal RBCs (haemolysis) because the body views them as foreign. Fetal problems are uncommon in the first pregnancy; however, in subsequent pregnancies the destruction of fetal RBCs results in fetal anaemia and can lead to haemolytic disease of the newborn.

COVID-19

SARS-CoV-2 (COVID-19) and other similar respiratory viruses are not known to be transmitted via blood products (Australian Red Cross Lifeblood 2021). Screening procedures do not allow anyone with symptoms of illness to donate blood. SARS-CoV2 convalescent plasma was collected in Australia from May 2020 until 31 March 2021 to see if it had potential to treat cases, but international evidence indicates there is no benefit (Australian Red Cross Lifeblood 2021).

ZIKA VIRUS

Women may be concerned about the safety of blood transfusions and effects on the fetus, such as microcephaly. In Brazil cases of transmission of the Zika virus during transfusion of whole blood have occurred (Pifer & Hicks 2017). The risk of contracting the Zika virus in Australia and New Zealand is very low. In Australia people who have had the Zika virus confirmed are not able to donate blood until 4 months after full recovery and may have to defer giving blood if they have travelled to a country where the Zika virus is present (Australian Red Cross Blood Service 2021).

SAFE TRANSFUSION PRACTICE: PRINCIPLES AND PROCEDURES

The Australian and New Zealand Society of Blood Transfusion (ANZSBT 2020) stresses the critical need to follow guidelines, policies and procedures to protect the safety of those receiving a blood transfusion and prevent human error resulting in compromised health. In Australia in 2017–18, there were 488,617 transfusion-related adverse events reported to the national haemovigilance program, with febrile non-haemolytic transfusion reactions (43%), allergic reactions (21%) and transfusion-associated circulatory overload (10.7%) the most common (NBA 2020). Human error contributes to adverse events, with failure to give the correct blood component occurring in 4.7% of serious adverse events (NBA 2020). Factors contributing to adverse events include transfusion in an emergency setting and not adhering to hospital transfusion guidelines (NBA 2020).

Identification and documentation

Accurate identification is essential for safety and the woman should be included as an active participant whenever possible (Stout & Joseph 2016). When blood samples are collected for pre-transfusion testing (cross-match, group and hold) the woman must be correctly identified; there is zero tolerance for errors. Failure to correctly identify the woman at any stage could result in the wrong woman being transfused and this is a major cause of morbidity and mortality (ANZSBT 2019). The transfusion request form must be signed by a medical officer (or authorised health professional in New Zealand).

The woman must be identified with three unique patient identifiers, which must be the same on the request form and the specimen label. The ANZSBT (2020) indicates that the three unique identifiers should be:

- full name (both family and given name or names)
- date of birth
- medical record number (MRN) in Australia or the national health index (NHI) number in New Zealand.

Request forms for pre-transfusion testing (including requests to upgrade existing blood samples to a pre-transfusion request) must have a signature confirming identification processes have been followed. The ANZSBT (2020) indicates all requests should include the following information:

- gender and location
- test(s) requested
- signature (or other traceable identifier) and contact details of phlebotomist (person who collected the blood specimen)
- date and time of specimen collection
- name and contact details of requesting practitioner
- type of blood product(s) with number of units or dose
- special requirements (e.g. irradiated or cytomegalovirus [CMV] seronegative)
- clinical diagnosis and indication for transfusion
- date, time and location of transfusion
- previous transfusions including any adverse reactions
- relevant history (red cell antibodies, obstetric history including receipt of RhD-Ig).

In an emergency situation, such as when a person is unconscious and their identity is unknown, temporary or emergency identifiers must be used until identity is confirmed (Australian and New Zealand Society of Blood Transfusion [ANZBT] 2020). The capacity for a verbal face-to-face or telephone request for blood is available in an emergency and must follow institutional policies (ANZBT 2020).

CONSENT

Informed consent means the woman and the person prescribing the blood have discussed the reason for the transfusion, the nature of the transfusion, the risks (such as the risk of alloimmunisation) and the benefits and other appropriate management strategies (ANZSBT 2019). All questions should be answered and an interpreter used if necessary.

The midwife must check verbal or written consent has been given and is documented before the blood is transfused (except in an emergency situation). In an emergency situation the next-of-kin are asked to give consent; the woman should be fully informed retrospectively. When a woman is unable to give consent and no next-of-kin or authorised patient advocate is available, a clinical decision to transfuse can be made (if there is no written advance directive declining blood transfusion). The reason for transfusion and a summary of the information given is recorded in the woman's medical records. The decision can be documented in the clinical record retrospectively. Some women will refuse consent for specific blood products; this should be clearly documented and refusal of consent for a blood product transfusion must also be documented (ANZSBT 2019).

PREPARATION FOR BLOOD PRODUCT TRANSFUSION

- Adequate staffing levels are important to ensure appropriate care. Ideally non-urgent transfusions/infusions take place during the day.
- The IV cannula is patent and the correct size for a blood transfusion. A single-lumen standard IV cannula can be used for blood (unless a rapid blood transfusion is needed).
- The medical infusion device should be maintained as for any medical device and the rate checked throughout the transfusion/infusion. It is not necessary to prime the IV administration set

with any other IV fluids, just the blood to be administered (0.9% sodium chloride can be used).

- In Australia, blood is not considered a medicine and is authorised rather than prescribed. In New Zealand, a blood product is prescribed as it is classified as a medicine (ANZBT 2019).
- All blood transfusions should be completed within 4 hours. Before obtaining blood products, check the woman is ready (with correct ID in place) so the transfusion can be commenced promptly.
- Warming is not necessary for standard-rate blood transfusions.
- The blood may be delivered to the ward and received by midwifery, nursing or medical staff, or collected from the laboratory fridge, depending on local protocol.
- Ensure the woman's ID and blood product details match exactly. If any discrepancies are found, contact the haematologist.
- Blood is transported promptly in the approved carrier. A single unit of blood is delivered to avoid wastage, except in an emergency (e.g. critical haemorrhage).
- The transfusion should commence within 30 minutes of the blood leaving the laboratory fridge (blood unrefrigerated for > 30 minutes should be reported to the haematologist to determine if it is safe to proceed).
- As an unconscious woman will not be able to report any reactions, additional vigilance is needed (vital signs, non-verbal observations and urine output).

SKILL 24.1 Blood transfusion

1. Perform hand hygiene.
2. Ensure informed consent is documented.
3. Gather equipment:
   - IV administration set with 170–200-micron filter (Fig 24.1)
   - blood product
   - blood product prescription/order blood transfusion checklist
   - personal protective equipment
   - alcohol wipes
   - blood warmer if applicable (e.g. massive transfusion)
   - approved observation chart and/or transfusion chart
   - fluid balance chart.
4. Confirm the correct blood product has been delivered and check the expiry date.
5. Complete identification with a second authorised person (e.g. midwife, registered nurse, medical officer). This must be at the woman's bedside. Ask her to state her name and date of birth. Check her full name, date of birth and medical record number/national health index number. All data must be identical to the woman's ID band and the compatibility tag on the blood product and the prescription/order. Both staff members must sign the appropriate documentation.
6. Check blood group and blood unit numbers on the compatibility label, match the manufacturer's label on the blood. Ensure compliance with order (e.g. irradiated, CMV negative).
7. Check if any actions, such as use of a blood warmer, are required.
8. Inspect the pack to ensure it is not leaking and there is no evidence of haemolysis, unusual colouring or the presence of large clots. Nothing should be added to the blood.
9. Prime the giving set with the blood product or sodium chloride 0.9%.
10. Connect the giving set to the infusion pump (blood must not be piggybacked onto another line) and attach a blood warmer if required.
11. Program the infusion pump.
12. Using aseptic non-touch technique (ANTT), attach the IV line to the cannula.
13. Take vital signs (temperature, heart rate, respiratory rate, blood pressure, oxygen saturation and level of consciousness) prior to commencing the transfusion to ensure baseline data (Cortez-Gann 2017).
14. Review the symptoms of an adverse transfusion reaction before commencing the transfusion and instruct the woman to report them immediately; ensure the call bell is within easy reach.
15. Commence infusion at the appropriate rate as outlined in the local guidelines (blood must be completed within 4 hours). The rate may differ for RBCs, platelets, FFP and cryoprecipitate.
16. Serious reactions can occur rapidly; therefore, the woman must be observed for the first 30 minutes of the transfusion. Monitor her frequently during the transfusion as a large variation in the time period for a reaction exists, with an average of 92 minutes (Cortez-Gann 2017).
17. Record vital signs after 15 minutes and then repeat if there are any changes from baseline. Follow local protocols as there is no consensus on the frequency of observations.
18. If a second unit of blood is being given, this can be commenced after appropriate checks; if not, the transfusion is discontinued and the woman's condition reassessed. The IV giving set is changed after 12 hours and at the end of the transfusion.

Continued

SKILL 24.1 Blood transfusion—cont'd

19. If no reactions have been observed, the blood bag can be disposed of as clinical waste. If a reaction is observed or suspected, return the blood product pack to the laboratory.
20. Complete documentation, including the date and the time transfusion commenced and was completed, identification check and the rate infused on the required forms and in the clinical record. Documentation must be thorough at every stage of the process.
21. If the woman is being discharged, ensure she knows that a reaction is possible in the next 24 hours. If hospitalised, vital signs should be completed 4-hourly.
22. Haematological screening is completed, often the following day (e.g. full blood count and urea and electrolytes).

CAUTIONS

The following cautions should be noted, according to the ANZSBT (2019).

- Platelets must not be transfused in a giving set previously used for red blood cells.
- In the context of critical bleeding, use a large-gauge cannula.
- The only IV fluid compatible with all blood components is 0.9% sodium chloride.
- Incompatible fluids may result in clotting in the infusion line.
- No medications can be added to blood or the blood administration set.

The rate of infusion is dependent on the clinical situation. In the context of critical haemorrhage, rapid transfusion may be required; however, if there is risk of circulatory overload, the transfusion rate will be slower. The typical infusion rates for stable adults without bleeding suggested by the ANZSBT (2019) are listed in Table 24.3.

MANAGEMENT OF TRANSFUSION REACTIONS

Despite careful screening, there is the possibility of disease or antibody transmission. Hindley (2016) indicates the most common serious adverse reactions are:

- transfusion incompatibility (haemolysis due to ABO incompatibility)

TABLE 24.3 TYPICAL INFUSION RATES IN ADULTS

Red blood cells	60–180 minutes per unit
Platelets	15–30 minutes in Australia 30–60 minutes in New Zealand
Fresh frozen plasma	30 minutes per unit
Cryoprecipitate	30–60 minutes per unit

Source: Australian and New Zealand Society of Blood Transfusion (ANZSBT) and Royal College of Nursing Australia: Guidelines for the administration of blood products, 3rd ed., revised 2019, 2019. Online 11 April 2021. Available: anzsbt.org.au/guidelines-standards/anzsbt-guidelines/.

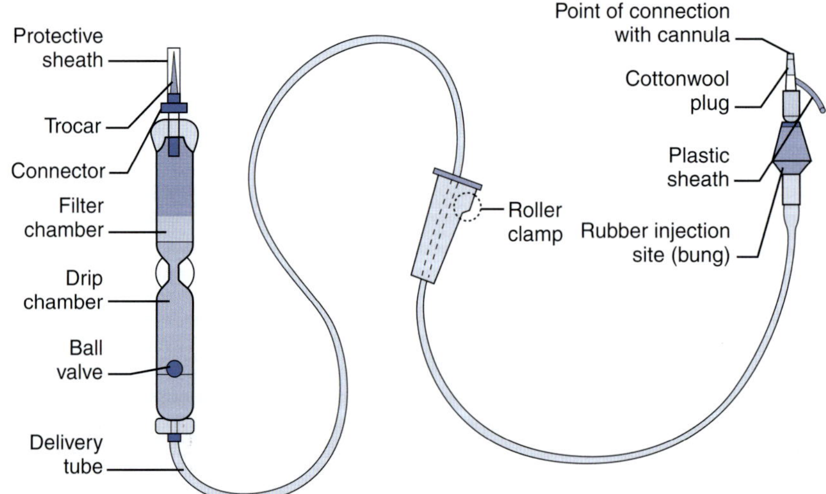

FIGURE 24.1 **Blood transfusion administration set; note the filter and double chambers.**
Source: Adapted with kind permission from Jamieson EM, McCall JM, Whyte LA: Clinical nursing practices, 4th ed., Churchill Livingstone, Edinburgh, 2002.

- circulatory overload
- acute transfusion reactions
- delayed transfusion reactions.

Transfusion incompatibility

Signs of haemolytic reactions in the conscious woman include flushing, shivering, loin and abdominal pain (Watson & Denison 2014), headache, chest pain, tachycardia, tachypnoea, hypotension, haematuria, haemorrhage, oliguria, anxiety and possible death. Usually it is a rapid reaction, occurring after a few millilitres of transfusion. An unconscious woman is likely to demonstrate hypotension, tachycardia and a bruised appearance—bleeding into the skin (Norfolk 2013).

Action: Stop transfusion, maintain venous access with 0.9% normal saline (new cannula), call medical aid urgently, resuscitate the woman using the ABC approach (see Chapter 42). Intensive care may be required.

Circulatory overload

Women have an increased blood volume in pregnancy (1.5 L extra) making it easier to overload their circulatory system if they are not hypovolaemic; fluid gathers in the lungs (pulmonary oedema) resulting in dyspnoea, hypertension, tachycardia, cough, decreased oxygen saturation and raised central venous pressure may be seen during or after transfusion.

Action: Stop transfusion, call medical aid, administer oxygen and diuretic. Transfusion-associated circulatory overload (TACO) is a serious complication and a major cause of morbidity and mortality (Henneman et al 2017).

Febrile reaction

As much as possible, white cells are removed from donated blood, but after a large transfusion, women can have a significant febrile reaction. This includes hyperpyrexia, rigors, sweating and tachycardia. Onset is often within 30–90 minutes and can mimic a haemolytic reaction.

Action: Stop transfusion, call medical aid, exclude haemolytic reaction. If transfusion is to continue, antihistamines and steroids may be needed. A mild febrile reaction (a temperature rise of up to 1.5°C) is often seen; antipyretics may be given, and care should always be taken to ensure that a 'mild' reaction is not the onset of a major reaction. Among the more significant signs and symptoms experienced by those given a transfusion are febrile reactions (46%), hives and itching (23%), tachycardia (18%), chills (18%), dyspnoea (17%), hypotension (14%) and hypoxemia (12%). Other minor reactions include flushing, nausea, back and chest pain, cyanosis and shock (Cortez-Gann 2017).

Allergic reaction

The severest type of reaction is anaphylaxis (Chapter 18); it can occur within 30 minutes, exhibiting rash, wheezing, shortness of breath and hypotension.

Action: Stop transfusion, call for assistance (urgently if clearly anaphylaxis), resuscitate using adrenaline (epinephrine).

Other reactions

Thrombophlebitis, air embolism, iron overload, hypothermia, excess potassium and reduced calcium are other dangers that can occur, either with or following the transfusion. If any reaction is observed, request medical assistance.

IRON INFUSION

The most common reason for anaemia in pregnancy is iron deficiency (Esen 2017). For treatment of anaemia during pregnancy, IV iron is preferable if oral iron is poorly absorbed or not well tolerated (NBA 2015) and if iron stores need to be restored rapidly (Mayson et al, 2016). Anaemia during pregnancy is associated with morbidities for the mother and neonate, including preterm birth and low birth weight (Mayson et al 2016). Women with iron-deficiency anaemia have an increased risk of PPH (Luis et al 2016). The use of IV iron reduces anaemia and increases haemoglobin more rapidly than oral iron (Esen 2017). Iron infusions are effective in increasing haemoglobin and serum ferritin levels with minimal side effects (Lewkowitz et al 2019). Treatment of anaemia with iron in the third trimester reduces maternal morbidity (Oskovi-Kaplan et al 2021).

In Australia and New Zealand, the following iron preparations are available: iron sucrose, iron polymaltose and ferric carboxymaltose. In Australia these can be obtained at a subsidised rate from the Australian Pharmaceutical Benefits Scheme (PBS).

Iron infusions should only be given during the second and third trimester of pregnancy and when the benefits of treatment outweigh the risk to the fetus. Parenteral iron preparations can cause allergic or anaphylactic reactions. An allergic reaction can occur in patients who have received the same iron preparation previously. Having received IV iron previously does not mean the next administration will be reaction-free. Resources for cardiopulmonary resuscitation and administration of adrenaline must be available. If allergic reactions or signs of intolerance occur during administration, stop the treatment immediately.

A test dose is no longer required, although some preparations are commenced at a very slow rate. Anaphylactic reactions are most frequent in the first several minutes and may include sudden onset of respiratory difficulties, tachycardia and hypotension. For mild reactions, antihistamines can be given.

Oral iron supplements should be ceased 24 hours prior to iron infusions and are not recommended for 1 week after the infusion, because concomitant administration reduces the absorption of oral iron.

CAUTIONS

- **WARNING:** Parenteral iron preparations are NOT interchangeable. Each type of iron preparation has a different infusion rate and maximum dose.

- Iron preparations must only be mixed with sterile 0.9% sodium chloride as there is the potential for precipitation or interaction with other agents. A dedicated IV line (giving set) is used and no other medications or solutions must be added.
- Iron preparations should be administered with an infusion pump (or a syringe driver for Ferrinjet). Inspect ampoules for sediment and do not use if sediment is present.
- Paravenous infiltration must be avoided; brown staining of the skin may be permanent if iron leaks into the tissue. If paravenous infiltration occurs, the infusion must be discontinued immediately; apply ice to cause local vasoconstriction and decrease absorption. Do not massage; iron leakage at the injection site can cause pain, inflammation, tissue necrosis, sterile abscess and brown discolouration of the skin.
- Protect the iron preparation from light by covering it with the black cover supplied and use a light-sensitive IV infusion set.
- Women should be observed for at least 30 minutes after an iron infusion.

CONTRAINDICATIONS

Parenteral iron should not be administered if severe inflammation or acute infections are present because elemental iron can accumulate in inflamed tissues. This is not an exhaustive list of contraindications and the product information should be reviewed for each iron preparation.

Contraindications for all iron preparations are:

- hypersensitivity to the iron preparation
- anaemia not caused by iron deficiency
- first trimester of pregnancy
- iron overload
- haemochromatosis
- bacteraemia, acute infection or severe inflammation.

Other contraindications exist specific to the type of iron and these should be reviewed (Table 24.4).

TABLE 24.4 IRON FORMULATIONS: ADMINISTRATION, PRECAUTIONS AND SIDE EFFECTS

Iron sucrose (Venofer) **Supplied in glass ampoule, 5 mL with concentration of 20 mg/mL**	
IV infusion, dilute 500 mg iron sucrose in 500 mL sterile normal saline. (May be administered in smaller doses, for dilution see product information.) Maximum dose 500 mg per infusion and per week; therefore, intermittent doses are necessary if more than 500 mg is required. Infuse 500 mg of iron sucrose (25 mL Venofer) in 500 mL sterile 0.9% sodium chloride. Infuse the first 20 mg over 15 minutes. If tolerated can be increased to a maximum rate of 100 mg over 15 minutes. Some protocols advise a maximum rate of 50 mg over 15 minutes if the first 20 mg is tolerated. Women who have a history of asthma, eczema or other atopic allergies may be at increased risk of allergic reaction. Dose of iron sucrose is determined by a calculation. Check vital signs prior to the infusion, then every 5 minutes for 15 minutes, then every 30 minutes and when completed. (TGA 2021c)	Side effects include: • transient taste perversion • nausea • flushing, fever • hypotension
Iron polymaltose (Ferrosig) **supplied in ampoules in concentration of 100 mg/2 mL (equivalent to 50 mg/mL)**	
Infuse the first 50 mL slowly (5–10 drops/minute). Observe the woman carefully. If the initial 50 mL is well tolerated the rate can be increased to 30 drops/minute. When iron infusion is complete, flush the IV line by infusing 50 mL of sterile 0.9% sodium chloride. Dose is calculated using a formula. Pre-pregnancy weight (or ideal weight if obese) is required to determine the dosage. Check vital signs prior to the infusion, after 5–15 minutes, then every 15 minutes for the first 2 hours and then hourly until 30 minutes after completion of the infusion. (TGA 2021b)	Side effects: • headache • nausea • joint pain • tachycardia • flushing, sweating • chest and back pain • urticaria • bronchospasm with dyspnoea • hypotension, dizziness

TABLE 24.4 IRON FORMULATIONS: ADMINISTRATION, PRECAUTIONS AND SIDE EFFECTS—cont'd

Ferric carboxymaltose (Ferinject) 100 mg/2 mL, 500 mg/10 mL and 1000 mg/20 mL	
Do not administer more than 1000 mg per week. IV infusion 500–1000 mg (maximum single dose is1000 mg), with 100 mL sterile 0.9% sodium chloride in 15 minutes (maximum amount 250 mL). Use as soon as possible after preparation OR use syringe driver 500–1000 mg in 20 mL, then flushed with 20 mL sterile 0.9% sodium chloride. (TGA 2021a)	Side effects: • headache • dizziness • nausea • abdominal pain • rash • injection site reactions • low blood phosphate levels

Source: Therapeutic Goods Administration (TGA): Australian product information—Ferinject® (ferric carboxymaltose) solution for injection, 2021a. Online 29 August 2021. Available: www.ebs.tga.gov.au/ebs/picmi/picmirepository.nsf/pdf?OpenAgent&id=CP-2011-PI-02557-3&d=20210828172310101. Therapeutic Goods Administration (TGA): Ferrosig injection (iron polymaltose compound), consumer medicine information, 2021b. Online 29 August 2021. Available: www.ebs.tga.gov.au/ebs/picmi/picmirepository.nsf/PICMI?OpenForm&t=&q=iron%20polymaltose. Therapeutic Goods Administration (TGA): Australian product information—Venofer (iron sucrose), 2021c. Online 29 August 2021. Available: www.ebs.tga.gov.au/ebs/picmi/picmirepository.nsf/PICMI?OpenForm&t=pi&q=Venofer.

SKILL 24.2 Iron infusion

As with blood transfusion, iron infusions should be given during the day if possible and when adequate staffing is available.

1. Perform hand hygiene.
2. Ensure informed consent is documented.
3. Gather equipment:
   - IV giving set—for light-sensitive medications (usually orange colour) (Fig 24.2)
   - iron product
   - iron prescription
   - medication label
   - personal protective equipment
   - alcohol wipes
   - syringe driver (for Ferinject) or IV infusion pump
   - approved observation chart
   - fluid balance chart.
4. Confirm the correct iron product has been delivered and check the expiry date.
5. Complete identification with a second authorised person (e.g. midwife, registered nurse, medical officer). Ask the woman to state her name and date of birth and check her full name, date of birth and medical record number.
6. Inspect the iron ampoule to ensure no sediment is present. Most IV iron will be prepared in the pharmacy (check expiry date, usually less than 24 hours). If preparing: draw up iron using an 18-gauge BD blunt filter needle 5 microns). Iron should be used immediately after preparation.
7. Prime the giving set with the iron product.
8. Connect the giving set to infusion pump (iron must not be piggybacked onto another line) OR prepare syringe driver.
9. Program infusion pump OR syringe driver if used.
10. Using ANTT, attach IV line to cannula.
11. Take vital signs (temperature, heart rate, respiratory rate, blood pressure, oxygen saturation, level of consciousness and fetal heart rate during pregnancy) prior to commencing the infusion to ensure baseline data.
12. Review the symptoms of an adverse infusion reaction before commencing the infusion and instruct the woman to report them immediately. Ensure call bell is within easy reach.
13. Commence infusion at an appropriate rate (local guidelines will vary and should be followed); suggested rates are as follows.
    - *Iron polymaltose:* 20–40 mL/hour for the first 50 mL, then increase to 120 mL/hour for reminder of infusion.
    - *Iron sucrose:* 500 mg can be infused in 500 mL of 0.9% normal saline over 3.5 to 4 hours.
    - *Ferric carboxymaltose:* Syringe driver with 20 mL syringe, infuse iron over 15 minutes, then give 20 mL normal saline.
14. Serious reactions can occur rapidly; the woman must be observed for the first 15 minutes of infusion.
15. Record her vital signs every 15 minutes for the first 30–60 minutes, then every 30 minutes for 60 minutes, then every 30–60 minutes for the remainder of the infusion. Follow local protocols. During pregnancy check the fetal heart rate following the infusion.
16. Discontinue infusion. Disconnect if no further IV fluids required, or replace giving set and commence fluids as ordered.
17. Complete documentation, including the date and time infusion commenced and was completed, identification check and rate infused on the required forms and in the clinical record.
18. Observe the woman for 30 minutes after infusion has been completed.

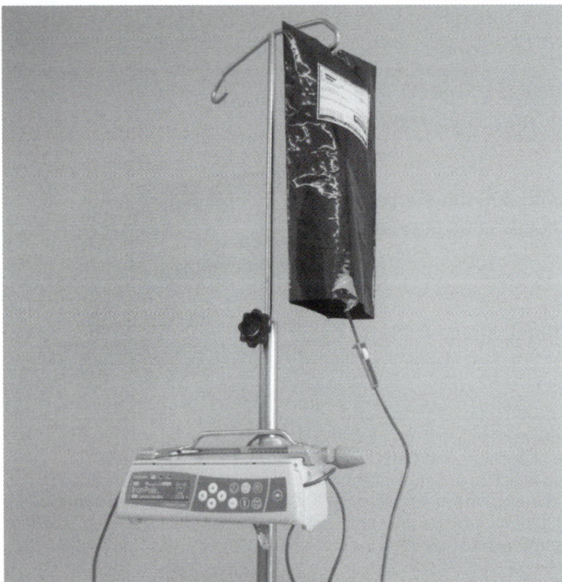

FIGURE 24.2 **Light protective cover and tubing for iron infusion.**

Role and responsibilities of the midwife

These can be summarised as:

- undertaking the procedure competently at every stage, maintaining up-to-date knowledge and skills with regard to safe transfusion practice
- understanding the administration of an iron infusion
- contemporaneous and thorough record keeping at every stage
- instigating appropriate referral when necessary.

SUMMARY

- Blood transfusion is valuable in saving lives; the whole process of blood transfusion should be robust; for the midwife, this starts with the booking history and initial blood-taking. Thorough checking, particularly of patient identity, is highlighted at every stage.
- There are dangers associated with blood transfusions and iron infusions; the midwife should maintain careful observation of the woman.

Self-assessment exercises

The answers to the following questions may be found in the text.

1. What is a blood transfusion?
2. When may a blood transfusion be necessary?
3. Which blood group and Rh factor is the universal donor? Why is this?
4. Describe the process that protects the woman from receiving an incompatible transfusion.
5. Describe how the midwife would recognise that haemolysis was occurring.
6. When does the midwife assess vital sign observations during a transfusion?
7. Under what circumstances would an iron infusion be indicated?

Resources

Australian Red Cross Lifeblood: www.lifeblood.com.au.

Australian and New Zealand Society of Blood Transfusion (ANZBT): anzsbt.org.au.

National Blood Authority Australia: www.blood.gov.au.

NZBLOOD: NZblood.co.nz.

References

Arnlind M, Fryklund L, Vitols S, Bertilsson, G: Biosimilar erythropoiesis-stimulating agents and the risk of developing anti-drug antibodies—a systematic review, European Journal of Clinical Pharmacology 72(10):1161, 2016.

Australian and New Zealand Society of Blood Transfusion (ANZSBT) and Royal College of Nursing Australia: Guidelines for the administration of blood products, 3rd ed., revised 2019, 2019. Online 11 April 2021. Available: anzsbt.org.au/guidelines-standards/anzsbt-guidelines/.

Australian and New Zealand Society of Blood Transfusion (ANZSBT): Guidelines for transfusion and immunohaematology laboratory practice, 2020. Online 10 April 2021. Available: anzsbt.org.au/guidelines-standards/anzsbt-guidelines.

Australian Commission on Safety and Quality in Health Care (ACSQHC): National safety and quality health service standards. 2nd ed.—version 2. 2021. Available: www.safetyandquality.gov.au/sites/default/files/2021-05/national_safety_and_quality_health_service_nsqhs_standards_second_edition_-_updated_may_2021.pdf.

Australian Red Cross Blood Service: Zika virus update, 2016. Online 11 April 2021. Available: transfusion.com.au/node/725.

Australian Red Cross Lifeblood: Coronavirus disease (COVID-19) and the impact on blood supply, 2021. Online 11 April 2021. Available: transfusion.com.au/coronavirus.

Bullock S, Hales M: Principles of pathophysiology, Pearson, Melbourne, 2018.

Centre for Epidemiology and Evidence: New South Wales mothers and babies 2017, NSW Ministry of Health, Sydney, 2018. Online 11 April 2021. Available: www.health.nsw.gov.au/hsnsw/Publications/mothers-and-babies-2017.pdf.

Collis R, Guasch E: Managing major obstetric haemorrhage: pharmacotherapy and transfusion, Best Practice & Research: Clinical Anaesthesiology 31:107–124, 2017.

Cortez-Gann J: Blood transfusion vital sign frequency: what does the evidence say? Medsurg Nursing 26:89–92, 2017.

Department of Health: Clinical practice guidelines: pregnancy care, Australian Government, Canberra, 2020.

Dills H, McLemore M, Tran R, Curry, M: 616: Evaluation of erythropoiesis-stimulating agents in acutely anemic Jehovah's Witnesses, Critical Care Medicine 44(12, Suppl 1):230, 2016.

Esen U: Iron deficiency anaemia in pregnancy: the role of parenteral iron, Journal of Obstetrics and Gynaecology 37(1):15–18, 2017.

Flood MM, Pollock WE, McDonald SJ, Davey, M-A: Monitoring postpartum haemorrhage in Australia: opportunities to improve reporting, Women and Birth S1871–5192(17):30006–9, 2017.

Frass KA: Postpartum hemorrhage is related to the hemoglobin levels at labor: observational study, Alexandria Journal of Medicine 51:333–337, 2015.

Henneman EA, et al: Transfusion-associated circulatory overload: evidence-based strategies to prevent, identify, and manage a serious adverse event, Critical Care Nurse 37:58–66, 2017.

Hindley C: Blood transfusion in the context of maternity care, British Journal of Midwifery 24:838–844, 2016.

Hunt BJ, Allard S, Keeling D, et al: A practical guideline for the haematological management of major haemorrhage, British Journal of Haematology 170(6):788–803, 2015.

Jones A, Heyes J: Processing, testing and selecting blood components, Nursing Times 110(37):20–22, 2014.

Kerr R, Eckert L, Winikoff B, et al: Postpartum haemorrhage: case definition and guidelines for data collection, analysis and presentation of immunization safety data, Vaccine 34:6102–6109, 2016.

Kidson-Gerber G, Kerridge I, et al: Caring for pregnant women for whom transfusion is not an option. A national review to assist in patient care, The Australian and New Zealand Journal of Obstetrics and Gynaecology 56(2):127–136, 2016.

Lewkowitz A, Gupta A, Simon L, et al: Intravenous compared with oral iron for the treatment of iron-deficiency anemia in pregnancy: a systematic review and meta-analysis. Journal of Perinatology 39(4): 519–532, 2019.

Lowe J, Rieger R, Moss N, et al: Impact of erythropoiesis-stimulating agents on behavioral measures in children born preterm, The Journal of Pediatrics 184:75-80.e1, 2017.

Luis J, Fadel M, Lau G, et al: The effects of severe iron-deficiency anaemia on maternal and neonatal outcomes: a case–control study in an inner-city London hospital, Journal of Obstetrics and Gynaecology 36(4):473–475, 2016.

Mayson E, Ampt A, Shand A, et al: Intravenous iron: barriers and facilitators to its use at nine maternity hospitals in New South Wales, Australia, The Australian and New Zealand Journal of Obstetrics and Gynaecology 56(2):162–172, 2016.

McDonnell NJ, Browning R: How to replace fibrinogen in postpartum haemorrhage situations? (Hint: Don't use FFP!), International Journal of Obstetric Anesthesia 33:4–7, 2017.

National Blood Authority (NBA): Australian Haemovigilance Report data for 2017–18, 2020. Online 11 April 2021. Available: www.blood.gov.au/haemovigilance-reporting.

National Blood Authority (NBA): Patient blood management guidelines: Module 5 obstetrics and maternity, 2015. Online 11 April 2021. Available: www.blood.gov.au/pbm-module-5.

Norfolk D: Handbook of transfusion medicine, 5th ed., TSO, Norwich, 2013.

NSW Health: Postpartum haemorrhage (PPH), 2021. Online 28 August 2021. Available: www1.health.nsw.gov.au/pds/ActivePDSDocuments/GL2021_010.pdf.

Oskovi-Kaplan Z, Kilickiran H, Buyuk G, et al. Comparison of the maternal and neonatal outcomes of pregnant women whose anemia was not corrected before delivery and pregnant women who were treated with intravenous iron in the third trimester. Archives of Gynecology and Obstetrics 303(3):715–719, 2021.

Pifer LW, Hicks W: Blood transfusion safety and the challenge of Zika virus, Journal of Continuing Education Topics and Issues 19:36–41, 2017.

Scharman C, Burger D, Shatzel J, et al: Treatment of individuals who cannot receive blood products for religious or other reasons, American Journal of Hematology 92(12):1370–1381, 2017.

Seto S, Itakura A, Okagaki R, et al: An algorithm for the management of coagulopathy from postpartum hemorrhage, using fibrinogen concentrate as first-line therapy, International Journal of Obstetric Anesthesia 32:11–16, 2017.

Stout L, Joseph S: Blood transfusion: patient identification and empowerment, The British Journal of Nursing 25:138–143, 2016.

Watson D, Denison C: Recognising and managing transfusion reactions, Nursing Times 110(39):18–21, 2014.

Watson D, Hearnshaw K: Understanding blood groups and transfusion in nursing practice, Nursing Standard 24(30):41–48, 2010.

World Health Organization (WHO): Haemoglobin concentrations for the diagnosis of anaemia and assessment of severity, 2011. Online 19 Feb 2018. Available: apps.who.int/iris/bitstream/10665/85839/3/WHO_NMH_NHD_MNM_11.1_eng.pdf?ua=1.

CHAPTER 25

INHALATION

Learning outcomes

Having read this chapter, the reader should be able to:

- describe the safe and effective use of nitrous oxide
- identify the signs and symptoms of adverse reactions and discuss appropriate management
- detail the role and responsibilities of the midwife when administering nitrous oxide.

Nitrous oxide is widely used as an inhalation analgesic during labour in Australia, New Zealand, Europe, the United Kingdom (UK) and increasingly the United States. Nitrous oxide inhalation was certified for use and endorsed for administration by midwives in the UK for labour analgesia in 1936 (O'Sullivan 1989). Nitrous oxide was first evaluated in labour by Dr Stanislav Kliclowicz in Russia in 1880 (Eley et al 2015). Nitrous oxide use has increased in other areas of healthcare including paediatrics, trauma and dentistry.

According to some hospital protocols, nitrous oxide can also be used for difficult intravenous insertion, external cephalic version, intracervical balloon placement, perineal repair, manual removal of the placenta and for women with opioid dependency (Migliaccio et al 2017).

Nitrous oxide is self-administered by women under the supervision of a midwife. Inhaled nitrous oxide is the most common pain relief method and was used in labour by 53% of Australian women (Australian Institute of Health and Welfare [AIHW] 2021). This chapter reviews the safe use of inhalational analgesia in the context of the role and responsibilities of the midwife as they care for women during labour and birth.

UNDERSTANDING NITROUS OXIDE

Nitrous oxide (N_2O) is a colourless gas with a slightly sweet odour and is an N-methyl-D-aspartate (NMDA) receptor antagonist (Brown & Sneyd 2016). Nitrous oxide is also known as dinitrogen oxide, dinitrogen monoxide, Entonox and laughing gas. Nitrous oxide is classified as a dissociative anaesthetic (National Drug & Alcohol Research Centre [NDARC] 2021) Entonox (N_2O_2) is premixed and contains 50% oxygen and 50% nitrous oxide. Nitrous oxide can be supplied in portable cylinders (with white and blue shoulders) or piped (tubing has a blue and white stripe). Cylinders are labelled by name as well as colour. Nitrous oxide is piped into birth rooms via a blender, which can be adjusted to alter the ratio of oxygen to nitrous oxide from zero to a maximum concentration of 70% nitrous oxide with 30% oxygen. In Australia and New Zealand nitrous oxide is a schedule 4 medication.

Nitrous oxide is purported to work via stimulation of endogenous opioid release in the brain stem which moderates pain impulse processing in the spinal cord (Collins 2014). The complex mechanism of action also involves potassium channel inhibition in the central nervous system and possible N-methyl-D-aspartate (NMDA) receptor antagonism (Baysinger 2019). Nitrous oxide increases dopamine and noradrenaline (Illuzzi et al 2018). Nitrous oxide increases cerebral blood flow and has an analgesic action similar to morphine (Grant 2020). Case reports indicate that women find nitrous oxide has anxiolytic properties (Collins 2014). The anxiolytic effect may involve gamma aminobutyric (GABA) receptors (Baysinger 2019) and is similar to benzodiazepines (Alai 2017). Nitrous oxide has poor solubility in blood and does not bind to protein. It is absorbed rapidly by diffusion in the lungs, where it spreads through the lining of the arterial alveolar membrane. Because metabolisation and elimination occur mostly through the lungs, the effects are reversed rapidly when discontinued and there is no associated nephrotoxicity or hepatotoxicity (Alai 2017). The half-life is around 5 minutes and less than 0.004% is metabolised; therefore, it is eliminated in a non-metabolised (unaltered) state (Alai 2017).

The National Institute for Health and Care Excellence (NICE) recommends that nitrous oxide be available in all birth settings (NICE 2017). Inhaled nitrous oxide reduces pain intensity without increasing operative birth, or adversely affecting fetal wellbeing and provides a useful non-invasive addition to pain relief options during labour (Fig 25.1) (Klomp et al 2012). Nitrous oxide is accessible at short notice, decreases pain perception, provides an anxiolytic effect, is inexpensive, is easily discontinued, preserves mobility and avoids interventions such as catheterisation and intravenous infusion (Likis et al 2014). Nitrous oxide does not disrupt uterine contractions or the normal physiological process of labour (Vallejo & Zakowski 2019).

The effects of nitrous oxide are transient, with a rapid onset and offset of approximately 1–2 minutes (Collins 2017). The effects cease rapidly once inhalation ceases and there are no residual effects (Alai 2017). Maternal sedation is minimal and fetal heart rate patterns are not compromised (Bobb et al 2016). The Apgar score of newborns whose mothers used nitrous oxide has not been significantly different to newborns whose mothers used no analgesia (Attar et al 2016, Bobb et al 2016, Koyyalamudi et al 2016, Likis et al 2014, Parsa et al 2017). Rates of neonatal resuscitation are not increased. Nitrous oxide is lipid soluble and crosses the placenta, reaching concentrations of 80% of maternal values (Jordan 2010). However, it is rapidly eliminated from the newborn's lungs after birth (Likis et al 2014), which avoids excretion via the less mature liver and kidneys (Jordan 2010).

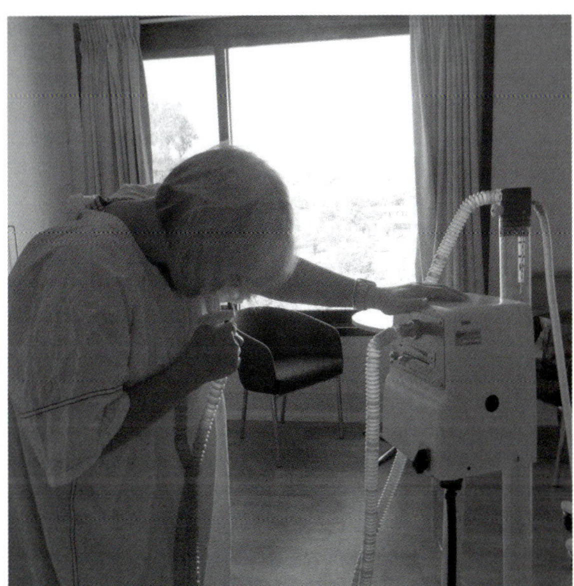

FIGURE 25.1 **Using nitrous oxide.**

Nitrous oxide has a positive effect on labour satisfaction and breastfeeding, possibly related to reduced stress, and higher levels of endorphins and prolactins which are beneficial for lactogenesis (Zanardo et al 2017). The anxiolytic effect may help reduce the negative effects of fear and anxiety (Collins 2014). Nitrous oxide does not alter uterine contractions (Collins 2017) as it has no effect on smooth muscle (Jordan 2010) and endogenous oxytocin and normal labour physiology are not disrupted (Rooks 2012). A shorter duration of labour has been reported with its use (Attar et al 2016, Parsa et al 2017).

Nitrous oxide appears to provide better short-term pain relief than pethidine without causing neonatal respiratory depression or feeding difficulties; in additional, maternal cardiorespiratory parameters are barely altered, although women complain of a dry mouth (Mobaraki et al 2016). According to the manufacturer's information, 50% nitrous oxide is equivalent to 100 mg of pethidine (BOC 2015). Epidural anaesthesia is more efficacious than nitrous oxide (Koyyalamudi et al 2016, Likis et al 2014). Women using nitrous oxide rate their pain as less severe (Attar et al 2016, Koyyalamudi et al 2016). A concentration of 25% provides a marked reduction in pain (BOC 2017); a 50:50 oxygen–nitrous oxide blend has minimal sedation and anxiolytic effects with negligible adverse effects (Migliaccio et al 2017). For a woman to become unconsciousness, a concentration of around 70% is required (BOC 2008).

Nitrous oxide does not eliminate the sensation of contractions, but reduces the level of pain and anxiety. The effect is often described by women as 'taking the edge off' the contraction. Women using nitrous oxide are as likely to be satisfied with their choice as women receiving an epidural (Collins 2017). Midwives are responsible for ensuring women are informed about the effects, advantages and disadvantages of nitrous oxide. Advantages include the ability to self-administer nitrous oxide, which places control in a woman's hands (Collins 2017, Smith et al 2021). Women who wish to avoid interventions can use nitrous without requiring intravenous fluid, continuous fetal heart-rate monitoring and catheterisation (Illuzzi et al 2018). Women continue to experience contractions and can remain mobile. Self-administration is important for safety and avoiding overdosage. As a woman inhales using the mouthpiece or mask, a negative pressure is created allowing the demand valve to open and release nitrous oxide. The demand valve closes during exhalation, so no gas is delivered. If the woman becomes drowsy she is unable to achieve a negative pressure during inhalation; the demand valve snaps shut and no nitrous oxide is released. The sound of the demand valve opening and closing is audible. The apparatus should remain in place during expiration to avoid exposing others to exhaled nitrous oxide. Exhaled nitrous oxide is eliminated unchanged from the lungs (Patel et al 2018). Therefore, breathing in exhaled nitrous oxide is almost the same as breathing in nitrous oxide directly from the apparatus.

The apparatus also includes a microbiological filter to prevent cross-infection. It has a slightly sweet smell and taste (Nagele et al 2014). Women can rapidly adjust their use as desired and if side effects occur (Collins 2017). Reported side effects include nausea and vomiting, dizziness and drowsiness (Attar et al 2016, Koyyalamudi et al 2016). Nausea occurs in 5–40% of women, vomiting in around 5% and dizziness in 3–5% (Grant 2020).

The analgesic effects can be achieved within a few breaths (25–35 seconds) and last for approximately 60 seconds after inhalation ceases (Jordan 2010). For the most effective use, inhalation of nitrous oxide commences as soon as a contraction is felt. In the second stage of labour, nitrous oxide may help women waiting for the presenting part to descend before actively pushing. It can be used effectively for examining the perineum and for suturing at the end of the third stage of labour.

Use of nitrous oxide analgesia is appropriate for women with mild-to-moderate asthma and is considered safe when used correctly. Unfortunately, its use as an illicit recreation drug has increased, leading to serious adverse effects, including lung damage, neuropathy, respiratory distress, myocardial infarction and seizure (Alai 2017). Nitrous oxide can induce vitamin B_{12} deficiency (Stockton, Simonsen & Seago 2017).

During self-administration of nitrous oxide, women may hyperventilate during a contraction to achieve maximum pain relief. This may be followed by hypoventilation between contractions. Excessive breathing (hyperventilation) results in a reduction of carbon dioxide; this commences a cascade of effects that can include dizziness, fetal hypoxia and tetany. Tetany may result in spasm of the larynx and airway obstruction; early signs include involuntary spasms in the muscles of the extremities. Jordan (2010) recommends the breaths taken when using nitrous oxide should be slow and with reasonable depth. Dizziness, tingling or twitching in the hands are all suggestive signs of hyperventilation. Nitrous oxide should not be used for women with respiratory compromise or oxygen saturation less than 95% (Grant 2020).

Nitrous oxide, like all anaesthetic gases, depresses the nervous system. Sedation, obvious detachment from the situation (often with hallucinations) and inability to respond to verbal commands would suggest a deeper stage of anaesthesia has been reached than is desired. The nitrous oxide should be stopped and medical assessment organised.

Concomitant administration of nitrous oxide with centrally acting medications (morphine derivatives, benzodiazepines, fentanyl) may increase sedation. If used concomitantly, the level of sedation, respiratory rate and depth should be monitored. The manufacturers specifically caution against the use of nitrous oxide with a high dose of fentanyl as the two can cause a reduction in heart rate and cardiac output (BOC 2017).

CONTRAINDICATIONS

Nitrous oxide should not be used if women have any condition where gas may be trapped within the body, including pneumothorax in the past 6 weeks, ocular surgery utilising intraocular gas, increased intraocular pressure, recent middle ear surgery and head injuries with impaired consciousness (BOC 2017).

Nitrous oxide is contraindicated during episodes of asthma with wheezing or if significant respiratory compromise is present (Alai 2017).

Potential complications and precautions for use

The potential exists for diffusion hypoxia to occur at the end of an anaesthetic procedure when nitrous oxide administration ceases and the gas diffuses into the alveoli (Bullock & Manias 2017). This is generally a transient situation. Administering more oxygen before the end of the procedure will avoid this situation. Oxygen should be available to administer to the woman or neonate should this occur.

Nitrous oxide should not be used for longer than 24 hours (BOC 2017). For some labours, this means commencing it when labour is established, rather than in the latent phase.

Prolonged use of nitrous oxide inactivates vitamin B_{12} (a cofactor in methionine synthase), disrupts folate metabolism and consequently impairs DNA synthesis (BOC 2017). Using nitrous oxide in the setting of low vitamin B_{12} levels represses methionine synthase production, increasing the risk of megaloblastic anaemia (Collins 2017). Both vitamin B_{12} and folic acid deficiency are associated with neural tube defects, miscarriage and premature birth (Ahmadi et al 2017, Finkelstein et al 2015). It is beneficial to check a woman's vitamin B_{12} during pregnancy and whether symptoms of vitamin B_{12} deficiency are present (Nash 2016). Women with Crohn's or coeliac disease, pernicious anaemia or a gastric bypass and women on a vegetarian diet are at increased risk of low vitamin B_{12}. Folic acid supplements taken to reduce the risk of neural tube defects can mask vitamin B_{12} deficiency (NHS Choices 2016). Metformin can also disrupt vitamin B_{12} metabolism (Nash 2016). Nitrous oxide is best avoided in women with vitamin B_{12} deficiency or pernicious anaemia.

Existing pathology

The effectiveness of nitrous oxide as an analgesic will potentially be impaired for some groups of women. This includes any compromise to the cardiovascular system (e.g. pre-eclampsia), nervous system damage (e.g. muscular sclerosis) and haematology changes (e.g. sickle cell anaemia). Anyone with known sinus or ear problems should use nitrous oxide with caution. Nitrous oxide should not be used for more than 24 hours (BOC 2017).

SAFETY PRECAUTIONS

Nitrous oxide is non-flammable, but like oxygen, supports combustion. Oils or grease should not be used for lubrication on any parts, and sources of ignition must be avoided.

Nitrous oxide needs to be stored in such a way that the two gases do not separate. At −6°C for cylinders, or piped at −30°C, the gas separation means pure oxygen would be administered first, followed by pure nitrous oxide. Both are life-threatening situations. Nitrous oxide cylinders should be stored horizontally and at room temperature (at least > 10°C) to prevent this separation. Australian Standards AS2896—Medical Gas Systems covers the safety requirements for non-inflammable medical gas pipeline systems used for patient care (Australian Business Licence and Information Service [ABLIS] 2011). In New Zealand, adverse reactions are reported to the New Zealand Pharmacovigilance Centre (see Resources section).

Occupational exposure

Exposure to nitrous oxide is a consideration for midwives, although it is difficult to identify the risks accurately. Associations between chronic occupational exposure and reproductive issues, such as decreased fertility, spontaneous abortion and preterm birth, have been reported (Alai 2017). The Centers for Disease Control and Prevention (CDC) indicate that workers exposed to nitrous oxide may have effects to the central nervous system, bone marrow and the peripheral nervous system and it may cause reproductive toxicity (National Institute for Occupational Safety and Health [NIOSH] 2014).

Midwives need to be aware of the signs of vitamin B_{12} deficiency. Nash (2016) recommends midwives have their vitamin B_{12} levels checked annually if they are frequently exposed to nitrous oxide.

Safety practices should be in place so midwives and other staff are not exposed to excessive levels. The implications for midwives who are exposed to nitrous oxide on a daily basis are unknown. Nitrous oxide should be administrated in rooms with adequate ventilation and a scavenging system (Fig 25.2) (Nash 2016). Modelling of nitrous oxide levels in clinical situations indicates that it does not accumulate at floor level despite having a higher density than air; instead, it shows a plume distribution related to heat generated by people. Older studies showing exposure to nitrous oxide above recommended levels were in rooms without scavenging systems and with poor ventilation (Likis et al 2014).

If adequate safety measures are followed, such as well-ventilated rooms, demand valves and short-term usage, the nitrous oxide levels should remain below

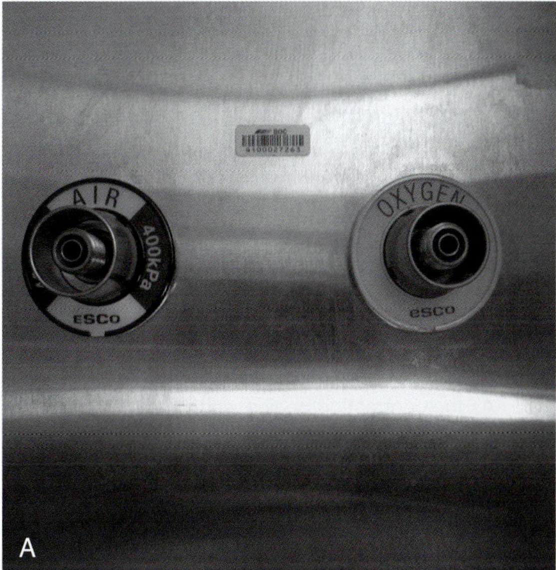

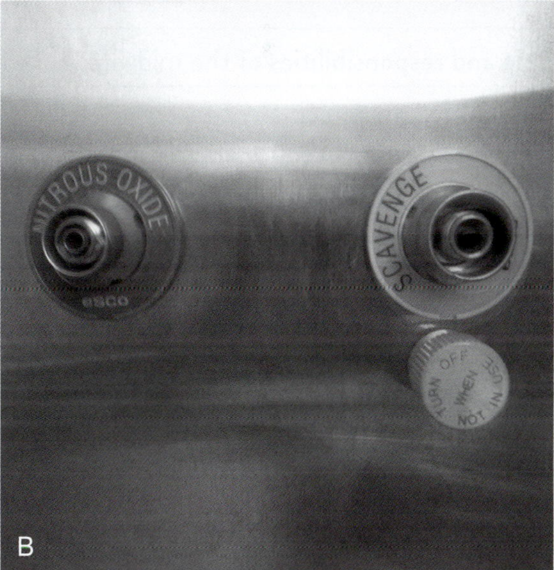

FIGURE 25.2 **Outlets for nitrous oxide, including scavenger outlet. A, Air and oxygen outlets, B, Nitrous oxide and scavenger outlets.**

the occupational exposure limit (Pecheli et al 2016). In birth areas, nitrous oxide use is intermittent and concentrations are lower than those found in the operating theatre (Migliaccio et al 2017).

Occupational exposure to nitrous oxide has been limited in the UK to 100 ppm over an 8-hour period (Likis et al 2014). WorkSafe standards in Australia and New Zealand indicate scavenging of waste nitrous oxide gas should take place to ensure rooms have a level of nitrous oxide below 25 ppm (Safe Work Australia 2021). Scavenging systems appear to decrease occupational exposure risks (Buhre et al 2019).

SKILL 25.1 Using nitrous oxide in labour

1. Ensure the equipment is working correctly.
2. Review the woman's history to ensure no contraindications are present.
3. Ensure every woman is provided with information and understands how nitrous oxide is used safely prior to giving informed consent.
4. Explain how to use the mouthpiece or mask in place so a seal is obtained. Explain the importance of only the woman holding the mouthpiece. An adequate seal is necessary to allow opening of the negative pressure valve to release the nitrous oxide.
5. As the contraction begins, encourage the woman to breathe through the mouthpiece, taking in the gas by taking slow breaths with reasonable depth.
6. When exhaling, the woman should exhale into the mouthpiece and not into the room, so the scavenging system is able to access the nitrous oxide.
7. Observe each woman's response and any side effects, particularly as time passes.
8. Monitor all vital sign observations as for care in labour, ensuring that respiration rate and depth are noted. Pulse oximetry is considered if any observations are outside normal parameters.
9. Understand and observe for the possible effects/side effects of multiple pharmacology (e.g. use of opioid analgesics concurrently).
10. Document contemporaneously; include the duration of use, effects and side effects.
11. Ensure all apparatus is disposed of, cleaned and serviced, and ready to use again on completion.

Role and responsibilities of the midwife

These can be summarised as:

- if appropriately trained in its use, the midwife can administer nitrous oxide to labouring women during all stages of labour
- the midwife having a significant role in ensuring women understand how to use nitrous oxide safely and effectively
- monitoring respiration rate and depth (in addition to monitoring the woman's vital signs as part of labour care), encouraging the woman to breathe slowly but with reasonable depth; action should be taken if there are any signs or symptoms of overdose, hyperventilation or hypoxia
- keeping full and contemporaneous records
- the midwife being fully aware of how to use, store and clean the apparatus (particularly if using a portable cylinder) and of how to ensure potential faults are corrected
- upholding health and safety at work regulations with regard to nitrous oxide use; midwives should consider their own safety.

SUMMARY

- Nitrous oxide achieves an analgesic effect with few serious side effects for the mother and fetus.
- The side effects for the woman are transitory and there are no documented negative effects (at this time) for the fetus.
- The midwife is responsible for ensuring nitrous oxide is stored, serviced and used correctly. The midwife should be alert to any signs of adverse reactions with its use.
- Working in environments where nitrous oxide is used extensively may pose health threats to employees. Health and safety regulations should be upheld.

Self-assessment exercises

The answers to the following questions may be found in the text.

1. Describe how a midwife should support a woman to use nitrous oxide effectively in the first and second stages of labour.
2. Discuss the advantages and disadvantages of nitrous oxide as a labour analgesic.
3. Summarise the role and responsibilities of the midwife when caring for a woman using nitrous oxide in labour.
4. List the vital signs and observations to be undertaken regularly when a woman is using nitrous oxide.

Resources

New Zealand Pharmacovigilance Centre: nzphvc.otago.ac.nz/reporting/.

References

Ahmadi R, Ziaei S, Parsay S: Association between nutritional status with spontaneous abortion, International Journal of Fertility & Sterility 10:337–342, 2017.

Alai AN: Nitrous oxide administration, Medscape, 2017. Online 11 April 2021. Available: emedicine.medscape.com/article/1413427-overview.

Attar AS, Feizabadi AS, Jarahi L, et al: Effect of Entonox on reducing the need for pethidine and the relevant fetal and maternal complications for painless labor, Electronic Physician 8:3325–3332, 2016.

Australian Business Licence and Information Service (ABLIS): Australian Standard AS2896, Medical gas systems. Installation and testing of non-flammable medical gas pipelines systems. Australian Government,

2011. Online 11 April 2021. Available: ablis.business.gov.au/service/vic/australian-standard-as-2896-2011-medical-gas-systems-installation-and-testing-of-non-flammable-medical-gas-pipeline-systems/24526.

Australian Institute of Health and Welfare (AIHW): Australia's mothers and babies, cat. no. PER 101, AIHW, Canberra, 2020. Online 5 September 2021. Available: www.aihw.gov.au/reports/mothers-babies/australias-mothers-babies.

Baysinger C: Inhaled nitrous oxide analgesia for labor, Current Anesthesiology Reports 9(1):69–75, 2019.

Bobb L, Farber M, McGovern C, Camann, W: Does nitrous oxide labor analgesia influence the pattern of neuraxial analgesia usage? An impact study at an academic medical center, Journal of Clinical Anesthesia 35:54–57, 2016.

BOC: ENTONOX the essential guide, 2015. Online 11 April 2021. Available: www.bochealthcare.co.uk/en/index.html.

BOC: New Zealand Data Sheet. Medical nitrous oxide, 2017. Online 11 April 2021. Available: www.medsafe.govt.nz/profs/Datasheet/e/entonoxgas.pdf.

BOC: Nitrous oxide medical EP grade, 2008. Online 5 September 2021. Available: www.boc-healthcare.com.au/en/images/Product%20Information%20Compressed%20Nitrous%20Oxide_tcm350-72398.pdf.

Brown SM, Sneyd JR: Nitrous oxide in modern anaesthetic practice, BJA Education 16:87–91, 2016.

Bullock S, Manias E: Fundamentals of pharmacology, 8th ed., Pearson, Melbourne, 2017.

Buhre W, Disma N, Hendrickx J, et al: European Society of Anaesthesiology Task Force on Nitrous Oxide: a narrative review of its role in clinical practice, British Journal of Anaesthesia: BJA 122(5):587–604, 2019.

Collins M: A case report on the anxiolytic properties of nitrous oxide during labor, JOGNN 44:87–92, 2014.

Collins M: Nitrous oxide utility in labor and birth: a multipurpose modality, The Journal of Perinatal & Neonatal Nursing 31(2):137–144, 2017.

Eley V, Callaway L, Van Zundert A: Developments in labour analgesia and their use in Australia, Anaesthesia and Intensive Care 43:12–21, 2015.

Finkelstein JL, Layden AJ, Stover PJ: Vitamin B-12 and perinatal health, Advances in Nutrition 6:552–563, 2015.

Grant G: Pharmacologic management of pain during labor and delivery, UpToDate, Wolters Kluwer, 2020. Online 5 September 2021. Available: www.uptodate.com.

Illuzzi JL, Telfer ML, Rubin P: Nitrous oxide's revival in childbirth, Contemporary Ob/gyn 63(5):7–11, 2018.

Jordan S: Pain relief. In Jordan S, editor: Pharmacology for midwives, 2nd ed., Palgrave Macmillan, Basingstoke, 2010.

Klomp T, van Poppel M, Jones L, et al: Inhaled analgesia for pain management in labour, Cochrane Database of Systematic Reviews (9):CD009351, 2012.

Koyyalamudi V, Sidhu G, Cornett E, et al: New labor pain treatment options, Current Pain and Headache Reports 20(2):11.s, 2016.

Likis FE, Andrews JC, Collins MR, et al: Nitrous oxide for the management of labor pain: a systematic review, MIDIRS Midwifery Digest 24:486, 2014.

Migliaccio L, Lawton R, Leeman L, et al: Initiating intrapartum nitrous oxide in an academic hospital: considerations and challenges, Journal of Midwifery & Women's Health 29 May 2017.

Mobaraki N, Yousefian M, Seifi S, et al: A randomized controlled trial comparing use of enthonox with pethidine for pain relief in primigravid women during the active phase of labor, Anesthesiology and Pain Medicine 6(4):E37420, 2016.

Nagele P, Duma A, Kopec M, et al: Nitrous oxide for treatment-resistant major depression: a proof-of-concept trial, Biological Psychiatry 78:10–18, 2014.

Nash S: Vitamin B12 deficiency, British Journal of Midwifery 24(11):763–764, 2016.

National Drug & Alcohol Research Centre (NDARC): Nitrous oxide, 2021. Online 11 April 2021. Available: https://ndarc.med.unsw.edu.au/resource/nitrous-oxide-0.

National Institute for Health and Care Excellence (NICE): Intrapartum care: pain relief in labour, 2017. Online 11 April 2021. Available: www.nice.org.uk.

National Institute for Occupational Safety and Health (NIOSH): Nitrous oxide, 2014. Online 11 April 2021. Available: www.cdc.gov/niosh/topics/nitrousoxide/default.html.

NHS Choices: Vitamin B12 or folate deficiency anaemia, 2016. Online 11 April 2021. Available: www.nhs.uk/conditions/Anaemia-vitamin-B12-and-folate-deficiency/Pages/Introduction.aspx.

O'Sullivan EP: Dr Robert James Minnitt 1889–1974: a pioneer of inhalational analgesia, Journal of the Royal Society of Medicine 82(4):221–222, 1989.

Parsa P, Saeedzadeh N, Roshanaei G, et al: The effect of nitrous oxide on labour pain relief among nulliparous women: A randomized controlled trial, Journal of Clinical and Diagnostic Research 11(3):QC8–QC11, 2017.

Patel HH, Pearn ML, Patel PM, Roth, D: General anesthetics and therapeutic gases. In Brunton LL, Hilal-Dandan R, Knollmann BC, editors: Goodman & Gilman's: The pharmacological basis of therapeutics, 13th ed., McGraw-Hill, New York, 2018.

Pecheli M, Billoet C, Callibotte G: Modelling levels of nitrous oxide exposure for healthcare professionals during EMONO usage, Annals of Occupational and Environmental Medicine 28:30, 2016.

Rooks JP: Labor pain management other than neuraxial: what do we know and where do we go next? Birth 39(4):318–322, 2012.

Safe Work Australia. 2021. Hazardous Chemical Information System (HCIS): Exposure standard documentation, nitrous oxide, 2021. Online 5 September 2021. Available: hcis.safeworkaustralia.gov.au/ExposureStandards/Document?exposureStandardID=453.

Smith A, Laflamme E, Komanecky C, Pain management in labor, American Family Physician 103(6):355–364, 2021.

Stockton L, Simonsen C, Seago S: Nitrous oxide-induced vitamin B12 deficiency, Baylor University Medical Center Proceedings 30(2):171–172, 2017.

Vallejo M, Zakowski M: Pro-con debate: nitrous oxide for labor analgesia, BioMed Research International (1):1–12, 2019.

Zanardo V, Volpe F, Parotto M, et al: Nitrous oxide labor analgesia and pain relief memory in breastfeeding women, The Journal of Maternal–Fetal and Neonatal Medicine 1–22, 2017.

SECTION 6

SKILLS FOR SUPPORTING ANTENATAL WELLBEING

CHAPTER 26

BUILDING A THERAPEUTIC RELATIONSHIP

Learning outcomes

Having read this chapter, the reader should be able to:

- discuss the benefits of a trusting midwife–woman relationship
- discuss the features of a trusting relationship
- describe the steps in developing a trusting midwife–woman relationship.

The relationship a woman has with her midwife is a fundamental aspect of her feeling satisfied with her care (Lundgren & Berg 2007), and a woman-centred relationship wherein her values, preferences and power are taken into account, is advocated (Freeman & Griew 2007). Trust is the key element (Davison et al 2015), regardless of the practice setting (Bradfield et al 2019), because a trustful midwife–woman relationship can 'strengthen a woman's self-esteem and give her security' (Lundgren & Berg 2007). In this chapter, the skills of establishing and maintaining a trusting relationship with a woman that facilitates her to stay in control of decisions regarding her care are considered.

ESTABLISHING A TRUSTING RELATIONSHIP WITH WOMEN

At the heart of its philosophy, the International Confederation of Midwives (ICM) advocates for midwifery care to be provided in partnership with women, and to recognise women's right to self-determination. Midwifery is stated by the ICM to be respectful, personalised and non-authoritarian (ICM 2014), and the value of presence—defined as 'being there' or 'being with'—and of compassion in midwifery have also been identified (Pembroke & Pembroke 2008, Menage et al 2020). This view of how midwifery care should occur provides the basis for how midwives should relate to the women they care for. Since the 1980s the nature of the midwife–woman relationship has been recognised as of paramount importance in ensuring maternal satisfaction (Tinkler & Quinney 1998). Thomson and Downe (2013) concluded that women have more positive experiences when maternity services are designed to maximise authentic relationships based on mutual trust and respect between caregivers, and a midwife–woman relationship itself with trust at its heart has more recently been described as being 'everything' to some women (Davison et al 2015). There can, however, be costs to midwives who develop an empathetic connection with those in their care (see for example Leinweber & Rowe 2010), and this phenomenon is addressed in Chapters 51 and 53.

FEATURES OF A TRUSTING MIDWIFE–WOMAN RELATIONSHIP

Three decades have now passed since Kirby and Slevin (1992) identified the key elements, namely authenticity of being, conscience, commitment, presence, compassion, empathy and empowerment, that are encompassed in effective therapeutic relationships. According to Kirkham (2000), for women the relationship with their midwife or midwives is 'about feeling safe and able', and for midwives it is about enabling women to feel safe and to 'take up their power' (p. 227). More recently, women's perception of a 'good' midwife has been reported to be one who possesses the attributes of 'theoretical knowledge, professional competencies, personal qualities, communication skills and moral values' (Borelli et al 2016, p. 106). The vital importance of a safe, enabled, trusting relationship between midwife and woman is clearly evident when the alternative is considered: in a study exploring the antecedents of emotionally traumatic birth, for example, Thomson and Downe (2008) found fragmented, inadequate and abusive care led to women feeling that their personal values and self-knowledge were not acknowledged; in turn, this resulted in a sense of helplessness and isolation among participants that ultimately left them disconnected from their childbearing experience. Egan (2014, pp. 46–48) asserts that respect must be the foundational value of any trusting relationship, and that to achieve it, the professional should specifically commit to the following respect-demonstrating behaviours:

- doing no harm through either being unprincipled or incompetent
- not rushing to judge
- being committed and competent
- being genuine
- making it clear you are 'for' the client (woman): this is not the same, according to Egan (2014, p. 47) as taking their side; rather it is about taking their point of view seriously
- assuming the client's (woman's) goodwill
- keeping the client's (woman's) agenda in focus
- being empathetic.

As well as being trustworthy, being motivating, empowering and energetic are additional behaviours that have been proposed as valuable strengths for establishing and maintaining trusting relationships, as have the ability to establish rapport, a capacity for impression management, being able to manage emotional intensity, using touch judiciously, and practising cultural competence (Taylor 2008, pp. 21, 177).

Demonstrating respect is also achieved through the practice of active listening, which focuses the attention on the speaker and requires the listener to paraphrase what they have heard in their own words to check their understanding; the effect is to communicate to the listener that they have really been heard and understood (Boyd & Dare 2014, pp. 72–73). The actively listening midwife should:

- face the speaker (see the SOLER skill checklist in Skill 26.1)
- maintain eye contact
- respond appropriately to show understanding by using statements that validate and show support
- minimise external distractions as far as possible to give the speaker full attention
- minimise internal distractions in order to listen with focus to what is being said
- focus solely on the speaker and what they are saying
- engage by asking questions for clarification
- keep an open mind (Boyd & Dare 2014, pp. 74–75).

SKILL 26.1 Establishing a trusting relationship with a woman

Arguably, the most fundamental skill set for conveying respect for the other party in a healthcare relationship is that summarised by the acronym 'SOLER' (Egan 2014, p. 77–78). In midwifery, this means that on meeting with a woman, whatever the context, the midwife should practise these SOLER skills.

1. Face the client (woman) **S**quarely.
2. Adopt an **O**pen posture.
3. Remember that it is possible at times to **L**ean towards the other.
4. Maintain good **E**ye contact (even with women who are visually impaired, who will be able to detect voice direction).
5. Try to be relatively **R**elaxed or natural in the above behaviours.

WORKING WITH WOMEN WITH ADDITIONAL COMMUNICATION NEEDS

Most midwives' practice now includes working with women for whom English is a second language (ESL); midwives may also have women in their care who use sign language due to severe hearing impairment, and occasionally women will attend with both a language and a hearing barrier. In most cases, midwives working with these women will need to use an accredited interpreter (not a family member or friend) to help establish and maintain a relationship (Adams 2002, Kaur et al 2014) and to minimise the increased risk of medical errors and of poor health outcomes to which those with communication barriers are susceptible (Kaur et al 2014). It is also incumbent on all health professionals, including midwives, to demonstrate cultural sensitivity to all those in their care (Cioffi 2004, p. 441), and to be mindful that some refugee and migrant women whose first language is not English may be torture or trauma survivors (Correa-Velez & Ryan 2011). Despite the obvious benefits of using interpreters in healthcare, Kaur et al (2014) note an array of challenges to doing so, which include:

- complication of the relationship between the healthcare service user and the health professional
- the woman being talked about in the third person and excluded from the conversation
- lack of interpreter availability
- cost.

Additionally, although accredited telephone interpreting is likely to be suitable for non-English speaking women, it will not work for those who are hearing impaired; these women require eye contact, clear expression and non-verbal gestures that can only be facilitated by a physically present, face-to-face interpreter (Lieu et al 2007). Regardless of whether the interpreter is present by telephone or in person, there are a number of key messages and points for the health professional to consider (Edwins 2009, p. 125), which are reflected in Skill 26.2.

SKILL 26.2 Working with an interpreter

1. Brief the interpreter before the consultation so they know its purpose and can prepare.
2. Confirm how much time the interpreter has.
3. Establish the terms of confidentiality and who will be told what during and about the consultation. Make sure the woman is aware that everything she says will be heard and passed on to you (and anyone else in the room) by the translator, and that the interpreter will only give advice if they have been asked to pass on that advice provided by you or another health professional who is present.
4. Establish clear boundaries between yourself and the interpreter, as outlined above, and ensure the interpreter reports these to the woman.
5. If it is a face-to-face conversation, ensure the seating is arranged so that you can practise SOLER skills and active listening with the woman.
6. Address the woman, not the interpreter.
7. If you must perform an examination or test, ask the interpreter to explain that you may be quiet or silent for a little while as you do so, but that you will explain your findings once you have finished.

Role and responsibilities of the midwife

These are summarised as:

- knowing and applying best practice
- undertaking the processes of establishing trust and engaging an interpreter correctly
- using SOLER skills appropriately to establish a trusting relationship with women and regularly practising/updating this skill
- maintaining woman-centred care by using an accredited interpreter with women who have an aural barrier to communication
- maintaining woman-centred care by using an accredited interpreter with women who have a language barrier to communication
- performing accurate contemporaneous record keeping.

SUMMARY

- The relationship a woman has with her midwife is a fundamental aspect of the woman feeling satisfied with her care.
- Since the 1980s the nature of the midwife–woman relationship has been recognised as of paramount importance in ensuring maternal satisfaction.
- For women, the relationship with their midwife or midwives is reportedly about feeling safe and able.
- Respect is the foundational value of the midwife–woman relationship.
- On meeting with a woman, whatever the context, the midwife should practise the SOLER skills to convey respect.
- The use of an accredited interpreter is essential when working with women who have a language-related or a hearing-related communication barrier.

Self-assessment exercises

The answers to the following questions may be found in the text.

1. Discuss the features of a trusting midwife–woman relationship.
2. Summarise the role and responsibilities of the midwife in relation to establishing an effective midwife–woman relationship.
3. Describe the different components of the SOLER skill set.
4. Discuss the challenges of using an interpreter with women who have communication difficulties.
5. Describe how to work with an interpreter.

References

Adams K: Making the best use of health advocates and interpreters, British Medical Journal 325(7355):S9a, 2002.

Borelli S, Spiby H, Walsh D: The kaleidoscopic midwife: a conceptual metaphor illustrating first-time mothers' perspectives of a good midwife during childbirth. A grounded theory study. Midwifery, 39:103–111, 2016.

Boyd C, Dare J: Communication skills for nurses, John Wiley & Sons, Chichester, 2014.

Bradfield Z, Kelly M, Hauck Y, Duggan R: Midwives 'with woman' in the private obstetric model: where divergent philosophies meet. Women and Birth: Journal of the Australian College of Midwives April, 32(2):157–167, 2019.

Cioffi J: Caring for women from culturally diverse backgrounds: midwives' experiences, Journal of Midwifery and Women's Health 49(5):437–442, 2004.

Correa-Velez I, Ryan J: Developing a best practise model of refugee maternity care, Women and Birth 25(1):13–22, 2011.

Davison C, Hauck Y, Bayes SJ, et al: The relationship is everything: women's reasons for choosing a privately practising midwife in Western Australia, Midwifery 31:772–778, 2015.

Edwins J: Community midwifery practice, John Wiley & Sons, Chichester, 2009.

Egan G: The skilled helper: a problem-management and opportunity-development approach to helping, 10th ed., Brooks/Cole Cengage Learning, Belmont, CA, 2014.

Freeman L, Griew K: Enhancing the midwife–woman relationship through shared decision making and clinical guidelines, Women and Birth 20:11–15, 2007.

International Confederation of Midwives (ICM): CD2005_001 Core document: Philosophy and model of midwifery care, ICM, The Hague, 2014.

Kaur R, Oakley S, Venn P: Using face-to-face interpreters in healthcare, Nursing Times 110(21):20–21, 2014.

Kirby C, Slevin O: A new curriculum for care. In Slevin O, Buckenham M, eds. Project 2000: The Teachers Speak—Innovations in the Nursing Curriculum, pp. 57–88, Campion Press, Edinburgh, 1992.

Kirkham M: How can we relate? In Kirkham M, ed.: The mother–midwife relationship, Palgrave Macmillan, Basingstoke, 2000.

Leinweber J, Rowe HJ: The costs of 'being with the woman': secondary traumatic stress in midwifery. Midwifery 26(1):76–87, 2010.

Lieu CC, Sadler GR, Fullerton JT, Stohlmann PD: Communication strategies for nurses interacting with deaf patients, Medsurg Nursing 16(4):239–245, 2007.

Lundgren I, Berg M: Central concepts in the midwife–woman relationship, Scandinavian Journal of Caring Sciences 21(2):220–228, 2007.

Menage D, Bailey E, Lees S, Coad J: Women's lived experience of compassionate midwifery: human and professional, Midwifery 85:102662–102662, 2020.

Pembroke, NF, Pembroke, JJ: The spirituality of presence in midwifery care. Midwifery 24(3):321–327, 2008.

Taylor RR: The intentional relationship: occupational therapy and use of self, FA Davis Company, Philadelphia, 2008.

Thomson G, Downe S: A hero's tale of childbirth, Midwifery 29(7):765–771, 2013.

Thomson G, Downe S: Widening the trauma discourse: the link between childbirth and experiences of abuse, Journal of Psychosomatic Obstetrics and Gynaecology 29:268–273, 2008.

Tinkler A, Quinney D: Team midwifery: the influence of the midwife–woman relationship on women's experiences and perceptions of maternity care, Journal of Advanced Nursing 28(1):30–35, 1998.

CHAPTER 27

ABDOMINAL EXAMINATION DURING PREGNANCY

Learning outcomes

Having read this chapter, the reader should be able to:

- outline the reasons for abdominal examination in pregnancy and labour
- specify the elements of an abdominal examination and the rationale for each
- describe how the fetal heart may be auscultated
- outline the midwife's role and responsibilities in relation to this skill.

Abdominal examination is a skill that is used to assess fetal growth during pregnancy, to determine the presentation, position and lie as the pregnancy progresses towards term and at the onset of labour and to auscultate the fetal heart sounds. Palpation of uterine contractions during labour also involves abdominal palpation (see Chapter 31). This chapter considers the skills of abdominal examination during pregnancy, focusing on how and why this is undertaken and the significance of the information obtained. The different ways of assessing the fetal heart rate will also be discussed.

ANTENATAL ABDOMINAL EXAMINATION

At the time of writing (January 2021), both the Department of Health in Australia (2018) and the Royal Australian and New Zealand College of Obstetricians and Gynaecologists (RANZCOG 2019) recommend that antenatal care should include assessment to determine abnormal fetal growth. The Australian Department of Health asserts that a core practice in antenatal care is to 'assess fetal growth' (Department of Health 2018, p. 8), while RANZCOG holds that 'measurement and recording of SFH [symphysial-fundal height] should be a routine part of antenatal visits' and propose this occurs as part of 'routine palpation' (RANZCOG 2019, p. 6). Although research suggests serial symphysis–fundal height assessment is beneficial, there is no strong evidence to recommend it over abdominal palpation for assessing fetal growth, therefore the midwife can use their discretion. Palpation to determine fetal presentation, however, is recommended to be reserved for 36 weeks gestation or later, when it is likely to influence plans for birth (Department of Health 2018). For example, detection of a breech presentation at 36 weeks enables the woman to consider whether she would like to have an external cephalic version attempted at 37 weeks gestation.

Some women may want to know more about which way round the baby is earlier than 36 weeks gestation, and the midwife can provide this information by palpating the abdomen rather than simply measuring SFH, but needs to discuss the significance of doing so at an earlier gestation than recommended and the possibility of the information changing as the pregnancy moves towards term.

Although there is no evidence that auscultation of the fetal heart as part of the abdominal examination at each antenatal visit is beneficial, it is supported in Australia to be offered to women via Doppler from 12 weeks gestation and either Doppler or Pinard stethoscope from 28 weeks' gestation (Department of Health 2018). Regardless of whether the fetal heart is auscultated or not, ongoing discussion with the woman about the importance of them monitoring fetal movements as an indicator of fetal wellbeing should be initiated early in pregnancy, and repeated at every visit thereafter (Department of Health 2018).

To summarise, the recommended components for abdominal examination during pregnancy are assessment of:

- fetal growth by abdominal palpation and/or symphysis–fundal height measurement
- fetal presentation at and beyond 36 weeks.

Antenatal abdominal examination should be conducted:

- as part of each antenatal assessment
- before the fetal heart is auscultated.

Contraindications

Abdominal palpation can stimulate uterine contractions. Therefore, caution should be exercised if the woman is experiencing:

- placental abruption
- preterm labour.

ABDOMINAL EXAMINATION: PRINCIPLES

This examination is not undertaken in isolation but involves consideration of the woman and how she is looking and feeling, and what is revealed through discussion. For example, if the woman describes experiencing indigestion, breathlessness and the fetus pushing under her ribs, the midwife may wonder if the fetus is in a breech presentation.

The procedure should be explained to the woman, particularly that there may be some discomfort associated with it and the rationale for undertaking the procedure, so that her informed consent is obtained. The examination should begin with an exploration of the woman's perception of the growth and movement of the fetus/es, as this is a two-way sharing of information (Blee & Dietsch 2012). The discussion should be continued throughout so the woman is aware of what will be happening and what has been identified, and she is given the opportunity to feel where the head or buttocks are and the position the fetus/es. Nishikawa and Sakakibara (2013) found that this helped increase maternal awareness of the fetal position(s) and increased maternal–fetal attachment. When the procedure is complete, there should be a full discussion of the findings and, if further investigations are required, what they are and why they are needed. The findings and discussion should be documented in the woman's notes.

The woman should be asked to empty her bladder prior to the procedure, as this will be more comfortable for her, and then to lie semirecumbent on an examining couch or similar firm surface. It is preferable for the woman not to lie completely flat because of the risk of aortocaval compression. If for some reason she does need to be flat, a wedge should be placed under her right hip. The woman needs to be comfortable with her arms stretched out and relaxed by her side so that her abdominal muscles relax. This is helped if the room is warm and privacy is ensured; also, the woman may choose to have family or friends present at this time. The woman will need to reposition her clothes so that access to all of her abdomen is possible.

The midwife should wash and dry their hands before and after touching the woman's abdomen; other standard precautions are usually unnecessary unless contact with body fluids is expected. This may also help to warm the midwife's hands, which is more comfortable for the woman.

Visual appearance of the abdomen

The abdomen is inspected at the beginning of the examination as a lot of information can be gleaned from this.

- The size of the abdomen is considered and this can be affected by maternal obesity, lax abdominal muscles causing a pendulous abdomen, multiple pregnancy, poly- and oligohydramnios, fetal size and lie, uterine fibroids and gestation period. The enlarging uterus is often seen abdominally from around 12 weeks and will increase in size as the fetus grows and the amount of amniotic fluid increases.
- The fetal position or presentation may be evident in the shape of the abdomen. For example, a saucer-shaped dip over the woman's umbilicus suggests the fetus is lying with their occiput posteriorly; if the 'bump' is low and broad, it may indicate a transverse lie. Nulliparous women may have a more ovoid appearance to their abdomen than multiparous women, but this can also be very individual. The abdomen often appears symmetrical in shape.
- Observe for any skin changes, such as the linea nigra, stretch marks (new ones, 'striae gravidarum', appear pink/red, while older ones, 'striae albicantes', are silvery-white coloured), signs of previous abdominal surgery (particularly for caesarean section), presence of rashes or itching.
- Fetal movements may be seen.
- Signs of potential domestic abuse (e.g. bruising) may be observed.

Measuring fundal height

Traditionally the **fundal height** was assessed against landmarks on the maternal body—symphysis pubis,

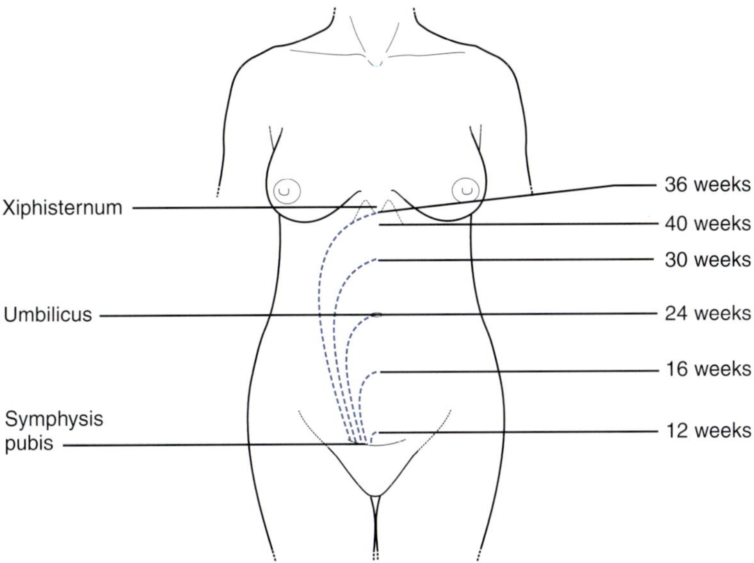

FIGURE 27.1 **Fundal height at different stages during pregnancy.**
Source: Johnson R, Taylor W: Skills for midwifery practice, 4th ed., Elsevier, London, 2016.

umbilicus and xiphisternum (Fig 27.1). This provides an approximation of gestational age, but can be affected by the individual shape of the woman. Serial measurements of the distance between the symphysis pubis and the fundus have been shown to be effective in determining fetal growth, and so this practice is now recommended to be incorporated into routine antenatal care. Despite the evidence for it not being strong, RANZCOG (2019) supports serial measurement of symphysis–fundal height measurement as a routine part of antenatal visits, along with targeted ultrasound where it is deemed necessary. The plotting of these serial measurements on customised charts is practised in other healthcare systems (see, for example, the 'GROW' charts listed under Resources at the end of the chapter), but this is not the case in Australia or New Zealand at the time of writing. Serial measurement of SFH is also recommended to occur at each antenatal appointment by the United Kingdom's Royal College of Obstetricians and Gynaecologists (RCOG 2013) 'from 24 weeks as this improves prediction of a **SGA** [**small for gestational age**] neonate' (p. 2). According to Wright and colleagues (2006) the SFH measurement should ideally be undertaken by the same person each time to reduce inter-observer variation; however, Roex and colleagues (2012) found this not to matter in their study: a significantly higher detection rate of SGA by using serial plotting of SFH measurements was found, even when multiple practitioners with varying levels of experience obtained these measurements.

The SFH is measured in centimetres and each centimetre of growth is commonly thought to equate to an additional week of gestation, with a margin of error of ±2–3 cm. However, Morse and colleagues (2009) caution that this is an erroneous assumption as it does not represent a reliable correlation. For women where this measurement may be inaccurate (e.g. BMI > 35, polyhydramnios, large fibroids), serial assessment of fetal size via ultrasound rather than by SFH is recommended (RCOG 2013).

A fundal height that is higher than expected may indicate:

- inaccurate dates
- that the fetus is larger than expected
- that the amount of amniotic fluid might be greater than expected—polyhydramnios
- multiple pregnancy
- uterine mass (e.g. fibroid, cyst or tumour)
- poor technique.

A fundal height that is shorter than expected may indicate:

- inaccurate dates
- that the fetus is smaller than expected
- that the amount of amniotic fluid is less than expected—oligohydramnios
- abnormal lie (e.g. transverse)
- poor technique
- intrauterine death.

The RCOG (2013) recommend the use of ultrasound measurement for fetal size if there is a single SFH below the 10th centile or if serial measurements demonstrate slow or static growth by crossing centiles. This is important as clinical estimation of fetal weight for babies > 4.0 kg or < 2.5 kg by palpation is not very accurate (Levin et al 2011).

SKILL 27.1 Obtaining the symphysis–fundal height measurement

1. Discuss the procedure with the woman and gain her informed consent.
2. Encourage the woman to empty her bladder.
3. Gather equipment:
   - single-use tape measure
   - sheet, if needed
   - antenatal record.
4. Ask the woman to lie semirecumbent with her arms relaxed at her sides, knees slightly bent, and expose her abdomen, using the sheet to cover her legs if necessary and ensuring privacy.
5. Wash and dry your hands.
6. Locate the top of the fundus and place a non-stretchable tape measure facedown to avoid observer bias, so that 0 cm is on the top of the fundus.
7. Keeping the tape measure in contact with the skin, place it along the longitudinal axis of the uterus, without correcting to the midline of abdomen, until the top of the symphysis pubis is reached.
8. Note where this is on the tape measure and record the measurement in centimetres.
9. The measurement should only be taken once and documented on the customised growth chart.
10. Assist the woman to recover and adopt a comfortable position.
11. Wash and dry hands.
12. Discuss the findings with the woman and refer as necessary.

Palpation

As pregnancy progresses, or upon maternal request, a full abdominal palpation comprising a fundal, lateral and pelvic palpation can be undertaken to assess the presentation, lie and position of the fetus and, if requested, to auscultate the fetal heart sounds. The order of the palpation can vary; however, many midwives begin at the fundus, undertake the lateral palpation and end with the pelvic palpation, whereas others will palpate the fundus, then the pelvic palpation with the lateral palpation last. The order is less important than the technique.

Fundal palpation

Fundal palpation is undertaken to determine which pole is in the upper part of the uterus—usually the breech is felt here when the presentation is cephalic, and if the breech is presenting, the head will be felt in the fundus. The woman continues to lie in the position adopted for measuring the SFH. The midwife should be facing the woman so that she can make eye contact and assess verbal and non-verbal communication for signs of discomfort. The midwife places her hand on the top of the woman's abdomen, below the xiphisternum, as described earlier, to find the top of the fundus. When the fundus is felt, the palmar sides of the fingers of both hands are placed on either side of the fundus and gentle pressure applied as the fingers curve around to palpate what is beneath them (Fig 27.2). The buttocks often appear broad, irregular, softer, bulkier and difficult to move, whereas the head is firm, smooth, more rounded and ballotable; that is, it can be moved gently from side to side between the hands (this will not happen if there is a breech presentation with extended legs). If no pole is felt in the fundus, it is likely to be due to a transverse lie (Fig 27.3).

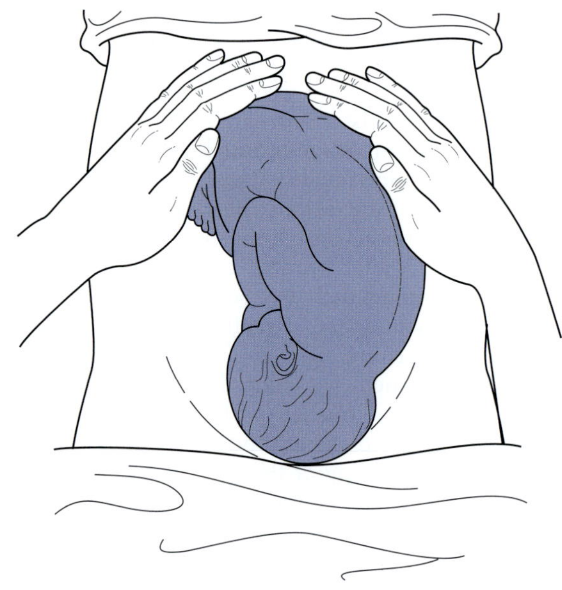

FIGURE 27.2 **Fundal palpation.**
Source: Johnson R, Taylor W: Skills for midwifery practice, 4th ed., Elsevier, London, 2016.

Pelvic palpation

The presentation is the part of the fetus lying in the lower segment of the uterus, at or within the pelvic brim. This is determined by **pelvic palpation**, which may also assess the degree of flexion or extension (in conjunction with the lateral palpation), the degree of engagement and if the presenting part has not engaged, whether or not it is movable (Fig 27.4A & B).

There are five main presentations (Fig 27.5) and two methods of performing a pelvic palpation. Care should be taken to avoid causing the woman discomfort; it

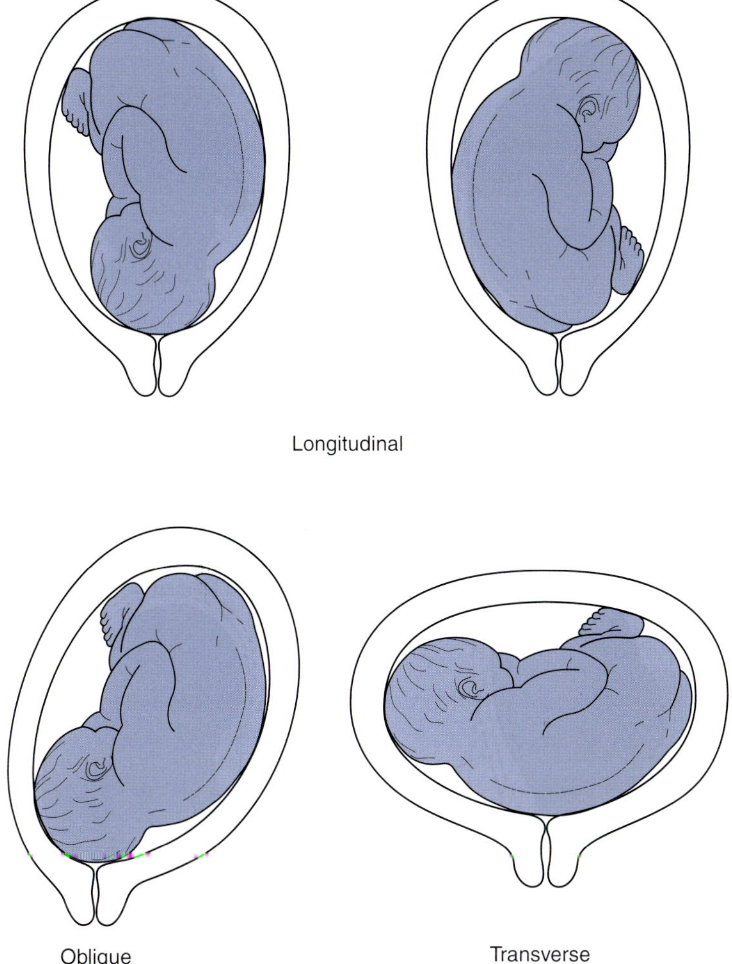

FIGURE 27.3 **The lie of the fetus.**
Source: Johnson R, Taylor W: Skills for midwifery practice, 4th ed., Elsevier, London, 2016.

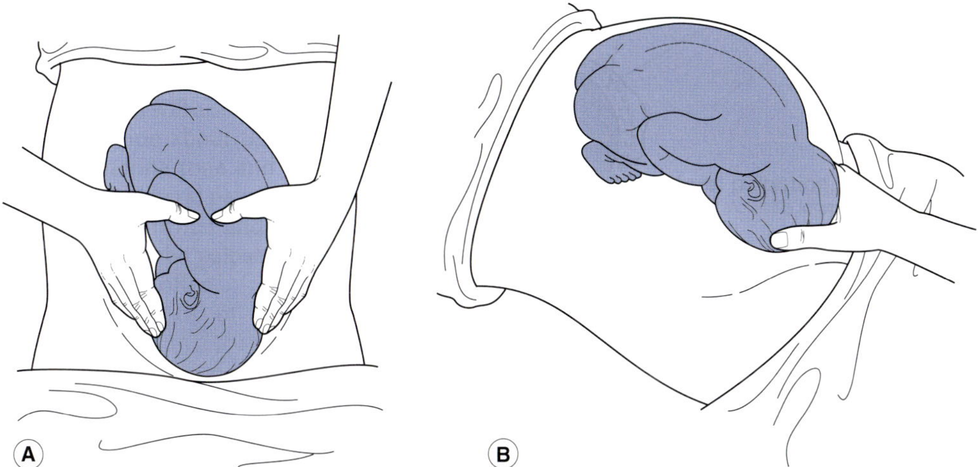

FIGURE 27.4 **A, Pelvic palpation: the fingers are directed inwards and downwards. B, Pawlik's manoeuvre.**
Source: Johnson R, Taylor W: Skills for midwifery practice, 4th ed., Elsevier, London, 2016.

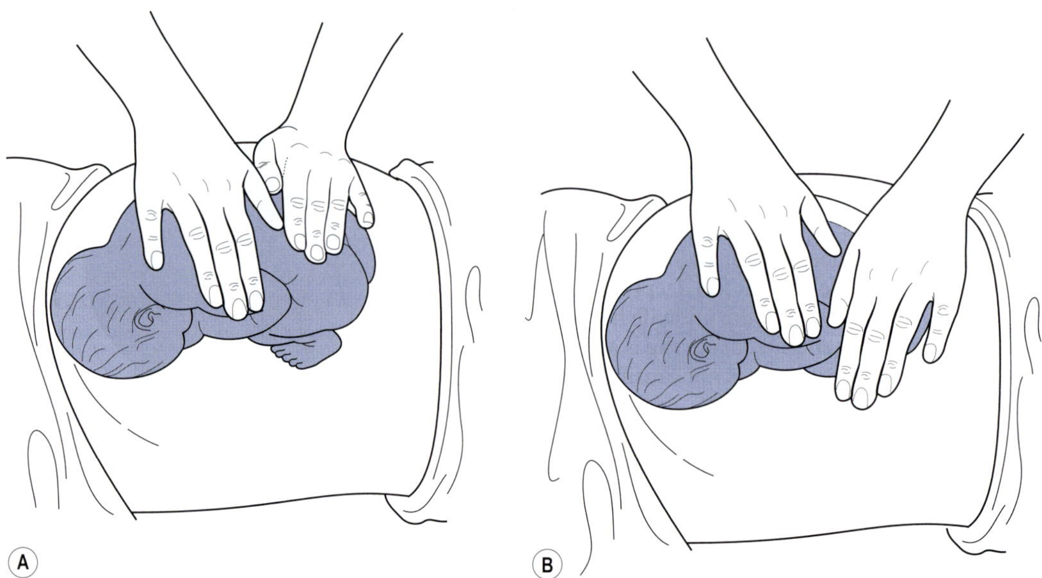

FIGURE 27.7 **'Walking' the fingertips across the abdomen to locate the fetal back.**
Source: Johnson R, Taylor W: Skills for midwifery practice, 4th ed., Elsevier, London, 2016.

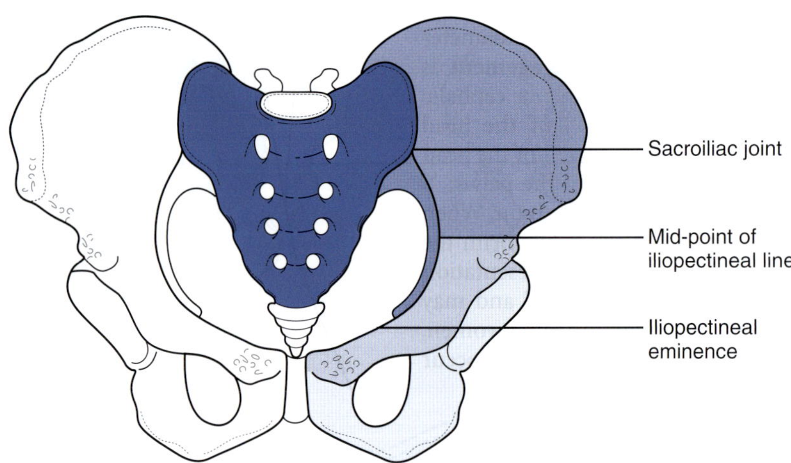

FIGURE 27.8 **Relevant landmarks on the pelvic brim.**
Source: Johnson R, Taylor W: Skills for midwifery practice, 4th ed., Elsevier, London, 2016.

The position is defined according to the position of the fetal denominator (a fixed point on the presentation; e.g. occiput for cephalic presentation, sacrum for breech presentation) to a pelvic landmark. Figure 27.8 indicates the relevant landmarks on the pelvic brim. For example, if the occiput is in apposition with the iliopectineal eminence of the pelvis, the position is described as occipitoanterior (Fig 27.9). It is further defined according to whether it is on the maternal left or right. If the occiput is in apposition with the sacroiliac joint, it is described as occipitoposterior. For occipitolateral, the occiput is found midway on the iliopectineal line (Fig 27.9). The occiput may also be at the front or back of the pelvis—referred to as a direct occipitoanterior or direct occipitoposterior position.

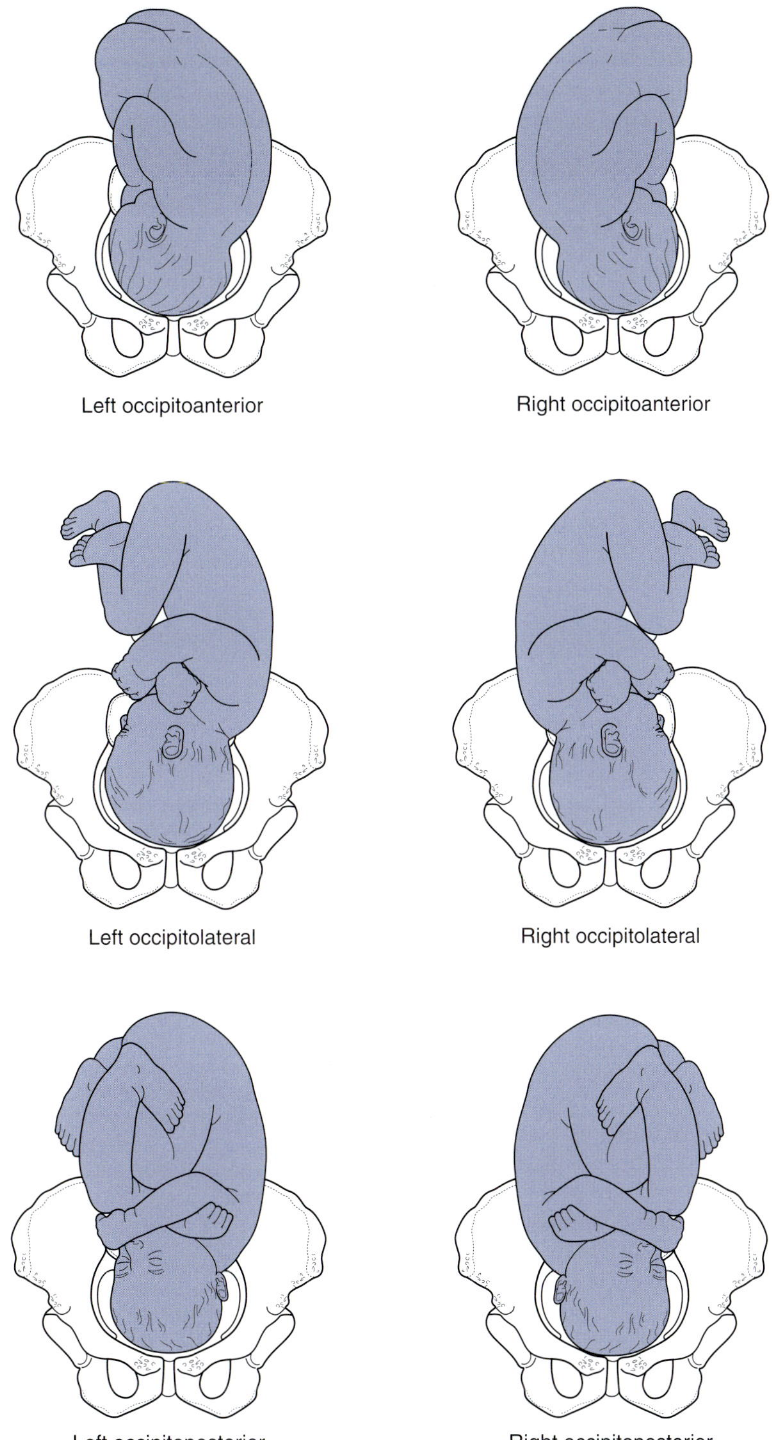

FIGURE 27.9 **Six positions in a vertex presentation.**
Source: Johnson R, Taylor W: Skills for midwifery practice, 4th ed., Elsevier, London, 2016.

SKILL 27.2 Abdominal examination

1. Establish the woman's health and wellbeing; discuss her thoughts (e.g. fetal movements, growth, possible position).
2. Discuss the procedure with the woman and gain her informed consent.
3. Encourage the woman to empty her bladder.
4. Gather equipment:
   - single-use tape measure
   - if needed, watch with a second-hand
   - Pinard stethoscope or fetal Doppler
   - conduction gel
   - tissues
   - sheet, if needed
   - antenatal record.
5. Ask the woman to lie semirecumbent with her arms relaxed at her sides, knees slightly bent, and expose her abdomen, using the sheet to cover her legs if necessary and ensuring privacy.
6. Wash and dry hands.
7. Undertake fundal palpation and use the tape measure to assess symphysis–fundal height (see earlier); undertake lateral and pelvic palpations if gestation > 36 weeks or maternal request (see earlier).
8. If requested or indicated, auscultate the fetal heart while simultaneously palpating the maternal radial pulse (described in the next section).
9. Assist the woman to replace her clothing and to move into a comfortable position then discuss the findings with her.
10. Wash and dry your hands.
11. Document the findings and act accordingly.

Auscultation of the fetal heart

In the presence of normal fetal movements, there is limited value in routinely auscultating the fetal heart rate during the antenatal visit. However, during pregnancy auscultation should be undertaken for 1 full minute:

- prior to the application of a CTG monitor
- to determine fetal life in the event of absence of fetal movements
- upon maternal request.

During pregnancy, if there is an indication to auscultate the fetal heart sounds, this can be undertaken using a Pinard stethoscope, with Doppler ultrasound or, where continuous monitoring is indicated, through the use of a CTG.

The heart rate should be recorded as a single rate rather than a range and any accelerations or decelerations heard should be noted. In the presence of a fetal heart rate abnormality (e.g. deceleration, bradycardia) the maternal pulse should be palpated to determine whether fetal or maternal heart rate sounds are heard.

Ideally, an abdominal palpation should precede fetal heart auscultation, as this will assist with locating the best position to listen to the fetal heart. Maternal anxiety will be unnecessarily heightened if the midwife 'guesses' where to place the equipment to hear the fetal heart and has to keep moving it around because an abdominal palpation was omitted. The clearest fetal heart sounds are heard though the fetal shoulder (scapula), although they can sometimes be heard through the fetal chest wall depending on the fetal position. The fetal heartbeat is heard as a rapid double beating (often rather like a tapping sound) between 110–160 beats per minute (bpm) with increases in the rate noted with fetal movements.

Skills for auscultating the fetal heart by Pinard stethoscope, by Doppler ultrasound and by CTG are found in Chapter 33.

Role and responsibilities of the midwife

These can be summarised as:

- knowing and applying current evidence-based practice
- undertaking all procedures correctly
- performing appropriate abdominal examination procedures and regularly practising/updating this skill
- educating, advising and supporting the woman
- undertaking accurate contemporaneous record keeping
- seeking consultation and referral for deviations from normal.

SUMMARY

- Abdominal assessment antenatally and in labour is a skill from which significant information can be gained.
- Accurate measurement of the symphysis–fundal height and plotting this on a customised chart can help to detect slow or static fetal growth.
- The midwife has a responsibility to undertake the abdominal examination competently and sensitively, document the findings and make a referral when necessary. It is more uncomfortable for women when in labour.
- The fetal heart can be auscultated using a Pinard stethoscope, fetal Doppler or CTG monitor. It is always preceded by an abdominal examination.

- CTG monitors should be applied correctly and the trace interpreted accordingly.
- Palpation of uterine contractions in labour assesses the frequency, strength, length and resting tone of the uterus. It is a significant aspect of labour care.

Self-assessment exercises

The answers to the following questions may be found in the text.

1. Describe the different components of an abdominal examination.
2. Discuss the rationale for each aspect of an abdominal examination.
3. Describe how to measure the symphysis–fundal height.
4. Discuss the different ways the fetal heart rate is auscultated.
5. Summarise the role and responsibilities of the midwife in relation to abdominal examination.

Resources

Perinatal Institute, Fetal growth: 'GROW' charts 2018. Available: www.perinatal.org.uk.

References

Blee D, Dietsch E: Women's experience of the abdominal palpation in pregnancy; a glimpse into the philosophical and midwifery literature, New Zealand College of Midwives Journal 46:21–25, 2012.

Department of Health, Clinical practice guidelines: Pregnancy care (2019 Edition), Australian Government, Department of Health, Canberra, 2018. Online 26 January 2021. Available: www.health.gov.au/sites/default/files/pregnancy-care-guidelines_0.pdf.

Levin I, Gamzu R, Buchman V, et al: Clinical estimation of fetal weight: is accuracy acquired with professional experience? Fetal Diagnosis and Therapy 29(4):321–324, 2011.

Morse K, Williams A, Gardosi J: Fetal growth screening by fundal height measurement, best practice and research, Clinical Obstetrics and Gynaecology 23:809–818, 2009.

Nishikawa M, Sakakibara H: Effect of nursing intervention program using abdominal palpation of Leopold's maneuvers on maternal-fetal attachment, Reproductive Health 10:12, 2013.

Roex A, Nikpoor P, van Eerd E, et al: Serial plotting on customised fundal height charts results in doubling of the antenatal detection of small for gestational age fetuses in nulliparous women, Australian and New Zealand Journal of Obstetrics and Gynaecology 52:78–82, 2012.

Royal Australian and New Zealand College of Obstetricians and Gynaecologists (RANZCOG): Routine antenatal assessment in the absence of pregnancy complications, RANZCOG, East Melbourne, 2019. Online 26 January 2021. Available: www.rcog.org.uk/en/guidelines-research-services/guidelines/gtg31/

Royal College of Obstetricians and Gynaecologists (RCOG): Green-top Guideline No. 31 2013, The investigation and management of the small–for–gestational–age fetus. Online 23 March 2018. Available: www.rcog.org.uk/globalassets/documents/guidelines/gtg_31.pdf.

Wright J, Morse K, Kady S, et al: Audit of fundal height measurement plotted on customized growth charts, MIDIRS Midwifery Digest 16(3):341–345, 2006.

CHAPTER 28

INTERPROFESSIONAL WORKING TO OPTIMISE WOMEN'S ANTENATAL CARE

Learning outcomes

Having read this chapter, the reader should be able to:

- discuss the role of the interprofessional team in providing optimum care for the woman in the antenatal period
- describe the professional role of the midwife in the process of collaboration, consultation and referral of a childbearing woman
- explain the process of collaboration, consultation and referral of a childbearing woman.

Childbearing is a normal physiological event; however, for some women it may be or become physiologically, socially and/or psychologically complicated. Where this is the case, the midwife may need to refer to or consult with another healthcare professional. The interprofessional team then works together to provide the woman with care throughout her pregnancy and beyond if necessary. This chapter will outline the interprofessional collaboration between midwives, childbearing women and other members of the healthcare team; potential barriers to interprofessional antenatal care; and the possible implications for the childbearing woman and her fetus.

WHAT IS INTERPROFESSIONAL CARE?

Interprofessional care, collaborative care and multidisciplinary team care in relation to pregnancy are all interchangeable terms and simply refer to a group of healthcare professionals working together to provide a woman and her family with holistic care (Chamberlain-Salaun et al 2013). As well as midwives, other healthcare professionals that may be involved in a woman's care include an obstetrician, general practitioner (GP), social worker, physiotherapist, dietitian and/or clinical psychologist.

Interprofessional care may be required throughout a woman's pregnancy. The need for consultation with or referral to another healthcare professional may occur at any time in the pregnancy when complex issues arise. In this case, where the midwife has been the primary or lead caregiver, they remain so, while working closely with the interprofessional team to provide the woman with optimum care (Australian College of Midwives [ACM] 2021).

INTERPROFESSIONAL MIDWIFERY CARE

All women have the right to receive accurate, unbiased, evidence-based information to enable educated choices to be made about their maternity care. All women have the right to accept or decline care or referral. The Pregnancy Care Guidelines published by

Australia's Department of Health (2020) endorse the need, as identified by the Australian Health Ministers' Advisory Council (AHMAC) in 2008, 'for maternity services to work within collaborative and consultative frameworks, to more closely match services to women's needs, preferences and expectations'. The guidelines cite the National Health and Medical Research Council (NHMRC 2010) definition of collaboration as 'a dynamic process of facilitating communication, trust and pathways that enable health professionals to provide safe, woman-centred care [and that] enables women to be active participants in their care'. The NHMRC (2010) document from which the Australian Department of Health draws its pregnancy care guidance details nine principles of maternity collaboration.

1. Maternity care collaboration places the woman at the centre of her own care, while supporting the professionals who are caring for her (her carers). Such care is coordinated according to the woman's needs, including her cultural, emotional, psychosocial and clinical needs.
2. Collaboration enables women to choose care that is based on the best evidence and is appropriate for themselves and for their local environment.
3. Collaboration enables women to make informed decisions by ensuring that they are given information about all of their options. This information should be based on the best evidence, and agreed to and endorsed by professional and consumer groups.
4. Collaborating professionals, regardless of the model of care, establish a clearly defined and inclusive reciprocal communication strategy using sensitive language to support professional trust.
5. Collaboration has an underpinning safety and quality framework that includes monitoring health outcomes for mothers and babies, regular multidisciplinary discussions about how the collaboration is working (involving women who have used the service) and public reporting.
6. Collaborating professionals respect and value each other's roles, provide support to each other in their work and provide education to meet each other's needs.
7. Collaboration is committed to joint education and training, following a consistent, agreed care plan and research focused on improving outcomes.
8. Collaboration aims to maximise a woman's continuity of care and carer, throughout pregnancy, birth and the early postnatal period.
9. Collaboration aims to maximise a woman's continuity of carer by providing a clear description of roles and responsibilities to support the person that a woman nominates to coordinate her care (her 'maternity care coordinator') (NHMRC 2010, p. 2).

The NHMRC document also lists a number of key elements of maternity care collaboration (NHMRC 2010, p. 2). These include:

- woman-centred care and communication
- communication among professionals
- awareness of disciplines and autonomy
- responsibility and accountability
- cooperation and coordination
- mutual trust and respect
- policy, procedures and protocols
- interprofessional learning
- organisational support systems.

In New Zealand, the lead maternity carer (LMC) or midwifery-led model was established in the Section 88 Primary Maternity Services Notice in 2007 and updated in 2021 (Ministry of Health 2021). The responsibilities of the LMC are specified in the Primary Maternity Services Notice 2021 (New Zealand Government 2021). Currently, each pregnant woman chooses her LMC, who can be a midwife, GP or specialist, such as an obstetrician; in most cases it is state-funded. The LMC is responsible for the coordination of care in pregnancy, labour and birth and up to 6 weeks postnatal. In this role, the midwife will act as the case manager and provide care in collaboration with specialists in low- and high-risk situations (New Zealand Government 2021).

Midwifery care is bound by core competency standards. The Midwife Standards for Practice (Australia) (Box 28.1) (National Midwifery Board of Australia [NMBA)] 2018) and the Competencies for Entry to the Register of Midwives (New Zealand) (Box 28.2) (Midwifery Council of New Zealand [MCNZ)] 2007) are used to assess performance and enable initial and ongoing registration as a midwife. The competency standards are specific to interprofessional collaboration.

GUIDELINES FOR AUSTRALIAN MIDWIVES WHO NEED TO CONSULT OR REFER

Midwives in Australia

Guidance for Australian midwives in relation to consultation and referral was first developed by the Australian College of Midwives in 2004; their purpose was, and remains, to assist midwives to integrate clinical judgement in providing evidence-based midwifery care to women in the public and private sectors. The guidelines were well received and are now used across most maternity services across Australia. The latest version of the guidelines (September 2021), like previous versions, is the result of review by a range of stakeholders.

The Australian National Midwifery Guidelines for Consultation and Referral (2021) are intended to:

> provide clear guidance to midwives across all practice contexts. They detail the clinical indications for engagement of other health care professionals in the care of women, babies and families. Importantly, they reflect the scope of the midwife and the importance of midwives in maintaining high-quality maternity

Box 28.1 Midwife Standards for Practice (Australia)

Standard 2

Engages in professional relationships and respectful partnerships

The midwife establishes and maintains professional relationships with the woman by engaging purposefully in kind, compassionate and respectful partnerships. The midwife will also engage in professional relationships with other health practitioners, colleagues and/or members of the public. These relationships are conducted within a context of collaboration, mutual trust, respect and cultural safety.

The midwife:

2.1 supports the choices of the woman, with respect for families and communities in relation to maternity care
2.2 partners with women to strengthen women's capabilities and confidence to care for themselves and their families
2.3 practises ethically, with respect for dignity, privacy, confidentiality, equity and justice
2.4 practises without the discrimination that may be associated with race, age, disability, sexuality, gender identity, relationship status, power relations and/or social disadvantage
2.5 practises cultural safety that is holistic, free of bias and exposes racism
2.6 practises in a way that respects that family and community underpin the health of Aboriginal and/or Torres Strait Islander Peoples
2.7 develops, maintains and concludes professional relationships in a way that differentiates the boundaries between professional and personal relationships, and
2.8 participates in and/or leads collaborative practice.

Source: National Midwifery Board of Australia (NMBA): Midwifery Standards for Practice, 2018. Available: www.nursingmidwiferyboard.gov.au/codes-guidelines-statements/professional-standards/midwife-standards-for-practice.aspx. Please see www.nursingmidwiferyboard.gov.au for the most up-to-date information.

Box 28.2 Competencies for Entry to the Register of Midwives (New Zealand)

Competency 2

The midwife applies comprehensive theoretical and scientific knowledge with the affective and technical skills needed to provide effective and safe midwifery care.

Selected performance criteria:

The midwife:

2.3 assesses the health and wellbeing of the woman/wāhine and her baby/tamaiti throughout pregnancy, recognising any condition which necessitates consultation with or referral to another midwife, medical practitioner or other health professional
2.6 identifies factors in the woman/wāhine or her baby/tamaiti during labour and birth which indicate the necessity for consultation with, or referral to, another midwife or a specialist medical practitioner
2.7 provides and is responsible for midwifery care when a woman's/wāhine pregnancy, labour, birth or postnatal care necessitates clinical management by a medical practitioner
2.12 assesses the health and wellbeing of the woman/wāhine and baby/tamaiti throughout the postnatal period and identifies factors which indicate the necessity for consultation with or referral to another midwife, medical practitioner, or other health practitioner
2.18 collaborates and cooperates with other health professionals, community groups and agencies when necessary.

Source: Midwifery Council of New Zealand (MCNZ): Competencies for Entry to the Register of Midwives, 2007, pp. 2–3. Available: www.midwiferycouncil.health.nz/common/Uploaded%20files/Registration/Competencies%20for%20entry%20to%20the%20Register.pdf.

> care. Furthermore, they highlight that a midwife's engagement in the care of women and families is always indicated.
>
> (ACM 2021, p. 4)

The Guidelines are organised into four sections:

1. Indications at the commencement of care
2. Clinical indications developed or identified during the antepartum period
3. Clinical indications during the intrapartum period
4. Clinical indications during the postpartum period (ACM 2021, p. 17).

Guidelines for New Zealand midwives were first appended to the Section 88 Maternity Service Notice 2002 (Ministry of Health 2021). The Guidelines for Consultation with Obstetric and Related Specialists Medical Services (Referral Guidelines) were developed in 2007 by the Ministry of Health, and revised and updated in 2012 with the assistance of a working group that included midwives, researchers, the midwifery advisers and representatives from the consumer council and various medical colleges (Ministry of Health 2012). The referral guidelines are 'based on best practice and are informed by available evidence, expert opinion and current circumstances in New Zealand' (Ministry of Health 2012, p. 1).

The guidelines are organised into four sections:

1. a primary condition
2. a consultation condition
3. a transfer condition
4. an emergency condition (Ministry of Health 2012, p. 5).

Three levels of consultation and referral: Australia

The guidelines (ACM 2021) provide for promotion of care based on the principle of close mutual cooperation between primary-, secondary- or tertiary-level maternity caregivers and the woman involved. When a variance from normal is identified during a woman's care, the ACM (2021) recommends that the midwife uses their clinical judgement and the guidance to determine the appropriate course of action. There are four levels of consultation and referral.

- **A/A*—Discuss.** When a woman presents with indications listed under Level A or A*, care is provided by the midwife. 'Discuss' refers to the midwife's responsibility to initiate a (documented) discussion with the woman at the commencement of care to seek clinically relevant information, understand the woman's needs and preferences, and plan ongoing care. (Note: the midwife may discuss clinical situations with a midwifery colleague, medical practitioner and/or healthcare provider, but this is not indicated.)
- **B—Consult.** When a woman presents with indications listed under Level B, the midwife is guided to consult with a relevant medical practitioner or other healthcare provider with the woman's informed consent.
- **C—Refer.** When a woman presents with indications listed under Level C, the midwife is guided to refer her and/or her baby to a relevant medical practitioner or other healthcare provider with the woman's informed consent.
- **Appendix A** and **Appendix B** are provided for midwives' guidance and use when a woman declines proposed care, consultation or referral (ACM 2021, pp. 53–65).

Regardless of the nature or level of discussion, consultation or referral, communication between members of the multidisciplinary team about changes to care plans should always include the woman and be clearly documented and communicated to all parties involved (ACM 2021, pp. 21–23).

Case Study

You are an independent midwife and you have been contacted by Awhina who is a G1P0 (gravida 1 para 0; pregnant for first time and hasn't given birth) and has a body mass index (BMI) of 45 and would like to have a home birth. How do you approach this sensitive topic and fulfil your professional responsibilities as a midwife?

When a woman chooses care outside the guidelines: Australia

In keeping with a woman-centred approach to maternity care that has informed consent at its foundation, the Australian Guidelines also provide for women who decline suggested or recommended care. The final part in the document (Appendix A and B), is designed to assist midwives in continuing to provide midwifery care when a woman chooses a course of action against advice or outside the guidelines.

The guidelines also provide for a midwife to either continue care when a woman has chosen a course of action outside midwifery standards of practice, or to withdraw from the arrangement if she or he feels unable to continue (Australian College of Midwives 2021, pp. 53–65).

Case Study

Despite your best education and information, Awhina has decided against your recommended care. What do you do and what documentation would you need to complete?

NEW ZEALAND CONSULTATION AND REFERRAL GUIDELINES

In New Zealand, the Ministry of Health has developed Guidelines for Consultation with Obstetric and Related Medical Services (Referral Guidelines), similar to those of the Australian College of Midwives (Ministry of Health 2012). These provide LMCs with clear guidance on referral and consultation procedures and 'previously appended to the Section 88 Maternity Services Notice 2002, are to be used in conjunction with the Primary Maternity Services Notice 2007' (Ministry of Health 2012, p. i).

The Referral Guidelines are based on best practice and are informed by available evidence, expert opinion and current local circumstances. The stated purpose of the guidelines is an intention to:

1. improve maternity care safety and quality
2. improve the consistency of consultation, transfer and transport services

3. give confidence to women, their families and whānau, and other practitioners if a primary healthcare or specialist consultation, or a transfer of clinical responsibility is required
4. promote and support coordination of care across providers (Ministry of Health 2012, p. 1).

Four categories in consultation and referral: New Zealand

The Guidelines (Ministry of Health 2012) define four categories of referral and consequent action. These categories are primary, consultation, transfer and emergency. Primary referral refers to the LMC discussing with the woman that consultation with another healthcare provider, medical practitioner or midwife may be required. Consultation referral is where the LMC recommends to the woman that a consultation with a specialist is required; this may result in the transfer of clinical responsibility. Transfer referral is when the care is transferred to a specialist. Decisions must then be made as to the ongoing responsibility and the role of the LMC. Emergency referral is the immediate transfer of care in response to an emergency; this may result in the emergency transport of the woman or baby via road or air. At all times the woman must be involved in decisions with her care and all information must be documented.

Case Study

You are the LMC for Mary who is 38 weeks pregnant and she has recently confided in you that she has genital herpes. Is referral necessary? If so, what type?

When a woman chooses care outside the guidelines: New Zealand

The Code of Health and Disability Consumers' Rights in New Zealand (Parliamentary Counsel Office 1996) states in Right 7 Right to make an informed choice and give informed consent (p. 5) that consumers have the right to make an informed choice and give informed consent, including the right to refuse medical treatment. 'This means that a woman can choose to decline treatment, referral to another practitioner or transfer of clinical responsibility' and 'in the event a woman chooses to decline, the LMC must advise, explain, share and document' (Ministry of Health 2012, p. 18). The woman must be *advised* of her recommended care; have it *explained* to her to consider discussing her care with another midwife, specialist or experienced mentor; and the resulting outcome must be *shared* with the woman; and finally, the care, discussion, recommendations and decisions made all *documented* (Ministry of Health 2012, p. 18).

Case Study

Kikyo is a G2P3 (third pregnancy, two live babies) and is currently 41 weeks pregnant; as she will soon be 'post-dates' you have referred her to an obstetrician for review. Kikyo refuses to attend the appointment, telling you that all her other babies have come by themselves at 42 weeks. What do you do?

WHEN IS REFERRAL NECESSARY IN AUSTRALIA AND NEW ZEALAND?

Referral may take place at any stage of the woman's pregnancy (e.g. when there is PV [vaginal] bleeding); when in labour (e.g. prolonged rupture of membranes); during birth (e.g. postpartum haemorrhage [PPH]); or in the postpartum period (e.g. postnatal depression [PND]). The reasons for referral are extensive and can be found by accessing the Australian and New Zealand guidelines (see References).

MAKING A REFERRAL

When maternity care is referred to another healthcare professional, the woman must give consent prior to the transfer of care. The midwife may continue to provide midwifery care within their scope of practice in collaboration with the other healthcare professional. At all times, the woman must be involved in the changes to her care; this should be clearly communicated to her and documented.

When a referral is deemed necessary and consent has been given, it is recommended the midwife provide a referral letter. This letter should contain information regarding:

- demographics
- current clinical information
- past medical history if appropriate
- the midwife's contact details.

The midwife must also state that care will be continued by the midwife in a collaborative manner.

A sample referral letter can be found in Appendix B, National Guidelines for Consultation and Referral (Australian College of Midwives 2021).

Case Study

Sarah is a currently 24 weeks pregnant in her sixth pregnancy, having had five live-born babies previously (G6P5); she has an uneventful obstetric history, birthing all babies vaginally. She has contacted the rural Midwifery Group Practice (MGP) in the small country town where she lives, which is 2 hours away from the metropolitan area. Can the MGP accept her for midwifery-led care? If not, what level or category of your country's guidelines does Sarah fit into?

The MGP team decides that Sarah is not suitable for midwifery-led care. Write a referral letter to the metropolitan hospital, explaining your decision to transfer care.

SKILL 28.1 The process of referral

The steps midwives should take when referring a woman to another health professional are outlined in Figures 28.1 and 28.2.

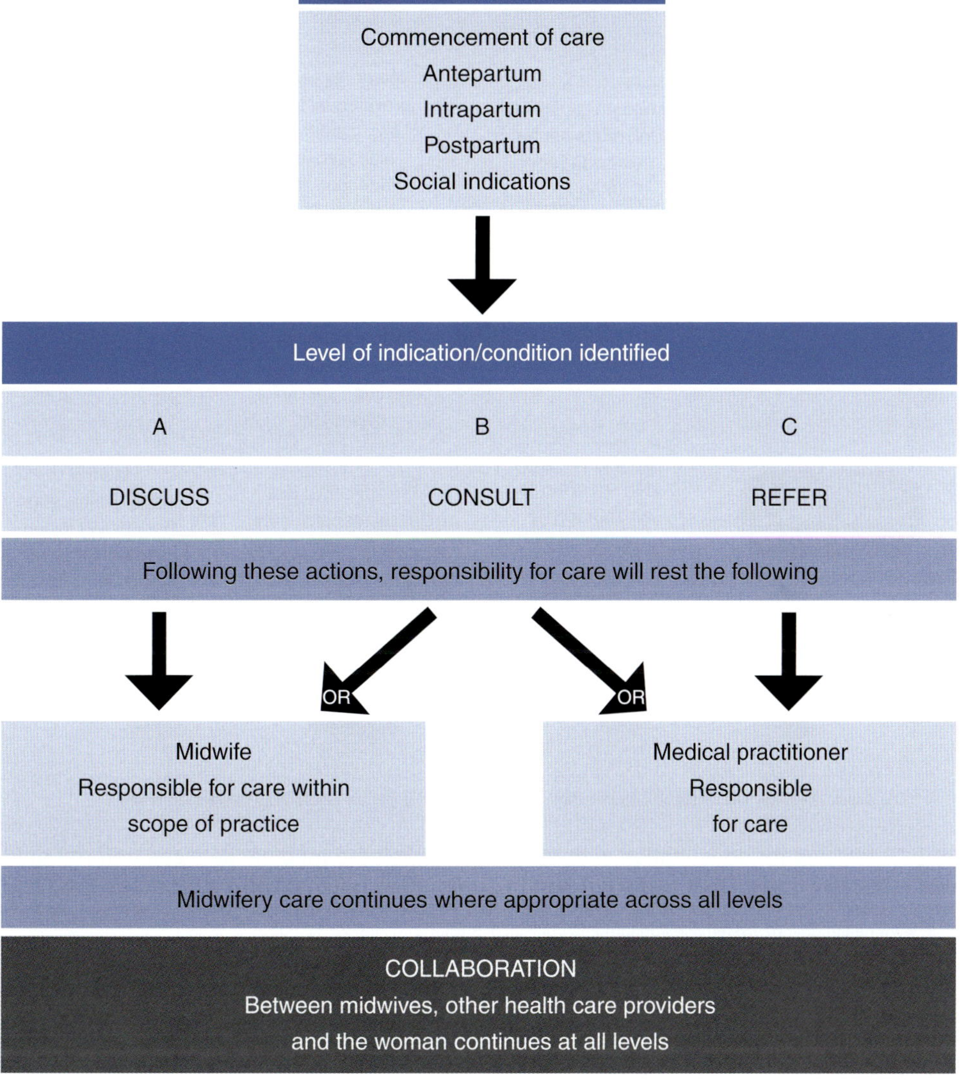

FIGURE 28.1 National Midwifery Guidelines for Consultation and Referral. Australian College of Midwives, 2021.

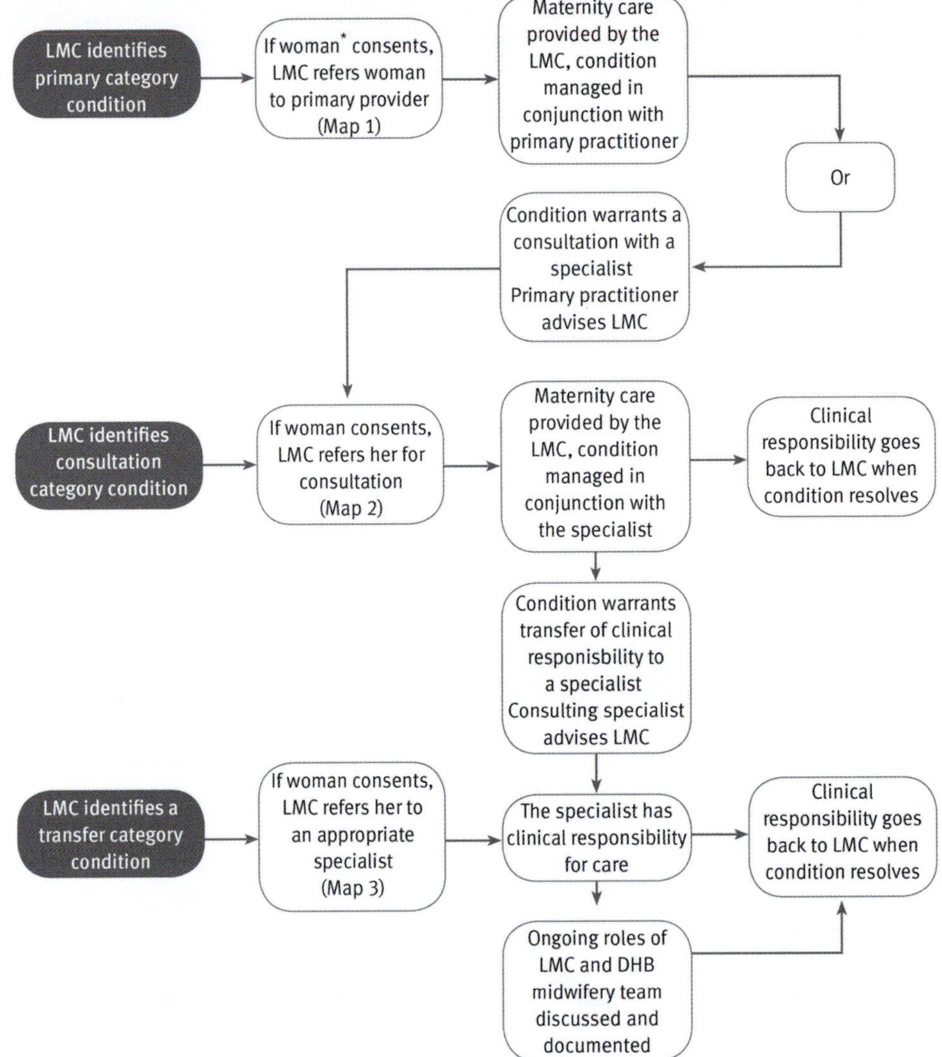

* The woman, her baby and family/whānau (as defined by the woman) are at the centre of all conversations and decisions about her care.

FIGURE 28.2 **Guidelines for consultation with obstetric and related medical services (referral guidelines). LMC = lead maternity carer; DHB = district health board. (See original source for maps 1–3.)**
Source: Ministry of Health: Guidelines for Consultation with Obstetric and Related Medical Services (Referral Guidelines), 2012. Online 6 June 2018. Available: www.health.govt.nz/system/files/documents/publications/referral-glines-jan12.pdf.

Role and responsibilities of the midwife

These can be summarised as:

- identifying the need for interprofessional collaboration
- advising and educating the woman of the care recommended
- documenting the process
- discussing and planning future care.

SUMMARY

- Interprofessional collaboration between midwives, childbearing women and other healthcare team members throughout pregnancy, labour and the postnatal period is often required when care changes from low risk to a high-risk status
- Midwives must be able to recognise when the care required is outside the midwife's scope of practice.
- Midwives need to understand the process of collaboration, consultation and referral.

Self-assessment exercises

The answers to the following questions may be found in the text.

1. What are three conditions that may arise in pregnancy that may require referral?
2. What is the process of referral?
3. What is the midwife's responsibly if the woman declines referral?

References

Australian College of Midwives (ACM): National Midwifery Guidelines for Consultation and Referral, ACM, Canberra. 2021. Accessed 22 September 2021. Available: www.midwives.org.au/sites/default/files/uploaded-content/website-content/acm_cr_guidelines_a5_final_v3.pdf.

Australian Health Ministers' Advisory Council (AHMAC): Primary Maternity Services in Australia: a Framework for Implementation. Prepared by NSW Health, on behalf of the Maternity Services Inter-jurisdictional Committee, NSW Health, Sydney 2008.

Chamberlain-Salaun J, Mills J, Usher K: Terminology used to describe health care teams: an integrative review of the literature, Journal of Multidisciplinary Healthcare 6:65, 2013.

Department of Health: Clinical Practice Guidelines: Pregnancy Care, 2020. Canberra: Australian Government. Online 22 September 2021. Available: www.health.gov.au/resources/publications/pregnancy-care-guidelines.

Midwifery Council of New Zealand (MCNZ): Competencies for Entry to the Register of Midwives, 2007. Online 22 September 2021. Available: www.midwiferycouncil.health.z/common/Uploaded%20files/Registration/Competencies%20for%20entry%20to%20the%20Register.pdf.

Ministry of Health: Guidelines for Consultation with Obstetric and Related Medical Services (Referral Guidelines), 2012. Online 6 June 2018. Available: www.health.govt.nz/system/files/documents/publications/referral-glines-jan12.pdf.

Ministry of Health: Primary Maternity Services, 2021. Online 22 September 2021. Available: www.health.govt.nz/our-work/life-stages/maternity-services/primary-maternity-services.

National Health and Medical Research Council (NHMRC): National Guidance on Collaborative Maternity Care, 2010.

New Zealand Government: Primary Maternity Services Notice 2021, 2021. Online 22 September 2021. Available: https://gazette.govt.nz/notice/id/2021-go2473?stageDraft.

Nursing and Midwifery Board of Australia (NMBA): Midwife standards for practice, 2018. Online 14 June 2018. Available: www.nursingmidwiferyboard.gov.au/Codes-Guidelines-Statements/Professional-standards/Midwife-standards-for-practice.aspx.

Parliamentary Counsel Office: New Zealand legislation. Health and Disability Services Commissioner (Code of Health and Disability Services Consumers' Rights) Regulations 1996, 1996. Online 6 June 2018. Available: www.legislation.govt.nz/regulation/public/1996/0078/latest/whole.html.

SECTION 7

SKILLS FOR PREPARING WOMEN FOR LABOUR, BIRTH AND EARLY PARENTING

CHAPTER 29

FACILITATION OF LEARNING IN EXPECTANT AND NEW PARENTS

Learning outcomes

Having read this chapter, the reader should be able to:

- identify pregnancy as a 'teachable moment'
- discuss the need to underpin education during the childbearing episode with adult learning principles
- discuss the range of ways in which teaching and learning during pregnancy might be facilitated
- explain the midwife's role and responsibilities in relation to each of these aspects of care.

A fundamental aspect of the midwife's role is the provision of new information to the women in their care to strengthen their capacity to make decisions about the myriad options that are presented to them during pregnancy, in labour and birth and through the puerperium. This chapter considers the childbearing episode, but especially pregnancy, as an optimal time for the assimilation of new information and for behavioural change. It also outlines skills for effectively facilitating childbearing women to learn new information.

PREGNANCY AS A 'TEACHABLE MOMENT'

Having a baby is said to engender an urge in women to learn about the physical and emotional changes that occur during this period (Atkinson et al 2016, Herman et al 2012). Pregnancy has been termed a 'teachable moment'; that is, a naturally occurring life transition or health event that motivates individuals to spontaneously adopt risk-reducing health behaviours (Phelan 2010). McBride and colleagues (2003) characterised teachable moments as times in life when perceptions of personal risk and outcome expectancies are increased, prompting strong affective or emotional responses, and redefining one's self-concept or social roles. It has been recognised that teachable moments offer health professionals an opportunity to capitalise on this increased motivation (Atkinson et al 2016).

Group antenatal education seemingly has a protective effect against antenatal and postnatal birth fear, depression, anxiety and stress symptoms, and is associated with increased childbirth self-efficacy and a higher likelihood of vaginal births compared to women who do not participate (Çankaya & Şimşek 2020). It cannot be said, however, to have a completely beneficial impact on physiological birth outcomes: in a literature review by Ferguson and colleagues published in 2013, it was found to reduce anxiety and false labour admissions, but it was also found to effect higher labour induction and epidural use rates. It is also well known to benefit pregnant women's 'social agenda'—the wish to meet other women going through pregnancy at the same time, which is a high priority (Nolan 2009), to the point where not having the opportunity to attend antenatal classes has been identified as a source of distress (Redshaw et al 2007). Since the last edition, many maternity services have moved their antenatal classes online, and at the time of writing (January 2021), evidence about the effectiveness of this format is limited and suggests that although it is associated with participants reporting a reduction in anxiety towards pregnancy and birth, feeling closer to the baby and having an increased intention to breastfeed compared to non-attenders (Shahid & Johnson 2018), online education may not effectively address the needs of non-English speaking participants (Chedid et al 2018).

Regardless of the delivery mode for antenatal education, the application of adult learning theory can optimise the effect of midwives' efforts to engender these outcomes.

CHARACTERISTICS OF ADULT LEARNERS

It has long been recognised that adults and children learn differently. To effectively teach adults new information, midwives are therefore advised to underpin their education efforts with adult learning principles. The most widely known and referenced set of adult learning principles was developed by Malcolm Shepherd Knowles, and educator from the United States. Knowles (1980) originally identified four characteristics of adult learners, and added a fifth several years later (Knowles 1984) (Box 29.1).

FACILITATING LEARNING IN CHILDBEARING WOMEN

In keeping with the women-centred midwifery philosophy that underpins this text, the term 'facilitation', which implies empowerment, is preferred over the term 'education', which has paternalistic connotations. According to Prendiville (2004), facilitation of learning 'is a developmental educational method that encourages people to share ideas, resources and opinions and to think critically in order to identify needs and find effective ways of satisfying those needs'. Along with the addition of his fifth characteristic of adult learners, Knowles also proposed four principles that should underpin adult learning (1984). First, educators of adults need to include them in the planning and evaluation of their instruction. Second, learners' experience (including mistakes) should be recognised to provide the basis for the learning activities. Third, it should be acknowledged that adults are most interested in learning subjects that have immediate relevance to and impact on their job or personal life. Fourth, the concept that adult learning is problem-centred rather than content-oriented should be taken into account (Kearsley 2010). As well as optimising women's learning capacity through the application of Knowles' characteristics and principles, midwives who lead group antenatal education should bear in mind the seminal work on adult education by Daines and colleagues (2006), who proposed that the optimal class size is between 12 and 20 participants. This enables facilitators to create a climate where interaction can flourish, where people can participate in safety, and where they can learn both with and from others.

The aspects listed under Skill 29.1 all apply in group teaching situations, as well as learning and teaching episodes with individual women. As well as optimal group size, there are also some additional considerations when supporting more than one woman at a time to learn new information and skills. According to Prendiville (2004), groups formed for a specific purpose undergo three stages once the preparatory stage is completed (wherein practical issues, such as agreeing on a common aim and basic rules, are established); these are labelled 'Nurturing', 'Individuating' and 'Cohesiveness'. Knowing them will help facilitators understand the behaviours occurring in their group (see Box 29.2, Skill 29.2).

Box 29.1 Knowles' five characteristics of adult learners

1. *Self-concept:* As a person matures, his/her self-concept moves from one of being a dependent personality towards one of being a self-directed human being.
2. *Adult learner experience*: As a person matures, he/she accumulates a growing reservoir of experience that becomes an increasing resource for learning.
3. *Readiness to learn*: As a person matures, his/her readiness to learn becomes oriented increasingly to the developmental tasks of his/her social roles.
4. *Orientation to learning*: As a person matures, his/her time perspective changes from one of postponed application of knowledge to immediacy of application. As a result, his/her orientation towards learning shifts from one of subject-centredness to one of problem-centredness.
5. *Motivation to learn:* As a person matures, the motivation to learn is internal.

Source: Knowles M: The adult learner: a neglected species, 3rd ed., Gulf Publishing, Houston, 1984, p. 12.

SKILL 29.1 Teaching adults

1. Ask the woman what she wants to know, rather than making assumptions about what she needs to know; include her in designing her learning.
2. Make reference to the woman's experience during learning and teaching episodes.
3. Ensure the content of the learning and teaching episode has immediate relevance to and impact on the woman's experience.
4. Focus on relating learning and teaching to situations the woman recognises or will face, rather than imparting abstract information.

Box 29.2 Three stages of groups

1. Nurturing

This is the stage where security and trust are established. It involves setting up a safe place for the group, both emotionally and physically, creating conditions of acceptance, understanding, mutual support, confidentiality and nurturing.

2. Individuating

This stage involves moving on from the nurturing stage, so that individuals can stand independently within the group. People find a sense of themselves again. Members can and do confront each other, and give and receive honest feedback. People learn to analyse, to differentiate and separate at this stage. It relates to the critical, intellectual side of being in a group.

3. Cohesiveness

At this stage, people acknowledge both their individuality and their commitment/belonging to the group. This phase acknowledges the interrelatedness of each of the members to one another. Each individual is equal, can lead and be led, is active in decision-making, problem-solving and the work of the group generally. There is a balance of task and process, with people expressing their interdependency and satisfaction with being in the group. People will be able to move to the end of the group well, or to continue by renewing the group.

Source: Prendiville P: Developing facilitation skills: a handbook for group facilitators, Combat Poverty Agency, Meitheal, Republic of Ireland, 2004, pp. 29–30. Online 14 May 2018. Available: www.academia.edu/37232772/Developing_Facilitation_Skills_A_Handbook_for_Group_Facilitators.

SKILL 29.2 Teaching groups

1. Ensure group size is between 12 to 20 participants.
2. Introduce yourself and ask group members to do the same.
3. Establish the aim of the session or course. For example, the aims of a session on facilitating women and their partners to make the best decision for them about which model of maternity care to choose might be stated as follows.
   - Understand the range of models of maternity care available in (the area).
   - Recognise the implications of each model of maternity care for the pregnancy and birth experience.
   - Identify your own priorities and expectations for your pregnancy and birth and of maternity caregivers.
   - Decide which model of maternity care will most likely facilitate the pregnancy and birth experience you would like.
4. Establish participants' expectations.
5. Agree on basic rules (e.g. respect for each other's opinions, confidentiality).
6. Utilise the elements of Skill 29.1 and also provide opportunities for members to learn from each other.
7. Facilitate forward movement through the class content if participants become 'stuck' on a topic, by bringing the group to attention and saying, for example, 'Let's move on now to ...'.
8. Conduct a review at the end of the session to ensure all aims and expectations have been met.

Role and responsibilities of the midwife

These can be summarised as:

- knowing and using current evidence-based practice to inform the learning of expectant parents
- maintaining a woman-centred philosophy to facilitate learning
- ensuring group workshops contain no more than 20 participants.

SUMMARY

- The childbearing episode and especially pregnancy are teachable moments.
- The midwife's role includes facilitating learning in the women she works with.
- The use of adult learning principles will optimise women's capacity to learn new information and skills.
- Supporting groups of women to learn requires additional skills that recognise how groups work.

Self-assessment exercises

The answers to the following questions may be found in the text.

1. Describe the known benefits and disadvantages of antenatal education for women's birth outcomes.
2. Describe Knowles' five characteristics of adult learners.
3. Define facilitation.
4. What must adult learning facilitators include in the preparatory stage of group formation?

References

Atkinson L, Shaw RL, French DP: Is pregnancy a teachable moment for diet and physical activity behaviour change? An interpretative phenomenological analysis of the experiences of women during their first pregnancy, British Journal of Health Psychology 21:842–858, 2016.

Çankaya S, Şimşek B: Effects of antenatal education on fear of birth, depression, anxiety, childbirth self-efficacy, and mode of delivery in primiparous pregnant women: a prospective randomized controlled study, Clinical Nursing Research, 2020. Available: https://doi.org/10.1177/1054773820916984.

Chedid RA, Terrell RM, Phillips KP: Best practices for online Canadian prenatal health promotion: a public health approach, Women and Birth 31(4):e223–e231, 2018.

Daines J, Daines C, Graham B: Adult learning, adult teaching, 4th ed., Welsh Academic Press, Cardiff, Wales, 2006.

Ferguson S, Davis D, Browne J: Does antenatal education affect labour and birth? A structured review of the literature, Women and Birth: Journal of the Australian College of Midwives 26(1):e5e8, 2013.

Herman JW, Rogers S, Ehrenthal D: Women's perceptions of centering pregnancy: a focus group study, Maternal-Child Nursing 37:19–28, 2012.

Kearsley G: Andragogy (M. Knowles). The theory into practice database, 2010. Online. Available: http://158.132.155.107/posh97/private/TIP/12.htm.

Knowles M: The adult learner: a neglected species, 3rd ed., Gulf Publishing, Houston, 1984.

Knowles MS: The modern practice of adult education: from pedagogy to andragogy, Prentice Hall/Cambridge, Englewood Cliffs, 1980.

McBride CM, Emmons KM, Lipkus IM: Understanding the potential of teachable moments: the case of smoking cessation, Health Education Research 8(2):156–170, 2003.

Nolan M: Information giving and education in pregnancy: a review of qualitative studies, The Journal of Perinatal Education 18(4):21–30, 2009.

Phelan S: Pregnancy: a 'teachable moment' for weight control and obesity prevention, American Journal of Obstetrics and Gynecology 202(2):135, 2010.

Prendiville P: Developing facilitation skills: a handbook for group facilitators, Combat Poverty Agency, Meitheal, Republic of Ireland, 2004. Online 14 May 2018. Available: www.academia.edu/37232772/Developing_Facilitation_Skills_A_Handbook_for_Group_Facilitators.

Redshaw M, Rowe R, Hockley C, Brocklehurst P: Recorded delivery: a national survey of women's experience of maternity care 2006, National Perinatal Epidemiology Unit, Oxford, 2007.

Shahid A, Johnson, R: Evaluation of an online antenatal course 'Understanding pregnancy, labour, birth and your baby' by the Solihull Approach, Evidence Based Midwifery September, 16(3):101–106, 2018.

PART 2

WORKING WITH THE WOMAN AND BABY DURING LABOUR AND BIRTH

Section 8: Monitoring wellbeing in early labour

Section 9: Monitoring wellbeing in established labour

Section 10: Monitoring wellbeing during the expulsive phase

Section 11: Monitoring wellbeing during and after the third stage

SECTION 8

MONITORING WELLBEING IN EARLY LABOUR

CHAPTER 30

PRINCIPLES OF INTRAPARTUM SKILLS: FIRST-STAGE ISSUES

Learning outcomes

Having read this chapter, the reader should be able to:

- discuss what is meant by the latent phase and active/established phase of the first stage of labour and how this affects subsequent assessment of progress
- discuss the different positions a woman may adopt during the first stage of labour and when each of these may be recommended
- list the indications for undertaking a vaginal examination (VE) during labour
- discuss the information that may be obtained from a VE and how this assesses progress
- describe the procedures for VE, amniotomy and the application of a fetal scalp electrode.

The first stage of labour consists of two phases, which have been identified as the latent phase and the active/established phase. The transition between the two phases is difficult to objectify as they are variable and no definition will apply to all women. The first stage commences with the onset of labour contractions and is completed when the cervix is no longer detectable. This chapter focuses on a selection of the skills used by the midwife when caring for a woman during the first stage of labour (some of which may also be used at other times; e.g. second stage of labour). The chapter begins with a discussion of the definition of latent and active phase as progress is assessed on the basis of how these are defined. The use of different positions the woman can adopt follows and the chapter concludes with some of the skills used during the first stage of labour. The skills reviewed are examination per vaginam, often referred to as a vaginal examination (VE), amniotomy (artificial rupture of membranes [ARM]) and application of a fetal scalp electrode (FSE) which may occur during a VE. It is recognised that the midwife uses other important skills during labour, in particular communication with and observation of the woman, as much information can be gleaned from this. However, this is not discussed within this text.

THE LATENT AND ESTABLISHED PHASES OF THE FIRST STAGE OF LABOUR AND PROGRESS OF LABOUR

While the first stage of labour is classified as having two phases: the **latent phase** and **active phase**, otherwise known as established labour, there is no universal agreement as to when one phase ends and the other begins, which makes assessing progress difficult. The latent phase has been described as a period of time, possibly intermittent periods, associated with irregular painful contractions and some cervical effacement and dilation less than 4 cm (NICE 2014) to 6 cm (Zhang et al 2010). Women who present to hospital in the latent phase are often encouraged to go home and wait for labour to establish. NICE (2014) provides a very clear definition of the latent phase based around whether painful contractions are regular and whether the cervix is dilated from and beyond 4 cm. However, some multiparous women are assessed as being in the latent phase when they have painful contractions every 15 minutes and their cervix is 4 cm dilated as this may be considered a 'multiparous os'. The woman herself may consider she is in labour and not wish to go home. Equally, some women will never have regular contractions, yet still birth their baby, and when, if ever, they were in a discernible latent or established phase at any point will never be known. A medicalised definition of when the different phases of labour begin and end is often very different to the woman's perception of her labour (Royal College of Midwives [RCM] 2012b) (Fig 30.1).

There is no consensus in the literature on what constitutes the length of a normal latent phase.

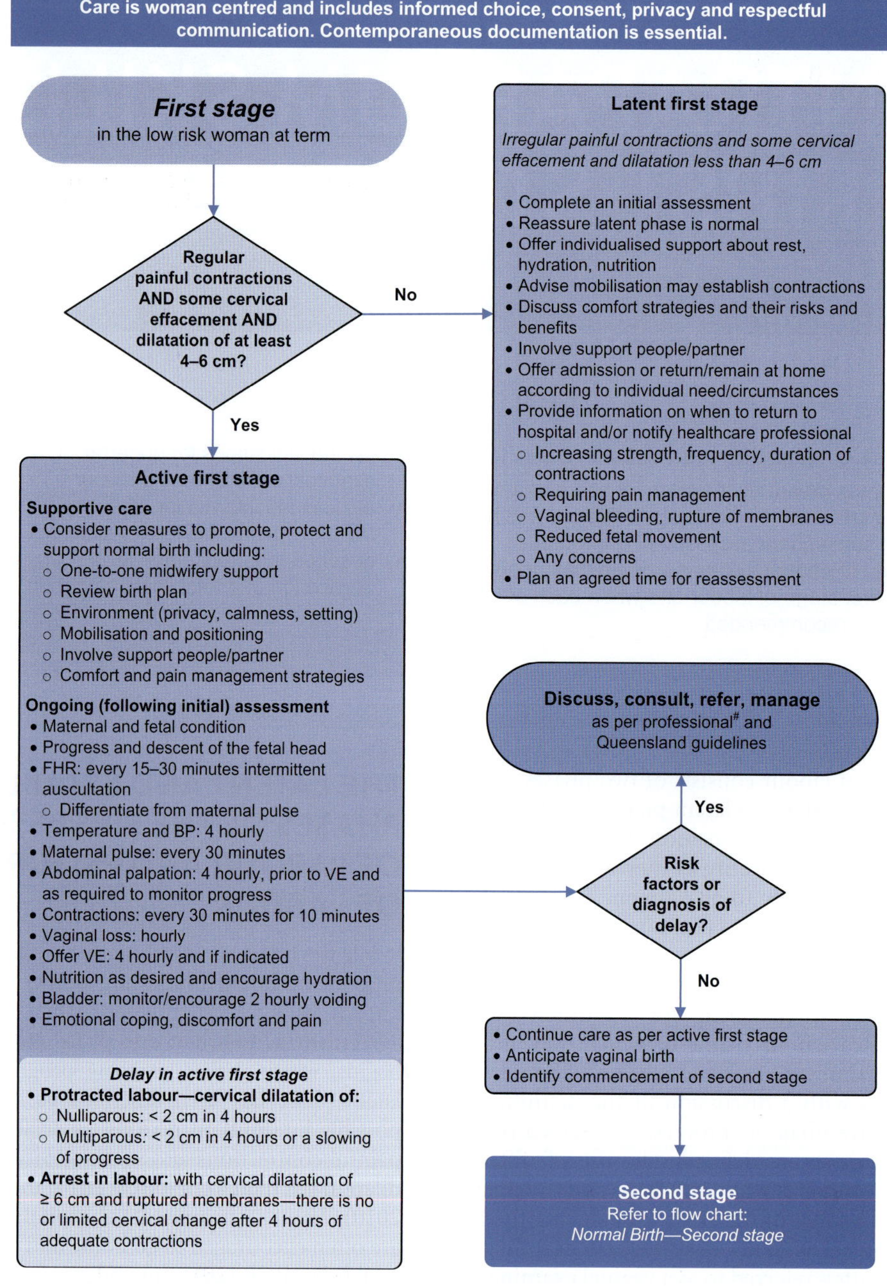

FIGURE 30.1 **Normal birth—first stage.**
Source: Queensland Clinical Guidelines (QCG): Normal birth.
Maternity and Neonatal Clinical Guidelines, 2017. Online 14 May 2018. Available: www.health.qld.gov.au/__data/assets/pdf_fi le/0014/142007/g-normalbirth.pdf.

Definitions vary from 6 to 8 hours (NICE 2014) up to 24 to 36 hours (Stables & Rankin 2010). Confusing the latent phase with a poorly progressing active phase can lead to inappropriate and unnecessary interventions that may affect the outcomes for mother and baby (Kobayashi et al 2017).

NICE (2014) suggests the average length of time for the duration of established labour (following the latent phase) for primiparous women is around 8 hours, and it is unusual for it to last longer than 18 hours, whereas for multiparous women the duration is around 5 hours and is unlikely to last over 12 hours. This would indicate the expectation that the duration of labour between primiparous and multiparous women is different. However, NICE (2014) classifies a suspected delay in the first stage where there is cervical dilatation of < 2 cm in 4 hours for both primiparous and multiparous women. They also both state that the amount of descent and rotation of the presenting part and any changes in the strength, duration and frequency of uterine contractions should be considered (NICE 2014). However, a reduction in the frequency of contractions and slowing of cervical dilatation may be experienced as part of normal labour. Schmidt and Downe (2010) suggest the woman will undergo a number of transition phases during labour, which include a period when the cervix is dilated to 5–6 cm and again around 8–9 cm. During these transition periods, for some women, contractions slow and labour can slow down, perhaps even stop. According to Schmidt and Downe (2010), this is a time when the woman can restore her physical energy and, as such, should not be considered abnormal, otherwise unnecessary intervention will occur. Zhang and colleagues (2010) found it can take > 6 hours for the cervix to dilate from 4 to 5 cm and over 3 hours to move from 5 to 6 cm and suggest that with both primiparous and multiparous women the progress of cervical dilatation is the same up to 6 cm, after which the multiparous labour often progresses more rapidly than the first labour. They argue that, particularly for primiparous women, labour does not progress in a consistent manner (Zhang et al 2010) yet women can birth their babies vaginally without adverse outcomes to the mother or the baby, which is a view supported by Incerti and colleagues (2011). They also suggest that the established phase of labour should not be considered to begin until cervical dilatation is ≥ 6 cm, as before then it is often normal for there to be no change in cervical dilatation (Zhang et al 2010).

Grasek and colleagues (2014) studied the descent of the fetal head during term labour and calculated the median station for each centimetre of cervical dilatation for primiparous and multiparous women. Primiparous women had a median station of −3 at 0–1 cm, −2 at 2–3 cm, −1 at 4–5 cm, 0 at 6–8 cm, +1 at 9 cm and +2 at 10 cm, whereas multiparous had a slower descent of −3 at 0–3 cm, −2 at 4–5 cm, −1 at 6 cm, 0 at 7–9 cm and +2 at 10 cm (Grasek et al 2014). Descent time between each of the stations was significantly quicker in multiparous women, except for descent between +2 and +3.

When assessing progress, the midwife should consider more than cervical dilatation; they should also consider whether the position of the cervix has moved from a posterior to a central or anterior position, whether it has ripened (softened), whether it has become effaced (thinned out) and whether the presenting part has rotated, flexed and descended (RCM 2012a). The midwife should also consider where the woman is in her labour, what is happening with the contractions, whether the woman has entered a transition phase (as may be noted by her changing behaviours) and what definition of latent and established labour and 'progress' is being used. One advantage of assessing progress is that it allows time to transfer the woman to a facility with a higher level of care if delay is suspected (Downe et al 2013).

MATERNAL POSITIONING

Women should be encouraged to adopt whichever positions they find comfortable during the first stage of labour (Leap & Hunter 2016). Lawrence and colleagues (2013) suggest that, given the freedom to do so, women will change position throughout labour and a change in positions should be encouraged to avoid the occurrence of pressure ulcer formation (see Chapter 47). For some women, changing position is more difficult due to constraints such as epidural anaesthesia or continuous fetal heart rate monitoring; however, the midwife can still enable the woman to make some positional changes, such as side-lying. The RCM (2012c) suggests midwives should be proactive in demonstrating and encouraging different positions in labour, particularly for women with challenges such as continuous fetal heart rate monitoring and intravenous therapy. The environment is often the key to freedom of movement; one without a variety of furniture and props to encourage positional changes is more likely to have women who remain semireclined on the bed (Cutler 2012, RCM 2012c). When the bed is the dominant feature in the room women are likely to adopt this position; it is also a convenient position for the midwife when certain procedures are required (e.g. abdominal palpation, examination per vaginam). Lawrence and colleagues (2013) suggest many women will be upright throughout labour but within the Western world, there is a preference for lying down when the cervix is around 5–6 cm. This would tie in with the transitional phase that occurs around this time in labour and at a time when the woman needs to recharge her energy. Once this has happened the woman should be encouraged to be upright again. Cutler (2012) cautions midwives not to guide the woman onto the bed for their own convenience. Equally, after procedures such as abdominal palpation and VE are undertaken with the woman on the bed, the midwife should encourage her to adopt her previous position.

Positions adopted can vary from upright (including walking, sitting, kneeling, squatting, all-fours) to recumbent (including supine, semirecumbent, lateral or side-lying). Upright positions appear more comfortable than sitting positions (Chapman 2009, RCM, 2012c). Upright positions encourage the fetus to descend into the pelvis (Lawrence et al 2013) and may also result in a shorter first stage, less severe pain and less narcotic and epidural use (RCM 2012c). Leap and Hunter (2016) encourage women to keep moving in labour and also advocate: rocking against the wall; holding onto an open door; swaying; walking around, up and down stairs; and using a birthing ball to remain upright. Simkin and colleagues (2017) support the use of upright positions, suggesting moving around during labour can help the pelvic bones accommodate the fetus during its travels through the pelvis. Baker (2010) agrees, suggesting upright positions optimise the changes that occur within the pelvic joints during the end of pregnancy and labour (increasing pelvic diameters and causing slight changes in pelvic shape). Midwives advocate the use of stair walking or lifting one leg onto a surface so that the woman's knee is higher than the other where labour appears to be slowing or asynclitism is present. The National Childbirth Trust (NCT 2011) suggests that if a woman has been mobilising but is getting tired she could try kneeling or if she wants to sit, to ensure her feet are lower than her pelvis.

Squatting makes use of gravity and the pelvic changes (Sanderson 2012), but Cutler (2012) cautions that women in the Western world find it hard to maintain a squatting position as a result of shortening of the Achilles tendon from the use of chair sitting, wearing heeled shoes and not using squatting toilets. For a woman to use squatting during labour, it is worth discussing this during pregnancy and encouraging her to practice, particularly if her partner is going to support her in the squat.

All-fours

Hunter and colleagues (2007) found that women who were labouring with fetuses in an occipitoposterior position experienced less backache when adopting an all-fours position. This may also be achieved by leaning over a birthing ball to relieve pressure on the woman's arms. It may be more comfortable for the woman if she has support/cushioning under her knees (e.g. pillow, padded mat). Hanson (2009) suggests that an open knee–chest position (the buttocks are high, with the thighs at right angles to lower legs) can help to reduce the premature urge to push, while a closed knee–chest position (the buttocks are lower to the ground, with knees and hips flexed and abducted beneath the abdomen) is useful if the cervix is oedematous.

Lateral (side-lying)

Simkin and colleagues (2017) recommend women with an occipitoposterior position lie on their side, ensuring it is the same side as the position of the fetal spine, to encourage fetal rotation to an occipitoanterior position (e.g. lie on right side for right occipitoposterior position). This was found to increase the incidence of spontaneous vaginal delivery, decrease the length of labour and reduce the risk of caesarean section compared with lying on the opposite side or any other position (Ridley 2007). This may be a way of alternating the position of a woman with restricted mobility (e.g. with epidural use) and relieving pressure from the buttocks, sacral area and heels.

Supine

Women should be discouraged from lying supine. When the woman lies flat, the weight of the pregnant uterus can compress the major blood vessels (aortocaval compression), which can compromise maternal cardiac function and uterine blood flow. This reduces fetal oxygenation and causes alterations in the fetal acid–base status. If a woman wishes to lie supine, it is advisable to place a wedge under her right side to relieve the pressure off the major vessels. Contractions can appear to be less strong in the supine position, compared to upright or lateral positions, but if the woman becomes upright again, the contractions should return to their previous state (Lawrence et al 2013).

Semirecumbent

Kerrigan (2006) suggests there is little evidence to support use of this position; however, some women may need to rest and adopt this position periodically during labour.

EXAMINATION PER VAGINAM

A VE is an intimate, invasive procedure with the potential to cause distress and pain to the woman; thus, it should only be undertaken when there is a clear clinical indication. Hassan and colleagues (2012) remind us that for women, VE is a living experience that they may feel empowers them by increasing their self-confidence and belief in their childbearing ability or, equally, increase their feeling of vulnerability. In a more recent study, 35% of women associated VE with pain, embarrassment, not being able to relax, not feeling respected and not feeling able to stop the examination (de Klerk et al 2018). While it is often undertaken to assess progress, VE is imprecise when performed by different clinicians (RCM 2012a). There is also a risk of ascending infection with multiple examinations, particularly once the membranes have ruptured, although Cahill and colleagues (2012) suggest the risk of maternal fever is not significantly increased by the number of VEs. While Lewin and colleagues (2005) found women experience an average of three VEs during labour, some women will have far more than this: Shepherd and Cheyne (2013) found the number of VEs undertaken increased as the length of time in labour in hospital increased, with 52% of women undergoing three or more VEs during labour with the most common rationale given by midwives being that it was to assess labour progress.

Dixon and Foureur (2010) suggest VE is an intervention which disrupts the woman's concentration and interferes with the labour rhythm, particularly as the woman may be required to change her position. There is no research-based information on which to make a recommendation for the timing and frequency of VEs during labour (RCM 2012a). Hassan and colleagues (2012) caution that a VE should be done only when necessary and consideration should be given to the woman's feelings and experiences during a VE. However, NICE (2014) recommends it should be undertaken 4-hourly if there is concern about progress or in response to the woman's wishes. An abdominal palpation should be undertaken prior to the VE so the results of each can be correlated.

Indications

A VE may be undertaken prior to labour as part of an induction of labour procedure to insert a prostaglandin pessary or gel (Chapter 20) or to perform a membrane sweep (Chapter 32).

During labour, the midwife may undertake a VE to:

- confirm the onset of labour
- identify the presentation and position
- assess progress during labour
- perform an ARM
- apply an FSE
- exclude cord prolapse following spontaneous rupture of the membranes where there is an ill-fitting or high presenting part
- confirm the onset of the second stage of labour, especially with a breech presentation and multiple pregnancy.

Contraindications

The midwife should not undertake a VE when there is:

- no consent from the woman
- active bleeding
- placenta praevia
- suspected preterm labour
- pre-labour rupture of the membranes.

This can be a very distressing procedure for some women and it is important the procedure is discussed with the woman before the VE is undertaken. Her informed consent should be obtained and the VE not undertaken if the woman does not agree. The discussion should include the rationale for the procedure, what will happen, what is required of the woman and confirmation that the VE will be stopped at any point if requested by the woman. The ideal time for much of this discussion is before the onset of labour, but it should be repeated each time a VE is indicated. The discussion should also occur in a manner that allows the woman to ask questions and refuse the examination. Verbal and non-verbal communication should be continued during the procedure, not only to provide the woman with information about what is happening, but also so the midwife can recognise when the woman is experiencing discomfort or pain and requires the VE to end (Dixon & Foureur 2010).

INFORMATION GAINED FROM UNDERTAKING AN EXAMINATION PER VAGINAM

External genitalia

Prior to performing the VE the external genitalia should be observed for abnormalities such as varicosities, oedema, warts, signs of infection and scarring, particularly if indicative of previous perineal or labial trauma or female genital mutilation. NICE (2014) indicates a VE, catheterisation and application of an FSE may be very difficult in the presence of infibulated genital mutilation. If this circumstance is noted, a discussion should occur with the woman to inform her of the risks around delay in the second stage of labour, spontaneous 'perineal' trauma, the need for an anterior episiotomy and possibly defibulation in labour (NICE 2014), although this discussion should ideally take place during pregnancy.

If there is any discharge or bleeding from the vagina, the colour, consistency, amount and odour should be recorded. If the membranes have ruptured, amniotic fluid may be seen and the colour and odour should be noted. Clear liquor with a non-offensive odour is normal.

Vagina

The vagina should feel warm and moist, with soft distensible walls. A hot, dry vagina could be indicative of dehydration, infection or obstructed labour and a vagina that feels 'tense' may be associated with fear or previous scarring. The presence of varicosities, a cystocele or rectocele should be noted. A full rectum may be felt through the posterior vaginal wall, which may lead the midwife to suggest the use of suppositories or an enema.

Cervix

The cervix is assessed for position, consistency, effacement, dilatation and application to the presenting part. The cervix is usually in a central or posterior position, firm, non-effaced with the os closed (unripe) during pregnancy. However, during the latter weeks of pregnancy and early labour, the structure and position of the cervix alters as the cervix 'ripens', causing the cervix to feel less rigid and adopt an anterior position. A soft and stretchy 'ripe' cervix is often associated with good dilatation of the os uteri, whereas a tight unyielding unripe cervix at term is more likely to be associated with prolonged labour. An unripe cervix requires three to four times more uterine effort than a ripe cervix (Burnhill et al 1962).

With the primigravid woman, effacement usually precedes dilatation, but they can occur simultaneously with the multigravid woman. Effacement is assessed by the length of the cervix and the degree to which it protrudes into the vagina. A non-effaced cervix feels long and tubular, with the os closed or partly dilated. The cervix thins out and becomes shorter with effacement, as the lower uterine segment 'takes it up' (Fig 30.2). A fully effaced cervix feels continuous with the lower uterine segment and does not protrude into the vagina.

In the primigravid woman, the os uteri is usually closed until labour begins, but with a multigravid woman the os may allow one or two fingers through before labour, commonly referred to as a 'multip's os'. With a breech presentation the fetal anus should not be mistaken for a closed cervix as the anus will be traumatised if fingers are inserted through it (Warwick et al 2013).

Dilatation of the os uteri, measured in centimetres, is assessed by inserting one or both fingers through the external os and parting the fingers to assess the diameter. In early labour, when the cervix is less than 2 cm dilated, usually only one finger can be inserted. It may be easier to feel around the remaining rim of the cervix towards the end of the first stage to estimate dilatation; for example, a rim of 1 cm equates to a dilatation of 9 cm, as there is 1 cm of cervix remaining. When feeling a rim of the cervix that is stretchy, it is important to assess dilatation without stretching; this may be easier to achieve by using fingertips on the edge of the cervix. Full dilatation occurs when the cervix can no longer be felt and is equal to 10 cm. This is the point at which the fetal head can pass through the cervix; although for the preterm fetus this may happen before full dilatation. If the presentation is breech, the foot and leg can protrude through the cervix before it is fully dilated (footling breech). Dilatation of the os uteri should occur progressively throughout the first stage of labour and is one factor in determining progress.

A cervix that is well applied to the presenting part is associated with good uterine activity (Blackburn 2013). The reverse may also be true, that a poorly applied cervix is associated with less efficient uterine activity and slower progress. For example, when the fetus is in an occipitoposterior position, the head is not pushed directly onto the cervix; rather, it is directed downwards and forwards against the back of the symphysis pubis, leading to a decrease in the effectiveness of uterine contractility, slower cervical dilatation and prolonged labour (Chamberlain 1993). The application of the cervix to the presenting part can be assessed by feeling between them.

The membranes

The membranes should be felt to determine if they are intact or ruptured. Intact membranes can be felt as a shiny surface over the presenting part but may be difficult to feel, especially in early labour or when the forewaters are shallow with the membranes tightly pressed against the presenting part. In this situation they may be mistaken for ruptured membranes. Bulging forewaters may be felt when the cervix is poorly applied to the presenting part as amniotic fluid is positioned between the membranes and the presenting part. During a contraction the pressure within the forewaters increases, causing the membranes to feel tense with a predisposition to rupturing spontaneously. This is more likely to occur if the presenting part is poorly applied (e.g. high or ill-fitting presenting part, malposition or malpresentation). Occasionally the membranes are

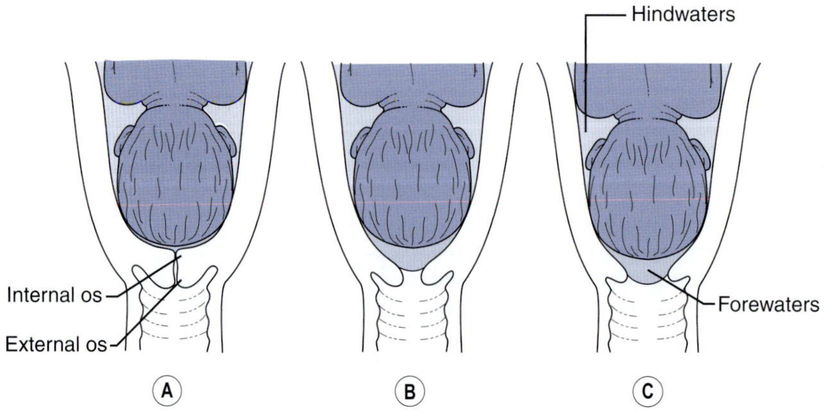

FIGURE 30.2 **Effacement of the cervix.**
Source: Johnson R, Taylor W: Skills for midwifery practice, 4th ed., Elsevier, London, 2016.

intact but amniotic fluid is leaking; this is most likely caused by a hindwater leak. Care should be taken not to rupture the membranes (unless there is an indication to do so and consent obtained), particularly if a pulsation is felt beneath the membranes, as this could be due to either a cord presentation or vasa praevia. Referral should be sought as an emergency caesarean section may be indicated to prevent cord prolapse or fetal haemorrhage from ruptured vasa praevia.

Presentation

The information gained from the abdominal examination is used in conjunction with the landmarks identified on the presenting part to confirm the presentation.

- A cephalic presentation will feel smooth, round and firm, and sutures or fontanelles may be felt, which can help confirm the position and the degree of flexion. Moulding can be assessed by the degree of overlapping of the bones of the vault. No moulding is when there is normal separation of the bones with open sutures; 1+ occurs when the bones are touching each other; 2+ occurs if the bones overlap but can be separated with gentle digital pressure; 3+ (severe moulding) occurs when the bones are overlapping and cannot be separated with gentle digital pressure. Caput succedaneum may also be felt as a soft or firm mass on the presenting part, which can make the identification of sutures and fontanelles more difficult.
- Both the breech and face presentation feel soft and irregular. With the breech presentation, the sacrum may be palpable as a hard bone, with the anus close by and the landmarks of the ischial tuberosities and sacrum located in a straight line. A finger inadvertently inserted into the anus will be gripped and no gum margins will be felt. Fresh meconium is also likely to be present.
- With a face presentation, the orbital ridges may be felt, a finger inserted into the mouth may be sucked and gum margins felt, the landmarks of the malar bones and mouth are located in a triangular position and an ear may be felt. If a face presentation is suspected or confirmed, care should be taken to avoid damaging the eyes; application of an FSE is not recommended and obstetric cream should not be used, as it could initiate a chemical conjunctivitis.
- When the cord presents, the pulsations may be palpated through the membranes; the membranes should not be ruptured due to the danger of cord prolapse. If a cord is felt without membranes, the emergency procedure for managing cord prolapse should be instigated while the examining midwife keeps her fingers in the vagina and attempts to push the presenting part off the cord.

Level of the presenting part

The level of the **presenting part** is determined by assessing the distance between the presenting part and the ischial spines in centimetres (Fig 30.3). The ischial spines are referred to as zero station, with the presenting part being above (−cm) or below (+cm) this. The ischial spines may be difficult to palpate; thus, this becomes a subjective measurement. The midwife should ensure it is the level of the presenting part being assessed and not caput succedaneum. Descent of the presenting part is one indicator of progress during labour and the assessment should correlate with the

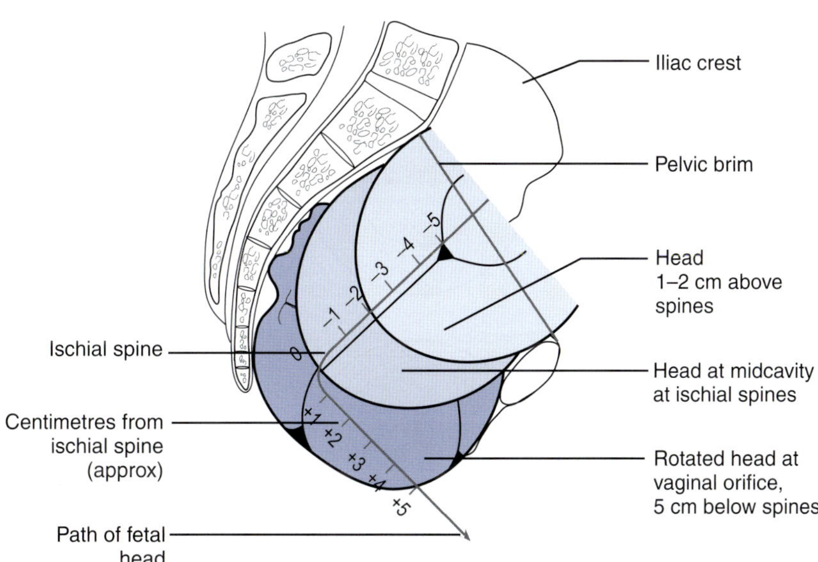

FIGURE 30.3 **Level of presenting part in relation to the ischial spines.**
Source: Johnson R, Taylor W: Skills for midwifery practice, 4th ed., Elsevier, London, 2016.

findings from the degree of engagement assessed during the abdominal examination.

Position

With a cephalic presentation, identification of sutures and fontanelles will confirm the position and attitude. The sagittal suture is easily identified as a long straight suture; its position is taken in relation to the maternal pelvis, moving from back to front.

- If it is in the anteroposterior diameter, it is indicative of a direct occipitoanterior or occipitoposterior position.
- A sagittal suture in the right oblique (felt moving from the posterior right quadrant of the maternal pelvis obliquely forwards to the left anterior quadrant) (Fig 30.4) is indicative of left occipitoanterior or right occipitoposterior position. If in the left oblique diameter, it is indicative of a right occipitoanterior or a left occipitoposterior position.
- Where the sagittal suture is in the transverse diameter, it is indicative of a right or a left occipitolateral/transverse position.
- A sagittal suture that does not run centrally through the pelvis but is located more to one side than the other may be indicative of asynclitism.

The posterior fontanelle is felt as a small triangular area with three sutures running from it and is indicative of a well-flexed cephalic presentation, usually occipitoanterior position if felt in the upper quadrant of the pelvis. As labour progresses the posterior fontanelle may close due to moulding and it may not be possible to feel three sutures if a caput succedaneum is present.

The anterior fontanelle is felt as a larger, diamond-shaped area, with four sutures running from it. However, if a caput succedaneum is present, it may not be possible to feel all four sutures. Palpation of the anterior fontanelle is usually associated with a deflexed head, often with an occipitoposterior position (where it will be felt in the upper quadrant of the pelvis). If felt centrally, it could be indicative of a brow presentation.

Progress is indicated where there is progressive flexion (or extension with a face presentation), descent and rotation. Comparing thc position of the landmarks from all previous VEs should demonstrate this. Some midwives will draw what they felt and this will also reflect the changing attitude and rotation.

Pelvic outlet

The adequacy of the pelvis for the size of the baby can be assessed as part of the VE. However, this is a subjective assessment and the pelvis is a dynamic structure with measurements that can vary according to the position of the woman. The assessment of the size of the fetus may also be considered a 'best estimate'; even the use of ultrasound scans to assess weight gives a weight range. For the midwife undertaking the VE, usually two assessments of pelvic adequacy are undertaken which give an indication of whether the pelvic outlet is narrowed. The first is to assess the distance between the ischial spines. Ischial spines are difficult to palpate; if they are prominent and easily felt, the transverse diameter of the outlet is reduced, which could affect progress, particularly in the second stage of labour. The second assessment is of the subpubic angle and is assessed by moving the top

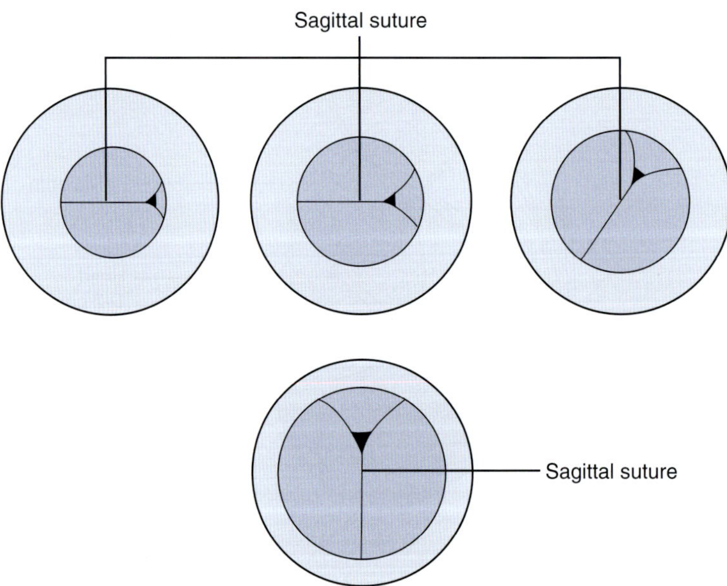

FIGURE 30.4 **Rotation of a cephalic presentation felt on examination per vaginam.**
Source: Johnson R, Taylor W: Skills for midwifery practice, 4th ed., Elsevier, London, 2016.

part of the two examining fingers towards the pubic arch. Two fingers should fit snugly under the pubic arch, indicating an angle of 90° or greater. A reduced subpubic angle is often found with prominent ischial spines and may be associated with an android pelvis. This can result in more pressure being placed on the perineum and perineal trauma, as well as delay in the second stage. Care should be taken when assessing the subpubic angle to avoid pressing on the clitoris, which can be painful.

SKILL 30.1 Examination per vaginam (VE)

A VE should be carried out using an aseptic non-touch technique (ANTT) with the wearing of sterile gloves providing the non-touch component. Sterile VE packs and lotions to wash the genital area are no longer used in labour wards as NICE (2014) advises tap water is sufficient for perineal cleansing where it is required. In support of this, Ohlsson and colleagues (2014) and Lumbiganon and colleagues (2014) found the use of chlorhexidine did not reduce the incidence of maternal and neonatal infection; the midwife should refer to the hospital policy for local requirements on perineal cleansing. The procedure for perineal cleansing follows this procedure. If an assistant is present, she can open packs and equipment for the midwife.

1. Confirm the woman's identity if she is not known to the midwife.
2. Discuss the procedure fully with the woman and gain informed consent.
3. Recognise and discuss religious and cultural considerations with the woman.
4. Ensure privacy.
5. Gather equipment:
   - apron
   - sterile gloves
   - lubricant (e.g. water-soluble lubricant, obstetric cream [the latter should not be used with a face presentation])
   - disposable sheet
   - alcohol-based hand rub
   - other equipment as necessary (e.g. amnihook, FSE)
   - Pinard stethoscope or Sonicaid.
6. Encourage the woman to empty her bladder if she is not catheterised.
7. Wash and dry hands.
8. Perform an abdominal palpation to determine the lie, presentation, position and degree of engagement, and auscultate the fetal heart.
9. Ask the woman to adopt an almost recumbent position (use a wedge to avoid aortocaval occlusion if necessary), with her knees flexed and parted, and ankles together (be aware of the difficulty experienced by women with pelvic girdle pain when opening their legs).
10. Place the disposable sheet beneath her buttocks.
11. Ask the woman to remove any sanitary towels or underwear, while keeping the genital area covered with a modesty sheet (assistance may be required, particularly in the case of epidural analgesia).
12. Wash and dry hands and apply an apron.
13. Open the equipment to be used, including the lubricating gel.
14. Apply alcohol-based hand rub, allow it to dry and then put on gloves.
15. Ask the woman to lift up the modesty sheet to allow access to the genital area.
16. Lubricate the first two fingers of the dominant hand with lubricant/antiseptic cream.
17. Advise the woman that she will feel her labia being touched and with the thumb and forefinger of the non-examining hand, part the labia, observing the condition of the vulva.
18. Assess for any fluid loss evident on the maternity pad, bedding or vaginal area.
19. Inform the woman of what is about to happen; then, if no contraction is present, gently insert the first two fingers of the examining hand into the vagina, in a downwards and backwards direction along the anterior vaginal wall, ensuring the thumb does not come into contact with the woman's clitoris or anus.
20. Locate the cervix and determine the position, tone, consistency, degree of effacement and dilatation and application to the presenting part (if the cervix is not located, ask the woman to place her clenched hands under her buttocks, tilting her pelvis upwards).
21. Gently move the fingers through the cervical os to ascertain the presence/absence of the forewaters, the presentation, position, degree of flexion and level of the presenting part, the presence of caput succedaneum and the degree of moulding.
22. If necessary and consent has been gained prior to the examination, rupture the membranes (see next section) and/or apply an FSE (p. 305).
23. Withdraw the fingers gently, assessing the pelvic outlet.
24. Auscultate the fetal heart.
25. Assist the woman into a comfortable position, reapply sanitary pad if required and discuss the findings.
26. Dispose of equipment appropriately, removing the gloves then apron.
27. Wash and dry hands.
28. Document the findings in the notes (also the partogram and or cardiotocograph [CTG] if being used) and act accordingly.

AMNIOTOMY (ARTIFICIAL RUPTURE OF MEMBRANES)

Intact membranes provide a cushion for the presenting part, providing protection from compression and infection. They also apply an even pressure on the cervix to assist with effacement of the cervix. Vincent (2005) suggests bulging membranes at the introitus help to prestretch the perineum prior to crowning.

Over two-thirds of women can reach full dilatation prior to the membranes rupturing spontaneously (Romano 2008); however, for many women this is not achieved, as the membranes have been ruptured artificially. While many midwives would not rupture the membranes without a clear clinical indication, **artificial rupture of membranes (ARM)** remains one of the most commonly performed procedures in both obstetric and midwifery practice (Smyth et al 2013).

A disposable sterile amnihook or an amnicot should be used for the procedure. The **amnihook** is a crochet-like, long-handled hook with a very sharp tip that is pressed against the chorion with the intention of tearing a hole in the membranes. The **amnicot** is a latex fingercot with a hook attached that is placed over the pulp of the middle or index finger of a gloved hand. The hook is used to gently scratch the membranes to rupture. The amniotic fluid can leak out through the hole increasing its size, or the membranes can be torn apart digitally.

ARM should not be undertaken with a labour that is progressing normally, as removing the cushion of the intact membranes means the presenting part will press directly onto the cervix. The RCM (2012d) argue that an ARM can have a negative impact on the woman by altering her ability to cope, and recommend using benign measures (e.g. positional changes) to increase the strength of contractions if progress is considered 'slow'. An ARM, 'breaking the waters', is not part of physiological labour and can disrupt the normal process of labour, often leading to other interventions (Andrees & Rankin 2007, Svardby et al 2007), such as continuous electronic fetal monitoring (CEFM). However, NICE (2014) is clear that ARM alone for suspected delay in labour is not an indication for CEFM. Prostaglandin PGE_2 is released by the amnion and cervix, while the chorion produces prostaglandin dehydrogenase (PDHG), an enzyme that prevents the cervix from ripening (Smyth et al 2013). It has been proposed that the part of the chorion in contact with the cervical os at term releases less PDHG, thus allowing PGE_2 to exert its effect. However, if an amniotomy is performed early in labour (< 3 cm) this effect is lost and labour may slow down (Smyth et al 2013). Olsen and colleagues (2010) caution that the risk of endometritis increases approximately 1.7-fold within 1 hour following amniotomy; thus it is important to monitor the woman for signs of this if an ARM is undertaken.

Amniotomy is often undertaken to 'speed up' labour by increasing the frequency of contractions, possibly by releasing prostaglandins and oxytocin. NICE (2014) concurs, advising an ARM shortens labour length by 1 hour, but the strength of contractions will intensify, increasing the degree of pain felt. However, Smyth and colleagues (2013) found no evidence indicating this was a significant outcome from performing an ARM.

The RCM (2012d) caution that fetal heart rate abnormalities can be seen after ARM, which can result in intervention with an increased risk of caesarean birth. The fetal heart should always be auscultated/recorded following an ARM. Dilbaz and colleagues (2006) suggest there is an increase in variable decelerations with early amniotomy. These changes may be a result of fetal haemodynamic changes. Fok and colleagues (2005) found there was a significant reduction in the impedance of the fetal middle cerebral artery (MCA) and renal artery, which they attribute to being a response to fetal stress and release of vasoactive substances following ARM. Amniotic fluid embolism (anaphylactoid syndrome of pregnancy) is a rare side-effect associated with ARM (Mato 2008).

Indications

- Induction of labour
- Augmentation of labour
- Application of FSE and/or assessment of liquor colour
- Maternal request
- Often prior to birth of second twin

Contraindications

- No maternal consent
- High presenting part (risk of cord prolapse)
- Preterm labour
- Known vaginal infection
- Maternal HIV-positive status
- Caution is taken with polyhydramnios or any malposition or malpresentation
- Placenta praevia
- Vasa praevia

If the presenting part is high and ballotable, it is unwise to perform an ARM. However, the obstetrician may choose to perform a controlled ARM and the midwife may be asked to apply light pressure to the fundus to encourage the presenting part to engage in the pelvis as the membranes rupture. The obstetrician ensures the fluid has drained and no cord has prolapsed before removing the hand. Cord prolapse does occur following ARM; Dilbaz and colleagues (2006) suggest this is more likely to occur if there is a malpresentation, multiparity, low birth weight, prematurity or polyhydramnios, but it may still be unexpected. Thus, it is important the midwife feels for the presence of cord following the ARM and takes appropriate steps if it is found.

Standard precautions should be followed and the sharpness of the amnihook or amnicot means the midwife must take care to avoid personal injury and dispose of the hook into a sharps box. It is also important to confirm the membranes are intact, as trauma to the fetal scalp or anus (if a breech presentation) (Warwick et al 2013) can occur if the membranes have already ruptured and the amnihook or amnicot is scraping the fetal skin. This can be difficult to ascertain when the membranes are tight across the presenting part and no liquor is draining. It may be easier to rupture the membranes when a contraction is present and the membranes are bulging under the pressure; however, this is not an absolute necessity.

SKILL 30.2 Artificial rupture of the membranes

1. Discuss the indication with the woman and gain her informed consent.
2. Auscultate the fetal heart or review CTG if in progress.
3. Gather equipment:
   - equipment as for VE
   - amnihook or amnicot.
4. Undertake a VE as detailed in Skill 30.1, maintaining sterility of the amnihook or amnicot. With the examining hand, locate the cervix and ensure conditions are favourable for an ARM to be performed (e.g. descent of presenting part, no pulsation felt beneath the examining fingers).

For amnihook

a. Holding the amnihook with the non-examining hand, slide it carefully between the examining hand and anterior vaginal wall with the point of the hook pointing downwards.
b. Use the examining hand to guide the amnihook into position with the hook pressed against the membranes.
c. Use the non-examining hand to twist the amnihook slightly to tear the membranes.
d. Withdraw the amnihook gently while retaining the fingers in the cervix as the amniotic fluid drains out (ensuring the amniotic fluid does not come into contact with the midwife's clothing).
e. The examining fingers can then locate the tear and digitally increase the size of the opening.

For amnicot

a. Apply the amnicot over the middle or index finger.
b. Ensure the hook is facing the palm.
c. So that the hook remains in position during use, roll the amnicot up tight and pull it tightly over the finger for at least 1 cm.
d. Complete rolling the amnicot firmly to the base of the finger. Define the presenting part and absence of contraindications by inserting one finger through the cervix.
e. Without removing the hand from the vagina, remove the examining finger and insert the finger with the amnicot through the cervix.
f. Gently scratch the membranes to rupture.
g. Remove the amnicot from the finger.

5. Reassess the cervix, fetal descent and position, and feel for the presence of the umbilical cord.
6. If indicated, an FSE can be applied at this point (see below).
7. Withdraw the hand and auscultate the fetal heart.
8. Assist the woman with regard to hygiene, comfort and position.
9. Discuss the findings with the woman.
10. Dispose of equipment correctly and wash and dry hands.
11. Document the indications for ARM with the findings and act accordingly.

APPLICATION OF A FETAL SCALP ELECTRODE

A **fetal scalp electrode (FSE)** can be used when continuous CTG monitoring is indicated to ensure continuity of contact. Fetal cardiac electrical activity is detected through the FSE to a transducer, usually located on the woman's thigh. This is then attached to the electrocardiograph (ECG) port on the monitor. The sound of the fetal heart is continuous regardless of maternal or fetal position and movement, and is not accompanied or confused by sounds of fetal movement or uterine blood flow. Harper and colleagues (2013) found a decrease in caesarean section birth with FSE use which they attribute to an improved ability to monitor fetal heart tones compared with external monitoring. However, it is an invasive procedure for both the woman and the fetus; the electrode is secured under the fetal scalp, with either a clip or spiral connection. It is assumed that the fetus experiences some pain from its application and the transfer of viruses such as HIV and herpes simplex from mother to child is more likely (Baker 2007) (both are contraindications to FSE use). Skin infection or long-term scarring on the baby's scalp can also occur. Harper and colleagues (2013) did not find an increase in maternal infection with FSE use.

Needs and colleagues (1992) found clip electrodes performed better than other types with regard to attachment. The clip is applied by rotating the end of the electrode: anticlockwise rotation causes the clip to recede into the electrode head while clockwise rotation causes it to emerge from the electrode head and be caught on the scalp. It is usually spring-loaded and therefore rarely requires an active rotation clockwise to apply the clip. The Copeland FSE is commonly used and is considered to reduce the risk of needlestick injury as it has a protecting penetrating needle; this also controls the depth of penetration, reducing the risk of fetal injury to the skull (Cutlan 2006). If using a spiral electrode, it is rotated in the direction of the spiral, usually clockwise, until caught under the scalp.

Accuracy of scalp electrodes depends on their correct application. If the membrane is between the electrode and the scalp the tracing is likely to be unreliable, sometimes known as 'artefact' and interpretation of the trace is impossible. The electrode should not be placed near or through a fontanelle or suture line, the cervix or vagina; it should be positioned on the skin folds of the scalp. It can be used on the buttocks of a breech presentation, but causes obvious scarring. It should not be used with a face presentation.

SKILL 30.3 Application of a fetal scalp electrode

1. Discuss the indication with the woman and gain her consent.
2. Ensure that the monitor has an ECG facility and the correct leads and attachments.
3. Gather equipment:
   - equipment as for VE with amnihook or amnicot if membranes are intact
   - sterile FSE.
4. Perform a VE, as detailed in Skill 30.1.
5. Undertake an ARM (Skill 30.2) if membranes intact.
6. With the examining hand, locate the fetal scalp; ensure that sutures and fontanelles are avoided.
7. Slide the FSE (using the non-examining hand) between the examining hand and vaginal wall.
8. Use the examining hand to guide the electrode into place and support the head of the electrode against the scalp.
9. With the non-examining hand, turn the end of the electrode anticlockwise, then release to attach to the scalp, maintaining support of the electrode against the scalp.
10. The electrode should be attached to the scalp; a gentle pull will confirm whether it is attached.
11. An assistant may attach the leads to the transducer and the transducer to the monitor while the examining hand remains in place; if the electrode is not working, reapplication may be attempted.
12. Before withdrawing the examining hand, check that the electrode is securely placed over an appropriate area of the scalp.
13. Apply conductive gel to the transducer or the appropriate fastening and attach around the woman's thigh using a small belt or attach to the monitor on the woman's abdomen if appropriate (e.g. EZIplug 3 attaches to either the leg or the abdomen [Cutlan 2006]); ensure that monitoring is occurring satisfactorily.
14. Assist the woman with regard to hygiene, comfort and position.
15. Explain the differences in the fetal heart sounds heard.
16. Dispose of equipment correctly, wash and dry hands.
17. Document the indications for FSE with other aspects of the examination and act accordingly.

Removal of the FSE

It is important that the FSE is removed from the baby's scalp at or just before birth. This is particularly important to remember if the woman has an emergency caesarean section to avoid trauma to the fetal scalp as the baby is removed from the uterine cavity while the FSE is attached to the external monitor. It is imperative that the FSE is also removed from the woman's vagina to avoid it being retained within her body (Valenzuela 2006).

To remove the clip-style FSE, the electrode head is held against the scalp while the end is rotated anticlockwise. While an anticlockwise rotation can remove the spiral electrode, it is quicker to take hold of the two wires hanging from it and pull them apart; this will cause the clip to rotate and come loose from the scalp as the wires unravel. Care should be taken not to create any trauma while removing it. Any obvious puncture marks should be noted on the initial birth examination. The electrode should be disposed of in the sharps box.

Role and responsibilities of the midwife

These can be summarised as:

- encouraging and supporting the woman in the use of appropriate positions to enhance her comfort and labour progress
- undertaking a competent examination per vaginam in which all the information is gained without causing distress to the woman
- undertaking an amniotomy correctly, when indicated
- undertaking appropriate application of an FSE, when indicated
- recognising deviations from normal and instigating referral

- providing education, explanations and support to the woman
- undertaking appropriate record keeping.

SUMMARY

- Progress in labour is individual and can be assessed using a variety of indicators.
- Women should be encouraged and supported to change position during the first stage of labour and use those positions that are most comfortable, while avoiding the supine position.
- There is a need for more high-quality evidence regarding the advantages and disadvantages of the different positions used.
- An examination per vaginam is an invasive procedure, but one that can yield valuable information in relation to the assessment of progress in labour.
- Amniotomy should not be undertaken routinely in a labour that is progressing normally.
- Fetal scalp electrodes offer continuity of contact if continuous fetal monitoring is indicated.
- The risk of ascending infection is high; an aseptic non-touch technique should be used throughout.

Self-assessment exercises

The answers to the following questions may be found in the text.

1. How is progress assessed during the first stage of labour?
2. What advice can the midwife give to a woman regarding positioning during the first stage of labour?
3. For what reasons would the midwife undertake an examination per vaginam during labour?
4. What should be discussed with the woman to gain her informed consent regarding an examination per vaginam?
5. How would you perform an examination per vaginam?
6. How could the midwife identify a flexed cephalic presentation?
7. What information can be gained from an examination per vaginam and what is the significance of it?
8. Describe how to perform an amniotomy and apply a fetal scalp electrode.
9. What are the role and responsibilities of the midwife in relation to an examination per vaginam, artificial rupture of the membranes and application of a fetal scalp electrode?

References

Andrees M, Rankin J: Amniotomy in spontaneous, uncomplicated labour at term, British Journal of Midwifery 15(10):612–616, 2007.

Baker D: Consequences of herpes simplex virus in pregnancy and their prevention, Current Opinion in Infectious Diseases 20(1):73–76, 2007.

Baker K: Midwives should support women to mobilise during labour, British Journal of Midwifery 18(8): 492–497, 2010.

Blackburn ST: Maternal, fetal and neonatal physiology: a clinical perspective, 4th ed., Saunders, St. Louis, 2013, pp. 119–130.

Burnhill MS, Donezis J, Cohen J: Uterine contractility during labour studied by intra-amniotic fluid pressure recordings, American Journal of Obstetrics & Gynecology 83:561–571, 1962.

Cahill AG, Duffy CR, Odibo AO, et al: Number of cervical examinations and risk of intrapartum maternal fever, Obstetrics & Gynecology 119(6):1096–1101, 2012.

Chamberlain GVP: Obstetrics by ten teachers, 16th ed., Arnold, London, 1993.

Chapman V: Slow progress and malpresentations/ malpositions in labour. In Chapman V, Charles C, eds: The midwife's labour and birth handbook, 2nd ed., Wiley-Blackwell, Chichester, 2009, pp. 106–134.

Cutlan C: Electronic fetal monitoring and infection control, British Journal of Midwifery 14(10):584–585, 2006.

Cutler L: A consideration of the positions women adopt for labour, British Journal of Midwifery 20(5):346–350, 2012.

de Klerk HW, Boere E, van Lunsen RH, Bakker JJH: Women's experiences with vaginal examinations during labor in the Netherlands, Journal of Psychosomatic Obstetrics and Gynaecology 39(2):90–95, 2018.

Dilbaz B, Ozturkoglu E, Dilbaz S, et al: Risk factors and perinatal outcomes associated with umbilical cord prolapse, Archives of Gynecology and Obstetrics 274:104–107, 2006.

Dixon L, Foureur M: The vaginal examination during labour: is it benefit or harm? NZCOM Journal 42(May):21–26, 2010.

Downe S, Gyte GML, Dahlen HG, et al: Routine vaginal examinations for assessing progress of labour to improve outcomes for women and babies at term, Cochrane Database of Systematic Reviews (7):Art. No.: CD010088, 2013.

Fok WY, Leung TY, Tsui MH, et al: Fetal hemodynamic changes after amniotomy, Acta Obstetricia Gynecologica Scandinavia 84:166–169, 2005.

Grasek A, Tuuli M, Roehl K, et al: Fetal descent in labor, American College of Obstetricians and Gynecologists 123(3):521–526, 2014.

Hanson L: Second stage labor: challenges in spontaneous bearing down, Journal of Perinatol & Neonatal Nursing 23(1):31–39, 2009.

Harper LM, Shanks AJ, Tuuli MG, et al: The risks and benefits of internal monitors in laboring patients, American Journal of Obstetricians and Gynecologists 209(38):e1–e6, 2013.

Hassan SJ, Sundby J, Husseini A, et al: The paradox of vaginal examination practice during normal childbirth: Palestinian women's feelings, opinions, knowledge and experiences, Reproductive Health 9:16, 2012.

Hunter S, Hofmeyr GJ, Kulier R: Hands and knees in late pregnancy or labour for fetal malposition (lateral or posterior), Cochrane Database of Systematic Reviews (4):Art. No.: CD001063, 2007.

Incerti M, Locatelli A, Ghidini A, et al: Variability in rate of cervical dilation in nulliparous women at term, Birth (Berkeley, Calif.) 38(1):30–35, 2011.

Kerrigan A: The mother-midwife partnership: a critical analysis of intrapartum care, British Journal of Midwifery 14(6):346–350, 2006.

Kobayashi S, Hanada N, Matsuzaki M, et al: Assessment and support during early labour for improving birth outcomes, Cochrane Database of Systematic Reviews (4):Art No.: CD011516, 2017.

Lawrence A, Lewis L, Hofmeyr GJ, et al: Maternal positions and mobility during the first stage of labour, Cochrane Database of Systematic Reviews (10):Art. No.: CD003934, 2013.

Leap N, Hunter B: Supporting women for labour and birth: a thoughtful guide, Routledge, Abingdon UK, 2016.

Lewin D, Fearon B, Hemmings V, et al: Informing women during vaginal examination, British Journal of Midwifery 13(1):26–29, 2005.

Lumbiganon P, Thinkhamrop J, Thinkhamrop B, et al: Vaginal chlorhexidine during labour for preventing maternal and neonatal infections (excluding Group B streptococcal and HIV), Cochrane Database of Systematic Reviews (9):Art. No.: CD004070, 2014.

Mato J: Suspected fluid embolism following amniotomy: a case report, AANA Journal 76(1):53–59, 2008.

National Childbirth Trust (NCT): Positions for labour and birth, 2011. Online 14 May 2018. Available: www.nct.org.uk/sites/default/files/related_documents/NCT%20Positions%20for%20labour%20birth.pdf.

National Institute for Health and Care Excellence (NICE): Intrapartum care. Care of healthy women and their babies during childbirth, 2014. Online 14 May 2018. Available: www.nice.org.uk.

Needs L, Grant A, Sleep J, et al: A randomised controlled trial to compare three types of fetal scalp electrode, British Journal of Obstetric Gynaecology 99(4): 302–306, 1992.

Ohlsson A, Shah VS, Stade BC: Vaginal chlorhexidine during labour to prevent early-onset neonatal group B streptococcal infection, Cochrane Database of Systematic Reviews (12):Art. No.: CD003520, 2014.

Olsen MA, Butler AM, Willers DM, et al: Risk factors for endometritis after low transverse cesarean delivery, Infection Control and Hospital Epidemiology 31(1): 69–77, 2010.

Ridley RT: Diagnosis and intervention for occiput posterior malposition, Journal of Obstetric Gynecology Neonatal Nursing 36(2):135–143, 2007.

Romano AM: Research summaries for normal birth, Journal of Perinatal Education 17(1):48–52, 2008.

Royal College of Midwives (RCM): Evidence-based guidelines for midwifery-led care in labour. Assessing progress in labour. RCM, London, 2012a.

Royal College of Midwives (RCM): Evidence-based guidelines for midwifery-led care in labour. Latent phase. RCM, London, 2012b.

Royal College of Midwives (RCM): Evidence-based guidelines for midwifery-led care in labour. Positions for labour and birth. RCM, London, 2012c.

Royal College of Midwives (RCM): Evidence-based guidelines for midwifery-led care in labour. Rupturing membranes. RCM, London, 2012d.

Sanderson TA: The movement of the maternal pelvis: a review, MIDIRS Midwifery Digest 22(3):319–326, 2012.

Schmidt V, Downe S: Midwifery skills for normalizing unusual labours. In Walsh D, Downe S, eds: Essential midwifery practice intrapartum care, Wiley-Blackwell, Chichester, 2010, pp. 159–190.

Shepherd A, Cheyne H: The frequency and reasons for vaginal examination in labour, Women and Birth: Journal of the Australian College of Midwives 26(1):49–54, 2013.

Simkin P, Hason L, Ancheta R: The labor progress handbook: early interventions to prevent and treat dystocia, 4th ed., Blackwell, Oxford, 2017.

Smyth RMD, Markham C, Dowsell T: Amniotomy for shortening spontaneous labour, Cochrane Database of Systematic Reviews (6):Art. No.: CD006167, 2013.

Stables D, Rankin J: Physiology in childbearing with anatomy and related biosciences, 3rd ed., Baillière Tindall Elsevier, Edinburgh, 2010.

Svardby K, Nordstrom L, Sellstroni E: Primiparas with or without oxytocin augmentation: a prospective descriptive study, Journal of Clinical Nursing 16(1):179–184, 2007.

Valenzuela P: Removal of a fetal scalp electrode lodged in the vagina of a patient for 23 years, Journal of Obstetric Gynecology 26(7):704–705, 2006.

Vincent M: Amniotomy: to do or not to do? Midwifery 8(5):228, 2005.

Warwick A, Strachan B, McNally J: The bottom line: iatrogenic fetal anal trauma in undiagnosed breech presentation, British Journal of Midwifery 21(7):481–483, 2013.

Zhang J, Landy HJ, Branch DW, et al: Contemporary patterns of spontaneous labor with normal neonatal outcomes, Obstetric Gynecology 116(6):1281–1287, 2010.

CHAPTER 31

ABDOMINAL EXAMINATION DURING LABOUR

Learning outcomes

Having read this chapter, the reader should be able to:

- discuss the indications for abdominal examination during labour
- discuss the different components of an abdominal examination, indicating the nature of the information sought and the rationale for it
- describe how uterine contractions are palpated in labour, why this is undertaken and the significance of the findings
- explain the midwife's role and responsibilities in relation to each of these aspects of care.

The presentation, position and lie of the fetus at the onset of and throughout labour is used to determine engagement and descent of the presenting part and the optimal position to auscultate the fetal heart. Palpation of contractions during labour also involves abdominal examination. This chapter considers the skills of abdominal examination during labour, focusing on how and why this is undertaken and the significance of the information obtained.

ABDOMINAL EXAMINATION IN LABOUR

Abdominal palpation during labour is conducted to determine if there are any deviations from normal. They should always be carried out before a vaginal examination. During labour when the uterus is contracting, the abdomen may be more sensitive and thus this may be more uncomfortable for the woman and harder to do, but it is an aspect of care that supports and informs other aspects of care. The procedure should not be undertaken unnecessarily and should be completed promptly between contractions to minimise discomfort and make it easier to palpate the fetus. Caution is advised in relation to the accuracy of abdominal palpation intrapartum: in one study involving 508 women, there was disagreement about abdominal fetal head station between abdominal assessors by 1 cm in almost half of the cases, and this was not influenced by years of professional experience (Buchmann & Libhaber 2008). Further, Webb and colleagues (2011) found that determining the position, specifically left occipitoanterior, at the onset of labour is not very accurate. This confirms the suggestion made by Peregrine and colleagues (2007) that the lateral palpation assesses the position of the fetal spine, which does not always correspond to the position of the fetal head.

This procedure requires the woman to be in a semirecumbent position, which is not ideal for labour. Thus the midwife should ensure that the woman is encouraged to adopt a more upright position following the examination, whenever possible. It is undertaken to gain a baseline on which care is provided and subsequent progress is assessed by:

- determining the gestation, lie, position, presentation and engagement
- assessing uterine activity (length, strength and frequency of contractions)
- monitoring progress in labour by assessing descent and rotation of the presenting part
- prior to auscultation of the fetal heart or commencing monitoring using cardiotocograph (CTG)
- prior to undertaking an examination per vaginam
- with multiple births, following the birth of each baby, to determine the lie, position and presentation of the remaining fetuses.

Role and responsibilities of the midwife

These can be summarised as:

- displaying knowledge and application of current evidence-based practice
- undertaking all procedures correctly
- providing education, advice and support to the woman
- undertaking accurate contemporaneous record keeping (see also Chapter 27)
- referring for deviations from normal.

SUMMARY

- Abdominal assessment in labour is a skill from which significant information can be gained.
- The midwife has a responsibility to undertake the abdominal examination competently and sensitively, document the findings and make a referral when necessary. It is more uncomfortable for women when in labour.
- An abdominal examination always precedes auscultation of the fetal heart using a Pinard stethoscope, fetal Doppler or CTG monitor.
- Palpation of uterine contractions in labour assesses the frequency, strength, length and resting tone of the uterus. It is a significant aspect of labour care.

Self-assessment exercises

The answers to the following questions may be found in the text.

1. Describe the different components of an abdominal examination, discussing the rationale for each aspect.
2. Demonstrate how to palpate uterine contractions in labour.
3. Summarise the role and responsibilities of the midwife in relation to abdominal examination and use of electronic fetal monitoring.

References

Buchmann E, Libhaber E: Interobserver agreement in intrapartum estimation of fetal head station, International Journal of Gynecology and Obstetrics 101(3):285–289, 2008.

Peregrine E, O'Brien P, Jauniaux E: Impact on delivery outcome of ultrasonographic fetal head position prior to induction of labour, Obstetrics and Gynecology 109(3):618–623, 2007.

Webb AA, Plana MN, Zamora J, et al: Abdominal palpation to determine fetal position at labor onset: a test accuracy study, Acta Obstetricia et Gynecologica Scandinavia 90:1259–1266, 2011.

CHAPTER 32
MEMBRANE SWEEP

Learning outcomes

Having read this chapter, the reader should be able to:

- discuss the indications for membrane sweeping
- discuss the current evidence available
- describe how the procedure is performed
- discuss what the midwife can do if the cervix is closed
- summarise the role and responsibilities of the midwife.

The majority of women will go into spontaneous labour by 42 weeks. In Australia in 2018 over 91% of babies were born at term, 37–40 weeks (Australian Institute of Health and Welfare [AIHW] 2020). When pregnancy extends beyond 42 weeks the risk of fetal macrosomia, low APGAR scores, non-reassuring cardiotography (CTG), meconium aspiration and fetal acidaemia increase (Heilman & Sushereba 2015). Membrane sweeping decreases the rate of pregnancies extending beyond 42 weeks and reduces the need for formal induction (Avdiyovski et al 2019, Heilman & Sushereba 2015). Membrane sweeping is also referred to as a 'stretch and sweep' or 'stripping' the membranes. This chapter considers the skill of membrane sweeping.

MEMBRANE SWEEPING

Membrane sweeping refers to the use of a circular movement of the finger to separate the chorioamniotic membranes from the lower uterine segment during a vaginal examination (Kabiri et al 2015). The midwife uses her fingers to gently dilate (stretch) the cervical os and then separate the membranes from the lower segment (sweep). Membrane sweeping requires entry of the fingers through the cervix; therefore, the cervix must be soft enough to dilate or be beginning to dilate. If the cervix is not dilated, cervical massage can be undertaken instead (Heilman & Sushereba 2015, South Australian Maternal and Neonatal Clinical Network 2014). A closed cervix can be stretched and massaged by using the forefinger and middle fingers to make circular pushing and massaging movements on the surface of the closed cervix for 15–30 seconds duration (Yildirim et al 2010). The cervix can also be massaged around the vaginal fornices (Chodankar et al 2017).

Membrane sweeping promotes labour by causing the cervix and lower uterine segment to release endogenous prostaglandins, PGF2 α (Al-Harmi et al 2015), phospholipase A and oxytocin (Heilman & Sushereba 2015, p. 467). Sweeping the membranes increases the local production of prostaglandins and prostaglandin metabolites within the maternal circulation (Boulvain et al 2005, Yildirim et al 2010). The release of hormones and stretching of the cervix facilitates ripening of the cervix and uterine contractions. Sweeping the membranes has not been shown to increase the incidence of complications for mother or fetus (Boulvain et al 2005) or to increase risk of operative birth or caesarean section (Rizzo et al 2021). A Cochrane Review found membrane sweeping may reduce the number of formal labour inductions and women may be more likely to have a spontaneous onset of labour (Finucane et al 2020).

In Australia, the most common reasons for induction are diabetes (14%), prolonged pregnancy (12%) and prelabour rupture of membranes (10%) (AIHW 2020). In New Zealand, prolonged pregnancy is also a common reason for induction of labour. The rates of induction have been increasing, with approximately 33% of women having an induction of labour in New Zealand (Wise et al 2014). In Australia in 2018, the number of babies born after 40 weeks had decreased, with fewer than 0.4% of newborns post-term, which is defined as ≥ 42 weeks gestation (AIHW 2020). The World Health Organization (WHO 2018) notes there is insufficient evidence for induction of labour for women less than 41 weeks gestation with uncomplicated pregnancies. A 2018 Cochrane review noted labour induction (compared to expectant management) is associated with fewer infant deaths, fewer caesarean sections and more assisted vaginal births. The review concluded further investigation is warranted to determine the optimal time to offer induction of labour to women at or beyond term (Middleton et al 2018).

Membrane sweeping appears to decrease the incidence of prolonged pregnancy (Adams et al 2017, Kabiri et al 2015). Therefore, once a woman's pregnancy passes 40 weeks gestation, it is appropriate to discuss the advantages and disadvantages of membrane sweeping (NSW Health 2014). Each woman requires individual assessment related to her preferences, health and fetal wellbeing (NSW Health 2014). Women should also be provided with the opportunity to have their questions answered (Department of Health 2020). The National Institute for Health and Care Excellence (NICE) recommends discussing the options for managing prolonged pregnancy at the 38-week antenatal visit (NICE 2021a). According to a Cochrane Review (Boulvain et al 2005), eight women would need to have membrane sweeping to prevent one induction of labour.

Local protocols may vary, with NSW Health (2014) recommending discussion of membrane sweeping after 40 weeks gestation and offering the procedure after 41 weeks gestation. Queensland induction of labour guidelines (Queensland Health 2017) suggest discussing membrane-sweeping antenatally and offering a membrane sweep prior to induction. The *Clinical Practice Guidelines: Pregnancy Care* (Department of Health 2020) and NICE (2021b) recommend discussing the option of membrane sweeping for women with prolonged pregnancy. In New Zealand, the *National Women's Guidelines: Induction of Labour* recommend offering women the option of membrane sweeping from 38 weeks gestation, with a plan for membrane sweeping at 40 weeks (Auckland District Health Board 2015). The Canadian *Guidelines for the Management of Pregnancy at 41+0 to 42+0 weeks* (Delaney & Roggensack 2017) recommend discussing and offering membrane sweeping commencing at 38 to 41 weeks.

Women with prolonged pregnancy and those scheduled for an induction of labour can be offered membrane sweeping (Department of Health 2020). Sweeping of the membranes should be avoided for women with increased risk of group B streptococcus (GBS), who are less than 40 weeks gestation (Department of Health 2020). Women who request membrane sweeping prior to 41 weeks gestation should be provided with information about its risks prior to 41 weeks gestation (pain, bleeding, irregular contractions, labour does not commence) and the discussion and any intervention documented (NSW Health 2014). Membrane sweeping is the most popular natural method for induction of labour (Andrusiak et al 2014).

The frequency of membrane sweeping is still subject to debate. A randomised controlled trial involving sweeping the membranes of women with an unfavourable cervix at 39 weeks once a week or twice a week concluded that the frequency does not alter the likelihood of birth prior to 41 weeks (Putnam et al 2011). According to Avdiyovski and colleagues (2019), membrane sweeping appears to be effective from 38 weeks gestation, with one membrane sweep probably as effective as multiple sweeps. A study by Ugezu and colleagues (2020) found spontaneous labour occurred in 79% of women who received a membrane sweep, 73% of nulliparas and 76% of multipara gave birth within 7 days. The spontaneous labour rate was 97% for women with a Bishop's score > 6 (Ugezu et al 2020). Membrane sweeping appears to be more effective at later gestations (Rizzo et al 2021). The risk of incidental membrane rupture may be increased when the cervix is greater than 1 cm dilation at the time of membrane sweeping (Hill et al 2008).

A study examining the effect of membrane sweeping using ultrasound found women who gave birth within 24 hours of membrane sweeping were more likely to have a Bishop's score > 5, be multiparous, have a cervical dilation ≥ 2 cm and have a shorter cervical length ≤ 17.5 mm with an increased posterior cervical angle (Rizzo et al 2021).

The factors associated with birth within 24 hours of membrane sweeping have been noted as gestational age, multiparity and dilation of the cervix (Haj Yahya et al 2019). Using cervical ultrasound assessment, parity and gestational age have been used to predict the likelihood of birth within 24–48 hours after membrane sweeping (Rizzo et al 2021). New technology, such as elastographic imaging of the cervix, may provide further information on the stiffness or softness of the cervix and could help prevent failed induction (Swiatkowska-Freund & Preis 2017).

Benefits and risks

Overall, membrane sweeping appears to reduce the time to spontaneous onset of labour and the need for formal methods of induction; for example, prostaglandin (PGE_2) (Kabiri et al 2015, Mozurkewich et al 2011, NICE 2021b, Ugezu et al 2020). In an Irish population studied, having a membrane sweep resulted in spontaneous onset of labour for 79% of women (Ugezu et al 2020). For women with a Bishop's score greater than six, the rate of spontaneous labour was 97% (Ugezu et al 2020). Sweeping the membranes has been found beneficial for nulliparas who have an unfavourable cervix when labour induction is commenced; benefits include reduced induction-to-labour interval, lower doses of oxytocin and increased vaginal birth rate (Al-Harmi et al 2015). Women who had membrane sweeping prior to formal induction indicated they had more pain, but the time to birth was decreased, oxytocin infusions were of a shorter duration and women had higher satisfaction with the birth process and a higher rate of spontaneous vaginal birth (Heilman & Sushereba 2015). Women with one prior caesarean section were randomised to either membrane sweeping or no membrane sweeping; the women with membrane sweeping had higher rates of normal birth (Afzal et al 2015).

Maternal and neonatal outcomes are the same for women who had membrane sweeping or massage compared with those who did not (e.g. prelabour rupture of membranes, maternal and neonatal infection requiring antibiotic treatment, meconium-stained liquor, vaginal bleeding, instrumental and operative delivery, neonatal morbidity) (Boulvain et al 2005, de Miranda et al 2006, Hamdan et al 2009, Yildirim et al 2010).

Approximately 20–30% of women are colonised with *Streptococcus agalactiae* (GBS). The American College of Gynecologists (ACOG) and the Centers for Disease Control (CDC) discuss the potential risks of membrane sweeping, but do not consider GBS a contraindication to membrane sweeping (Kabiri et al 2015). The STRIP-G prospective cohort study found there was no increase in adverse maternal events or serious morbidity and no neonatal sepsis or serious neonatal morbidity when women were GBS-positive (Kabiri et al 2015). Sweeping of the amniotic membranes does not appear to increase adverse events in women who are GBS-positive; however, information is not available on the outcomes for women with HIV or hepatitis (Heilman & Sushereba 2015). According to the *Clinical Practice Guidelines: Pregnancy Care*, membrane sweeping can be performed when women are GBS-positive (Department of Health 2020).

Membrane sweeping is associated with increased maternal discomfort, contractions and vaginal bleeding following the procedure (Boulvain et al 2005, Heilman & Sushereba 2015). According to Ugezu et al (2020) the majority of women found membrane sweeping resulted in mild to moderate discomfort with 8% reporting severe discomfort; the least discomfort was reported when membrane sweeps were performed by midwives. Although membrane sweeping causes discomfort, 90% of women would recommend a membrane sweep to other women (Ugezu et al 2020). The membranes may be accidently ruptured during membrane sweeping. It is important a woman is aware of these factors before she consents to the procedure.

Contraindications

Contraindications to membrane sweeping are the same as those precluding normal birth and include malpresentations, low-lying placenta, vasa praevia or placenta praevia and obstructions to labour (Heilman & Sushereba 2015), as well as planned caesarean section (South Australian Maternal & Neonatal Clinical Network 2014). Contraindications also include pregnancy less than 38 weeks gestation and poor tolerance of vaginal examination.

Sweeping the membranes appears to be a safe procedure which may reduce the incidence of prolonged pregnancy. Provided there are no complications, or contraindications to labour or vaginal birth, membrane sweeping can be offered to women over 40 weeks gestation. Local protocols should be followed, but generally this procedure can be undertaken in an outpatient setting, such as the woman's home or the antenatal clinic. Asepsis should be maintained and the midwife should be trained in this aspect of care prior to undertaking the procedure.

The midwife should maintain contemporaneous records and document the discussion with the woman, that consent was obtained, when and how the procedure was undertaken and the findings from the vaginal examination.

SKILL 32.1 Membrane sweep

An antenatal assessment should be completed prior to sweeping the membranes. This includes abdominal palpation, history, pregnancy complications and fetal movements. If additional risk factors are present, such as reduced fetal movements of poor fetal growth, further consultation may be required and a CTG performed.

1. Discuss the procedure, including benefits and risks with the woman and gain informed consent.
2. Auscultate the fetal heart prior to sweeping the membranes.
3. Prepare for and undertake the examination per vaginam.
4. Undertake a Bishop's scoring (or similar) assessment (see Glossary) of the cervix.
5. Insert one or two fingers into the cervix to gently dilate the os, moving the finger(s) between the lower uterine segment and fetal membranes.
6. Using some inward pressure, move the finger(s) with a sweeping circular action through 360° (Fig 32.1). This should be undertaken fairly decisively as the woman will be uncomfortable, which will increase if the procedure is unnecessarily prolonged.
7. If the cervix is closed, perform cervical massage for 15–30 seconds using the fore- and middle fingers to make circular pushing and massaging movements on the cervix.
8. Remove the examining hand gently and remove gloves.
9. Auscultate the fetal heart for at least 60 seconds.
10. Assist the woman to dress and resume a comfortable position; discuss the findings.
11. Dispose of equipment appropriately and wash and dry hands.
12. Document findings and act accordingly.

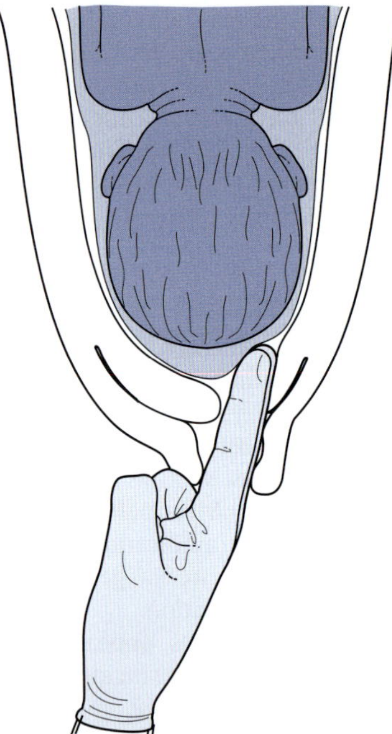

FIGURE 32.1 **Sweeping the membranes.**
Source: Johnson R, Taylor W: Skills for midwifery practices, 3rd ed., Churchill Livingstone, Edinburgh, 2010.

Role and responsibilities of the midwife

These can be summarised as:

- discussing the procedure with the woman and providing information on the benefits and risks
- encouraging the woman to relax
- ensuring the woman is appropriately covered
- undertaking the procedure correctly after gaining informed consent
- checking the fetal heart rate prior to and after the procedure
- completing contemporaneous documentation.

SUMMARY

- Sweeping the membranes involves gently dilating the cervical os and digitally separating the membranes from the lower uterine segment.
- Sweeping the membranes appears to reduce the need for formal induction for women with post-term pregnancy.

Self-assessment exercises

The answers to the following questions may be found in the text.

1. When should membrane sweeping be offered and undertaken?
2. When is membrane sweeping contraindicated?
3. What information would the midwife discuss with the woman to help her make an informed decision about whether or not to undergo membrane sweeping?
4. Discuss how membrane sweeping and cervical massage can be undertaken.
5. Summarise the role and responsibilities of the midwife in relation to this procedure.

References

Adams R, Lichorad A, Simmons J: Membrane sweeping to decrease rates of postdate induction, American Family Physician 95(1):35–36, 2017.

Afzal M, Asif U, Miraj B: Induction of labour; efficacy of sweeping of membranes at term in previous one c-section, Professional Medical Journal 22(4):385, 2015.

Al-Harmi J, Chibber R, Fouda M, et al: Is membrane sweeping beneficial at the initiation of labor induction, The Journal of Maternal-Fetal & Neonatal Medicine 28(10):1214–1218, 2015.

Andrusiak M, Gordon W, Hays K: Natural methods of induction of labour: use by certified professional midwives in an out-of-hospital setting, 2014. ProQuest Dissertations and Theses.

Auckland District Health Board: National Women's Guidelines: Induction of labour, 2015. Online 11 April 2020. Available: https://nationalwomenshealth.adhb.govt.nz/healthprofessionals/referrals-and-information/maternity/induction-of-labour/.

Australian Institute of Health and Welfare (AIHW): Australia's mothers and babies 2018: in brief. Perinatal statistics series no. 36. Cat. no. PER 108, AIHW, Canberra, 2020.

Avdiyovski H, Haith-Cooper M, Scally, A. (2019). Membrane sweeping at term to promote spontaneous labour and reduce the likelihood of a formal induction of labour for postmaturity: a systematic review and meta-analysis. Journal of Obstetrics and Gynaecology, 39(1), 54–62.

Boulvain M, Stan CM, Irion O: Membrane sweeping for induction of labour, Cochrane Database of Systematic Reviews (1):Art No.: CD000451, 2005.

Chodankar R, Sood A, Gupta J: An overview of the past current and future trends for cervical ripening in induction of labour, The Royal College of Obstetricians and Gynaecologists 19:219–226, 2017.

de Miranda E, van der Bom JG, Bonsel GJ, et al: Membrane sweeping and prevention of post-term pregnancy in low-risk pregnancies: a randomised controlled trial, British Journal of Obstetrics and Gynaecology 113(4):402–408, 2006.

Delaney M, Roggensack A, Clinical Practice Obstetrics Committee: No. 214 Guidelines for the management of pregnancy at 41+0 to 42+0 weeks, Journal of Obstetrics and Gynaecology Canada 39(8):e164–e174, 2017.

Department of Health, Clinical practice guidelines: pregnancy care, Australian Government, 2020. Online

11 April 2021. Available: www.health.gov.au/resources/pregnancy-care-guidelines

Finucane EM, Murphy DJ, Biesty LM, Gyte GML, Cotter AM, Ryan EM, Boulvain M, Devane D. Membrane sweeping for induction of labour. Cochrane Database of Systematic Reviews 2020, Issue 2. Art. No.: CD000451.

Haj Yahya R, Ezra Y, Berghella V, et al: Development of a nomogram for prediction of successful membrane sweeping, The Journal of Maternal-Fetal & Neonatal Medicine 32(9):1401–1406, 2019.

Hamdan ML, Sidhu K, Sabir N, et al: Serial membrane sweeping at term in planned vaginal birth after cesarean: a randomized controlled trial, Obstetrics and Gynecology 114(4):745–751, 2009.

Heilman E, Sushereba E: Amniotic membrane sweeping, Seminars in Perinatology 39(6):466–470, 2015.

Hill MJ, McWilliams GD, Garcia-Sur D, et al: The effect of membrane sweeping on prelabor rupture of membranes: a randomized controlled trial, Obstetrics and Gynecology 111(6):1313–1319, 2008.

Kabiri D, Hants Y, Yarkoni TR, et al: Antepartum membrane stripping in GBS carrieres, Is it safe? The STRIP-G Study, PLoS ONE 10(12):1–12, 2015.

Middleton P, Shepherd E, Crowther CA: Induction of labour for improving birth outcomes for women at or beyond term, Cochrane Database of Systematic Reviews 9 May 2018. Available: https://doi.org/10.1002/14651858.CD004945.pub4.

Mozurkewich EL, Chilimigras JL, Berman DR, et al: Methods of induction of labour: a systematic review, BMC Pregnancy and Childbirth 11:84, 2011.

National Institute for Health and Care Excellence (NICE): Antenatal care, NICE guideline [NG201], 2021a. Available: www.nice.org.uk/guidance/ng201.

National Institute for Health and Care Excellence (NICE): Induction of labour overview, NICE Pathways, 2021b. Online 29 August 2021. Available: http://pathways.nice.org.uk/pathways/induction-of-labour

NSW Health: Maternity—Management of pregnancy beyond 41 weeks gestation, 2014. Online 11 April 2021. Available: www1.health.nsw.gov.au/pds/ActivePDSDocuments/GL2014_015.pdf.

Putnam K, Magann EF, Doherty DA, et al: Randomized clinical trial evaluating the frequency of membrane sweeping with an unfavorable cervix at 39 weeks, International Journal of Women's Health 3:287–294, 2011.

Queensland Health: Queensland clinical guidelines: Induction of labour, 2017. Online 11 April 2021. Available: www.health.qld.gov.au/__data/assets/pdf_file/0020/641423/g-iol.pdf.

Rizzo G, Aloisio F, Yacoub M, et al: Ultrasound assessment of the cervix in predicting successful membrane sweeping: a prospective observational study, The Journal of Maternal-Fetal & Neonatal Medicine 34(6):852–858, 2021. Available: https://doi.org/10.1080/14767058.2019.1619689.

South Australian Maternal & Neonatal Clinical Network: Clinical guideline: Induction of labour techniques, 2014. Online 11 April 2021. Available: www.sahealth.sa.gov.au/wps/wcm/connect/ac7d37804ee4a27985598dd150ce4f37/Induction+of+labour_Clinical+Guideline_final_Dec14.pdf?MOD=AJPERES.

Swiatkowska-Freund M, Preis K: Cervical elastography during pregnancy: clinical perspectives, International Journal of Women's Health 9:245–254, 2017.

Ugezu CH, Corcoran P, Dunn EA, Burke C: Does membrane sweep work? Assessing obstetric outcomes and patient perception of cervical membrane sweeping at term in an Irish obstetric population: a prospective multi-centre cohort study, Irish Journal of Medical Science 189(3):969–977, 2020. Available: https://doi.org/10.1007/s11845-020-02191-w .

Wise M, Ansell L, Belgrave S, et al: Auckland consensus guideline on induction of labour, 2014. Online 11 April 2021. Available: nationalwomenshealth.adhb.govt.nz/assets/Uploads/Auckland-IOL-consensus-guideline.pdf.

World Health Organization. WHO recommendations: induction of labour at or beyond term. 2018. Online 11 April 2021. Available: apps.who.int/iris/bitstream/handle/10665/277233/9789241550413-eng.pdf?ua=1

Yildirim G, Güngördük K, Karadağ Öİ, et al: Membrane sweeping to induce labor in low-risk patients at term pregnancy: a randomized controlled trial, The Journal of Maternal-Fetal & Neonatal Medicine 23(7):681–687, 2010.

CHAPTER 33

FETAL HEART MONITORING

Learning outcomes

Having read this chapter, the reader should be able to:

- describe different fetal heart monitoring modalities
- discuss the decision-making pathway and criteria for intermittent auscultation
- explain the indications for using a cardiotocograph (CTG) machine, how it is applied and how to interpret the tracing
- describe the criteria used to identify normal and abnormal CTG tracings
- describe how uterine contractions are palpated in labour, why this is undertaken and the significance of the findings
- explain the midwife's role and responsibilities in relation to each of these aspects of care.

The monitoring of fetal wellbeing during labour and birth is an essential midwifery skill that uses a number of basic skills. These include: abdominal palpation to determine the fetal presentation, position, lie and descent and the frequency, length and strength of uterine contractions; and auscultation of the fetal heart rate, either intermittently or continuously. During pregnancy, women should be offered information on intrapartum fetal surveillance by those responsible for provision of maternity care (Royal Australian and New Zealand College of Obstetricians and Gynaecologists [RANZCOG] 2019). This chapter considers different fetal heart monitoring modalities and focuses on the decision-making process to support selection of the method of monitoring, interpretation of fetal monitoring and the actions that arise out of this interpretation.

AUSCULTATION OF THE FETAL HEART

Auscultation is the action of listening to the noises inside the body. When monitoring fetal wellbeing during labour and birth, it is the fetal heart that is being listened to. The purpose is to monitor changes in fetal heart rate (FHR) and rhythm that provide alert signals; or in other words, it is a screening tool for the detection of FHR abnormalities (Maude et al 2010). Intermittent auscultation (IA) is an appropriate method of intrapartum fetal monitoring in women without recognised risk factors (RANZCOG 2019).

Auscultation should be undertaken:

- prior to the application of a cardiotocograph (CTG) monitor
- throughout labour to monitor the fetal response to labour
- to determine fetal life in the event of absence of fetal movements
- if requested by the woman.

During labour, IA of the fetal heart sounds can be undertaken using a **Pinard stethoscope** or a **handheld Doppler device** (Fig 33.1). The Pinard stethoscope is a hollow wooden, plastic or metal cone-shaped device that amplifies the fetal heart sounds. The wide end of the Pinard is held against the woman's abdomen, while the midwife listens through the other end. The handheld Doppler device is a small battery-operated device that uses ultrasound technology to provide an audible simulation of the fetal heart sounds.

During the active first stage of labour, IA of the fetal heart is conducted according to a standardised protocol. For consistency, a standardised approach to fetal heart monitoring, interpretation and the language used to communicate the findings should be used in all maternity units. The RANZCOG fetal surveillance guideline (2019) should be uniformly applied in Australia and New Zealand. It recommends listening to and documenting

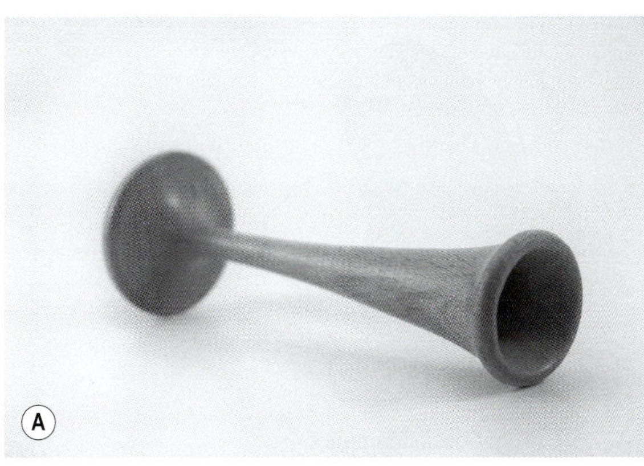

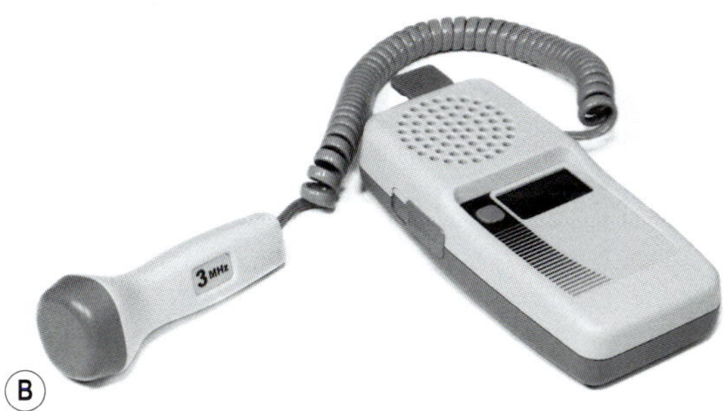

FIGURE 33.1 **Auscultation devices A, Pinard stethoscope. B, Handheld Doppler device.**
Source: iStockphoto/levil (Pinard); iStockphoto/thelastlight (Doppler).

the fetal heart every 15–30 minutes in the active phase of the first stage of labour and after each contraction, or at least every 5 minutes in the active second stage of labour. Each auscultation episode should commence towards the end of a contraction and be continued for at least 30–60 seconds after the contraction has finished (RANZCOG 2019). Fetal and maternal heart rates should be differentiated whatever the mode of monitoring used, ideally with monitors capable of simultaneously recording maternal and fetal heart rates (RANZCOG 2019). The counted fetal heart rate should be recorded as a single rate and any FHR increases or decreases heard (above or below the previously determined average FHR) should be noted. A decision-making flowchart, such as the intelligent structured intermittent auscultation (ISIA) framework, supports risk assessment at admission and throughout labour, choice of fetal heart monitoring method, conduct and interpretation of monitoring and advice on management of abnormal fetal heart findings (Maude et al 2014, 2016, Pairman et al 2018).

An abdominal palpation (see Chapter 27) should precede the auscultation as this will assist with locating the best position to listen to the fetal heart. Maternal anxiety will be unnecessarily heightened if the midwife 'guesses' where to place the equipment to hear the fetal heart and has to keep moving it around because an abdominal palpation was omitted. The clearest fetal heart sounds are heard through the anterior fetal shoulder (scapula) (Fig 33.2), although they can sometimes be heard through the fetal chest wall depending on the fetal position. The fetal heartbeat is heard as a rapid double beating (often described as a vibration or a tapping sound) between 110 and 160 beats per minute (bpm) with increases in the rate noted with fetal movements.

USING A PINARD STETHOSCOPE

Familiarity with the use of a Pinard stethoscope enables the midwife to confirm it is the fetal heart that has been heard. It can be difficult to use the Pinard stethoscope with some positions adopted by women in labour (e.g. hands and knees), and during water immersion. In these instances it may be preferable to use a handheld Doppler device in order to reduce disruption to the normal rhythms of labour.

Using the Pinard stethoscope effectively is a learned and practised skill which improves with continuing use, but it can be difficult to use to begin with. Wickham (2002) suggests the auscultated fetal heartbeat is more of a vibration than a sound, similar to listening to the Korotkoff sounds when taking a manual blood pressure. It is harder to hear if there are other external noises competing and it may be easier to listen with closed eyes and hands off the stethoscope. If the fetal heart is not heard where expected, the position of the Pinard should be changed but not rotated, and if it is still not detected, use the Doppler device. Midwives with hearing difficulties may find it easier to use the Doppler device.

SKILL 33.1 Using a Pinard stethoscope

1. Discuss the procedure with the woman and gain her informed consent.
2. Encourage the woman to empty her bladder.
3. Undertake an abdominal examination to determine the position of the fetus.
4. Position the Pinard stethoscope over the area where heart sounds are expected (Fig 33.3), with the widest part on the maternal abdomen and the midwife's ear over the hole in the earpiece. Apply gentle pressure; the woman can tell you if the pressure is comfortable. Do not hold onto the Pinard as this may interfere with clarity of sound.
5. Listen to and count the fetal heart for 1 minute, simultaneously palpating the woman's radial pulse to ensure it is the fetal heart being auscultated.
6. Compare the counted FHR with the previously established average rate and earlier recordings to determine whether it is in the normal range.
7. Discuss the results with the woman.
8. Document the time of listening, the device used, the FHR (as a single number), any other information obtained during monitoring and a plan for follow-up (if required).

Source: Johnson R, Taylor W: Skills for midwifery practice, 4th ed., Elsevier, London, 2016.

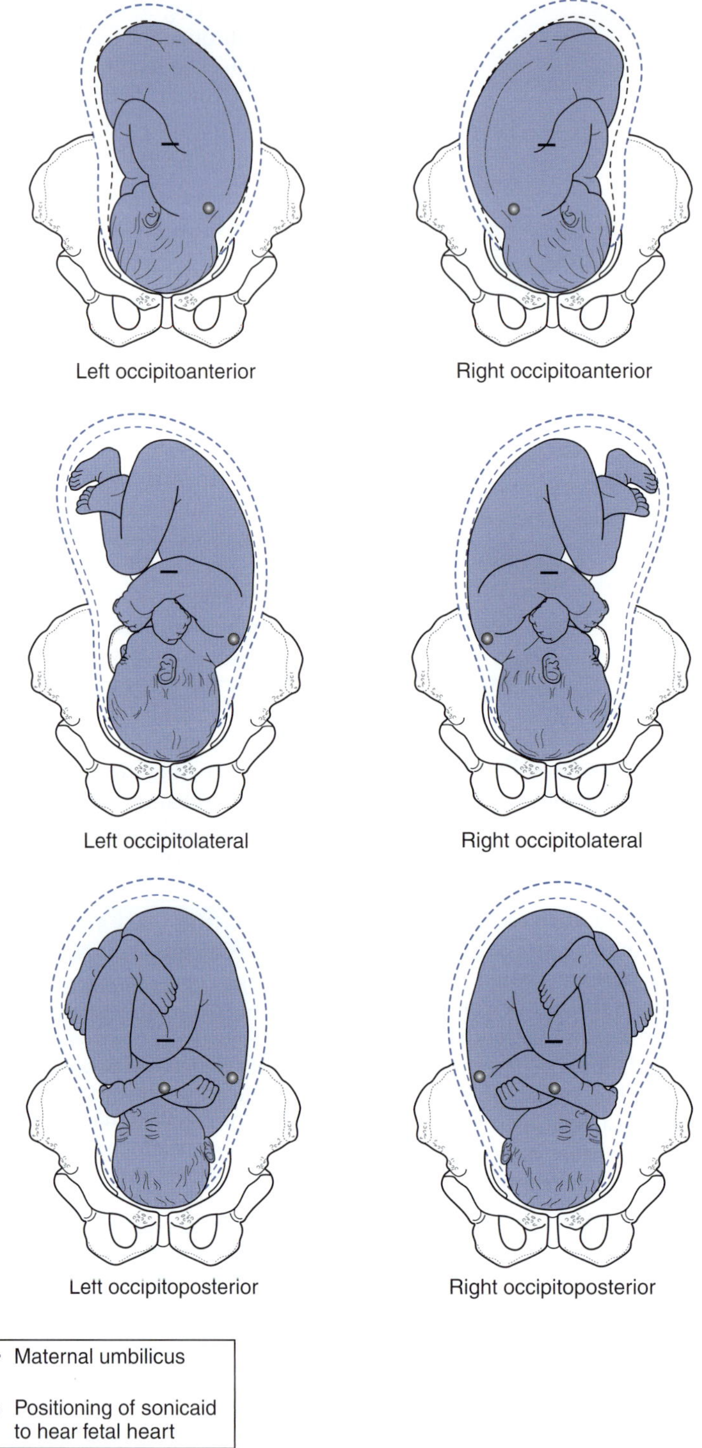

FIGURE 33.2 **Positioning of the auscultation device with a vertex presentation.**
Source: Johnson R, Taylor W: Skills for midwifery practice, 4th ed., Elsevier, London, 2016.

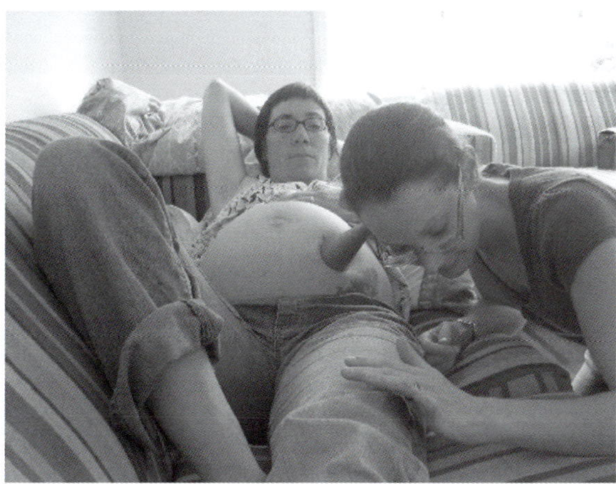

FIGURE 33.3 **Using a Pinard stethoscope.**
Source: Robyn Maude, 2010, permission granted.

USING AN ULTRASOUND DOPPLER DEVICE

A handheld Doppler device can also be used to auscultate the fetal heart. These devices use ultrasound technology to reflect and amplify sounds from the moving fetal heart walls and valves (Feinstein et al 2008). The Doppler device gives an audio-converted representation of the fetal cardiac cycle (Goodwin 2000), then changes this into a digital display and/or sound that can be heard by all in the room. This may be reassuring to the woman and her support people and other health professionals. The handheld Doppler device can be more physically comfortable for the woman and can easily be used in various positions and locations adopted by the woman during active labour (Lewis & Downe 2015).

The midwife should always be alert to the possibility of an absent fetal heart and therefore may choose to confirm its presence with a Pinard stethoscope first. The Doppler transducer should be placed directly over the fetal shoulder in order to hear the fetal heart. Identification of the correct placement of the transducer comes from careful abdominal palpation, as stated earlier. Less pressure is needed on the abdomen compared with a Pinard and some devices can be used in water. Other sounds (swooshing of blood through uterine vessels, fetal hiccoughs, fetal movements) can be heard and will need explaining to the listening woman and her support people.

SKILL 33.2 Using a handheld Doppler device

1. Discuss the procedure with the woman and gain her informed consent.
2. Encourage the woman to empty her bladder.
3. Undertake an abdominal examination and auscultate the fetal heart using a Pinard stethoscope.
4. Lubricate the Doppler ultrasound probe with a suitable conductive gel to facilitate ultrasound transmission.
5. Position the Doppler probe over the area where heart sounds are expected. If the fetal heart is not heard where expected shift the angle of the probe rather than moving the probe to a different place.
6. Count the heartbeat for 1 minute, as with Pinard auscultation. Do not rely on the number displayed on the screen as this can be inaccurate due to interference and loss of contact.
7. Simultaneously palpate the maternal radial pulse to ensure it is the fetal heart that is being heard.
8. Reassure the woman about the other sounds that can be heard.
9. Wipe the gel off with a tissue.
10. Discuss the results with the woman.
11. Document the time of listening, the device used, the FHR (as a single number), any other information obtained during monitoring and a plan for follow-up (if required).

CARDIOTOCOGRAPH (CTG)

The **cardiotocograph (CTG)** machine, using ultrasound technology, is a way to undertake continuous monitoring of the FHR over a specific period of time where there is potential for fetal compromise due to antenatal or intrapartum risk factors (Box 33.1). The use of admission CTG in labour is appropriate in the presence of risk factors, but careful consideration should be given to its use for well women with uncomplicated pregnancies due to its association with increased interventions and caesarean section (Devane et al 2012).

Alfirevic and colleagues (2013) caution that while the use of continuous CTG during labour is associated with a reduction in neonatal seizures, there are no significant differences in cerebral palsy incidence, infant mortality rates or other measures of neonatal wellbeing, but there is an increase in both the number of caesarean sections and instrumental births (Alfirevic et al 2013). There is the possibility that the maternal pulse rate is detected rather than the FHR, particularly

Box 33.1 Risk factors for continuous CTG monitoring

Antenatal and intrapartum factors that increase the risk of fetal compromise. Intrapartum cardiotocography (CTG) is recommended.

Antenatal risk factors

- Abnormal antenatal CTG
- Abnormal Doppler umbilical artery velocimetry
- Suspected or confirmed intrauterine growth restriction
- Oligohydramnios or polyhydramnios
- Prolonged pregnancy ≥ 42 weeks
- Multiple pregnancy
- Breech presentation
- Antepartum haemorrhage
- Prolonged rupture of membranes (≥ 24 hours)
- Known fetal abnormality which requires monitoring
- Uterine scar (e.g. previous caesarean section)
- Essential hypertension or pre-eclampsia
- Diabetes, where medication is indicated or poorly controlled, or with fetal macrosomia
- Other current or previous obstetric or medical conditions which constitutes a significant risk of fetal compromise (e.g. cholestasis, isoimmunisation, substance abuse)
- Fetal movements altered unless there has been demonstrated fetal wellbeing and return to normal fetal movements
- Morbid obesity (BMI ≥ 40)
- Maternal age ≥ 42
- Abnormalities of maternal serum screening associated with an increased risk of poor perinatal outcomes (e.g. low PAPP-A < 0.4 MoM [multiple of the median])
- Abnormal placental cord insertion
- Abnormal cerebroplacental ratio

Intrapartum risk factors

- Induction of labour with prostaglandin/oxytocin
- Abnormal auscultation or CTG
- Oxytocin augmentation
- Regional anaesthesia (e.g. epidural* or spinal) and paracervical block
- Abnormal vaginal bleeding in labour
- Maternal pyrexia ≥ 38°C
- Meconium or blood-stained liquor
- Absent liquor following amniotomy
- Prolonged first stage as defined by referral guidelines
- Prolonged second stage as defined by referral guidelines
- Preterm labour less than 37 completed weeks
- Tachysystole (more than five active labour contractions in 10 minutes, without fetal heart rate abnormalities)
- Uterine hypertonus (contractions lasting more than 2 minutes in duration or contractions occurring within 60 seconds of each other, without fetal heart rate abnormalities)
- Uterine hyperstimulation (either tachysystole or uterine hypertonus with fetal heart rate abnormalities)
- Following a decision to insert an epidural block, a CTG should be commenced to establish baseline features prior to the block's insertion

Conditions where a recommendation for intrapartum CTG are not indicated when the condition occurs in isolation, but if multiple conditions are present, a recommendation for intrapartum CTG should be considered.

Antenatal risk factors

- Pregnancy gestation 41.0–41.6 weeks gestation
- Gestational hypertension
- Gestational diabetes mellitus without complicating factors
- Obesity (BMI 30–40)
- Maternal age ≥ 40 and < 42 years
- Amniotic fluid index (AFI) 5–8 cm (or maximum vertical pocket [MVP] 2–3 cm)

Intrapartum risk factors

- Maternal pyrexia ≥ 37.8°C and < 38°C

Source: Royal Australian and New Zealand College of Obstetricians and Gynaecologists (RANZCOG): Intrapartum fetal surveillance, Clinical guideline, 4th ed., RANZCOG, Melbourne, 2019. Available: https://ranzcog.edu.au/RANZCOG_SITE/media/RANZCOG-MEDIA/Women%27s%20Health/Statement%20and%20guidelines/Clinical-Obstetrics/IFS-Guideline-4thEdition-2019.pdf?ext=.pdf.

during the second stage (Nurani et al 2012); thus, it is important to distinguish between the two. Newer machines have a probe that is placed over the woman's finger, which will record her pulse rate at the same time. While CTG can be a useful tool in assessing fetal wellbeing, it is not infallible and decisions about a woman's care, particularly in labour, should not be made on the basis of CTG findings alone (RANZCOG 2019). CTG monitoring should not be used as a substitute for adequate intrapartum midwifery care.

The CTG monitor can record the fetal heart and uterine pressure abdominally, with some having the ability to do this internally (Fig 33.4). There are two transducers, one placed over the fundus to sense the

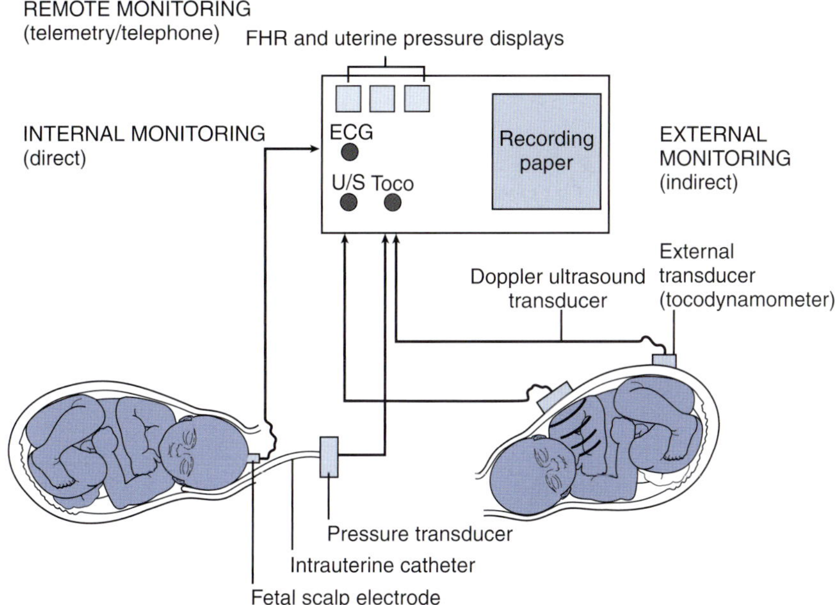

FIGURE 33.4 **Cardiotocography monitor. ECG = electrocardiograph; FHR = fetal heart rate; Toco = tocodynamometer; U/S = ultrasound.**
Source: Johnson R, Taylor W: Skills for midwifery practice, 4th ed., Elsevier, London, 2016.

changing pressure of the uterus (tocodynamometer) and one to listen to the FHR. Often they are secured in place with belts wrapped around the woman's abdomen. Internal monitoring of the FHR requires the application of a fetal scalp electrode and is more invasive (Fig 33.4).

The FHR and uterine contractions are printed out on graph paper, which should run at 1 centimetre per minute. The actual pressure changes in the uterus do not equate exactly with the printed strength of contractions; therefore, CTG should not replace regular abdominal palpation of uterine activity by the midwife. As the fetus moves, which may be accompanied by an increase in the heart rate, there may also be a loss of contact as the baby moves away from the sound beam. This should be annotated directly onto the trace.

The midwife should remain with the woman for the duration of CTG monitoring, providing one-to-one support and ensuring the focus of the care centres on the woman, not the CTG. RANZCOG (2019) recommends that auscultation in labour should be undertaken (whether by IA or CTG) and documented every 15–30 minutes in the active phase of the first stage of labour, and with each contraction or at least every 5 minutes in the active second stage of labour. It should be regularly recorded, either by written or electronic entry, in the medical record that the CTG has been reviewed. As well, any intrapartum events that may affect the FHR (e.g. vaginal examination, obtaining a fetal blood sample [FBS], insertion/top-up of an epidural), should be noted at the same time including date, time and signature.

Interpretation of the CTG is a skill that requires regular education and assessment, and for many midwives is part of their mandatory annual updating. Midwives are encouraged to use a 'fresh eyes' approach when interpreting CTG traces (Donnelly & Hamilton 2012, Fitzpatrick & Holt 2008); this means discussing the CTG trace with another midwife colleague and/or a medical colleague as recommended by RANZCOG (2019), which suggests that 'consideration should be given to a policy of a second clinician independently assessing the CTG periodically' (p. 23).

Cardiotocograph interpretation

CTG interpretation begins with knowledge of relevant maternal and fetal physiology, the woman's history and current clinical profile and that the monitor has been correctly applied. Any changes of maternal position, vomiting, vaginal examination, epidural analgesia and other such variables should be noted and considered. The presence (or absence) of uterine contractions should be noted for their frequency, strength and length. RANZCOG (2019) recommend four features of the fetal heart tracing are assessed during labour (in conjunction with uterine activity): baseline rate, baseline variability, accelerations and decelerations.

RANZCOG (2019) classifies each of these features and the overall trace as follows.

- Normal: low probability of fetal compromise (Fig 33.5)
  - Baseline rate 110–160 bpm
  - Baseline variability of 6–25 bpm

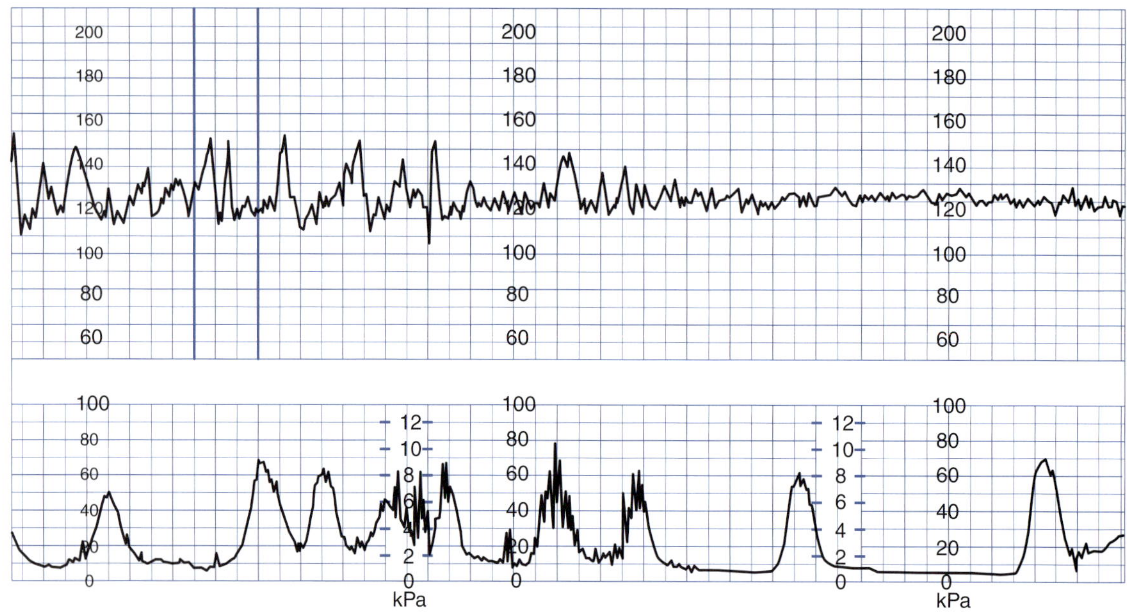

FIGURE 33.5 **A normal CTG tracing.**
Source: Johnson R, Taylor W: Skills for midwifery practice, 4th ed., Elsevier, London, 2016.

- Accelerations 15 bpm for 15 seconds
- No decelerations
- Abnormal but unlikely to be associated with fetal compromise when occurring in isolation
  - Baseline rate 100–109 bpm
  - Reduced or reducing baseline variability 3–5 bpm
  - Absence of accelerations
  - Early decelerations
  - Variable decelerations without complicating factors
- Abnormal and may be associated with significant fetal compromise and require further action
  - Baseline fetal tachycardia > 160 bpm
  - Rising baseline FHR (even when it remains within the normal range)
  - Complicated variable deceleration
  - Late decelerations
  - Prolonged decelerations
- Abnormal and likely to be associated with significant fetal compromise requiring immediate management, which may include urgent delivery.
  - Prolonged bradycardia (a fall in the baseline FHR > 5 minutes) > 160 bpm
  - Absent baseline variability < 3 bpm
  - Sinusoidal pattern
  - Complicated variable decelerations with reduced or absent baseline variability
  - Late decelerations with reduced or absent baseline variability

Baseline rate

The **baseline rate** is the mean level of the FHR when this is stable, excluding accelerations and decelerations and contractions. It is determined over a time period of 5 or 10 minutes and expressed in bpm. Preterm fetuses tend to have values towards the upper end of this range. A progressive rise in the baseline is important, as well as the absolute values (RANZCOG 2019). A normal FHR is between 110 and 160 bpm and is the rate to which the fetal heart returns after accelerations, decelerations or a period of activity or sleep. It should be assessed between contractions and where there is no current fetal activity or fetal sleep.

Baseline variability

Baseline variability refers to the three- to five-cycle per minute fluctuations around the baseline FHR. Variability reflects the balance between the sympathetic and parasympathetic nervous systems. Normal baseline variability indicates a well-oxygenated central nervous system and is considered the most important indicator of fetal wellbeing.

Variability may be reduced during fetal sleep periods and with the administration of certain drugs (e.g. magnesium sulfate). It is assessed by estimating the difference in bpm between the highest peak and the lowest trough of fluctuation in 1-minute segments of the trace between contractions. Normal baseline variation is described as 6–25 bpm at the baseline FHR. Baseline variability of between 3–5 bpm is described as *reduced baseline variability* and baseline variability less than 3 bpm is called *absent baseline variability*. Baseline variability of > 25 bpm is known as *increased baseline variability*. A serious abnormality of baseline variability is called *sinusoidal pattern*. This is seen as a regular oscillation of the baseline FHR resembling a sine wave. This smooth, undulating pattern is persistent, has a relatively fixed period of 2–5 cycles per minute and an amplitude of 5–15 bpm above and below the baseline. Baseline variability is absent and there are no accelerations.

Accelerations

Accelerations are transient increases in the FHR of 15 bpm or more above the baseline rate, lasting 15 seconds or more. Accelerations are a fetal response to stimulation and commonly occur with fetal movements and sometimes with contractions. During the fetal sleep cycle, often between 20–40 minutes at a time, accelerations are reduced or absent. Like baseline variability, accelerations can be caused by certain drugs and medications such as narcotics. The significance of reduced accelerations during labour in an otherwise normal CTG is unclear, and does not necessarily imply the fetus is compromised.

Decelerations

Decelerations are transient episodes of decrease in FHR below the baseline of more than 15 bpm lasting at least 15 seconds. They are classified as early, variable, complicated typical, prolonged and late.

- *Early decelerations* are usually insignificant and result from head compression. They are uniform, repetitive decreases in the FHR with slow onset early in the contraction and slow return to baseline by the end of the contraction. They often occur during fetal sleep cycle and around 4–8 cm cervical dilatation (Baker et al 2009).
- *Variable decelerations* are repetitive or intermittent decreases in the FHR with rapid onset and recovery. Time relationships with the contraction cycle may be variable, but most commonly occur simultaneously with contractions and vary in depth and duration. Variable decelerations may be affected by maternal position, cord entanglement, low liquor levels, fetal movements and abnormal uterine activity.
  - They are classified as variable decelerations if they drop at least 15 bpm from the baseline and last for 15 seconds.
  - The amplitude (depth) and duration reflect the degree and duration of cord compression rather than the fetal condition.
  - Persistent deep (> 60 bpm) and/or broad (> 60 seconds) variable decelerations indicate recurrent prolonged interruptions to the blood flow and therefore oxygenation.
  - Variable decelerations may be associated with shouldering, a transient increase in the FHR immediately before and/or after the deceleration.
- *Complicated variable decelerations* have the following additional features that increase the likelihood of fetal hypoxia:
  - rising baseline rate or fetal tachycardia
  - reducing or absent baseline variability
  - slow return of the deceleration to the baseline after the end of the contraction
  - a loss of shouldering where it previously existed
  - decelerations of large amplitude (> 60 bpm) and/or long duration (> 60 seconds)
  - presence of smooth post deceleration overshoots (temporary smooth increase in FHR above the baseline).
- *Prolonged decelerations* are a decrease of the FHR below the baseline for > 90 seconds but < 5 minutes in duration. They are caused by fetal hypoxia and by a change in the fetal environment, such as:
  - maternal hypotension, often associated with changes in maternal position or following administration of epidural analgesia
  - prolonged cord compression
  - prolonged uterine activity.
- *Late decelerations* are caused by contractions in the presence of hypoxia (Baker et al 2009). They are uniform and repetitive decreases of the FHR with, usually, slow onset mid-to-end-of contraction and nadir > 20 seconds after the peak of the contraction.
  - Late decelerations do not need to be ≥ 15 bpm below the baseline to be significant
  - Late decelerations can be shallow (saucer shaped) and may have a normal baseline rate
  - The presence of late decelerations warrants immediate assessment for delivery.

SKILL 33.3 Application of the CTG machine

1. Discuss the procedure with the woman and gain and record her informed consent.
2. Encourage the woman to empty her bladder.
3. Record baseline maternal observations of temperature, blood pressure and pulse, if not already undertaken.
4. Perform an abdominal examination and auscultation of the fetal heart.
5. Position the woman in a sitting or semirecumbent position; this can be changed once the monitor has been applied and is recording well.
6. Place the two belts in position behind and around the woman and ensure she is covered sufficiently.
7. Apply gel to the cardio transducer.

Continued

SKILL 33.3 Application of the CTG machine—cont'd

8. Place the cardio transducer over the area where heart sounds are expected; the signal will indicate when the positioning is good.
9. Secure the cardio transducer in position using an abdominal belt.
10. Check the date and time settings on the CTG printout, once it is turned on. Adjust the settings on the machine if they are incorrect.
11. Palpate the maternal pulse to ensure that it is different from the audible FHR.
12. Place the uterine pressure transducer on the fundus of the uterus and secure it with the other abdominal belt.
13. When the uterus is relaxed, adjust the setting on the machine to 20 mmHg, unless set automatically or local protocol suggests a different figure.
14. Start the paper printing (1 cm per minute) and annotate the trace (or apply label) with the date, time commenced, woman's name and ID number, indication for monitoring, all the maternal observations and any other relevant details on the trace (e.g. gestation, epidural analgesia, oxytocin); then sign and print your name.
15. Encourage the woman to record fetal movements if applicable.
16. Discuss what is being observed on the CTG and the significance of the two printouts, the sounds heard and what to do if loss of contact occurs.
17. For women receiving continuous CTG, the trace should be reviewed at least every 15–30 minutes and should be acted upon. Record, either by written or electronic entry, in the medical record that the CTG has been reviewed (RANZCOG 2019).
18. Ensure that all who review the CTG tracing record this on the tracing and in the maternal records, including the date, time and signature, and the findings of the recording (RANZCOG 2019).
19. Document all intrapartum events that may affect the FHR (e.g. vaginal examination, obtaining an FBS, insertion/top-up of an epidural) contemporaneously including date, time and signature (RANZCOG 2019).
20. Discontinue the CTG when satisfied the tracing is normal or when the baby is born, if continuous CTG was required during labour.
21. Wipe the gel from the woman's abdomen and remove both transducers and belts.
22. Sign and correctly store the tracing and record completion of the monitoring and the indications for care.
23. If birth has occurred, the date, time and mode of delivery should also be recorded on the tracing.
24. Discuss the results with the woman.
25. Clean, restock and store the equipment correctly.

DOCUMENTATION OF CTG FINDINGS

Maternity units will have guidelines for documentation, and health professionals must be aware of these in relation to fetal heart monitoring. Date and time settings on CTG machines should be validated whenever used.

- CTGs should be labelled with the mother's name, hospital number, date and time of commencement, indication for monitoring and gestation, and should include the maternal observations.
- Any intrapartum events that may affect the FHR (e.g. vaginal examination, obtaining an FBS, insertion/top-up of an epidural) should be noted contemporaneously on the CTG trace and in the medical record, including date, time and signature.
- For women receiving continuous CTG, the trace should be reviewed at least every 15–30 minutes and should be acted on. It should be regularly recorded, either by written or electronic entry, in the medical record that the CTG has been reviewed. Some maternity units use a sticky label or electronic template for interpreting the CTG.
- Health professionals should be aware that machines from different manufacturers use different vertical axis scales, and this can change the perception of FHR variability.

Role and responsibilities of the midwife

These can be summarised as:

- displaying knowledge and application of current evidence-based practice
- undertaking all procedures correctly
- undertaking appropriate IA and CTG interpretation and regular update of such skills
- providing education, advice and support to the woman
- undertaking accurate contemporaneous record-keeping
- referring for deviations from normal.

SUMMARY

- The fetal heart can be auscultated using a Pinard stethoscope, handheld Doppler device or cardiotocograph (CTG) monitor. It is always preceded by an abdominal examination.
- Fetal heart monitoring guidelines provide decision-making pathways for intermittent auscultation and

CTG monitoring.
- CTG monitors should be applied correctly, the trace interpreted accordingly and appropriate actions taken.
- Midwives should have ongoing education in the use and interpretation of fetal heart rate monitoring during labour.

Self-assessment exercises

The answers to the following questions may be found in the text.

1. Discuss the different ways the fetal heart rate is auscultated.
2. Describe the procedure when using intermittent auscultation (IA).
3. Describe the procedure when applying a CTG monitor.
4. Discuss the indications for use of IA and CTG monitoring.
5. Discuss which factors the midwife needs to consider when interpreting a CTG tracing.
6. If a CTG tracing was described as 'abnormal', what would this mean?
7. Summarise the role and responsibilities of the midwife in relation to fetal heart monitoring in labour.

References

Alfirevic Z, Devane D, Gyte GML: Continuous cardiotocography (CTG) as a form of electronic fetal monitoring (EFM) for fetal assessment during labour, Cochrane Database of Systematic Reviews (5):CD006066, 2013.

Baker LS, Beaves MC, Trickey DJ, et al: Fetal surveillance: a practical guide. Royal Australian and New Zealand College of Obstetricians and Gynaecologists (RANZCOG), 2009.

Devane D, Lalor JG, Daly S, et al: Cardiotocography versus intermittent auscultation of fetal heart on admission to labour ward for assessment of fetal wellbeing, Cochrane Database of Systematic Reviews (2):CD005122, 2012.

Donnelly L, Hamilton L: A 'fresh eyes approach'. Misinterpretation of CTG can be a common occurrence in practice, but using a simple buddy system can yield significant improvements, RCM Midwives Magazine 15(5):44, 2012.

Feinstein N, Sprague A, Trépanier M: Fetal heart rate auscultation, 2nd ed., Association of Women's Health, Obstetric and Neonatal Nurses (AWHONN), Washington, 2008.

Fitzpatrick T, Holt L: A 'buddy' approach to CTG: Theresa Fitzpatrick and Louise Holt from Leeds Teaching Hospitals NHS Trust describe an innovative way to reduce misinterpretation of cardiotocographs, RCM Midwives Magazine Oct–Nov:41, 2008.

Goodwin L: Intermittent auscultation of the fetal heart rate: a review of general principles, Journal of Perinatal and Neonatal Nursing 14(3):53–61, 2000.

Lewis D, Downe S: FIGO consensus guidelines on intrapartum fetal monitoring: intermittent auscultation, International Journal of Gynecological Obstetrics 131(1):9–12, 2015.

Maude R, Foureur M, Skinner J: Intelligent structured intermittent auscultation (ISIA): evaluation of a decision-making framework for fetal monitoring of low-risk women, BMC Pregnancy and Childbirth 14:184, 2014.

Maude R, Foureur M, Skinner J: Putting intelligent structured intermittent auscultation (ISIA) into practice, Women and Birth 29:285–292, 2016.

Maude R, Lawson J, Foureur M: Auscultation—the action of listening, New Zealand College of Midwives Journal 43:13–18, 2010.

Nurani R, Chandraharan E, Lowe V, et al: Misidentification of maternal heart rate as fetal on cardiotocography during the second stage of labor: the role of the fetal electrocardiograph, Acta Obstetricia et Gynecologica Scandinavia 91:1428–1432, 2012.

Pairman S, Tracy S, Dahlen HG, Dixon, L: Midwifery preparation for practice, 4th ed., Elsevier, Sydney, 2018.

Royal Australian and New Zealand College of Obstetricians and Gynaecologists (RANZCOG): Intrapartum fetal surveillance. Clinical guideline—fourth edition 2019, RANZCOG, Melbourne, 2019. Available: https://ranzcog.edu.au/RANZCOG_SITE/media/RANZCOG-MEDIA/Women%27s%20Health/Statement%20and%20guidelines/Clinical-Obstetrics/IFS-Guideline-4thEdition-2019.pdf?ext=.pdf.

Wickham S: Pinard wisdom tips and tricks from midwives, part 2, The Practising Midwife 5(10):35, 2002.

CHAPTER 34
NON-PHARMACOLOGICAL PAIN RELIEF

Learning outcomes

Having read this chapter, the reader should be able to:

- discuss non-pharmacological pain relief options for labour
- outline the benefits and limitations of non-pharmacological pain relief
- describe transcutaneous electrical nerve stimulation (TENS) and its underlying principles leading to effectiveness in labour
- discuss complementary and alternative medicine (CAM) therapies, including the philosophical approach and the different types of therapies commonly used
- explain the principles of hypnobirth
- summarise the midwife's responsibilities and role.

In this chapter various non-pharmacological pain relief options are discussed, reflecting the growing trend and changing appeal for women in labour. The midwife's responsibilities and role in applying or supporting the various options are considered.

COMPLEMENTARY AND ALTERNATIVE MEDICINES (CAM)

Complementary and alternative medicine (CAM) is defined by the World Health Organization (WHO) as 'a broad set of healthcare practices that are not part of that country's own tradition or conventional medicine and are not fully integrated into the dominant healthcare system' (World Health Organization [WHO] 2017). As such, this involves using therapies that complement other treatment or interventions that are being used in the care of a woman in labour. Common types of therapies include herbal medicines (raspberry leaves, evening primrose oil, blue and black cohosh, partridgeberry, lobelia motherwort), relaxation techniques, aromatherapy, homeopathy, massage, acupressure and acupuncture (Hall, McKenna & Griffiths 2012). These therapies have a strong historical origin and use in the care of women in labour. Australian data suggests that 48% of women consult a CAM practitioner in pregnancy, up to 74% of women use some form of CAM antenatally and 67% also use non-pharmacological pain relief in labour (Frawley et al 2013, Steel et al 2014). Midwives globally continue to use CAM in their practice, more so than other health professional groups (Kalahroudi 2014). An explanation for this is that women choose CAM due to the various benefits it offers. As for midwives, the underlying philosophical approach of CAM allows them to be woman-centred, wherein holistic care can be given, allowing them to be responsive to the woman's needs (Hall et al 2012). To assist the woman in labour, therefore, it is important for the midwife to have knowledge of the various therapies, attend workshops and become credentialled where necessary or work alongside the therapist providing the therapy.

Although we have some indication of how many women consult CAM (noted earlier), there is little evidence available to indicate the factors influencing use. In low-resourced countries it is suggested that a high proportion of woman use CAM (Kalahroudi 2014). This is possibly due to traditional non-pharmacological approaches to pain relief and poor accessibility to health facilities and resources. In high-resourced countries there is a greater emphasis on pharmacological approaches due to the deeply entrenched biomedical model, and therefore there is perhaps less use of

CAM. Other factors have been identified by Steel and colleagues (2015) in their study of Australian women in labour; these include demographic characteristics, health status, easy and ready availability of resources, medical staff, and personal views and beliefs about CAM. In their survey, the researchers found that in birth and community centres non-pharmacological pain relief was more likely to be used and found to be more favourable by woman in labour. Added to this, the healthcare providers within such a setting played an important role in influencing women on the use of a broad range of CAM therapies.

Notwithstanding the growing popularity for CAM among women and midwives, there remains a tension between the use of non-pharmacological and pharmacological pain relief methods among health practitioners. This is largely due to the dominance of the biomedical approach within hospitals in Australia and New Zealand. Working within such a landscape can be challenging for midwives, as revealed in Hall, McKenna and Griffiths' study (2012). Their findings showed that some midwives acknowledged CAM worked well in reducing the extent of medical interventions. However, many were conscious of the biomedical opposition in their practice. As a result, midwives found alternative strategies to overcome opposition, became successful at negotiating with the medical team or they struggled at times with the tension and potential for conflict. To avoid conflict, some midwives controlled the release of information or avoided open dialogue.

In order to ensure that CAM is an important part of midwifery practice in the care of childbearing women, midwives have developed their own position statements. While there is no national statement in Australia, the Policy on Complementary and Alternative Therapies in Nursing and Midwifery Practice (2018) developed by the New South Wales Nurses and Midwives' Association together with the New South Wales branch of the Australian Nursing and Midwifery Federation provides a useful resource for all midwives in that country. In New Zealand, midwives are expected to adhere to the New Zealand College of Midwives' Consensus Statement: Complementary and Alternative Therapies (2018). Some hospitals also have their own clinical guidelines on CAM, acknowledging its benefits in the care of childbearing women and the need for specific post-registration qualification on the right to practise a particular therapy (Betts et al 2016).

Acupuncture

The use of acupuncture stems from traditional Chinese medicine and has a longstanding history as a form of pain relief. The method involves the use of thin needles to penetrate the skin at specific points on the body. Each point is selected individually based on the need for treatment and the needles are usually manually stimulated to reach a special sensation where the feeling of heaviness, soreness or numbness is felt (Yelland 2005). These sensations indicate correctly placed needles (Fig 34.1).

Its use is gaining momentum in various European countries such as Sweden and Denmark. In Australia and more so in New Zealand, acupuncture is performed by either midwives who have a certificate in midwifery acupuncture or acupuncturists the women are referred to by midwives. Studies have shown that women's satisfaction levels are high when acupuncture is used as a non-pharmacological pain relief. A unique study by Betts and colleagues (2016) in New Zealand examined the use of acupuncture among maternity patients (during pregnancy and postpartum period) in the outpatient clinic of a public hospital. Treatment was given for back or pelvic pain and labour preparation. Findings showed that at least 80% of women reported a significant positive change to their pain. Another study by Hope-Allan and colleagues (2004) investigated women in the antenatal clinic and the circumstances for use of acupuncture. Results showed that acupuncture was used for back pain, symphysis pubic pain and sciatica. All the women reported an

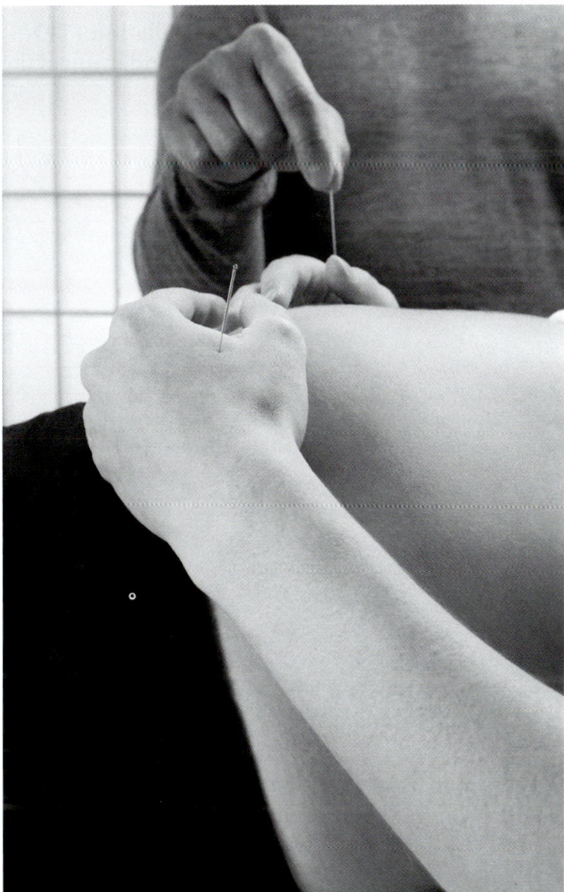

FIGURE 34.1 **Placing of acupuncture needles.**
Source: iStockphoto/under_score.

improved sense of wellbeing following treatment. Despite the positive results, more studies are needed to explore various other variables, such as influencing factors, demographic characteristics of the women and the level of involvement of midwives.

In terms of prebirth preparation, a series of acupuncture treatments in the last few weeks of pregnancy is known to be very effective. Betts (2004) and Betts and Lenox (2006) report that women spend less time in labour and are less likely to experience medical intervention. This may be related to the treatment, which prepares the cervix and pelvis for labour. The same preparation can also assist with pregnancy-induced hypertension, heartburn and haemorrhoids (Betts 2006). Although the benefits of acupuncture during pregnancy and childbirth are clear, it is important that safety for the mother and baby is ensured. Some acupuncture points are contraindicated as they may induce labour. However, Betts and Budd (2011) suggest that more research is needed in this area to ensure safe and best practice.

TRANSCUTANEOUS ELECTRICAL NERVE STIMULATION (TENS)

Transcutaneous electrical nerve stimulation (TENS) is frequently used by women in labour and involves the delivery of mild electrical impulses across the lower back to relieve pain (Johnson 2014). This technique is usually used under the guidance of a health practitioner, such as a physiotherapist or midwife. The device can be hired or purchased by the general public, with the manufacturer's instruction for self-administered treatment and use (Johnson 2014). This device is battery generated, portable and transmits biphasic pulsed electrical impulses in a repetitive manner. The strength of the impulses can be increased and controlled by the user. Electrical impulses typically are of 50–500 micron duration, with pulse rates of 1–200 per second, which may be of continuous or intermittent patterns. These impulses are delivered via the TENS device and through connecting wires to electrode pads. The electrode pads should ideally be placed at acupressure points rather than non-acupressure points over either side of the lower spine to achieve better results in reducing pain (Vance et al 2014). The impulse intensity should increase with pain intensity and decline as pain is reduced (Fig 34.2).

When used in labour, pain is relieved by stimulating the sensory nerve pathways to reduce pain-related activities within the nervous system. Sensations felt are often described as tingling or pleasant electrical vibrations (Tashani & Johnson 2009). Two mechanisms are involved to alter and relieve painful sensations. The

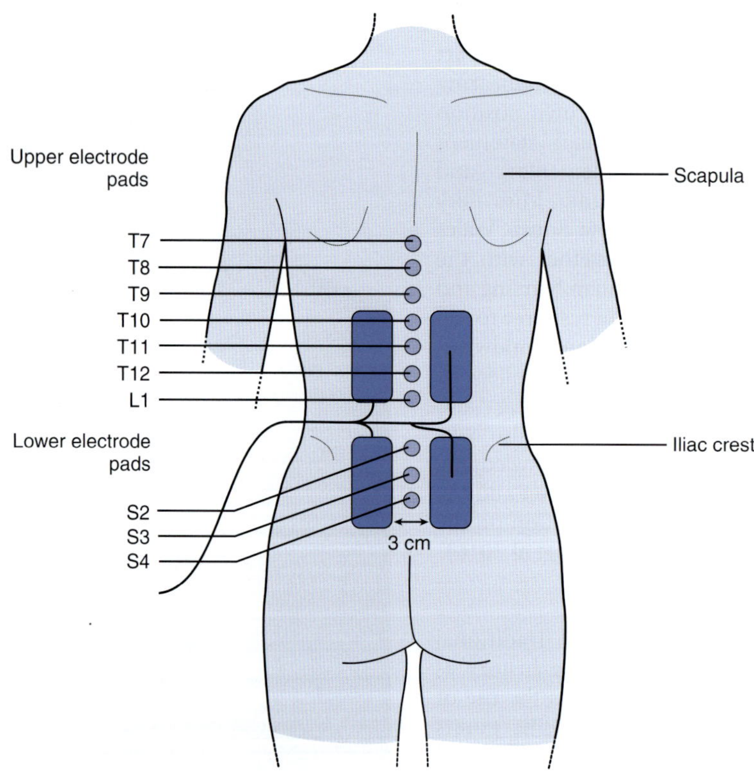

FIGURE 34.2 **Application of TENS during labour.**
Source: Johnson R, Taylor W: Skills for midwifery practice, 4th ed., Elsevier, London, 2016.

first mechanism is based on pain gate theory, which explains that pleasant and non-painful stimuli travel along the nerve pathways more rapidly than painful stimuli. As pleasant and non-painful stimuli reaches the base of the brain first, this blocks off painful stimuli from getting to the pain-sensing centres in the brain. The second mechanism is the release of the body's natural pain-inhibiting chemicals (e.g. endorphins, enkephalins and dynorphins) (Kaye 2019). To optimise these effects, TENS stimulation parameters need to be designed based on the woman's individual differences and needs; for example, adjusting the parameters of stimulation (current intensity, frequency, pulse width) according to the woman's evaluation of labour pain (Tang et al 2017).

Benefits of TENS

- Inexpensive, non-invasive and easy to use
- No side effects to mother or baby
- Has a distracting effect
- Reduces pain in early labour
- Postpones the need for pharmacological analgesia

Contraindications of TENS

- If the mother has a pacemaker, suffers from cardiac arrhythmias or has epilepsy
- Any skin irritation or damaged skin
- Earlier than 37 weeks of gestation
- No application to the abdomen
- When immersed in water (during waterbirth, shower or bath)

Despite the increasing use of TENS as a non-pharmacological pain relief, evidence in the literature is inconsistent. In a Cochrane Review, Jones and colleagues (2012) reported there was inadequate evidence to indicate whether or not TENS was an effective pain relief in labour. In another review by Bedwell (2011), the authors concluded there was little difference in pain relief between those who used TENS and those who did not. A review by DeSantana and colleagues (2008) indicated that adequate doses and intensity of electrical stimuli through the use of TENS was critical to pain relief. In a randomised controlled study, Santana and colleagues (2016) found that TENS not only significantly reduced labour pain, but also delayed the need for pharmacological analgesia. In a non-randomised control study, Peng and colleagues (2010) found that when TENS was used targeting specific acupoints, it led to effective pain relief during labour. This reported inconsistency may be due to the variation in application of TENS, which might render ineffectiveness of electrical stimulation (Francis 2014).

Suitability as a labour analgesic

Women increasingly are using non-pharmacological pain relief methods due to the many benefits they offer. TENS is generally used in early labour as it provides an opportunity for women to ease into the labouring process. In established labour, its effectiveness is diminished and the recommendation is that this method not be used (NICE 2014). However, in a study by Shahoei and colleagues (2017) findings showed that severity of labour pain among nulliparous women was significantly different between the experimental group and control group after TENS was used. These findings indicated that women receiving TENS had less pain than those who did not have TENS. Although the evidence around TENS and its effectiveness in pain relief is inconsistent, women reported that they would use TENS again in their next labour.

SKILL 34.1 Applying a TENS unit for a labouring woman

1. Support and assist the woman in her choice of pain relief method; review the benefits and limitations; discuss when the method is most effective; discuss what to expect; and establish that the contraindications do not apply.
2. Ensure the institution's guidelines are followed.
3. Check the device and attachments are safe and intact.
4. Wash hands and then assist the woman into an upright or sitting position. Gain access to her back.
5. Ensure the unit is switched off, but fully charged with electrodes connected and controls on the lowest possible setting.
6. Identify suitable positions for the electrodes and apply them to the skin as per the manufacturer's instructions.
7. Switch on the device so that tingling sensations can be felt. Demonstrate the boost of impulses and how to increase and decrease their intensity based on the severity of the pain.
8. Replace clothing and secure the device in a pocket if appropriate or tape it to clothing; expose the boost button for easy access.
9. Continue to monitor the woman and provide support in gaining maximum effectiveness from TENS through labour.
10. Ensure there is no electrical interference with any other items being used.
11. Document application and effect.
12. Discontinue the use of TENS at the end of labour or as needed by the woman.

HYPNOSIS, CALMBIRTH®

Hypnosis, hypnotherapy and hypnobirth are terms often used interchangeably, causing confusion. In this context, the terms refer to the same notion of a type of non-pharmacological pain relief used by women in labour, where a woman develops an intense sense of conscious awareness, like daydreaming; it involves concentrating in an inward-focusing way and a heightened responsiveness to suggestions (Madden and colleagues 2016). Under these situations, the woman can choose to overlook or reappraise various stimuli so that she can focus on the particular object of attention, which is the labour. The underlying principles include: removal of fear and allowing the body to relax; building confidence to birth; self-hypnotising to induce deep relaxation; utilising massage techniques to stimulate endorphins; and needing to visualise the situation to help feel serene and positive and to get the body and mind to work together efficiently and with ease. According to Watters (2015), this involves four techniques: breathing, relaxation, visualisation and deepening.

There are various hypnobirthing providers and programs based in Australia and New Zealand, through which prenatal hypnobirthing education is available. These include Hypnobirthing Australia, Hypnobirthing—The Mongan Method, and Australian Calmbirth®. Each program reflects the founder's profession, contemporary understanding of science and the subconscious. Several factors contribute to making hypnobirthing work, such as exercise, good nutrition, positioning and most importantly a supportive team of health practitioners (Fig 34.3) (Watters 2015).

Studies on hypnobirth have produced mixed results. As part of a randomised control study, Finlayson and colleagues (2015) undertook qualitative interviews of women to examine their experience of using hypnosis during labour and birth. The women mostly described feelings of calmness, empowerment and confidence. Abbasi, Ghazi, Barlow-Harrison and colleagues (2009) concurred with this positive experience in another qualitative study of Iranian women. In this study, women reported a sense of satisfaction, relief, confidence, decreased fear of giving birth, less tiredness and no anxiety. However, in a systematic review, Madden and colleagues (2016) found that there was no difference in coping capacity, satisfaction with pain relief and having a spontaneous vaginal delivery during labour for mothers in the hypnosis group compared to those in the control group. However, the authors concluded that although hypnosis helped reduce or delay the use of analgesia, this did not stop women from using an epidural.

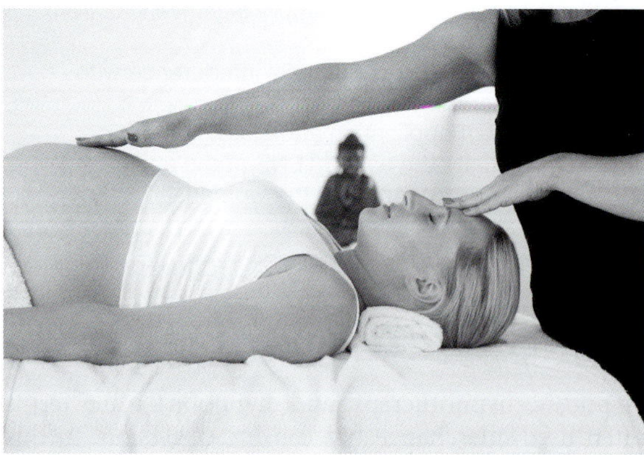

FIGURE 34.3 **Woman focusing on hypnobirth techniques.**
Source: iStockphoto/Dean Mitchell.

Role and responsibilities of the midwife

CAM

These can be summarised as:

- acquiring the necessary skills by participating in training programs on how to support the woman who opts to use CAM
- developing a sound understanding of the various therapies, their strengths and limitations
- appreciating how CAM fits in with the overall management of a woman in labour
- discussing with the woman the effectiveness and possible risks involved
- treating women with respect and dignity
- encouraging good and open communication
- being aware of guidelines for the use of CAM within the clinical setting.

TENS

These can be summarised as:

- supporting and assisting the mother in the use of TENS
- providing information as needed, so the woman can make informed decisions
- documenting the use and effectiveness of pain relief
- following the instructor's manual
- reporting and documenting any concerns.

Hypnobirth

These can be summarised as:

- being open-minded and receptive
- allowing the woman to utilise what works best for her
- being woman-centred and supportive
- working alongside her hypnobirth therapist.

SUMMARY

- Historically, women have used a variety of non-pharmacological pain relief to help them through labour.
- Midwives have a longstanding tradition of working with women and supporting them in choices regarding pain relief methods and assisting them through the birthing experience.
- There is much evidence to show why women favour non-pharmacological pain relief methods in labour; they enjoy the sense of control, satisfaction, empowerment and calmness.
- Systematic reviews provide mixed results, but have demonstrated that non-pharmacological pain

relief has no negative effect on maternal or infant outcome.

- Women-centred midwives need to become familiar with and knowledgeable about the various options for non-pharmacological pain relief, such as TENS, CAM and hypnobirth therapy so that they can support and assist women.

Self-assessment exercises

The answers to the following questions may be found in the text.

1. What is CAM?
2. Provide a definition for CAM.
3. In what way does CAM align with midwifery and its philosophy?
4. How can the midwife support a woman who has chosen to use CAM in labour?
5. Summarise the role and responsibilities of the midwife in relation to the use of CAM.
6. List four ways in which acupuncture may be useful in pregnancy and labour.
7. When in labour is TENS most effective?
8. When should TENS not be used?
9. Summarise the role and responsibilities of the midwife in relation to the use of TENS in labour.
10. What is hypnobirthing?
11. How would you as a midwife deal with tension in the workplace in relation to the use of TENS, CAM or hypnobirthing?
12. What are the roles and responsibilities of the midwife in the care of a woman who uses hypnobirthing techniques?

References

Abbasi M, Ghazi F, Barlow-Harrison A, et al: The effect of hypnosis on pain relief during labor and childbirth in Iranian pregnant women, The International Journal of Clinical and Experimental Hypnosis 57(2):174–183, 2009.

Bedwell C: Why do women use TENS equipment and how effective is it? British Journal of Midwifery 19(6):348–351, 2011.

Betts D: A review of research into the application of acupuncture in pregnancy, Journal of Chinese Medicine 80:50–55, 2006.

Betts D, Budd S: Forbidden acupuncture points in pregnancy: historical wisdom? Acupuncture in Medicine, 2011.

Betts D, Lenox S: Acupuncture for pre-birth treatment: an observational study of its use in midwifery practice, Medical Acupuncture 17(3):16–19, 2006.

Betts D, McMullan J, Walker L: The use of maternity acupuncture within a New Zealand public hospital: integration within an outpatient clinic, New Zealand College of Midwives Journal 52:45–49, 2016.

Betts D: The use of acupuncture as a routine pre-birth treatment, Journal of Chinese Medicine 76:5–8, 2004.

DeSantana J, Walsh D, Vance C, et al: Effectiveness of transcutaneous electrical nerve stimulation for treatment of hyperalgesia and pain, Current Rheumatology Reports 10(6):492–499, 2008.

Finlayson K, Downe S, Hinder S, et al: Unexpected consequences: women's experiences of a self-hypnosis intervention to help with pain relief during labour, BMC Pregnancy and Childbirth 15(229), 2015.

Francis R: TENS (Transcutaneous electrical nerve stimulation) for labour pain, Practice Midwife 15(5): 20–23, 2014.

Frawley J, Adams J, Sibbritt D, et al: Prevalence and determinants of complementary and alternative medicine use during pregnancy: results from a nationally representative sample of Australian pregnant women, Australian & New Zealand Journal of Obstetrics and Gynaecology 53(4):347–352, 2013.

Hall H, McKenna L, Griffiths D: Midwives' support for complementary and alternative medicine: a literature review, Women and Birth 25(1):4–12, 2012.

Hope-Allan N, Adams J, Sibbrit D, et al: The use of acupuncture in maternity care: a pilot study evaluating the acupuncture service in an Australian hospital antenatal clinic, Complementary Therapies in Nursing and Midwifery 10(4):229–232, 2004.

Johnson M: Transcutaneous Electrical Nerve Stimulation (TENS): research to support clinical practice, Oxford University Press, 2014.

Jones L, Othman M, Dowswell T, et al: Pain management for women in labour: an overview of systematic reviews, Cochrane Database System Reviews 14(3):CD009234, 2012.

Kalahroudi M: Complementary and alternative medicine in midwifery, Nursing and Midwifery Studies 3(2): e194–49, 2014.

Kaye K: Transcutaneous electrical nerve stimulation, Medscape, 2019. Online 28 September 2021. Available: https://emedicine.medscape.com/article/325107-overview.

Madden K, Middleton P, Cyna AM, et al: Hypnosis for pain management during labour and childbirth, Cochrane Review, 2016.

National Institute for Health and Clinical Excellence (NICE): Intrapartum care—care of healthy women and their babies during childbirth. Clinical guideline 1.10. Monitoring during labour; 2014. Online 28 September 2019. Available: www.nice.org.uk/guidance/cg190/resources/intrapartum-care-for-healthy-women-and-babies-pdf-35109866447557.

New South Wales Nurses and Midwives' Association and Australian Nursing and Midwifery Federation—NSW Branch: policy on complementary and alternative therapies in nursing and midwifery practice, 2018. Online 31 Jan 2021. Available: www.nswnma.asn.au/wp-content/uploads/2018/10/NSWNMA-Policy-on-Complementary-and-Alternative-Therapies-in-Nursing-and-Midwifery-Practice.pdf.

New Zealand College of Midwives: Consensus statement: complementary and alternative therapies, 2018. Online 31 Jan 2021. Available: www.midwife.org.nz/wp-content/uploads/2019/05/Complementary-and-Alternative-Therapies.pdf.

Peng T, Li X, Zhou S, et al: Transcutaneous electrical nerve stimulation on acupoints relieves labor pain: a non-randomized controlled study, Chinese Journal of Integrated Medicine 16(3):234–238, 2010.

Santana L, Gallo R, Ferreira C, et al: Transcutaneous electrical nerve stimulation (TENS) reduces pain and postpones the need for pharmacological analgesia during labour: a randomised trial, Journal of Physiotherapy 62:29–34, 2016.

Shahoei R, Shahghebi S, Rezaei M: The effect of transcutaneous electrical nerve stimulation on the severity of labor pain among nulliparous women: a clinical trial, Complementary Therapies in Clinical Practice 28:176–180, 2017.

Steel A, Adams J, Sibbritt D, et al: Managing the pain of labour: factors associated with the use of labour pain management for pregnant Australian women, Health Expectations 18(5):1633–1644, 2015.

Steel A, Adams J, Sibbritt D, et al: The influence of complementary and alternative medicine use in pregnancy on labor pain management choices: results from a nationally representative sample of 1835 women, Journal of Alternative and Complementary Medicine 20:87–97, 2014.

Tang ZY, Wang HQ, Xia XL, et al: [Mechanisms and applications of transcutaneous electrical nerve stimulation in analgesia], Sheng Li Xue Bao: [Acta Physiologica Sinica] 69(3):325–334, 2017.

Tashani O, Johnson MI: Transcutaneous electrical nerve stimulation (TENS): a possible aid for pain relief in developing countries? The Libyan Journal of Medicine 4(2):62–65, 2009.

Vance CGT, Dailey DL, Rakel BA, et al: Using TENS for pain control: the state of the evidence, Pain Management 4(3):197–209, 2014.

Watters Y: Hypnobirth: theories and practices for healthcare professionals, Rowman & Littlefield, Maryland, 2015.

World Health Organization (WHO): Traditional, complementary and integrative medicine, 28 September 2021. Available from: www.who.int/health-topics/traditional-complementary-and-integrative-medicine#tab=tab_1.

Yelland S: Acupuncture in midwifery, Elsevier, London, 2005.

CHAPTER 35 WATER IMMERSION FOR LABOUR AND BIRTH

Learning outcomes

Having read this chapter, the reader should be able to:

- discuss the benefits and safety of water use in labour
- discuss how to support a woman who uses water during labour and during birth
- discuss the midwife's role and responsibilities.

Water immersion for labour and birth is widely used internationally in all birth settings. It supports women to take back control of their labour and birth and to reduce the use of pharmacological pain relief and unnecessary, often routine, interventions (Plint & Davis 2016). Water immersion for labour and birth enables birthing women to have autonomy and offers midwives the opportunity to experience caring for women during physiological birth. Women and midwives can recount highly positive experiences of calm, straightforward births and women are highly satisfied using water immersion. While continuity of care(r) strongly supports informed decision-making, Charles (2013) believes that all midwives should be able to assist women to use water immersion during labour and birth. There is broad support from the Royal Australian and New Zealand College of Obstetricians and Gynaecologists (RANZCOG) in its position statement for warm water immersion during labour and birth (including for women at low risk of COVID-19 infection), and in the published evidence of efficacy and safety (Bovbjerg et al 2016, Burns et al 2012, Harper 2014, Nutter et al 2014, RANZCOG 2021, Taylor et al 2016). A Cochrane review confirms that '... women who are at low risk of complications who use water immersion during labour are probably no more or less likely to experience vaginal delivery and may be less likely to have to use regional analgesia, particularly when immersion occurs during the first stage of labour' and that there is '... no evidence of increased adverse effects to the neonate in terms of admissions to neonatal intensive care unit and infection rates' (Cluett et al 2018).

CONSIDERATIONS

Water has long been known for its therapeutic value, particularly its relaxing and pain-relieving properties. During pregnancy and early labour, women may choose to rest in the bath or take a shower to relieve pain. Immersion in deeper warm water during active labour is increasingly used for these benefits, but also for birthing. Intrapartum care providers should be familiar with the evidence of efficacy and safety of water immersion for labour and birth and have protocols that assist women and midwives to make informed decisions. Women's informed decision-making, informed choice and right to consent or refuse any aspects of care should be respected. Water used in this way may be in a home, birth centre or hospital setting, using deep baths or birth pools, which may be permanent or hired.

Water immersion for labour and birth is supported by midwifery principles, including a belief that pregnancy and birth are normal life events for most women; midwifery care is woman-centred and that continuity of care is desirable throughout (Pairman et al 2018). Water immersion during labour and birth provides midwives with the opportunity to exercise their autonomy while supporting physiological birth in partnership with informed women.

CONSIDERED BENEFITS AND SAFETY OF WATER IMMERSION

During the first stage of labour, water immersion can:

- aid descent of the fetal head and shorten the length of first stage
- promote an upright position and buoyancy which increases mobility
- provide a private and safe place, which aids relaxation and coping strategies
- reduce the need for pharmacological analgesia, risk of transfer before birth and medical intervention
- promote a relaxed, calm, less stressed and less fearful environment.

During the second stage of labour, water immersion can:

- facilitate spontaneous vaginal birth
- reduce perineal trauma, including the use of episiotomy
- reduce birth intervention
- provide a gentle transition to extra uterine life for the baby
- facilitate physiological placental birth.

Following birth in water, water immersion provides:

- immediate and sustained skin-to-skin contact
- increased satisfaction and feeling of being in control
- a positive birth experience.

(Burns et al 2012, Dahlen et al 2013, Garland 2011, Hall & Holloway 1998, Lukasse et al 2014, Maude & Foureur 2007, Maude & Caplice 2018, Nutter et al 2014, Young & Kruske 2012)

Both the Australian College of Midwives (ACM) (2013) and New Zealand College of Midwives (NZCOM) (2015), in light of currently available evidence, endorse the choice of access to water immersion facilities during labour and birth. RANZCOG (2021), however, takes a more conservative approach. This may be due to a lack of training and confidence in supporting physiological birth and in particular to the use of water immersion for labour and birth (Plint & Davis 2016). The RANZCOG position statement on water immersion during labour and birth supports it if the maternity service has protocols in place for candidate selection, infection control, work and safety procedures and exclusion/emergency criteria; if clinicians attending women labouring in water are appropriately trained and demonstrably competent to care for them; and if the woman has been enabled to make an informed choice (RANZCOG 2021). A key point of difference between the professional colleges' stand on water immersion for labour and birth appears to sit with the interpretation of the evidence. There are many good quality observational studies, but only a few randomised controlled trials (RCTs). An integrative analysis of peer-reviewed literature in 2014 included 38 studies (two RCTs and 36 observational) from 11 countries of over 31,000 waterbirths and report the existing evidence as reassuring (Nutter et al 2014). Further discussion on the use of water immersion for labour and birth can be found in Chapter 25 of *Midwifery: Preparation for Practice* (Pairman et al 2018).

CRITERIA FOR USE OF WATER FOR LABOUR AND BIRTH

In many situations the inclusion criteria for using water for labour and birth is the same as that for women planning to birth in a birth centre or at home: well women with uncomplicated pregnancies are suitable for intermittent auscultation in labour. However, any woman who has been given all the available information and wishes to use the pool should be considered. All decisions around care options during labour are individualised to each woman.

General inclusion criteria for pool use include:

- the woman's informed choice
- singleton fetus and cephalic presentation
- uncomplicated pregnancy of > 37 weeks gestation
- established labour
- no specific requirement for continuous fetal heart monitoring.

Situations in which the use of water is contraindicated include:

- maternal dislike
- maternal pyrexia > 37.5° C
- opiate use in labour of < 2 hours prior (NICE 2014)
- any known cause for concern for mother or fetus, particularly fetal compromise (presence of thick meconium included), maternal haemorrhage, oxytocin induction/augmentation, epilepsy, pre-eclampsia, breech presentation and twin pregnancy.

The following situations require individualised consideration.

- Known infection (e.g. group B streptococcus [GBS]). The use of universally applied standard precautions and adherence to cleansing protocols make this ban questionable. In a study comparing GBS-positive women who gave birth in water with those who gave birth on land found that babies born in water were less colonised. The authors concluded that being a GBS carrier is not a contraindication for birth in water (Zanetti-Dallenbach et al 2007).
- The need for continuous fetal heart monitoring. Equipment is available to monitor continually in water, but this raises a number of issues; as suggested above, the presence of fetal compromise prohibits delivery in water.
- Previous caesarean birth. However, McKenna and Symon (2014) record the successful use of water for women experiencing a vaginal birth after a caesarean section (VBAC).

- High body mass index. The woman may be more mobile and benefit from the buoyancy, but may be harder to remove from the pool in the event of an emergency.
- Prolonged rupture of membranes, for which no evidence is presented, although in some instances this may relate to the need for IV antibiotics.

Despite many women being in the low-risk group, the midwife should always be alert to any obstetric or neonatal emergency, facilitating the evacuation of the woman from the pool swiftly when necessary, and undertaking the correct management measures.

WHEN IS A GOOD TIME TO ENTER THE POOL?

Studies have investigated the effects of water immersion during labour on the length of the first, second and third stages. There is no clear agreement on whether water immersion reduces the length of the first stage of labour. This is likely related to the lack of definition of the period of time in the first stage that labour was measured. In some studies the time the woman was in the water was restricted (e.g. for 60 minutes only), making this a less reliable measure. The debate on early or late entry to the water came from one study of 200 women conducted in the 1990s (Eriksson et al 1997). Women in the 'early bath' group had longer labours and needed more augmentation and epidural analgesia, and led to Eriksson and team (1997) recommending that bathing should occur after 5 cm dilatation (Eriksson et al 1997). Cochrane reviewers Cluett and colleagues (2018), however, did not consider this sufficient evidence to make a definitive recommendation, and so this advice should be balanced around the needs of the woman. Water can both aid slow progress and cause labour to slow; consequently, the midwife should observe for contraction length, strength and frequency as for any and every labour and respond accordingly. The water can be used intermittently if that is the woman's choice.

WHEN SHOULD THE WOMAN GET OUT OF THE POOL?

- When she chooses.
- If choosing other analgesia (e.g. epidural).
- When ready after the birth.
- The midwife uses wise clinical judgment and discusses the following with the woman.
  - If labour progress slows (it is possible to mobilise for a while and return to the pool later).
  - If there are abnormalities to the fetal heart, suggestive of fetal compromise.
  - Any signs of haemorrhage, raised blood pressure or pyrexia. In the event of ante- or postpartum haemorrhage, the woman leaves the pool immediately and the protocol is followed as for any birth.
  - If the water is no longer clear. The reason for lack of clarity can be investigated (haemorrhage, bowel movement or meconium being the most likely); if no abnormality is found, the pool can be cleaned and refilled.
  - If there is a need to perform an episiotomy.
  - If delivery of the shoulders does not follow in the contraction after delivery of the head. The woman is assisted to stand and place one foot up on the side of the birth pool (equivalent to hyperflexion of the leg as in the McRoberts manoeuvre). Invariably, this movement is successful, but if the shoulders remain impacted the woman should be helped from the pool and the shoulder dystocia drill continued. Once the baby's head is in contact with air, the birth should continue in air.
  - If there is a tight nuchal cord which is not easily managed under water (as most are). The cord should not be clamped and cut under water.

SKILL 35.1 Supporting a woman during water immersion for labour and birth

1. Fill the pool/bath/tub to the level of the woman's breasts while she is in a sitting position.
2. Maintain the water temperature according to the woman's comfort (usually 33–37°C). Monitor water temperature every 30–60 minutes.
3. Ensure all required equipment is in the room (towels, sieve, torch, light source, mirror, protective clothing, delivery pack, oxygen, suction, oxytocics, waterproof Doppler or Pinard, Entonox, fan, foot stool, kneeling pad, bed/ mattress nearby).
4. Maintain an ambient room temperature which is comfortable for the woman and have supplies of cool water or ice chips and access to a fan.
5. Provide a continuous supportive presence while the woman is in the water.
6. Care of the woman and the baby should be as per unit protocols for low-risk women. The maternal temperature is recorded at least hourly. Fetal heart rate is recorded every 15–30 minutes.
7. Encourage the woman to explore different positions.
8. Encourage physiological or non-directed pushing.
9. Use the sieve to decontaminate the water as required.
10. Use a 'hands-off' approach to the birth of the baby.

Continued

CHAPTER 36
BIRTH AT HOME

Learning outcomes

Having read this chapter, the reader should be able to:

- discuss some of the evidence that relates to safety when birthing at home
- discuss the differences in skills and attitudes that the midwife utilises
- discuss the value and principles of good preparation for all the parties concerned
- list the equipment and information that the midwife needs to have available
- discuss the overall role and responsibilities of the midwife attending births at home
- discuss the initial assessment necessary if attending a birth that has already happened without medical assistance (born before arrival [BBA]).

This chapter focuses on the midwife's role and management of labour and birth in the home setting. It highlights the considerations for care at home, which are different from care in hospital; the reader may find it helpful to refer to Pairman and colleagues (2018, Chapter 6).

Some women will prefer to give birth in a hospital setting; this is as much their choice as homebirth is for other women. Safe homebirth is a team effort with the mother at the centre of the care. The immediate team includes the woman's chosen supporter(s), the midwife and backup midwife/midwives. The remainder of the 'team' needs to include the network of clinical support actioned if a transfer of care occurs. This network comprises the ambulance service, the lead midwife's colleagues, usually from the midwifery team with whom the midwife works, hospital midwifery and obstetrical colleagues and, if necessary, other medical professionals such as paediatricians.

PLANNED HOMEBIRTH

Homebirth is surrounded internationally by polarised opinion within and between different professional groups (Dahlen 2012, de Crespigny & Savulescu 2014, Roome et al 2016, Skinner & Foureur 2010). In Australia, in 2015 the rate of homebirth was 0.3% (Australian Institute of Health and Welfare [AIHW] 2017). In New Zealand, the rates of homebirth have remained stable at 3.7% from 2006 to 2015 (Ministry of Health 2017).

Safety

Concern for the safety of the woman and the baby is the driver for most debates about birth, and particularly out-of-hospital birth. A distinction needs to be made between planned births at home (often with low risk factors) and an unexpected birth at home where the mother had planned a hospital birth but unexpectedly gives birth at home or before arriving at the hospital (BBA). Planned homebirth is a choice made most often by women considered to be at low risk of obstetric complications.

A 2015 review of international research (Zielinski et al 2015) reached the following conclusion:

> While some studies suggest a small but significant increase in neonatal death and adverse outcomes, the majority of studies across a variety of countries have shown no increase in neonatal morbidity and mortality for planned homebirth. Additionally, maternal outcomes are consistently better for planned homebirth, including less intervention and fewer complications. Satisfaction with the birth experience is also high in the homebirth setting. (p. 374)

A study of publicly funded homebirths in Australia reported on the maternal and neonatal outcomes (Catling-Paull et al 2013). The results were similar to homebirth studies in other countries: 'Most studies of homebirth in other countries have found no statistically significant differences in perinatal outcomes between home and hospital births for women and babies at low risk of complications' (p. 618).

A systematic review by Australian researchers Scarf and colleagues (2018) has compared different places of birth in high-income countries using a recently developed analytical tool which was been specifically created to provide insights into the quality of research about place of birth. This systematic review sought to understand whether perinatal and maternal outcomes are 'significantly different from births planned at home, in birth centres or hospitals, for women with low-risk pregnancies' (Scarf et al 2018, p. 11). The authors found that 'combined maternal data from the selected studies indicated significantly lower odds of intervention and maternal morbidity, and significantly higher odds of normal vaginal births among planned homebirths compared to planned hospital births' (Scarf et al 2018, p. 26). Further, there were also lower odds of babies being admitted to neonatal intensive care units for those whose mothers planned a home rather than a hospital birth. Supporters of homebirth argue that birthing at home offers relative safety and a qualitatively better experience for the women who choose it (Dahlen 2012).

A 2012 New Zealand study (Miller & Skinner 2012) showed higher levels of intervention were experienced by nulliparous woman in hospital when compared with a matched sample of nulliparous women choosing homebirth, even when the same midwives were providing the care. In the Birthplace Study (Birthplace in England Collaborative Group 2011) low-risk women in hospital were three times more likely to have a caesarean section, twice as likely to have their baby born by forceps or vacuum extraction and twice as likely to require blood transfusion, have serious perineal trauma and/or be admitted to an intensive care unit than the women who birthed at home or in a midwife-led unit. Davis and colleagues (2011) also confirmed a similar increase in interventions for New Zealand women who chose a hospital birth, and reinforced the significant impact of the planned choice of birthplace on interventions in labour as well as the mode of birth.

From an ethical point of view, a woman has the right to make a choice about the place she gives birth. On the other hand, a midwife is not required to provide care that she thinks is unsafe. Consultation and referral guidelines in Australia and New Zealand provide a clear guide for discussion between midwives and women about those clinical indicators which carry risk and require an obstetrical consultation or transfer of care (see Table 36.1). The table contains two lists of factors,

TABLE 36.1 RISK FACTORS SUGGESTING PLANNED BIRTH AT OBSTETRIC UNIT

Type of condition	Unsuitable for homebirth	Requires careful discussion before planning homebirth
Medical	Systemic lupus erythematosus (SLE), severe connective tissue disorder, thrombophilia, severe cardiac disease, hypertension, (> 150/100), diabetes, cholestasis of pregnancy, severe hepatitis, oesophageal varices, haematological disorders (including anaemia < 90 g/L), infectious diseases, poorly controlled epilepsy, myasthenia gravis, spinal cord lesion, muscular dystrophy, brain aneurysm, acute unstable psychosis, glomerulonephritis, renal failure, previous kidney surgery, cystic fibrosis, organ transplant, severe respiratory condition, severe skeletal problems, current malignancy, cervical incompetence, severe abnormalities (pelvic floor, uterine, cervical, vaginal or vulval)	Inactive or mild connective tissue disorders, thrombophilia with no previous complications or thrombosis, milder cardiac condition, hypertension (> 140/90), diabetes controlled on diet, other endocrine conditions, cholelithiasis, active inflammatory bowel disease, chronic hepatitis, rubella, well-controlled epilepsy, multiple sclerosis, other mental health conditions, drug or alcohol dependence or abuse, chronic proteinuria, renal abnormality, asthma, dermatological problems requiring systemic treatment, previous malignancy, milder abnormalities (pelvic floor, uterine, cervical, vaginal or vulval)
Previous maternity history	Cervical incompetence	Caesarean section, previous placental abruption, previous hypertensive disease, large for gestational age, intrauterine growth restriction (IUGR), manual removal of placenta, perinatal death, primary postpartum haemorrhage (PPH), preterm birth (< 35 weeks), recurrent miscarriage, shoulder dystocia, sudden unexpected death in infancy (SUDI), 3rd- or 4th-degree tear, puerperal psychosis
Current pregnancy	Eclampsia, breech, transverse, oblique, unstable lie > 36 weeks, morbid obesity, multiple pregnancy, placenta previa, polyhydramnios, pre-eclampsia, preterm rupture of membranes without labour, prolonged pregnancy, premature labour (< 37 weeks)	Abnormal CTG, antepartum haemorrhage (APH), blood group antibodies, fetal abnormality, gestational proteinuria, intrauterine death, IUGR, large fetus, obesity (body mass index [BMI] > 35), oligohydramnios, reduced fetal movements, genital herpes, uterine fibroids, recurrent urinary tract infections (UTIs)

Source: Australian College of Midwives: National Midwifery Guidelines for Consultation and Referral, 2021; Ministry of Health: Guidelines for consultation with obstetric and related medical services (referral guidelines), Wellington, 2012.

one suggesting birth should be planned in hospital rather than at home and one where the risk requires careful discussion with the woman and her family and a specialist consultation.

Midwifery skills

The skills of the midwife supporting women to birth at home are technical, social and interpersonal. While working in the home environment might seem very relaxed, the midwife must know when to stay at home and when to propose transfer of care. The midwife's professional relationships are ideally collaborative, open and honest with the mother and her support team, but also with midwifery and hospital colleagues. Uncommonly, the midwife may need to act urgently and with skill to save a baby or a mother's life without the support of a hospital team. However, this team is a potential support in a crisis and with functioning relationships, can aid the midwife at the time by phone or later with debriefing.

While many midwives have limited experience of attending homebirths, those who do often regard it as a professionally enhancing experience. The relationship established during pregnancy enables the midwife/ midwives (or their backup) to enter the home and provide a knowledgeable, calming and caring presence. The tone of that presence is important; the midwife needs to be alert to what is going on and clearly document that detail, while quietly protecting the birth space.

The following additional skills are helpful.

- The ability to develop a trusting relationship and empower the woman to make informed decisions about her plans for birth at home.
- A full understanding of and confidence in labour physiology and a woman's ability to give birth naturally in her own environment.
- Fundamental midwifery skills using limited equipment (e.g. Pinard stethoscope or fetal Doppler sonicaid); supporting women in alternative positions for labour and birth; use of non-pharmacological pain relief (e.g. bath, birth pool, position changes, acupressure, hot towels, aromatherapy, massage, sounding).
- 'Active inactivity' (see Skill 36.1): women who have planned their birth at home often assume a greater level of control. A midwife may feel a little superfluous, but has, in fact, to remain 'with woman', to keep alert to, for example, signs of the labour progressing, while appearing to be relatively inactive.
- Flexibility and adaptability while, for example, continuing to maintain standard precautions, following aseptic guidelines and maintaining health and safety protocols.
- Ability to manage unexpected or emergency situations without immediate support, including resuscitation, haemorrhage, shoulder dystocia and breech birth.

SKILL 36.1 Active inactivity

Active inactivity is a skill which requires the midwife to have confidence and the ability to:

- generate a tone of calm, reassurance and encouragement
- maintain respect for the woman as the centre of care
- provide support as needed and not assume an active role
- quietly make and document accurate assessments and judgments throughout labour
- share details of the labour with a second midwife who will come to the birth
- be confident in their knowledge of the normal process of labour and birth
- make an initial baseline physical assessment after arriving when the woman indicates she is ready
- make regular assessments (fetal heart, pulse) and observations throughout labour and birth
- individualise care while being alert to deviations from normal
- perform internal examinations if and when necessary using an aseptic non-touch technique (ANTT)
- articulate concerns without a fuss when the process of labour deviates from normal
- unobtrusively prepare equipment for the birth
- manage emergencies professionally if and when necessary.

Equipment

Equipment (Box 36.1) should be stored, used, serviced, cleaned and restocked correctly. The midwife should be confident about its location and use, keeping items together (e.g. equipment for treatment of primary postpartum haemorrhage [PPH] or resuscitation). This means they are readily accessible and easily moved around the home with the woman. Access to the required drugs will either be prescribed by an endorsed midwife or by dependent prescribing under local protocols in Australia (Australian Government 2009, Nursing and Midwifery Board of Australia 2017). The Midwifery Council of New Zealand expects that all registered midwives are able to demonstrate competence in independent prescribing (Midwifery Council of New Zealand 2007).

Box 36.1 Equipment suggested for managing labour and birth at home

- Antenatal equipment includes a watch with a second-hand, Pinard stethoscope and/or fetal Doppler (waterproof) and gel, relevant spare batteries, sphygmomanometer, thermometer and bath thermometer, venepuncture equipment, sharps box, swabs and medium, reagent sticks, blood and midstream specimen of urine (MSU) bottles, pen torch, scissors, tape measure, gloves (sterile and non-sterile) and documentation such as continuation sheets, blood forms and prescription pad.
- Labour equipment, including sterile birth, vaginal examination (VE) and suturing packs, urinary catheters (residual and Foley and bag), amnihook, speculum and lubricating gel, cannulation equipment, fluids and giving sets, suturing materials, torch (waterproof if possible), incontinence pads, drugs (see below), suppositories, container for placenta, rubbish bags, water thermometer, documentation for labour care (including birth notification emergency management cards) and mobile phone and charger.
- Drugs: uterotonics (Syntometrine, Syntocinon [third stage and PPH], and ergometrine), lignocaine 1% for suturing, vitamin K, oxygen, intravenous fluids (crystalloid and colloid); see Chapter 31 in Pairman and colleagues (2018).
- Resuscitation equipment for woman and baby, including oxygen (with tubings, airways, bags and masks), suction with neonatal and maternal suckers, stethoscope, stopwatch, towels, heat source, and depending on local protocol, blood glucose sticks and lancets.
- Postnatal equipment, including weighing scales, equipment for neonatal examination and documentation such as neonatal examination forms, child health record, postnatal exercises and advice, transfer of care documentation, cord clamp cutter, stitch cutter and baby labels (Dahlen 2012, Thorpe and Anderson, 2015).

Usually by 36 weeks gestation the midwife will have visited the woman's home. This allows for discussion of the practicalities including finding the house in the dark. Who else will be present? Is there a mobile phone signal? Where does the woman anticipate giving birth? Will there be children or animals present? What will the plan be if transfer is needed?

The Australian College of Midwives has published midwifery practice standards for birth at home and guidelines for transfer to hospital, including associated documentation and handover (see Resources at the end of the chapter). Similarly, the New Zealand College of Midwives provides comprehensive guidance in this situation (see Resources at the end of the chapter). When a transfer is required, consideration should be given to timeliness, handover and the impact of the transfer on the woman.

It is likely that some of the equipment will be stored in the woman's home. In Australia and New Zealand uterotonics are carried in a cold store box and can be put straight into the woman's refrigerator. Although midwives in New Zealand can prescribe opioids, this is not seen as appropriate practice in the homebirth setting. Non-pharmaceutical pain-relieving strategies such as the use of water, massage, position changes and acupressure are usual at a homebirth. The New Zealand College of Midwives Consensus Statement is unequivocal in this regard: 'The College strongly discourages the use of opioids during labour at home' (New Zealand College of Midwives 2014). This is a safety issue and applies to their use for women in a labour at home but also to the midwife whose safety may be compromised if she is carrying such drugs. The accepted wisdom is that if the woman needs pharmaceutical pain relief, she needs to be in hospital.

Professional and practice considerations

The following points expand on the professional and practice considerations of a midwife during the course of a homebirth.

- Ensure the woman knows how the midwife will be notified and whether there is a requirement to notify anyone else (e.g. second midwife).
- Assessment on arrival consists of history of labour, fetal and maternal wellbeing, abdominal palpation and vaginal examination as needed, decisions about further care documented.
- Establish a working area with space for equipment and resuscitation and a place to write records.
- Ongoing labour care is as for any labouring woman, including assessments for labour progress, particularly fetal and maternal wellbeing. It is likely that the woman will naturally be mobile and utilise the furniture and supporters around her for comfort and pain relief. She may also take regular baths, use a birth pool or shower, eat and drink as she feels appropriate, pass urine as needed and go for walks, have rests or use other activities to help and distract her. As labour progresses, the midwife is more likely to observe the 'in on self' effect as the woman has less conversation and needs a greater level of concentration. The midwife will utilise the 'active inactivity' described in Skill 36.1 and is likely to begin to intuitively understand how the woman is progressing. For further information on a water labour or birth see Chapter 25 of Pairman and colleagues (2018).
- Physiological pushing is likely to be aided using the furniture available; the midwife remains vigilant to fetal and maternal wellbeing and indicators of

progress (see Chapter 40 for greater detail). The second midwife should be called if they are not already present. The midwife should be mindful of her own care (e.g. back strain) when needing to adapt to the woman's position. This is also true of hospital births, but in the home sofas and beds are often low. A hot water bottle, tumble dryer or radiator can be used to warm up the towels prior to the baby's arrival (remove the hot water bottle before using the towels).

- Regarding birth of the placenta, many women may opt for expectant management at home; this requires that the midwife understand the physiology and is competent to undertake its management (see Chapter 22 of Pairman et al 2018). The placenta remains the woman's property; however, sometimes the parents ask that the midwife remove it from the home in a suitable container and dispose of it, as for hospital births. If the woman wishes to keep it, she should be encouraged to bury it deeply in the garden. For many Māori women burying the whenua (placenta) and pito (umbilical cord) has special cultural and spiritual significance (Manatū Taonga Ministry for Culture and Heritage 2017) and the woman and whānau's (family's) wishes should be discussed before the birth and planned accordingly.
- The midwife will need to examine the genital tract with sufficient light (head torch) and visibility; if suturing is required, chairs may be used to support her legs and something firm may be needed beneath the woman's buttocks. All equipment requiring sterilisation is later taken to the local hospital.
- There is little difference in the care of the newborn at home compared to the hospital. If resuscitation is required, the decision to call help is made swiftly and the midwife follows the Resuscitation Council guidelines (Australian and New Zealand Committee on Resuscitation 2017). Skin-to-skin care for the first hour is carried out, as for any other birth, with early breastfeeding encouraged as the feeding cues are seen. An initial postpartum check is done and is also followed by a full neonatal check within 24 hours of the birth. In Australia, it depends on local protocols: it is sometimes done by the authorised practitioner at the birth, which is typically a midwife, but in some circumstances it may be the general practitioner or a paediatrician. In New Zealand this would be done by the lead maternity carer (LMC).
- For transfer to hospital, the midwife will have referral systems and phone numbers in place to the nearest consultant birthing suite. Transfer to hospital is made using an ambulance (often paramedic) in the event of an emergency; a non-urgent transfer may be made using the woman's own transport. Most women will have participated in discussion about transfer during labour, in the pregnancy. It is appropriate to discuss the likely criteria with her in advance, as well as at the time. Building a relationship, and therefore trust, with the woman during pregnancy is likely to make a transfer a little easier, especially if the midwife accompanies her to hospital. If an emergency transfer occurs, it can be helpful to have a card written out (filling in the details at the last minute) that a member of the family can read if they are speaking to ambulance control. Leaving the front door open and a light on can save valuable time. If a paramedic attends, the attendants should be aware that the woman is still the midwife's responsibility. As previously noted, when transfer is recommended, consideration should be given to the impact of the transfer on the woman. It is likely to be deeply disappointing for the woman.
- Documentation is as thorough as for any hospital birth, including all discussions, referrals, actions and rationales. In New Zealand the maternity record is held by the mother and shared with the midwife. The midwife takes a copy of the notes to be her legal record of births she has attended. The parts of the records that require computerisation will be undertaken by the midwife as locally agreed on.
- Occasionally women may bring in their own assistants, such as a herbalist or a doula. The midwife should ensure that, as the professional responsible, if the midwife needs the therapy to stop, this is accepted by the woman and the assistant.
- The midwife generally leaves no less than two hours after the birth when:
  - the mother's vital sign observations are confirmed to be within normal limits
  - the mother's uterus is well contracted with the expected lochial loss; any suturing has been completed, urine passed and generally the woman has had a shower or bath
  - the baby has been fed, has a temperature within normal limits, and has made an uncomplicated adaptation to extrauterine life; the midwife visits the mother and baby within 24 hours and checks that the newborn is breastfeeding well and has passed urine and meconium
  - the family have been supplied with appropriate telephone numbers to call at any time about, for example, increasing pain, signs of vaginal haemorrhage or clots, any baby feeding difficulties, any changes in the baby's colour (pallor/cyanosis) or tone or any other concerns they may have
  - a phone call is arranged to organise the next visit
  - the midwife is confident that all is well, has completed the records and has cleared away all necessary equipment

- the midwife completes any required birth notifications within her jurisdiction.

- Quality assurance activities include self-appraisal, client feedback and Midwifery Practice Review (Australian College of Midwives 2017)/Midwifery Standards Review (New Zealand College of Midwives 2017a), which all aid midwives to appreciate the importance of their care and to review any areas that can be improved.
- Midwives providing homebirth care should maintain appropriate indemnity cover. The Australian College of Midwives advises that 'midwives should comply with the Professional Indemnity Insurance (PII) Registration Standard of the NMBA (Nursing and Midwifery Board of Australia), which provides details about the requirement under section 129(1) where appropriate. The National Law provides for an exemption to the requirement for PII cover in respect of intrapartum care at home provided by privately practising midwives. The Safety and Quality Framework has been approved by the NMBA to enable privately practising midwives to be exempted from PII arrangements under section 284 (1)(c)(ii) of the National Law' (Australian College of Midwives 2011).
- The New Zealand College of Midwives (2017b) provides indemnity insurance for its members, as does the New Zealand Nurses Organisation (2017). Currently the Minister of Health requires authorised practitioners who have an access agreement (a contract to access the facilities within the local hospital[s]) to maintain indemnity insurance. Midwives who attend women at home usually have an access agreement (and by extension indemnity insurance) in order to provide continuity of care if a transfer occurs.

UNPLANNED HOMEBIRTH OR BABY BORN BEFORE ARRIVAL (BBA)

When births occur at home but are unplanned the midwife may be called as well as the ambulance service. It is necessary to make some swift assessments.

- Baby: Does it need resuscitating? Is it cold? What is its gestation? Where was it born? Has it been fed?
- Mother: Was it a precipitate labour? Placenta in or out? Bleeding? State of perineum? Blood group? Vital signs?

Unexpected births at home (or other locations) can cause mothers, babies and other family members to feel a little stunned. Labour has often been rapid and there may be a danger of haemorrhage. The baby may be hypothermic and very likely the placenta is undelivered. The midwife should prioritise issues quickly and effectively before deciding whether transfer to hospital is recommended, remembering that the woman might decline to leave the home. This decision is made in conjunction with the woman and her family, particularly if staying at home is a possible option. The midwife takes the time to thoroughly establish that all is well before leaving this client. The birth notification is completed and should include a note that the birth occurred without any professional in attendance.

Role and responsibilities of the midwife providing birth-at-home care

These can be summarised as:

- collaborating with the woman effectively during pregnancy to plan for a safe and relaxed homebirth
- professional, thorough labour care planned in the woman's home and according to all rules and protocols that govern safe and effective evidence-based practice
- recognising deviations from the norm, responding, consulting, referring or proposing transfer into hospital as appropriate
- undertaking contemporaneous and comprehensive record keeping
- registering the birth as required by Australian or New Zealand jurisdictions
- maintaining quality assurance processes
- making indemnity arrangements.

SUMMARY

- Providing labour care at home for healthy women with a planned homebirth can be a highly satisfying experience for the midwife, the mother and her family.
- A range of new and existing skills are utilised; maintenance of skills, such as resuscitation and other emergency drills, is essential.
- Preparation by all parties involved contributes to the safety and delivery of care. This includes issues such as drugs, equipment, accessibility to other healthcare professionals and referral systems.
- Many aspects of home care mirror hospital care, but the midwife often needs to utilise her professional autonomy to the full. This is particularly the case when the unexpected occurs or the woman is outside of the low-risk criteria.
- Care should be taken to protect the midwife's personal safety.

Self-assessment exercises

The answers to the following questions may be found in the text.

1. Compile low-risk criteria to identify women suitable for homebirth.

2. Discuss the skills needed by the midwife to undertake safe homebirths.
3. List the items needed for a homebirth.
4. Summarise the differences between caring for a labouring woman at home or in hospital.
5. Who should a midwife refer to if a deviation from the norm occurs?
6. Discuss what assessments would be made initially on arrival at a BBA.

Resources

Australian College of Midwives: Australian College of Midwives Birth at Home Midwifery Practice Standards, 2016. Online. Available at: www.midwives.org.au/guidelines-and-standards.

Australian College of Midwives: Australian College of Midwives transfer from planned birth at home guidelines, 2016. Available at: www.midwives.org.au/guidelines-and-standards.

New Zealand College of Midwives: Professional Practice Standards, n.d. Online 28 September 2021. Available: www.midwife.org.nz/midwives/professional-practice/.

References

Australian and New Zealand Committee on Resuscitation: ANZCOR Guideline 13.1—Introduction to resuscitation of the newborn infant, 2017.

Australian College of Midwives: Guidance for midwives regarding homebirth Services, 2011.

Australian College of Midwives: What is MPR? Australian College of Midwives Incorporated Journal, 2017. Online 15 May 2018. Available: www.midwives.org.au/what-mpr.

Australian Government: *Health Practitioner Regulation National Law Act 2009*. Online 15 May 2018. Available: www.ahpra.gov.au/about-ahpra/what-we-do/legislation.aspx.

Australian Institute of Health and Welfare (AIHW): Australia's mothers and babies 2015—in brief, AIHW, Canberra, 2017.

Birthplace in England Collaborative Group: Perinatal and maternal outcomes by planned place of birth for healthy women with low risk pregnancies: the Birthplace in England national prospective cohort study, BMJ 343:d7400, 2011.

Catling-Paull C, Coddington RL, Foureur MJ, et al: Publicly funded homebirth in Australia: a review of maternal and neonatal outcomes over 6 years, Medical Journal of Australia 198(11):616–620, 2013.

Dahlen H: Homebirth: ten tips for safety and survival, British Journal of Midwifery 20(12):872–876, 2012.

Davis D, Baddock S, Pairman S, et al: Planned place of birth in New Zealand: does it affect mode of birth and intervention rates among low-risk women? Birth 38(2):111–119, 2011.

de Crespigny L, Savulescu L: Homebirth and the future child, Journal of Medical Ethics 40(12):807–812, 2014.

Manatū Taonga Ministry for Culture and Heritage: Whenua—the placenta, Te Ara Encyclopaedia of New Zealand, 2017. Online 15 May 2018. Available: https://teara.govt.nz/en/papatuanuku-the-land/page-4.

Midwifery Council of New Zealand: Competencies for entry to the register of midwives, 2007.

Miller S, Skinner J: Are first-time mothers who plan home birth more likely to receive evidence-based care? A comparative study of home and hospital care provided by the same midwives, Birth 39(2):135–144, 2012.

Ministry of Health: Report on maternity 2015, Ministry of Health, Wellington, 2017.

New Zealand College of Midwives: Consensus statement: prescribing and administration of opioid analgesia in labour, 2014.

New Zealand College of Midwives: Midwifery standards review, New Zealand College of Midwives, 2017a. Online 15 May 2018. Available: www.midwife.org.nz/quality-practice/midwifery-standards-review.

New Zealand College of Midwives: Professional indemnity insurance, 2017b. Online 15 May 2018. Available: www.midwife.org.nz/join/professional-indemnity-insurance.

New Zealand Nurses Organisation: Indemnity insurance, 2017. Online 15 May 2018. Available: www.nzno.org.nz/membership/indemnity.

Nursing and Midwifery Board of Australia: Registration and endorsement, 2017. Online 15 May 2018. Available: www.nursingmidwiferyboard.gov.au/Registration-and-Endorsement.aspx.

Pairman S, Tracy S, Dahlen H, Dixon L: Midwifery: preparation for practice, 4th ed., Elsevier, Sydney, 2018.

Roome S, Hartz D, Tracy S, Welsh AW: Why such differing stances? A review of position statements on home birth from professional colleges, BJOG: an International Journal of Obstetrics and Gynaecology February, 123(3):376–382, 2016.

Scarf V, Rossiter C, Vedam S, et al: Maternal and perinatal outcomes by planned place of birth among women with low-risk pregnancies in high-income countries: a systematic review and meta-analysis, Midwifery 62:240–255, 2018. Advance online publication. Online 15 May 2018. Available: https://doi.org/10.1016/j.midw.2018.03.024.

Skinner JP, Foureur M: Consultation, referral and collaboration between midwives and obstetricians: lessons from New Zealand, Journal of Midwifery & Women's Health 55(1):28–37, 2010.

Thorpe J, Anderson J: Supporting women in labour and birth. In Midwifery Preparatory Practice, Elsevier, Sydney, 2015.

Zielinski R, Ackerson K, Kane Low L: Planned home birth: benefits, risks and opportunities, International Journal of Women's Health 7:361–377, 2015. Online 15 May 2018. Available: https://doi.org/10.2147/IJWH.S55561.

SECTION 9

MONITORING WELLBEING IN ESTABLISHED LABOUR

and uterine activity simultaneously provides a high degree of sensitivity, but a low level of specificity (Baker et al 2016). When CTG features suggest or indicate likely fetal compromise and the abnormality persists after correcting reversible causes (cord compression or reduced placental perfusion, uterine hyperstimulation [tachysystole or hypertonus], maternal tachycardia or pyrexia, or inadequate quality of CTG), FBS should be considered during labour if vaginal birth is not imminent, in order to establish a definitive diagnosis of fetal compromise. As well as identifying the fetus at risk of compromise, this can also reduce caesarean section rates (Queensland Clinical Guidelines 2019).

Where continuous electronic fetal monitoring is being used, it is recommended the facility have access to FBS equipment and professionals trained in its use (RANZCOG 2019). Such professionals include a suitably trained and competent resident medical officer, registrar or consultant obstetrician.

Fetal scalp stimulation

A vaginal examination is required in order to perform FBS, as there is a need to exclude factors for fetal compromise, such as cord prolapse, and establish that active labour has commenced, birth is not imminent and the cervix is at least 4 cm dilated to enable the practitioner to perform the procedure. Fetal scalp stimulation is a non-invasive test which can be used in conjunction with CTG findings and prior to undertaking the FBS procedure, to provide reassurance of fetal wellbeing. A review by East and colleagues (2014) found an acceleration in fetal heart rate following fetal scalp stimulation had a likelihood ratio of 0.5 for having a low scalp pH. An acceleration arising from scalp stimulation can be regarded as a reassuring feature and should be taken into consideration when reviewing the whole clinical picture (National Institute for Health and Care Excellence [NICE] 2017). Initial studies demonstrate that fetal scalp stimulation is potentially a reliable alternative to FBS (Tahir Mahmood et al 2017) and the reader is encouraged to observe for further developments in this area.

Undertaking intrapartum fetal blood sampling

It is important to recognise that FBS requires the woman to undergo an invasive, intimate procedure that can potentially cause distress and pain, at a time when there are concerns for her unborn baby's wellbeing. Informed consent is vital, and the woman should be given ample opportunity to ask questions and express her concerns around the indication(s) for the procedure, the risks and possible outcomes, including that it may prevent a caesarean section or an assisted birth. Providing the woman with information and time to consider the proposed intervention will also enable her to make an informed decision to refuse the intervention if she wishes. Both before and during the procedure, the midwives caring for the woman should ensure they are aware of the woman's verbal and non-verbal communication, so they can provide the woman with information about what is happening during the process, but also identify whether she is experiencing discomfort or pain and requires the procedure to be discontinued (Stewart 2005).

FBS should be carried out using an aseptic non-touch technique (ANTT) with sterile gloves worn to provide the non-touch component.

Indications for the use of fetal blood sampling

Where an abnormal CTG persists despite the implementation of appropriate corrective actions during the first and second stage of labour, FBS is indicated. Such abnormalities may include complicated tachycardia, recurrent decelerations, prolonged loss of variability not corrected by fetal stimulation, undefined deceleration patterns and any non-specific concerns about fetal wellbeing. Additional factors including clinical history, parity, stage and rate of progress of labour, and evolution of the FHR pattern should also be considered when making the decision to propose intrapartum FBS (SAMNCN 2020).

Contraindications and risks of fetal blood sampling

RANZCOG (2019) lists the following contraindications to intrapartum FBS:

- gestational age of less than 34 weeks
- evidence of serious, sustained fetal compromise
- risk of fetal bleeding disorders (e.g. fetal thrombocytopenia, haemophilia)
- non-vertex presentation
- maternal infection* (e.g. HIV, hepatitis B, hepatitis C, active primary herpes and suspected fetal sepsis)

Interpretation of fetal blood sample results

When interpreting FBS results, consideration for the whole clinical picture is important. Any previous lactate or pH measurements, the clinical features of the woman and baby and the rate of progress in labour, all need to be taken into account (SAMNCN 2020). Lactate levels in fetal blood correspond with the length of labour, and a high level of lactate is more likely associated with fetal compromise, particularly in the case of dysfunctional labour, than a low pH level (Wiberg-Itzel & Akerud 2011).

---

* Note: Group B streptococcus carrier status does not preclude FBS. Although it is considered to be a relatively safe test (SAMNCN 2020), there are risks associated with carrying out FBS according to Queensland Clinical Guidelines (2019) and SAMNCN (2020). These include:

- eyelid laceration
- subarachnoid penetration
- acute meningoencephalitis
- neonatal scalp abscess and ulceration.

Fetal scalp blood lactate levels have been found to be more successful at assessing fetal wellbeing than pH estimation (East et al 2015).

Normal fetal pH is greater than or equal to 7.25 units, and lactate less than 4.2 mmol/L. Where these results are borderline (pH 7.21 units to 7.24 units and lactate 4.2 to 4.8 mmol/L) the sample should be repeated in 30 minutes. Birth should be expedited where abnormal pH levels of less than or equal to 7.20 units and or lactate of greater than 4.8 mmol/L are present (Queensland Clinical Guidelines 2019). Where the CTG remains abnormal despite normal scalp lactate levels, the FBS should be repeated in 30 minutes to 2 hours (Auckland District Health Board [ADHB] 2020, Queensland Clinical Guidelines 2019). The use of scalp lactate rather than pH is recommended because it is easier to perform, requires a smaller sample size and is a more affordable method of providing a definitive diagnosis of fetal compromise (RANZCOG 2019). This is an important consideration as insufficient samples have been suggested to be obtained in as many as 20% of attempts (East et al 2010).

Clinical guidelines around thresholds of acceptable lactate levels vary depending on location, and parameters for interpretation depend on these. Also of note is that results may vary between machines (Queensland Clinical Guidelines 2019, RANZCOG 2019); therefore, machine calibration and accurate transcription of results also play a role in the correct of the clinical situation (Queensland Clinical Guidelines 2019).

SKILL 37.1 Intrapartum fetal blood sampling

1. Confirm the woman's identity if she is not known to the midwife, obstetrician, resident or registrar who will be performing the procedure.
2. Discuss the procedure fully with the woman and gain informed consent.
3. Ensure the woman is aware that the procedure will require her to have an amnioscope inserted into her vagina, which is similar to a speculum.
4. Ensure privacy.
5. Gather equipment:
   - apron
   - sterile gloves
   - lubricant (e.g. water-soluble lubricant)
   - disposable sheet
   - alcohol-based hand rub
   - disposable fetal scalp blood sampling kit
   - amnioscope
   - gauze
   - chlorhexidine
   - sterile liquid paraffin
   - heparinised capillary tube
   - other equipment as necessary (e.g. amnihook)
   - pinard stethoscope or sonicaid
   - light source.
6. Encourage the woman to empty her bladder if she is not catheterised.
7. Wash and dry hands.
8. Perform an abdominal palpation to determine the lie, presentation, position and degree of engagement, and auscultate the fetal heart.
9. Ask the woman to adopt a left lateral position, preferably, with hips well flexed and the lower leg extended. The upper leg should be flexed (placed into a stirrup) and the woman's buttocks should be over the end of the bed in a position that provides adequate vision and access for the clinician. Alternatively, lithotomy (using a wedge to avoid aortocaval occlusion or supine hypotension if necessary) can be used. Be mindful of the difficulty experienced by women with pelvic girdle pain when having them adopt either of these positions.
10. Place the disposable sheet beneath her buttocks.
11. Ask the woman to remove any sanitary towels or underwear, keeping the genital area covered.
12. Wash and dry hands, apply apron.
13. Open the equipment to be used, including the FBS kit and lubricating gel. Pour chlorhexidine onto gauze.
14. Apply hand rub; allow to dry, then put on gloves.
15. Using ANTT, attach the fetal scalp blade to an introducer (depth of 2 mm).
16. Ask the woman to lift up the cover to allow access to the genital area.
17. Advise the woman that she will feel her labia being touched and part her labia.
18. Ensure the cervix is at least 4 cm dilated and membranes are ruptured.
19. Inform the woman of what is about to happen, then under direct vision, using a light source, insert the amnioscope into the posterior fornix, angled downwards, below the horizontal plane.
20. Pass the anterior lip of the cervix and angle the cone anteriorly in order to visualise the presenting part.
21. Clean the presenting part using the chlorhexidine gauze, then apply the sterile liquid paraffin to the fetal scalp. The use of the paraffin is to encourage beading of the fetal blood and form a non-wettable surface.
22. Use the fetal scalp blade attached to the introducer to make a quick stab on the presenting part.
23. As blood appears from the clean incision, touch the blood with the heparinised capillary

Continued

SKILL 37.1 Intrapartum fetal blood sampling—cont'd

tube, keeping the tube angled downwards, and allow the blood to flow by gravity.

24. Amount to collect (without air bubbles or liquor):
    - at least 2 cm of blood for pH
    - minimum of 5 microlitres of blood for lactate
    - two samples.
25. Pass the samples to an assistant for processing immediately, before applying pressure for the duration of the next two contractions to the fetal scalp, to ensure bleeding has stopped.
26. Withdraw the amnioscope gently.
27. Auscultate the fetal heart.
28. Assist the woman into a comfortable position, reapply sanitary pad if required and discuss the findings.
29. Dispose of equipment appropriately, removing the gloves then the apron.
30. Wash and dry hands.
31. Document the findings in the notes (also the partogram and or CTG if being used) and act accordingly.

Role and responsibilities of the midwife

These can be summarised as:

- recognising deviations from normal and instigating referral
- providing education, explanations and support for the woman
- displaying due diligence in FBS equipment calibration
- providing assistance to the obstetrician, resident or registrar during the process of obtaining a fetal blood sample
- undertaking appropriate record keeping.

SUMMARY

- Intrapartum fetal blood sampling is an invasive procedure, but one that can yield valuable, definitive information in relation to fetal wellbeing when fetal distress is apparent on CTG monitoring, ultimately aiding the decision to expedite birth or allow labour to progress.
- The risk of ascending infection is high; an aseptic non-touch technique should be used throughout.

Self-assessment exercises

The answers to the following questions may be found in the text.

1. For what reasons would fetal blood sampling (FBS) be undertaken during labour?
2. What should be discussed with the woman to gain her informed consent regarding FBS?
3. How would the midwife assist in intrapartum FBS?
4. What information can be gained from intrapartum FBS and what is the significance of it?
5. What are the role and responsibilities of the midwife in relation to intrapartum FBS?

References

Auckland District Health Board (ADHB): Fetal surveillance policy, 2020. Online 31 Jan 2021. Available: www.nationalwomenshealth.adhb.govt.nz/assets/Womens-health/Documents/Policies-and-guidelines/Fetal-Surveillance-Policy-.pdf.

Baker L, Beaves M, Wallace E: Assessing fetal wellbeing: a practical guide, RANZCOG & Monash Health, Melbourne, 2016.

East C, Begg L, Colditz P, et al: Fetal pulse oximetry for fetal assessment in labour, Cochrane Database of Systematic Reviews (10):Art. No.: CD004075, 2014.

East CE, Leader LR, Sheehan P, et al: Intrapartum fetal scalp lactate sampling for fetal assessment in the presence of a non-reassuring fetal heart rate trace, Cochrane Database of Systematic Reviews (5):Art. No.: CD006174, 2015.

East CE, Leader LR, Sheehan P, et al: Intrapartum fetal scalp lactate sampling for fetal assessment in the presence of a non-reassuring fetal heart rate trace, Cochrane Database of Systematic Reviews (3):Art. No.: CD006174, 2010.

National Institute for Health and Care Excellence (NICE): Intrapartum care. Care of healthy women and their babies during childbirth Clinical Guideline 190, 2017. Online 8 June 2018. Available: www.nice.org.uk.

Queensland Clinical Guidelines: Intrapartum fetal surveillance, 2019. Online 31 Jan 2021. Available: www.health.qld.gov.au/__data/assets/pdf_file/0012/140043/g-ifs.pdf.

Royal Australian and New Zealand College of Obstetricians and Gynaecologists (RANZCOG), 2019. Intrapartum fetal surveillance clinical guideline – 4th ed. 2019. Online 31 Jan 2021. Available: https://ranzcog.edu.au/RANZCOG_SITE/media/RANZCOG-MEDIA/Women%27s%20Health/Statement%20and%20guidelines/Clinical-Obstetrics/IFS-Guideline-4thEdition-2019.pdf?ext=.pdf.

South Australian Maternal and Neonatal Clinical Network (SAMNCN): Perinatal practice guideline:

fetal acid base balance assessment, 2020. Online 31 Jan 2021. Available: www.sahealth.sa.gov.au/wps/wcm/connect/4953cc804ee46e14bcb7bdd150ce4f37/Fetal+Acid+Base+Balance+Assessment_PPG_v5_1.pdf?MOD=AJPERES&CACHEID=ROOTWORKSPACE-4953cc804ee46e14bcb7bdd150ce4f37-noGY8LW.

South Australian Maternal and Neonatal Clinical Network (SAMNCN), 2015. Normal pregnancy, labour and puerperium management clinical guideline. Online 8 June 2018. Available: http://www.sahealth.sa.gov.au/.

Stewart M: 'I'm just going to wash you down': sanitizing the vaginal examination, Journal of Advanced Nursing 51(6):587–594, 2005.

Tahir Mahmood U, O'Gorman C, Marchocki Z, et al: Fetal scalp stimulation (FSS) versus fetal blood sampling (FBS) for women with abnormal fetal heart rate monitoring in labor: a prospective cohort study, Maternal Fetal Neonatal Medicine 1–6, 2017.

Wiberg-Itzel E, Akerud H: 651: fetal blood sampling in normal and dysfunctional labor, American Journal of Obstetrics & Gynecology 204(1):S257, 2011.

CHAPTER 38

EPIDURAL AND SPINAL ANAESTHESIA/ANALGESIA

Learning outcomes

Having read this chapter, the reader should be able to:

- outline the indications and contraindications for epidural and spinal anaesthesia/analgesia
- identify the side effects and complications of epidural and spinal anaesthesia/analgesia and how they are recognised and managed
- explain how epidural and spinal anaesthesia/analgesia are administered
- describe the safe removal of an epidural catheter
- detail the role and responsibilities of the midwife during and after epidural and spinal anaesthesia/analgesia administration.

Epidural and spinal anaesthesia/analgesia occurs through the administration of local anaesthetic, with or without an opioid analgesic, into the epidural space and/or into the cerebrospinal fluid.

In this chapter, the use of epidural and spinal anaesthesia/analgesia and the roles and responsibilities of the midwife are reviewed.

Epidural analgesia/anaesthesia is widely used and has been demonstrated to provide more effective pain relief in labour than all other pharmacological treatments (ANZCA 2020, Anim-Somuah et al 2018). However, it is associated with an increased incidence of maternal hypotension, motor blockade, fever, urinary retention, longer first and second stages of labour, and oxytocic augmentation (Anim-Somuah et al 2018) and with fetal bradycardia (RANZCOG n.d.).

Spinal anaesthesia/analgesia is commonly administered for caesarean section and on occasion in combination with epidural anaesthesia/analgesia for labour pain. This is called a combined spinal–epidural (CSE) anaesthesia/analgesia.

Although midwives who have undertaken relevant education to do so can administer medication via the epidural/spinal route once a catheter has been situated, it is a medical practitioner skilled in anaesthetics who sites the catheter if one is placed.

This chapter clarifies the terminology and details the procedures for epidural/spinal catheter insertion, intermittent bolus administration and removal of the catheter after the birth of the baby. The indications, contraindications, side effects, recognition and management of complications and the midwife's role and responsibilities are discussed.

The rate of regional anaesthesia in Australia in 2015 for relief of pain in labour was 40% (Australian Institute of Health and Welfare [AIHW] 2020). Rates for epidural use in labour in New Zealand are lower at 26% (Ministry of Health 2017). Information from several studies indicates a consistently higher availability and use of epidural anaesthesia for pain relief in labour in private hospitals than in public hospitals in Australia (de Rooy 2015). Rates for epidural use in labour in Australia and New Zealand, however, are much lower than in the United States, where the incidence in 2018 was recorded to be 71% (Butwick et al 2018).

THE EPIDURAL SPACE

Containing blood vessels and fatty tissue, the epidural space is approximately 4 mm wide at the lumbar region and is situated around the dura mater, with the spinal nerves passing through it. During pregnancy the epidural space is further reduced due to engorgement of the vessels in pregnancy, and in labour due to the uterine contractions and increased blood flow.

EPIDURAL ANAESTHESIA/ ANALGESIA

Epidural anaesthesia/analgesia is achieved by the administration of medications (a local anaesthetic with or without an opioid analgesic) through a small catheter into the epidural space by bolus injection or continuous infusion (ANZCA 2020). The concentration and volume of local anaesthetic and opioid used affects the onset of action, duration and degree of the block. The aim of epidural anaesthesia/analgesia is to remove the sensation of pain by blocking the transmission of signals surrounding the specific fibres of the spinal nerves in conjunction with the absorption into the systemic circulation via the epidural veins (Rankin 2017). Traditionally, local anaesthetics used for epidurals were administered in high concentrations, giving effective pain relief for most women but rendering them numb from the waist down.

Successful placement of the epidural catheter is essential if effective analgesia is to be achieved. The anaesthetist has to estimate the distance from the woman's skin to her epidural space, as this varies between women. The risk of a dural puncture occurring is increased if the distance to insert the epidural needle is overestimated. Ultrasound imaging is being used more frequently to determine the depth to the epidural space (Hasanin et al 2017).

Patient-controlled epidural analgesia

Popularity has increased for the method of the administration of epidural anaesthetic in the form of **patient-controlled epidural anaesthesia (PCEA)**, which enables the woman to control the amount of medication she receives, depending directly on her need for pain relief (Tracy & Hartz 2015). Using PCEA reduces the amount of local anaesthetic used, thus decreasing common side effects that may be experienced with a continuous epidural infusion (CEI) (Tracy & Hartz 2015). Dilute concentrations of local anaesthetic (ropivacaine and bupivacaine) with and without background infusion provide effective analgesia in labour.

Low-dose epidurals that provide effective analgesia without loss of motor function can be offered in hospital settings and may be referred to as 'mobile' or 'walking' epidurals.

Spinal anaesthesia/analgesia

Spinal anaesthesia/analgesia is quick, easy to perform and very effective, producing a total and sensory block below the target area (Rankin 2017). This is achieved by injecting a single bolus of drug/s through the epidural space, dura and arachnoid membranes, into the intrathecal (subarachnoid) space (Rankin 2017). Lower doses of the drug(s) can be used as it is placed directly into the cerebrospinal fluid (CSF) where the opioid can bind to the opioid receptor sites in the dorsal horn of the spinal cord. Onset of analgesia is rapid but not as long lasting as an epidural and therefore is rarely used for labour on its own (Institute for Quality and Efficiency in Health Care 2018). It is often the analgesia/anaesthesia of choice for emergency caesarean section where rapid anaesthesia is required or for an elective caesarean section.

Combined spinal–epidural anaesthesia/analgesia

Combined spinal–epidural (CSE) anaesthesia/analgesia has become popular due to the rapid onset of the subarachnoid block with the advantage of having an epidural catheter in place during labour if operative or instrumental birth is required (Tracy & Hartz 2015). Combined spinal–epidural analgesia includes both a single spinal injection and an epidural catheter which can be used for ongoing pain relief. This combination has the advantage of being able to provide a transition from intraoperative to postoperative analgesia (Klimek et al 2018). The CSE procedure is more time-consuming than a spinal block (Klimek et al 2018).

DRUGS

Local anaesthetics (e.g. bupivacaine, ropivacaine) cross the dura and arachnoid membranes, where they are in contact with the lumbar and sacral nerve roots, producing the effect of epidural blockade (Tracy & Hartz 2015). Bupivacaine and ropivacaine both have moderate onset of action with long duration, with the extent of duration often dependent on dosages received (Tracy & Hartz 2015). Ropivacaine is considered less potent than bupivacaine, providing a shorter motor blockade than bupivacaine when used for caesarean (Tracy & Hartz 2015). Bupivacaine does not cross the placental barrier in appreciable amounts, resulting in no effect on the fetus (Bullock & Manias 2014). Studies indicate there is no difference regarding mode of birth, maternal satisfaction or neonatal outcomes between bupivacaine and ropivacaine (Wang et al 2017).

Opioids

The combination of a local anaesthetic and a strong opioid in low doses infused into the epidural space is synergistic with the potential to produce regional analgesia without increasing the incidence of side effects seen when the drugs are administered separately at higher doses (Bowrey & Thompson 2008).

INDICATIONS FOR EPIDURAL ANALGESIA

- Effective pain relief in labour
- The woman's choice of pain relief
- Where there is likelihood of instrumental or operative birth (e.g. malposition, malpresentation, multiple pregnancy)
- Hypertensive conditions in pregnancy
- Prolonged labour
- Preterm labour, to avoid the use of narcotic drugs and reduce the urge to push prematurely
- Maternal cardiac and respiratory disease, neuromuscular and neurological diseases where effective pain control may have an increased safety benefit

- For women who have significant risk factors for general anaesthesia, including difficult airway management and morbid obesity (King Edward Memorial Hospital 2014, Rankin 2017).

CONTRAINDICATIONS

- Patient refusal
- Haemorrhagic disease or clotting disorder
- Low platelets
- Localised skin infection on the lower back or generalised sepsis
- Haemorrhage and cardiovascular instability
- Hypovolaemia or hypotension
- Known allergy to drugs used
- Raised intracranial pressure
- Abnormal spine anatomy or chronic back problems
- Some neurological disorders (e.g. multiple sclerosis or impaired consciousness and cooperation)
- Lack of availability of adequately trained staff (Canterbury District Health Service 2017, Rankin 2017).

SIDE EFFECTS OF EPIDURAL ANALGESIA

The most common side effects caused by epidural analgesia during labour for the woman include:

- hypotension
- motor blockade
- fever
- urinary retention
- longer first and second stages of labour (leading to increased need for oxytocic augmentation) (Anim-Somuah et al 2018).

Additionally, fetal bradycardia can ensue (RANZCOG n.d.)

MANAGEMENT OF SIDE EFFECTS OF EPIDURAL ANAESTHESIA

Hypotension

It is essential to establish a woman's baseline blood pressure prior to the epidural procedure to ensure accurate identification of hypotension post-epidural insertion and commencement. Epidural anaesthesia causes a drop in blood pressure in about 14 out of 100 women, resulting in associated dizziness or nausea (Institute for Quality and Efficiency in Health Care 2018). This results from the action of the local anaesthetic as it blocks both the motor and sensory nerves, directly affecting the sympathetic nervous system by causing vasodilation and a possible drop in the maternal blood pressure (Rankin 2017). In the event of this occurring, the woman should be placed in the left lateral position and treatment commenced by intravenous fluid replacement via a peripheral intravenous cannula. Oxygen administration should be administered via Hudson mask at 6–8 L/min (Jain et al 2016, O'Sullivan & Cockerham 2016). Vasopressor medications may be considered if these treatments do not increase maternal blood pressure (Rankin 2017). Correcting hypotension is important as the drugs cause a decrease in vascular resistance, directly affecting uterine and placental blood flow and causing a reduction in the fetal heart rate (Parer et al 2018).

Motor block and leg weakness

Motor block can be caused by the administration of local anaesthetics into the epidural space, resulting in an exaggerated impairment of sensation and movement (Royal Children's Hospital Melbourne 2016). The assessment of motor block is essential to determine the amount of motor function and to ensure that the woman is able to ambulate if appropriate. The assessment is also integral in detecting if an infusion rate is too high, preventing pressure injury, especially around the heels, and detection of the onset of complications, including epidural haematoma or abscess (Royal Children's Hospital Melbourne 2016). If there is any concern about a haematoma forming during labour the epidural infusion should be turned off and no further boluses given, leg strength should be assessed every 30 minutes—when an increase in leg strength occurs the infusion/bolus administration can recommence.

Urinary retention

Epidurals can affect urinary elimination, with about 15 out of 100 women experiencing difficulty in urination due to epidural analgesia (Institute for Quality and Efficiency in Health Care 2018). Routine insertion of indwelling catheters for drainage of urine from the bladder is often practised due to concerns of obstructing fetal descent during active labour. However, the use of indwelling catheters can increase the risk of urinary tract infections (UTIs) and the literature suggests intermittent catheterisation when necessary is preferable for bladder management for women who have epidural anaesthesia in labour (Wilson et al 2015). When epidural or spinal anaesthesia is used for operative caesarean delivery, an indwelling catheter is recommended during the procedure and for a minimum of 12 hours following birth (King Edward Memorial Hospital 2014).

Maternal fever

Epidurals cause fever in about 23 out of 100 women, potentially impacting labour and birth management, with women likely to receive antibiotics throughout labour or during caesarean delivery. Maternal fever during labour can often be associated with adverse neonatal outcomes (Curtin et al 2015, Institute for Quality and Efficiency in Health Care 2018). Although maternal fever can be caused by both inflammatory and infective processes during labour, incidence of fever within 6 hours of the onset of epidural administration with a progressive increase in maternal temperature may be related to local anaesthetic agents routinely used for epidural pain relief. Further epidemiologic studies are required due to the elusiveness of the mechanism of maternal fever associated with epidural use (Sultan et al 2016).

Nausea and vomiting

Low doses of opioids activate the mu opioid receptors in the chemoreceptor trigger zone (CTZ), which can result in nausea and vomiting, although the effects are not as evident as when opioids are administered intravenously. Not all women will experience nausea and vomiting, as higher doses of opioids can suppress vomiting by acting at receptor sites deeper in the medulla. Where it does arise, it is usually managed easily with the administration of an intravenous anti-emetic.

Pruritus (itching)

This occurs more commonly over the face, chest and abdomen. It may be a result of the opioids causing histamine release or a side effect from the activation of the mu opioid receptors. Treatment is administration of an antihistamine with or without a decrease in the infusion rate if a CEI is used, or if severe, administration of a small dose of naloxone; however, this will decrease the analgesic effect of the opioid.

COMPLICATIONS

Complications are associated with siting or removing the epidural catheter or problems that arise throughout epidural use. The associated signs and symptoms may occur immediately or be delayed for several days after removal of the epidural catheter. As some of these complications are extremely serious, it is important the midwife is vigilant, so that early referral and treatment can be provided. Fortunately serious complications, such as epidural abscess, spinal haematoma, high spinal and local anaesthetic toxicity, are rare. It is important to note that local anaesthetic toxicity does not always occur at the time of the initial injection.

Severe local anaesthetic toxicity can occur from inadvertent intravascular injection and will present as a sudden alteration in the woman's mental status accompanied by severe agitation and/or loss of consciousness with or without tonic-clonic convulsions and a metallic taste. Initially the woman may experience light headedness, drowsiness, restlessness, tinnitus and/or circumoral tingling. If toxicity is undetected and higher toxic levels occur, then convulsions, hypoventilation, arrhythmias, hypotension, tachycardia and cardiac arrest may occur. Cardiovascular collapse can occur with bradycardia (Sekimoto et al 2017).

Should this occur while the injection is being given, the anaesthetist will stop the injection. Help should be called for immediately; an emergency medical code should be called and assistance given to maintain the airway. If the anaesthetist is not present, they should be summoned urgently as intubation may be indicated. The woman will require oxygen administration to maintain oxygen saturation levels ≥ 95% and a second intravenous cannula should be sited. Observation of vital signs should be undertaken and fluids administered to reverse the effects of hypotension. If seizures continue, medication may be required. If circulatory arrest occurs, cardiopulmonary resuscitation should commence using a left tilt and boluses of intravenous lipid emulsion given. Lipids are an effective remedy for the cardiotoxic effects of lipid-soluble local anaesthetics, such as bupivacaine and ropivacaine (Sekimoto et al 2017).

Partial block ('breakthrough' pain)

Although failure of effective pain relief is often due to poor identification of the epidural space and site location, other obstetric causes of breakthrough pain, although rare, need to be considered, including uterine rupture and placental abruption (Ong et al 2016). Breakthrough pain may also be experienced when the woman has bladder distention from a full bladder or when backpain persists due to a fetus in an occipito-posterior position (Allman et al 2016). Therefore, in the event of breakthrough pain being experienced an assessment should be undertaken to determine the rate of progress of labour, including evaluation of cervical dilation. The epidural catheter should also be checked to ensure it still remains in the epidural space (Clark et al 2016). If pain is felt in the upper part of the abdomen, the basal rate of the infusion can be increased as per the anaesthetist's instructions or a bolus given. If there is a missed segment, a bolus can be given with the woman lying on the side where she feels the pain. If this does not help, the anaesthetist should review the woman and may want to consider pulling the catheter back slightly (the midwife should NOT attempt this), giving a bolus of a different drug or re-siting the epidural catheter. If the pain is unilateral it may be due to the tip of the catheter being lodged on one side of the epidural space during its insertion, resulting in the drugs preferentially bathing the nerve roots on that side. Withdrawing the catheter slightly (undertaken by the anaesthetist) may correct this.

Dural puncture

This occurs when the epidural needle or catheter accidentally punctures the dura mater, resulting in leakage of the CSF and reduced intracranial pressure. This causes traction on the innervated tissues around the brain and can result in a severe headache occurring, usually in the following few days. If drugs are given immediately following an inadvertent dural puncture, they will be administered into the intrathecal rather than the epidural space, resulting in a total spinal block. If the dural puncture is noticed before the epidural catheter is inserted, the anaesthetist is likely to re-site the epidural or insert an intrathecal catheter. If there is no headache, labour continues and the woman can push during the second stage.

Postdural puncture headache (PDPH)

During epidural placement, inadvertent puncture of the dura mater occurs at a rate of 1.5%, with more than half of these patients developing **postdural puncture headache (PDPH)**. In a recent study it was suggested that PDPH after dural puncture with an epidural needle could be as high as 76–85% (Kwak 2017).

PDPH classically presents as a dull, throbbing headache with distribution over the fronto-occipital region, exacerbated when standing or sitting and only alleviated, even if partially, once lying down in the supine position (Kwak 2017). Associated symptoms include neck stiffness, photophobia, nausea, vomiting, diplopia, hyperacusis, hearing loss and tinnitus (Kwak 2017). The headache usually begins around 24–48 hours post-puncture (although rarely it may happen immediately following the dural puncture) and can resolve spontaneously within 5–10 days (but may take up to 3 weeks); however, the symptoms can be very debilitating, necessitating treatment of an epidural blood patch (EBP).

Diagnosis of PDPH is usually made based on the symptoms alone, but if there is any doubt, magnetic resonance imaging (MRI) can be performed, which may also show other causes of the headache. Discussion with the anaesthetist is warranted as soon as PDPH is suspected. The anaesthetist will then review the woman on a daily basis and consider whether conservative management, such as adopting whatever posture is most comfortable, maintaining hydration and simple analgesia, will be sufficient. Caffeine may also be prescribed, as it will help to dilate the constricted intracranial veins.

Where conservative management does not work, an EBP can be used. It is not advisable to use this form of treatment if the woman is pyrexial or within the first 24–48 hours due to its lower success rate and higher risk of bacteraemia. The woman is usually positioned in the left lateral position, which is more comfortable but also decreases the risk of further CSF leakage. Twenty millilitres of blood are taken from the woman and, after a Tuohy needle has been inserted into the epidural space below or at the site of the dural puncture, the blood is slowly injected into the epidural space (see Figure 38.1). The woman may feel some relief immediately as the blood exerts a mass effect within the epidural space, which increases the CSF pressure. A clot forms and blocks the puncture site, stopping further leakage of CSF and allowing the CSF to regenerate and return to a normal volume. Following the procedure, the woman should lie flat for 2 hours and then begin to mobilise slowly. Over the next 48 hours the woman should avoid heavy lifting, excessive bending or straining when defecating. If the headache recurs, the EBP can be repeated, although Obstetric Anaesthetists' Association (2014) state that 60–70% of headaches are resolved within a few minutes to a few hours.

Catheter migration

This is an extremely rare complication where the catheter migrates into the CSF causing a total spinal block from an intrathecal injection or a blood vessel, resulting in an intravascular injection. Intravascular administration of the epidural drugs can result in sedation from excess opioids or local anaesthetic toxicity. If this occurs the woman may experience tingling, numbness, twitching, convulsions, apnoea and loss of consciousness. Occasionally the catheter

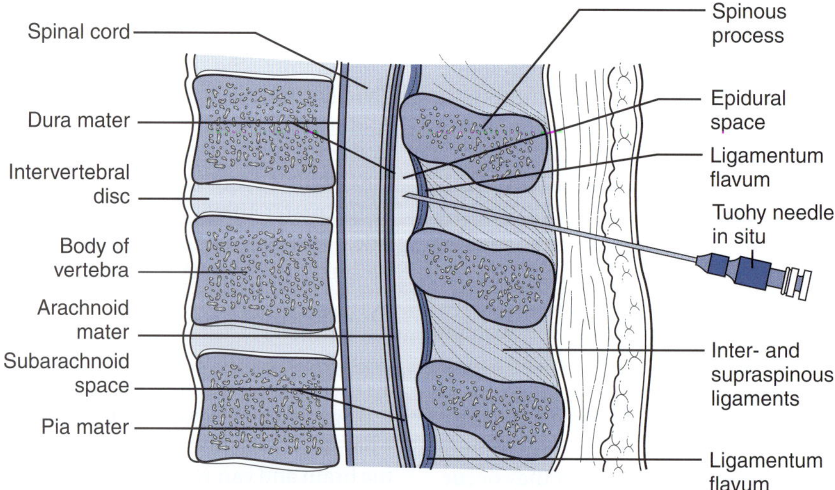

FIGURE 38.1 **Sagittal section of the lumbar spine with Tuohy needle in the epidural space.**
Source: Johnson R, Taylor W: Skills for midwifery practice, 4th ed., Elsevier, London, 2016.

falls out, causing an increase in pain and a feeling of wetness from leakage of the infusate.

Abscess formation

A rare but serious complication is the formation of an abscess within the epidural space. It usually occurs after the epidural catheter has been removed. The abscess can compress the spinal cord leading to nerve damage and paralysis, in addition to being the cause of sepsis. It manifests as back pain, tenderness and erythema around, and purulent discharge from, the insertion site; there may also be swelling around the insertion site. If the woman is pyrexial, a sample of the discharge should be sent for culture and sensitivity analysis. If this is noted before the epidural catheter is removed, the tip of the catheter should also be sent for analysis once it is removed.

Haematoma

This is fortunately also a very rare but serious complication. A haematoma forms as a result of trauma to the epidural blood vessels during catheter insertion or more likely, on removal. It is usually self-limiting and may be of no consequence. However, if the woman is receiving an anticoagulant, it can quickly become more serious. It presents as back pain and tenderness accompanied by sensory and/or motor weakness, particularly increasing leg weakness and bladder and/or bowel dysfunction. Untreated, an epidural haematoma can compress the spinal cord leading to permanent nerve damage and paralysis within 6–8 hours. Diagnosis should be made early with an MRI or computed tomography (CT) scan. The haematoma should be evacuated before permanent damage occurs.

High regional/total spinal anaesthesia

This is an excessively high block, above T4, and may occur due to inadvertent placement of the epidural catheter into the intrathecal rather than the epidural space and can cause paralysis of the intercostal respiratory muscles of the diaphragm. This results in rapid onset of analgesia accompanied by a dense motor block of the legs, symptomatic hypotension, dyspnoea, slurred speech and hoarseness, arm weakness/tingling, sedation/anxiety, high level of insensitivity to cold and touch and unconsciousness. Help should be called immediately, an anaesthetist or doctor specialising in tracheal intubation is necessary, as the woman will require intubation and ventilatory support and oxygen administered to maintain oxygen saturation levels ≥ 95%. If there is an epidural infusion running, it should be turned off. Hypotension should be corrected with intravenous fluids and vasoconstrictors (e.g. ephedrine, phenylephrine, metaraminol, adrenaline) to maintain blood pressure and reduce the risk of cardiac arrest. The woman should not be laid flat until the anaesthetist requests this, as it will result in the block becoming higher. Observations of pulse, blood pressure, respirations and oxygen saturation should be undertaken. The consultant obstetrician should be informed, as urgent delivery of the baby may be required once the woman's condition has stabilised; vaginal delivery may still be possible.

Meningitis

Fortunately, meningitis (an infection within the meninges and CSF) is an extremely rare complication of epidural. The woman may develop fever, headache, neck stiffness, photophobia, nausea and vomiting, and should be referred for urgent medical treatment to reduce the risk of complications.

EFFECT ON LABOUR

Epidural anaesthesia/analgesia has not been found to increase the rate of caesarean section overall or the rate of caesarean section for fetal distress (Schug et al 2020). The use of epidural analgesia can increase both the second stage of labour and the need for labour augmentation with oxytocic-assisted vaginal birth (Anim-Somuah et al 2018).

Traditionally, epidural use during labour was associated with an increased risk of instrumental delivery, caesarean section, oxytocin augmentation and lower Apgar scores. This may have been due to the high dose of local anaesthetic drugs that were used when epidural use was first introduced. Rankin (2017) suggests these drugs affect the pelvic autonomic and parasympathetic nerves, inhibiting oxytocin release and reducing the strength and frequency of contractions. During the second stage, the expulsive nature of contractions may be affected as the urge to push is lost due to the sensory blockade and a reduction in pelvic floor muscle tone, which can affect rotation of the presenting part. Different drugs and dosages have been used over time to reduce the adverse effects on labour, but epidural analgesia may still impact labour. Women are more likely to have a longer second stage, reduced mobility, hypotension, urinary retention, fever and an increased need for oxytocin augmentation and instrumental delivery.

The timing of the epidural does not appear to adversely affect the type of delivery. Sng and colleagues (2014) found there was no increase in the risk of caesarean section or instrumental delivery for women who had an early epidural (cervical dilatation ≤ 3 cm in comparison with those who had an epidural when the cervix was dilated to 4 cm or more) and suggest the epidural should be initiated when the woman requests it.

Cheng and colleagues (2014) agree that the second stage is longer with epidural use and propose that the definition of prolonged second stage should be reviewed for epidural use. Many intrapartum policies now provide for a longer second stage with delayed pushing. Cheng and colleagues (2014) suggest the length of the second stage for nulliparous women with an epidural should be 4 hours and 3 hours for multiparous women.

SKILL 38.1 Siting an epidural catheter and analgesia

Part of the informed consent process for epidural pain relief in labour involves the anaesthetist explaining to the woman the advantages, disadvantages and associated benefits and risks with epidural analgesia (Mahomed et al 2015). Written information, such as the fact sheet provided by the Australian and New Zealand College of Anaesthetists (n.d.), can be given to women to read prior to labour or on requesting an epidural for pain relief in labour.

1. Inform the anaesthetist and gather the equipment (this is often contained together on a trolley ready for use):
   - equipment for peripheral intravenous cannulation and intravenous infusion (usually crystalloid fluid)
   - cardiotocograph (CTG) monitor
   - trolley top or area for a sterile field to be set up
   - sterile gown and gloves
   - sterile dressing pack, with fenestrated drape and gauze
   - antiseptic lotion (e.g. chlorhexidine in 70% isopropyl alcohol)
   - epidural pack, usually containing a Tuohy needle with stylet, syringe, epidural catheter and antibacterial filter
   - sterile syringes and needles (these may be in the epidural pack)
   - local anaesthetics for the skin and epidural (e.g. lignocaine and bupivacaine)
   - opiate analgesia; if required this is usually combined with the local anaesthetic
   - tape/plastic skin dressing
   - appropriate documentation, often specific epidural chart and coloured stickers to differentiate epidural and intravenous lines.
2. Encourage the woman to empty her bladder.
3. If maternity service policy or guidelines permit, the midwife may cannulate the woman if competent to do so, and commence an intravenous infusion in accordance with standing orders.
4. Record baseline observations of blood pressure, pulse, respiration and temperature.
5. Position the woman according to her comfort and the anaesthetist's preference (two positions: either on her side or in a sitting position) to promote curvature of the spine so that access can be gained between the vertebrae.
   - In left lateral position with knees flexed and pulled up towards her chest with her head flexed forwards 'chin on chest'; this encourages anterior flexion of the vertebral column. The woman's back should be very close to the edge of the bed and a pillow placed under her head and another between her knees.
   - Sitting on the edge of the bed with feet supported on a chair/stool, shoulders hunched forwards with arms resting on a bed table or hugging a pillow and head resting on her arms to encourage anterior flexion of the spine.
6. Assist the anaesthetist to 'gown and glove' and to establish a critical aseptic field, pour the lotion, open the needles and syringes, hold ampoules of drugs for drawing up, etc.
7. Support the woman to remain still and keep her informed of what is happening while the epidural is sited by the anaesthetist.
   - The woman's back is cleansed, the drapes put in place and the local anaesthetic inserted into the skin.
   - While the woman is between contractions and very still, the Tuohy needle is inserted between the lumbar vertebrae to the ligamentum flavum where resistance is noted.
   - As the ligamentum flavum is punctured there will a sudden loss of resistance to pressure noted on the syringe plunger and the anaesthetist may feel a slight clicking sensation as the needle enters into the epidural space.
   - The stylet will be removed and normal saline injected to assess the resistance and ensure that the Tuohy needle is in the correct place.
   - When the anaesthetist is confident the needle tip is correctly placed, the epidural catheter is threaded through the needle 4–6 cm into the epidural space and the Tuohy needle removed over the catheter.
8. If used, spray plastic skin around the puncture site and/or secure the catheter with tape; the filter will be connected by the anaesthetist and this should be positioned for ease of access.
9. A small test dose is given and if satisfactory the first complete dose is given or a syringe driver/infusion pump attached for a CEI.
10. Assist the woman into the position advised by the anaesthetist for the initial 20 minutes after administration (often semirecumbent).
11. Record the woman's blood pressure, respiration and pulse every 5 minutes for the next 20 minutes and then every 30 minutes.
12. The woman's condition should also be observed, including her level of pain/block, respiratory rate, her warmth, safety, intravenous infusion, colour, sedation level and CTG changes.
13. After initial observations above are complete then hourly observations are required to check respiratory rate, blood pressure, heart rate, sensory block level, Bromage score (see Figure 38.2), and if CEI, the cumulative total in mL (SA Health 2017).
14. Temperature should be recorded 4-hourly. Notify the medical officer and record temperature hourly if outside the normal parameters (SA Health 2017).
15. The anaesthetist completes their contemporaneous records, including the controlled drug register if appropriate.
16. Refer to the anaesthetist if any observations give cause for concern (hypotension may be corrected by increasing the rate of the intravenous infusion, but the anaesthetist should always be informed).

SKILL 38.1 Siting an epidural catheter and analgesia—cont'd

17. Ensure the anaesthetist has disposed of the equipment correctly, including sharps.
18. Continue to monitor the fetal heart rate and uterine activity on the CTG.
19. If all observations are within normal limits after 20 minutes and the level of analgesia has been achieved, the woman can be assisted to change her position to a position of her choice (avoiding aortocaval compression).
20. Normal labour care continues, including care of the bladder, pressure-area care and the maintenance of contemporaneous records (ANZCA n.d.).
21. Administration of PCEA allows the woman to administer her own intermittent boluses with or without a low-dose background CEI, but will still require assessment of her vital signs and condition as described earlier following each bolus.

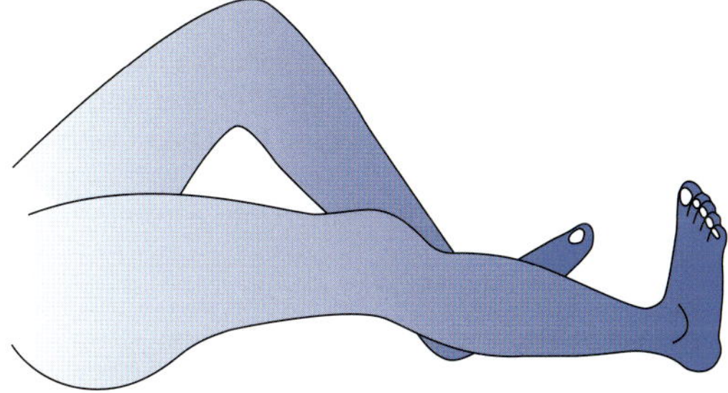

FIGURE 38.2 **Bromage score—assessment of motor block.**
Source: Adapted from Royal Children's Hospital: Assessment of motor block, 2016. Available: www.rch.org.au/anaes/pain_management/Assessment_of_motor_block/

CHECKING THE LEVEL OF THE BLOCK

The sensory level/block is assessed 20 minutes after the loading dose is administered, 20 minutes after each clinician-administered bolus dose and hourly otherwise. The level should be T6–T10: an effective labour epidural should have block levels of T10 or above, and block levels above T6 should be notified to the duty anaesthetist.

The upper level of the block should be determined bilaterally using a cold stimulus (e.g. an ice pack). The level at which the woman reports a change in sensation to cold is considered the block level. The dermatome level (see Figure 38.3) on each side at which the woman reports the change in sensation should be documented (Auckland District Health Board 2020).

The block level is checked using temperature change with an ice pack by initially testing an area well away from the possible dermatome (e.g. face/forearm), so the woman can feel the sensation of 'cold'. Proceed to the woman's torso or legs while moving the icepack up in intervals of 5 cm until the woman experiences the same cold sensation on her abdomen and chest that she experienced on her face or forearm.

The area is compared against a dermatome chart or map; if the block is too high (above L4), the duty anaesthetist should be called and the infusion stopped if it is continuous as there is a risk of respiratory arrest. When the level is too low, the woman is likely to be feeling pain and require a bolus or an increase in the basal infusion rate. If the woman is receiving a continuous infusion and the block is too low to be beneficial, the midwife should check that the catheter is still in situ and connected to the bacterial filter with no leaks in the tubing, and consider increasing the basal rate (as prescribed) before calling the anaesthetist, who may need to re-site the catheter.

Motor block is also assessed using the Bromage score (see Figure 38.2).

Intermittent epidural bolus administration

Boluses are used when CEI is not used (syringe top-ups), if there is breakthrough pain with a CEI or

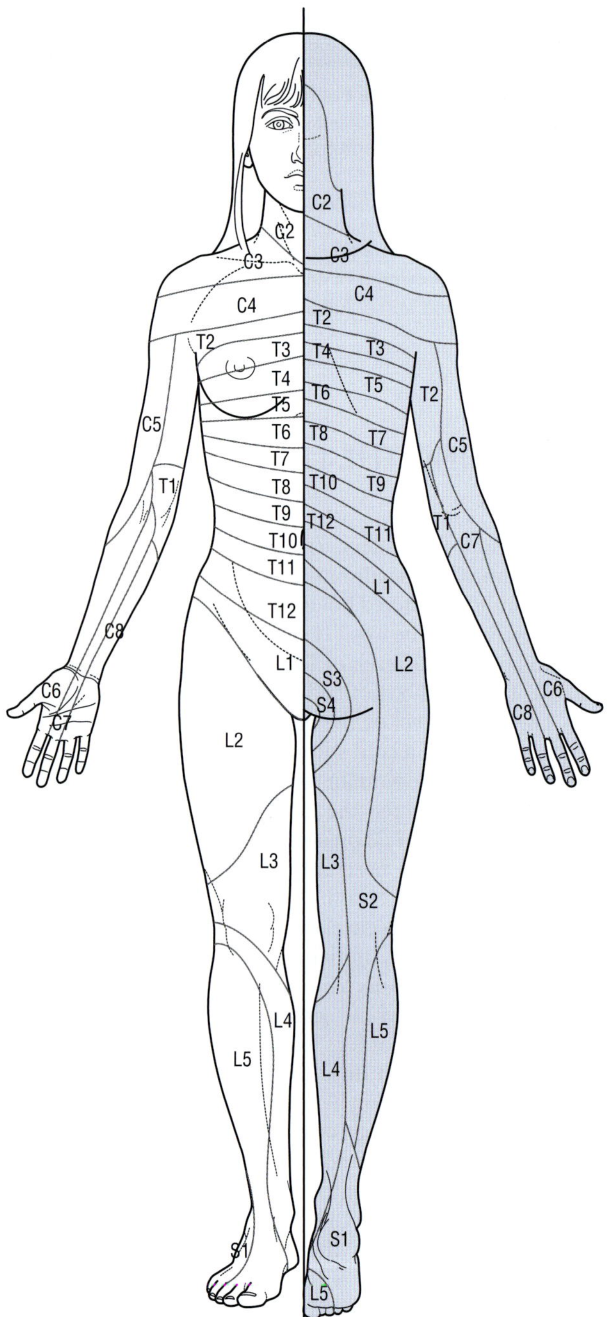

FIGURE 38.3 **Dermatome levels.**
Source: Adapted with kind permission from Walsh D: TENS: Clinical applications and related theory, Churchill Livingstone, Edinburgh, 1997.

if the woman administers a bolus with the PCEA. The anaesthetist prescribes the concentration and volume of the dose and the frequency with which a bolus can be administered. It is advisable to administer the dose in two halves with 5 minutes between them in case the catheter has migrated into the CSF. The observations recorded following a bolus also apply to a bolus administered via a PCEA pump by the woman. Observations should be assessed at 5-minute intervals for 20 minutes after each bolus is administered.

SKILL 38.2 Manual intermittent epidural bolus administration

1. Establish the need for the bolus, check the intravenous infusion is running correctly and gather equipment:
   - the prescribed drug(s)
   - the medicine administration chart and epidural chart
   - non-sterile gloves
   - sterile needle and syringe
   - locally approved cleanser.
2. Assist the woman into the position requested by the anaesthetist, either lateral or sitting.
3. Wash and dry hands, apply gloves, check the drugs with another midwife and draw up the correct dose using aseptic non-touch technique (ANTT).
4. Confirm the woman's identity on the medicine administration chart using at least three identifiers.
5. Following a contraction, remove the filter cap, scrub the tip of the port with the approved wipe, using up-and-down and side-to-side movements for at least 20 seconds using different parts of the wipe, then scrub the sides and allow to dry for at least 30 seconds.
6. Inject half of the medication at a rate of 5 mL per 30 seconds using an ANTT (if local protocol is to administer all the medication, do so).
7. Observe the woman throughout for adverse reactions, such as tinnitus, drowsiness and slurred speech.
8. Reapply the cap.
9. Observations of the maternal pulse, respiration, blood pressure and general condition are recorded as before: every 5 minutes for at least 20 minutes, every hour thereafter and with continuous monitoring of the fetal heart with cardiotocography.
10. If required, assist the woman into a comfortable position.
11. Dispose of equipment correctly.
12. Wash and dry hands.
13. Document the administration in all the relevant places and the effect of the drug(s).
14. Continue to observe for the effects, side effects and complications of the block; contact the anaesthetist if required.

SKILL 38.3 Removing an epidural catheter

The catheter is removed once the epidural is no longer required, usually once the third stage of labour is complete and the perineum is sutured. If the woman is on anticoagulants, the midwife should wait at least 12 hours after the last dose and 4–6 hours before the next dose before removing the catheter to decrease the risk of bleeding around the site. If there is any concern about the coagulation status of the woman, coagulation studies should be undertaken and the catheter removed only when agreed by the anaesthetist.

Discuss the procedure with the woman and gain informed consent.

1. Assist the woman into a suitable position (sitting or lying on her side with a flexed spine) and expose her back, ensuring privacy throughout.
2. Wash and dry hands.
3. Remove the tape/dressing and carefully and steadily withdraw the catheter.
4. Examine the tubing for completeness by visualising the blue catheter tip; checking with a second person may be required.
5. Administer an adhesive spray or a small dressing to the puncture site.
6. Document removal of the catheter and that the blue catheter tip was visualised.
7. Observe the woman for signs of haematoma formation.

POSTNATAL CARE

Until the effects of the epidural wear off, there will be a degree of numbness affecting the legs; thus mobilisation will be delayed. During this time the woman may require assistance to care for her baby and with breastfeeding. She will also need to be observed for signs of urinary retention and headache, two of the most common short-term side effects. Observations for backache may be needed in the longer term and women should be given written information regarding when and how to seek help should complications arise, particularly for women who have an early discharge from hospital (Obstetric Anaesthetists' Association 2013). When the woman feels ready to mobilise, the midwife should ensure she can weight bear first. Further observations, particularly of respiration, may be required in cases where the woman has had neuraxial analgesia (e.g. epidural, spinal) that includes opioids, because of the risk of delayed respiratory depression (Obstetric Anaesthetists' Association 2013).

Role and responsibilities of the midwife

These can be summarised as:

- completing and continuing the education required to maintain competence for the provision of boluses and/or the care of a CEI or a patient-controlled epidural anaesthetic
- educating the woman regarding the epidural procedure
- assisting and supporting the woman to assume the correct positioning for the siting of the epidural
- providing ongoing care, including appropriate observations of the woman and fetus
- recognising complications as they arise and responding appropriately
- removing the epidural catheter correctly, once the epidural is no longer required
- maintaining contemporaneous, thorough documentation of the epidural procedure, including observations undertaken, drugs given, effect of the epidural and removal of the epidural catheter.

SUMMARY

- Epidural analgesia can be a very effective form of labour analgesia, but it is not without potential complications.
- A local anaesthetic and an opioid are usually given together, either as a continuous infusion or as intermittent boluses.
- The side effects of an epidural generally relate to those of the drugs administered.
- The midwife has a responsible role at the time of siting the epidural, with the ongoing care and with the management of the infusion or intermittent bolus administration, both during labour and postnatally.
- Complications can be very serious and the midwife should be able to recognise these and respond accordingly.

Self-assessment exercises

The answers to the following questions may be found in the text.

1. Differentiate between epidural and spinal analgesia.
2. Outline the indications and contraindications for epidural analgesia.
3. Identify three complications of epidural analgesia and discuss how these are recognised and managed.
4. Describe the midwife's role throughout the epidural procedure.
5. Identify and explain the observations that should be undertaken on a woman who has an epidural in situ.

6. Outline the technique that a midwife can use to assess the level of the block once an epidural has been sited.
7. Describe how an intermittent epidural bolus is administered safely by a midwife.
8. Describe the procedure for safely removing an epidural catheter.

References/Acknowledgments

Allman K, Wilson I, O'Donnell A: Oxford handbook of anesthesia, Oxford University Press, Oxford, UK, 2016.

Anim-Somuah M, Smyth RMD, Cyna AM, Cuthbert A: Epidural versus non-epidural or no analgesia for pain management in labour, Cochrane Database of Systematic Reviews 5, Art. No.: CD000331, 2018. Online: 11 February 2021. Available: http://doi.org/10.1002/14651858.CD000331.pub4.

Auckland District Health Board: Epidural analgesia in labour – management and care clinical guideline: 2020. Online 3 October 2021. Available: www.nationalwomenshealth.adhb.govt.nz/assets/Womens-health/Documents/Policies-and-guidelines/Epidural-Analgesia-in-Labour-Management-and-Care.pdf.

Australian and New Zealand College of Anaesthetists: Pain relief and having a baby, 2020. Online 28 September 2020. Available: www.anzca.edu.au/patient-information/anaesthesia-information-for-patients-and-carers/pain-relief-and-having-a-baby.

Australian and New Zealand College of Anaesthetists: Patient information: pain relief and having a baby, n.d. Online 3 October 2021. Available: www.anzca.edu.au/getattachment/7df2e78d-7cec-42c8-b025-dd1150fbf457/Pain-relief-and-having-a-baby.

Australian Institute of Health and Welfare (AIHW): Australia's mothers and babies 2018: in brief. Perinatal statistics series no. 36. Cat. no. PER 108, AIHW, Canberra, 2020. Online 12 February 2021. Available: www.aihw.gov.au/getmedia/aa54e74a-bda7-4497-93ce-e0010cb66231/aihw-per-108.pdf.aspx?inline=true.

Bowrey S, Thompson J: Spinal opioids in postoperative pain relief 2: adverse effects, Nursing Times 104(31):28–69, 2008.

Bullock S, Manias E: Fundamentals of pharmacology, 7th ed., Pearson, Sydney, 2014.

Butwick AJ, Wong CA, Guo N: Maternal body mass index and use of labor neuraxial analgesia: a population-based retrospective cohort study, Anesthesiology 129:448–458, 2018. Available: https://doi.org/10.1097/ALN.0000000000002322.

Canterbury District Health Service (CDHS): Epidural analgesia in labour, Women's Health Service, Christchurch Women's Hospital: maternity guidelines, 2017. Available: www.cdhb.health.nz/Hospitals-Services/Health-Professionals/maternity-care-guidelines/Documents/GLM0007-Epidural-Analgesia-in-Labour.pdf.

Cheng YW, Shaffer BL, Nicholson JM, et al: Second stage of labor and epidural use, Obstetrics and Gynecology 123(3):527–535, 2014.

Clark V, Van de Velde M, Fernando R: Oxford textbook for obstetric anaesthesia, Oxford University Press, Oxford, UK, 2016.

Curtin WM, Katzman PJ, Florescue H, et al: Intrapartum fever, epidural analgesia and histologic chorioamnionitis, Journal of Perinatology 35(6):396–400, 2015.

de Rooy C: Epidural analgesia during labour: friend or foe? A reflection on medicine, midwives and Miranda Kerr, Australian Medical Student Journal (60):2, 2015.

Hasanin A, Mokhtar A, Amin S, et al: Preprocedural ultrasound examination versus manual palpation for thoracic epidural catheter insertion, Saudi Journal of Anaesthesia 11(1):62–66, 2017. Available: www.saudija.org/article.asp?issn=1658-354X;year=2017;volume=11;issue=1;spage=62;epage=66;aulast=Hasanin.

Institute for Quality and Efficiency in Health Care (IQWiG): Pregnancy and birth: epidurals and painkillers for labor pain relief, 2018. Available: www.ncbi.nlm.nih.gov/pubmedhealth/PMH0072751/.

Jain K, Makkar JK, Subramani Vp S, et al: A randomized trial comparing prophylactic phenylephrine and ephedrine infusion during spinal anesthesia for emergency cesarean delivery in cases of acute fetal compromise, Journal of Clinical Anesthesia 34:208–215, 2016.

King Edward Memorial Hospital (KEMH), 2014. Intrapartum care. Online 25 June 2018. Available: http://kemh.health.wa.gov.au/,/media/Files/Hospitals/WNHS/For%20health%20professionals/Clinical%20guidelines/OG/WNHS.OG.LabourFirstStageCareofthewoman.pdf.

Klimek M, Rossaint R, van de Velde M, et al: Combined spinal–epidural vs. spinal anaesthesia for caesarean section: meta-analysis and trial-sequential analysis, Anaesthesia 73(7):875–888, 2018.

Kwak K-H: Postdural puncture headache, Korean Journal of Anesthiology 70(2):136–143, 2017.

Mahomed K, Chin D, Drew A: Epidural analgesia during labour: maternal understanding an experience—informed consent, Journal of Obstetrics and Gynaecology: The Journal of the Institute of Obstetrics and Gynaecology 35(8):807–809, 2015.

Ministry of Health (MOH): Report on Maternity, 2017. Wellington Ministry of Health, 2019. Online. Available: www.health.govt.nz/system/files/documents/publications/report-on-maternity-2015-updated_12122017.pdf.

Obstetric Anaesthetists' Association (OAA): Headache after epidural or spinal injection—what you need to know, 2014. Available: www.labourpains.com/ui/content/content.aspx?ID=316.

Obstetric Anaesthetists' Association (OAA): OAA/AAGBI Guidelines for obstetric anaesthetic services 2013. Guideline no. 3, 2013. Online 3 October 2021. Available: www.oaa-anaes.ac.uk/assets/_managed/cms/files/Clinical%20Guidelines/obstetric_anaesthetic_services_2013.pdf.

Ong J, Kirthinanda D, Loh SKN, et al: Strategies to reduce neuraxial analgesia failure during labour, Trends in Anaesthesia & Critical Care 7(8):41–46, 2016.

O'Sullivan O, Cockerham R: Spinal-induced hypotension at caesarean section, Obstetric Anaesthesia 17(7):329–330, 2016.

Parer JT, King TL, Ikeda T: Electronic fetal heart rate monitoring: the five tier system, 3rd ed., Jones & Bartlett Learning, Burlington, MA, 2018.

Royal Australian and New Zealand College of Obstetricians and Gynaecologists. (RANZCOG): Pain relief in labour and childbirth, n.d. Online 12 February 2021. Available: https://ranzcog.edu.au/womens-health/patient-information-resources/pain-relief-in-labour-and-childbirth.

Royal Children's Hospital Melbourne: Assessment of motor block, 2016. Available: www.rch.org.au/anaes/pain_management/Assessment_of_motor_block/.

SA Health: Perinatal practice guidelines: analgesia for labour and birth (pharmacological). South Australia Maternal and Neonatal Clinical Community of Practice, 2017. Available: http://www.sahealth.sa.gov.au/wps/wcm/connect/052c4527-f3dd-4a18-809d-9d948302cdc9/Analgesia+for+Labour+and+Birth+%28Pharmacological%29_PPG_v1_0.pdf?MOD=AJPERES&CACHEID=ROOTWORKSPACE-052c4527-f3dd-4a18-809d-9d948302cdc9-m1FN0Qo.

Schug SA, Palmer GM, Scott DA, et al, SE Working Group of the Australian and New Zealand College of Anaesthetists and Faculty of Pain Medicine: Acute pain management: scientific evidence, 5th ed., ANZCA & FPM, Melbourne, 2020.

Sekimoto K, Tobe M, Saito S: Local anesthetic toxicity: acute and chronic management, Acute Medicine & Surgery 4:152–160, 2017.

Sng BL, Leong WL, Zeng Y, et al: Early versus late initiation of epidural analgesia for labour, Cochrane Database of Systematic Reviews (10):CD007238, 2014.

Sultan P, David A, Fernando R, et al: Inflammation and epidural-related maternal fever: proposed mechanisms, Anesthesia and Analgesia 122(5):1546–1553, 2016.

Tracy & Hartz: Interventions in pregnancy, labour and birth. In Pairman S, Pincombe J, Thorogood C, Tracy, S, eds: Midwifery: preparation for practice, 3rd ed., Elsevier, Sydney, 2015.

Wang TT, Sun S, Huang SQ: Effects of epidural labor analgesia with low concentrations of local anesthetics on obstetric outcomes: a systematic review and meta-analysis of randomized controlled trials, Anesthesia & Analgesia 124(5):1571–1580, 2017.

Wilson BL, Passante T, Rauschenbach D, et al: Bladder management with epidural anaesthesia during labor: a randomized controlled trial, MCN. The American Journal of Maternal Child Nursing 40(4):234–242, 2015.

SECTION 10

MONITORING WELLBEING DURING THE EXPULSIVE PHASE

CHAPTER 39

PRINCIPLES OF INTRAPARTUM SKILLS: SECOND STAGE

Learning outcomes

Having read this chapter, the reader should be able to:

- discuss the evidence and opinions surrounding the definition, recognition and duration of the second stage of labour, spontaneous pushing, maternal positions to facilitate normal birth, and the management of a nuchal cord
- discuss the preparation for, and conduct of, a birth
- discuss the role and responsibilities of the midwife during the second stage of labour.

INTRODUCTION

During the second stage of labour the baby descends and rotates through the pelvis; the symphysis pubis width increases (Rustamova et al 2009), contractions become expulsive, the perineum stretches and thins out and the baby is born. This chapter reviews the current evidence and clinical skills for the second stage of labour and includes a discussion on the definition and duration of the second stage, the effects of directed and spontaneous pushing, different maternal positions and the management of a nuchal cord. The chapter concludes with a discussion about preparing the birthing environment for second stage and the arrival of the baby, and swab and sharps management.

SECOND STAGE OF LABOUR DEFINITION

Traditionally, the **second stage of labour** has been viewed from a clinical perspective as the period from full dilatation of the os uteri to the complete birth of the baby. It is now recognised that this stage of labour has both a passive and an active phase (National Institute for Health and Care Excellence [NICE] 2017, Queensland Health 2017). Lai and colleagues (2009) acknowledge there is more to the second stage than cervical dilatation, with descent of the presenting part and maternal feelings also being important considerations. Recognition of the passive phase is important, so the woman is discouraged from pushing as soon as the cervix is fully dilated, as there is a perception that this can have adverse outcomes.

The **passive phase** describes the time from when the cervix is fully dilated but there is no strong urge to push; the presenting fetal part may still be high but is beginning to descend and rotate through the pelvis. It has been referred to as the 'rest and be thankful', 'rest and descent' and the 'pause for rotation' phase (Brancato et al 2008, Long 2006). The woman may feel drowsy and relaxed (Long 2006) and her contractions may appear less frequent and strong, giving the woman the opportunity to recharge and be ready for the active phase. Commonly, the woman is discouraged from pushing during the passive phase even if they feel the urge to, on the basis that it is perceived to be futile as well as fear that cervical damage will occur. However, it was reported in 2015 that there was no evidence to support this concern (Reed 2015) and there still appears to be none at the time of writing (April 2021); in fact, Reed (2015) says, 'downward pressure may assist the baby to rotate into an anterior position, or assist with cervical dilatation'. Conversely, directing women to push when they feel no urge to do so is essentially futile: Yildirim and Beji (2008) claim that women cannot push effectively when the urge to push is absent. Lai and colleagues (2009) argue that the fetus will descend more rapidly once it is approximately 1 cm past the ischial spines and has rotated to an occipitoanterior position.

Allowing the fetus to passively descend to the vulva allows for activation of oxytocin receptors and the pelvic nerve, releasing high doses of oxytocin. This activates the **Ferguson reflex**, which causes the fetus to descend into the vagina without maternal effort (Bonapace et al 2018).

The United Kingdom's NICE (2017) states that the **active phase** is when the woman experiences expulsive contractions with a strong urge to push; the cervix is fully dilated and the **presenting part** is visible. The urge to push occurs with the initiation of the Ferguson reflex as the fetus descends past the ischial spines onto the pelvic floor, stimulating the stretch receptors in the posterior vaginal wall (which, as noted previously, may occur in some women before the os uteri is fully dilated). This causes the posterior lobe of the pituitary gland to secrete more oxytocin creating a positive feedback mechanism. Lai and colleagues (2009) suggest the reflexive need to push hard in the active phase is three to four times higher when there has been descent of the presenting part. If the woman is pushing when the cervix is fully dilated but expulsive contractions are absent, NICE (2017) suggests this should also be considered the active phase.

There are reportedly advantages in the woman not pushing until the active phase has been reached, including: decreased maternal exhaustion; less perineal, bladder and pelvic trauma; reduced incidence of instrumental birth and fetal heart abnormalities; higher Apgar scores at 1 and 5 minutes and higher umbilical cord arterial pH levels; as well as an increased confidence and self-belief in the woman's ability to birth (Jansen et al 2013, Kopas 2014, Lai et al 2009).

RECOGNITION OF THE COMMENCEMENT OF SECOND STAGE

As the woman transitions from the first to the second stage, a number of signs may be seen. She may become quiet and withdrawn or particularly vocal and feel that she 'can't go on' or 'doesn't want to do this anymore'. Equally, she may feel renewed with energy. The Royal College of Midwives (2012) suggests there may be changes in facial expression and the woman will begin to breathe harder. A heavy blood-stained show may be noted as the **operculum** descends and a change in the nature of contractions is felt when the overwhelming urge to push occurs. As previously considered, there will be occasions when the urge to push does not signal the advent of the second stage, so if in doubt, a **vaginal examination (VE)** with the woman's consent may be considered. The contractions may slow initially, but then return more strongly and be more expulsive in nature. As the presenting part descends, pouting of the vulva and anus may be seen and the presenting part will become visible at the introitus. Other physical signs include a purple line extending up the anal cleft (Hobbs 1998), changes in abdominal shape (Burvill 2002), and/or a bulge at the sacral curve (rhombus of Michaelis) (Sutton 2003). Equally, in the absence of visible signs and expulsive contractions, the passive phase of the second stage may be diagnosed following a VE when the cervix is noted to be fully dilated. This is essential when the breech is presenting to avoid head entrapment where the body is birthed through a partially dilated cervix that the head cannot pass through. A VE may also reveal the presence of a **caput succedaneum** that is giving the appearance of a descending presenting part.

DURATION OF THE SECOND STAGE

While the Royal College of Midwives (2012) advises there is no good evidence to justify arbitrary time limits on the length of the second stage of labour, the Royal Australian and New Zealand College of Obstetricians and Gynaecologists (RANZCOG 2017b) asserts that normal second stage for primigravid women is up to 2 hours and for multigravida women up to 1 hour from the beginning of the active phase for most women. They advise referral for assessment by a medical practitioner if the second stage progresses past these time frames. The importance of recognising progress is also emphasised by NICE (2017); rotation and descent of the presenting part should be assessed if there is inadequate progress by 1 hour of active pushing for nulliparous women or 30 minutes for multiparous women, as a VE and amniotomy (Chapter 30) may need to be considered.

Downe (2011) considers the second stage extremely variable and may be extremely quick, particularly for the multiparous woman. The length of the second stage will be affected by factors such as maternal position and epidural anaesthesia, and the midwife should continue to observe for signs of normality and progress while recognising and managing any deviations from normal.

Despite providing time limits as above, RANZCOG (2017a) advises that the decision of the upper time limit for second stage should be made in each particular clinical circumstance and take the following aspects into consideration:

- prolonged pushing in the second stage, which is associated with an increased chance of fetal compromise
- maternal exhaustion and its effect on pushing
- increased risk of pelvic floor injury, including anal sphincter dysfunction, as the duration of the second stage increases.

The American College of Obstetricians and Gynecologists suggests the second stage is prolonged if birth has not occurred within 3 hours for nulliparous women with an epidural or 2 hours without, and for multiparous women, within 2 hours with an epidural and 1 hour without (Laughon et al 2014). However, Gillesby and colleagues (2010) found outcomes were better when women with an epidural delayed active pushing for 2 hours.

Hunt and Menticoglou (2015) found that 84% of primiparous women were spared an operative birth or difficult caesarean section when allowed a longer section stage. However, this was identified as carrying a greater risk of the baby suffering permanent neurologic handicap (Hunt & Menticoglou 2015). Cheng and colleagues (2007) found a second stage lasting longer than 3 hours for multiparous women was associated with increased risk of operative birth, increased maternal morbidity and lower Apgar scores.

A prolonged second stage of more than 3 to 4 hours has been reported in large retrospective and prospective observational studies as being associated with increased rates of intrapartum fever, uterine atony, postpartum haemorrhage, chorioamnionitis, hysterectomy and third- and fourth-degree tears (Kopas 2014, Laughon et al 2014).

Pushing

The Royal College of Midwives (2012) reminds us there is no good evidence for directed pushing using the **Valsalva manoeuvre**, and that women do not need to be instructed on how and when to push. Women should be encouraged to follow what their bodies are telling them to do and push when they have the urge (NICE 2017). The verbal communication used during the second stage is vital so the woman is empowered and able to take control of the birth. Borders and colleagues (2013) suggest this is achieved when the midwife uses affirmation, information sharing, direction (e.g. with changing position) and baby talk (talking to and about the baby). Active pushing accompanied by the Valsalva manoeuvre is accepted as having adverse consequences (Raynor & Catling 2017). As previously noted, once the woman's os uteri is fully dilated, a physiological resting phase occurs, during which her contractions may decrease in frequency, but become longer and stronger (Jansen et al 2013). Supporting this to occur gives the woman and the fetus time to rest before the active phase of the second stage, where the woman will develop a strong urge to push and will do so without instruction, often once the contraction has built up, rather than at the beginning of it (Jansen et al 2013). Delaying active pushing and waiting for the urge to push with descent of the fetus has been referred to as 'labouring down' (Borders et al 2013). This form of physiological spontaneous pushing uses a resting respiratory volume, not a deep breath, and short pushes lasting 3–6 or 5–7 seconds, three to five times during a contraction (Borders et al 2013). Spontaneous pushing has not been associated with a significant increase in the duration of the second stage of labour, with some evidence indicating that it may shorten it (Kopas 2014).

Directed pushing generally involves taking a deep breath and holding it, taking breaths quickly between pushes and giving three to four sustained pushes from when the contraction begins to when it ends. This is the Valsalva manoeuvre that was originally used to clear pus from the middle ear. It causes the glottis to close and increases intrathoracic pressure, which decreases venous return to the heart resulting in reduced cardiac output and blood pressure. This can result in reduced uterine blood flow and placental perfusion, increasing the likelihood of the fetus becoming hypoxic and acidotic (Prins et al 2011). Directed pushing is also associated with a significantly higher frequency and severity of perineal trauma, and may negatively affect urodynamic functioning (Kopas 2014). The woman may feel dizzy from holding her breath, which may cause her to gasp, allowing a sudden increase in the amount of blood returning to the heart and increasing blood pressure (Dempsey and colleagues 2014). Using the Valsalva manoeuvre can also result in a temporary reduction in vision and subconjunctival haemorrhage, which can occur as a result of transient subclinical retinal oedema (Connor 2010). Women who push in this way may experience more fatigue up to 24 hours post-birth, which can indirectly affect the physical and mental health of the new mother (Lai et al 2009).

In situations where the woman does not experience the urge to push for iatrogenic reasons (e.g. epidural anaesthesia), she may need some instruction on when and how to do so (Osborne & Hanson 2012). The principles of spontaneous pushing should be followed; for example, no breath-holding; short bursts allowing the contraction to build up first, and it is worth noting here that there are documented examples of women giving birth with no maternal effort at all, such as when they are in induced comas in intensive care settings.

A Cochrane review by Lemos and colleagues (2017) concluded that there was no conclusive evidence to support or challenge any specific style of pushing, with or without an epidural, as part of routine clinical practice. Additionally, there was an absence of strong evidence supporting a specific method or timing of pushing; therefore, the clinical context should be taken into consideration with the woman's comfort and preference to guide decisions as to which method is most appropriate.

Position

The position adopted by women during the second stage of labour is influenced by many factors, including cultural and societal norms. Meyvis and colleagues (2011) suggest the two most commonly adopted positions are horizontal and vertical (upright). Within many Western countries a semirecumbent position with legs on a support has been commonplace, which Meyvis and colleagues (2011) and Gupta and colleagues (2012) suggest was introduced to allow clinicians a good view of the perineum and facilitate manoeuvres such as assisted birth. De Jonge and colleagues (2007) consider routine use of the supine position as an intervention when used in normal labour. In traditional cultures, the vertical position is often favoured (Gupta et al 2012). While there may be advantages and disadvantages with each of the different positions, a woman should be able to birth in whichever position is comfortable for her (even with an epidural in situ). Given the choice, many women opt to use a variety of positions during labour and birth (Kemp et al 2013, Nieuwenhuijze et al 2013). Women should also be aware of the positive and negative effects of upright and horizontal positions to enable them to make an informed choice. Those who are able to choose and change positions appear to have a greater sense of control and less need for analgesia (Lawrence et al 2013). NICE (2017) agrees that women should be encouraged to use whichever position they choose, but advise they should be discouraged from lying supine or semisupine. The midwife has an important role in encouraging women to use different positions and supporting women in their choice. This is particularly important if a VE is performed during the second stage as De Jonge and Lagro-Janssen (2004) found women were more likely to remain supine following the VE.

A positive and supportive environment can promote a sense of competence and personal achievement (Gupta et al 2012). Cotton (2010) argues that a comfortable position will facilitate beta-endorphin production, thus enhancing analgesia at this time.

Sanderson (2012) suggests the pelvis should be viewed as a dynamic structure during birth and recommends a ‘sacrum-free’ position for birth to make use of the increased pelvic diameters. In 1969, Russell demonstrated an increase in both the transverse and anteroposterior diameters when a woman is in a squatting position (Russell 1969), and according to Sutton (2003), pelvic diameters also increase when a woman adopts a lateral position. These studies suggest that horizontal positions should be avoided where possible.

Horizontal positions include **lithotomy**, semirecumbent (sitting, semisitting) and left lateral (although it could be argued lateral positions are similar to vertical as there is no pressure on the sacrum). When the woman is sitting on her pelvis and the sacrum is unable to move, the pelvic diameters of the outlet are reduced. The woman may attempt to lift her buttocks off the bed, push her pelvis forwards and throw her arms back to rectify this (Downe 2011), although this practice is often discouraged unnecessarily. Downe (2011) suggests this is the opposite of the commonly encouraged semirecumbent position with the woman holding onto her thighs to pull her legs towards her and suggests it is more logical to allow the woman to follow her instincts. Bayes and White (2011) found lithotomy was used more when an instrumental birth was anticipated and argue this should be the only reason for its use as it is associated with an increased risk of third- and fourth-degree tears. Upright positions during labour are associated with greater levels of satisfaction with the birthing experience and lower reported levels of pain (Priddis et al 2012). When a semirecumbent position is used, Downe (2011) recommends the woman should be well supported by pillows and/or a wedge to prevent her from sliding into a dorsal position.

Vertical or upright positions include standing, squatting, kneeling and all-fours. Upright positions are thought to encourage descent of the presenting part, strong, efficient contractions, enhanced alignment of the fetus and assist the fetal ejection reflex (Cotton 2010). Pearson (2012) also claims the second stage is shorter, with fewer instrumental births and fetal heart abnormalities when an upright position is adopted.

Di Franco and colleagues (2007) consider upright positions make use of gravity and increase the pelvic diameters, but acknowledge they are more tiring than semirecumbent positions. To counteract this, they recommend using a supported squat, where the woman is supported under her arms. This results in less weight on her legs and feet, and lengthening of her trunk, which provides more space for the fetus to move through the pelvis.

When comparing the use of kneeling and sitting upright, Ragnar and colleagues (2006) concluded the outcomes do not differ significantly, although kneeling was associated with more favourable maternal experiences and reduced pain. Kneeling also allowed women the freedom to modify their position more easily, allowing them to feel more in control.

When adopting a supine, semirecumbent or prolonged squatting position, it is important to avoid excessive and prolonged thigh-holding, as this can cause compressive peroneal neuropathy (functional and/or pathological changes to the peroneal nerve which supplies the calf and foot). This presents with knee tenderness, foot drop and decreased sensation over the dorsum of the foot (Sahai-Srivastava & Amezcua 2007).

Midwives should therefore:

- inform and advise women about the advantages and disadvantages of the various positions that can be used in the second stage of labour
- encourage and support women to adopt the positions of their choice in which they are most comfortable, while remembering the advantages of an upright position (or lateral, where an epidural anaesthesia is present)
- show women and their birthing partners how to utilise upright positions together
- utilise available equipment such as beanbags, birthing balls/chairs/stools, etc.
- have confidence in their ability to facilitate safe births with women in different positions.

Asepsis

While it is often considered that the birth should be an aseptic procedure to reduce the incidence of postnatal infection for mother and baby, this is not always possible when the midwife is supporting the woman to give birth without the assistance of another health professional. In this situation the midwife should consider how they can reduce the risk of infection. Equipment used should be sterile at the onset of the birth and a sterile field established on the working surface and, with horizontal positions, the area of the woman's perineum. It is important to keep sterile and non-sterile equipment separate. Adaptations are necessary according to the environment and the position that the woman has adopted. Hand hygiene and use of personal protective equipment (PPE) are essential. Once the sterile gloves have been applied for birth, they should be kept sterile or changed as needed. An anal pad may be used to cover or remove any faeces that may escape from the anus in horizontal positions. **Hands-on** and **hands poised** approaches are discussed further in Chapter 40.

The nuchal cord

Checking for a **nuchal cord** around the baby's neck at birth has its origins in the medical textbooks of the late seventeenth century (Jefford et al 2009). Hutchon (2013) suggests a nuchal cord occurs in 20–30% of births and known risk factors include male sex, long umbilical cord, parity and being an infant of African American race (Nkwabong and colleagues 2018). There is no high-level evidence to support the practice of feeling around the baby's neck for the presence of the umbilical cord and Jefford and colleagues (2009) expressed concern that this will involve a VE for which the woman has usually not consented to and which is invasive and possibly painful.

If the nuchal cord is felt for, the next question is what to do with it: loop a loose cord over the baby's head, birth the baby through the cord or clamp and cut a tight cord? There is little evidence supporting these practices and the literature does not always distinguish between loose and tight cords (Reed et al 2009). The option of slipping a loose cord over the baby's head is favoured by midwives, but does involve handling the cord while the woman stops pushing. Clamping and cutting the cord severs the oxygen supply completely for the baby, which is detrimental should shoulder dystocia occur. Reed and colleagues (2009) suggest this could be the reason why babies have lower Apgar scores and pH levels in the studies reviewing the management of nuchal cords. It would appear to be preferable to leave the cord intact and facilitate the birth of the baby with the nuchal cord in place as placental blood flow can resume once the baby is born. This approach ensures there is no spasm of the umbilical vessels from handling the cord and the baby has the advantage of the additional blood volume from delayed cord clamping (DCC) (Hutchon 2013).

To birth the baby through the nuchal cord, the **somersault manoeuvre** is used, whereby both shoulders are birthed slowly without handling the cord, and as the shoulders birth the baby's head is flexed, using the palm of the clinician's hand on the baby's occiput to push the baby's face close to the mother's thigh (Hutchon 2013) (Fig 39.1). Then, keeping the baby's head flexed and close to the mother's perineum, the rest of the baby's body is encouraged to flex, allowing the baby to somersault out of the vagina and unwrap the cord (Hutchon 2013).

Management of the nuchal cord at birth remains a contentious issue with little evidence to support a particular management option. However, with the risk of shoulder dystocia and the advantages of DCC it would appear prudent not to clamp and cut the cord unless the birth is prevented by a tight, short cord. Therefore, it may be unnecessary to feel for a nuchal cord unless there is a clear clinical indication.

PREPARATION OF THE ENVIRONMENT

The support, communication, physical care, observations and record keeping that have extended through the first stage of labour should continue throughout the second stage using either a Doppler device or a Pinard stethoscope. It was determined in a recent scoping review that abnormal fetal heart rates are detected more often using a Doppler than with a Pinard stethoscope but that the difference is not statistically significant (Blix et al 2019). RANZCOG (2019) recommends fetal heart rate auscultation every 15 minutes during the passive phase of the second stage and immediately after a contraction for at least 1 minute, every 5 minutes during the active phase. In normal labour, maternal blood pressure and temperature should be taken every 4 hours (and temperature taken every 30 minutes when using water immersion), maternal pulse taken with fetal heart rate auscultation to ensure differentiation every 30 minutes during the passive phase and every 15 minutes during the active phase. Contractions should be assessed continuously throughout the second stage, along with vaginal loss. Observations should be increased in frequency if clinically indicated (Queensland Health 2017). VEs should only be undertaken during the second stage with the woman's consent, as clinically indicated to aid in decision-making (Queensland Health 2017), and should only occur after abdominal palpation and assessment of vaginal loss has been undertaken (NICE 2017). Passage of urine should be recorded, and encouraged frequently (NICE 2017, Queensland Health 2017).

The environment of the second stage should:

- include a midwife who is present throughout, with an assistant for birth (depending on local protocol, but ideally a second midwife)
- be calm and relaxed
- be warm and ready to receive the baby

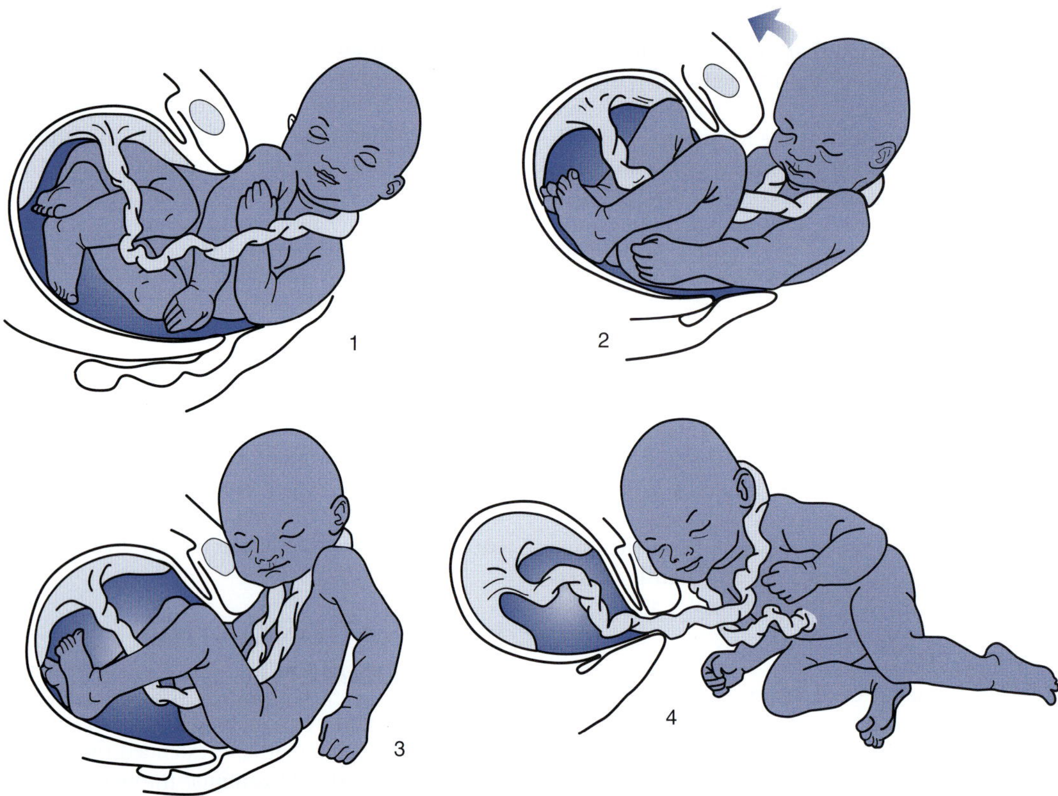

FIGURE 39.1 **The somersault manoeuvre. 1–2, Both shoulders are birthed slowly without handling the cord, while flexing the baby's head to push his face close to his mother's thigh. 3–4, Keeping the head next to the perineum, assist the baby to somersault out of the vagina.**
Source: Mercer JS, Skovgaard RL, Peareara–Eaves J, et al: Nuchal cord attachment and nurse–midwifery practice, Journal of Midwifery and Women's Health 50(5):373–379, 2005.

- contain all that is required for the birth
- have a recognised system for calling emergency assistance
- be equipped to begin emergency management for mother or baby; all equipment should be checked and the midwife must be competent in its use.

Swabs and sharps

All swabs and sharps opened should be counted and recorded and the count repeated after the birth with an entry in the woman's notes to record they are both correct. Double counting, out loud, with a colleague is best practice and swabs should be separated during the counting. The swabs should be woven gauze with a radiopaque thread throughout, so they are detectable on X-ray. When soaked in blood, swabs can be difficult to identify and may occasionally be left inside the vagina by mistake leading to fever, infection, pain, secondary postpartum haemorrhage and psychological harm (Lamont and colleagues 2010).

SKILL 39.1 Normal birth

Adaptations are made according to the birth environment and position of the woman. Note should be taken of the discussions in this chapter. Undertake a VE with the woman's consent to confirm second stage if there is a clear clinical indication (e.g. if breech presentation has been detected on abdominal palpation).

1. Prepare the environment and gather equipment:
   - alcohol-based hand rub
   - trolley or clean surface to work from
   - sterile birth pack, including warm towels to dry/wrap the baby in
   - sterile gloves
   - PPE: apron, eye protection
   - disposable sheets, non-sterile gloves and sanitary towels
   - extras: indwelling urinary catheter, amnihook,

SKILL 39.1 Normal birth—cont'd

lignocaine, needles and syringes, uterotonic agent
- an infectious waste refuse bag should be available, usually a floor bin
- for births occurring in a hospital environment, the Resuscitaire should be switched on and checked it is working; in a low-resource setting (e.g. the woman's home), resuscitation equipment should be checked and within reach).

2. Ensure that the room temperature is warm (21–24°C) and draughts excluded.
3. Continue to provide ongoing reassurance and explanations to the woman, supporting her with spontaneous pushing, choice of position and analgesia and maintaining maternal and fetal observations.
4. Position the disposable sheets strategically in the area of the perineum, while wearing non-sterile gloves.
5. When the birth is imminent, put on an apron and eye protection, wash and dry hands and open the outer covering of the birth pack.
6. Place all other sterile items onto the birth pack using aseptic non-touch technique (ANTT). (If there is an assistant present, they can do this.)
7. Apply alcohol-based hand rub, allow to dry and then put on the sterile gloves.
8. Count the swabs and sharps, and check the instruments in the birth pack, preferably with the assistant as a second checker.
9. Organise the birth trolley/surface in a way that suits, having cord clamps and a receiver for the placenta close by.
10. Keep observing the advancing presenting part while carrying out these procedures as some women experience short second stages.
11. Position any sterile drapes appropriately to provide a sterile field.
12. If being used with the woman's consent, place a warm compress on the perineum.
13. If being used with the woman's consent, place the anal pad in position.
14. Have a warm towel close by to dry the baby.
15. The perineum will stretch as the fetus reaches the perineum; this may sting and feel sore, so continue to encourage and support the woman. She may wish to see her baby in a mirror and/ or reach down to touch her/him and/or guide the birth; the baby's other parent may also wish to become directly involved in facilitating the birth with the woman's consent at this point.
16. As the head crowns, apply gentle pressure to it with one hand to slow the birth and 'guard' the perineum with the other hand if adopting a hands-poised approach; otherwise remain hands-off.
17. Encourage the woman to breathe slowly and give less forceful pushes if she can as the head extends and emerges. Note the time. Do not feel around the neck for a nuchal cord.
18. Restitution will be seen, followed by external rotation of the head as the shoulders rotate internally.
19. The next contraction usually occurs within 1–3 minutes and the woman will have the urge to push again. If a hands-poised approach is being taken, apply traction to the anterior shoulder (in a direction away from the symphysis pubis), followed by traction in the opposite direction to facilitate the birth of the posterior shoulder; otherwise allow the shoulders to emerge spontaneously if hands-off.
20. The body and limbs of the baby are birthed by lateral flexion in a 'hands-on' approach, following the curve of the birth canal, in an upward direction towards the woman's abdomen. The midwife may encourage the woman and/or her partner to assist the baby at this point if they haven't already done so.
21. Note the time of birth.
22. Ideally the baby is placed skin-to-skin with their mother and dried completely, with the wet towel replaced with a dry warm one; parents or midwife will check the gender.
23. Drying acts as stimulation, during which time the baby will take its first breath and cry; assess the Apgar score (see Chapter 48) at 1 minute. Act swiftly (before 1 minute) if it is obvious that resuscitation is required (see Chapter 48).
24. Clamping and cutting of the cord is generally attended after allowing time for the baby to receive iron-rich blood from the placenta and in accordance with the parents' wishes and chosen management of the third stage of labour (Chapter 43). Breastfeeding may be facilitated at this point (Chapter 49).
25. Share in the joy of the moment, but stay alert to the clinical situation.
26. Care moves into management of the third stage of labour; this may have included the administration of an intramuscular or intravenous uterotonic during the birth of the baby.

Role and responsibilities of the midwife

These can be summarised as:

- providing safe, evidence-based care for the woman and baby
- supporting and encouraging the woman to adopt a safe, comfortable position
- recognising and managing deviations from normal; referring as necessary
- undertaking contemporaneous record keeping.

SUMMARY

- The second stage has a passive and an active phase; the passive phase may be a time to rest while pushing occurs in the active phase.
- Restricting the length of the second stage is inappropriate providing there is progress and maternal and fetal wellbeing.
- Spontaneous pushing is safer than directed pushing and should be encouraged.
- The woman should be encouraged and supported to adopt a comfortable, preferably upright, position.
- Birth of the baby may be 'hands-on' or 'hands-off', although controlling the speed of birth of the head, support of the perineum and lateral flexion to the shoulders may result in less perineal pain in the short term.

Self-assessment exercises

The answers to the following questions may be found in the text.

1. What might lead you to suspect the woman has reached the second stage of labour?
2. Discuss when, whether and how you would encourage the woman to push and why.
3. Compare and contrast the various positions used during the second stage. Which would you encourage the woman to use?
4. Demonstrate how a normal birth is conducted, including management of the equipment and positioning of the hands.
5. Summarise the role and responsibilities of the midwife when providing complete care during the second stage of labour.

References

Bayes S, White C: Use of the lithotomy position for low-risk women in Perth, Australia, British Journal of Midwifery 19(5):285–289, 2011.

Blix E, Maude R, Hals E, Kisa S, Karlsen E, Nohr EA, et al: Intermittent auscultation fetal monitoring during labour: a systematic scoping review to identify methods, effects and accuracy, PLoS ONE 14(7):e0219573, 2019. Available: https://doi.org/10.1371/journal.pone.0219573.

Bonapace J, Gagné G, Chaillet N, et al: No. 355-physiologic basis of pain in labour and delivery: an evidence-based approach to its management, Journal of Obstetrics and Gynaecology Canada 40(2):227–245, 2018.

Borders N, Wendland C, Haozous E, et al: Midwives' verbal support of nulliparous women in second-stage labor, Journal of Obstetric, Gynecologic, and Neonatal Nursing 42:311–320, 2013.

Brancato RM, Church S, Stone PW: A meta-analysis of passive descent versus immediate pushing in nulliparous women with epidural analgesia in the second stage of labor, Journal of Obstetric, Gynecologic, and Neonatal Nursing 37(1):4–12, 2008.

Burvill S: Midwifery diagnosis of labour onset, British Journal of Midwifery 10(10):600–605, 2002.

Cheng YW, Hopkins LM, Laros RK Jr, et al: Duration of the second stage of labor in multiparous women: maternal and neonatal outcomes, American Journal of Obstetrics and Gynecology 196(6):585.e1–585.e6, 2007.

Connor A: Valsalva-related retinal venous dilation caused by defaecation, Acta Ophthalmologica 88(4):e149, 2010.

Cotton J: Considering the evidence for upright positions in labour, MIDIRS Midwifery Digest 20(4):459–463, 2010.

De Jonge A, Lagro-Janssen AL: Birthing positions: a qualitative study into the views of women about various birthing positions, Journal of Psychosomatic Obstetrics and Gynaecology 25(1):47–55, 2004.

De Jonge A, Teunissen DAM, van Diem MT, et al: Women's positions during the second stage of labour: views of primary care midwives, Journal of Advanced Nursing 63(4):347–356, 2007.

Dempsey J, Hillege S, Hill R: Fundamentals of nursing and midwifery: a person-centred approach to care, 2nd ed. Australian and New Zealand Edition, Lippincott, Williams & Wilkins, Sydney, 2014, pp. 1132–1168.

Di Franco JY, Romano AM, Keen R: Care practice #5: spontaneous pushing in upright or gravity-neutral positions, The Journal of Perinatal Education 16(3):35–38, 2007.

Downe S: Care in the second stage of labour. In McDonald S, Magill-Cuerden J, eds: Mayes' midwifery, 14th ed., Baillière Tindall, London, 2011, pp. 510–514.

Gillesby E, Burns S, Dempsey A, et al: Comparison of delayed versus immediate pushing during second stage of labor for nulliparous women with epidural anesthesia, Journal of Obstetric, Gynecologic, and Neonatal Nursing 39:635–644, 2010.

Gupta JK, Hofmeyr GJ, Shehmar M: Position in the second stage of labour for women without epidural anaesthesia, Cochrane Database of Systematic Reviews (5):Art No.: CD002006, 2012.

Hobbs L: Assessing cervical dilatation without VEs—watching the purple line, The Practising Midwife 1(11):34–35, 1998.

Hunt J, Menticoglou S: Perinatal outcome in 1515 cases of prolonged second stage of labour in nulliparous women, Journal of Obstetrics and Gynaecology Canada: Journal d'obstétrique et gynécologie du Canada: JOGC 37(6):508–516, 2015.

Hutchon DJR: Management of the nuchal cord at birth, Journal of Midwifery & Reproductive Health 1(1):4–6, 2013.

Jansen L, Gibson M, Bowles BC, et al: First do no harm: interventions during childbirth, The Journal of Perinatal Education 22(2):83–92, 2013.

Jefford E, Fahy K, Sundin D: Routine vaginal examination to check for a nuchal cord, British Journal of Midwifery 17(4):246–249, 2009.

Kemp E, Kingswood CJ, Kibuka M, et al: Positions in the second stage of labour for women with epidural anaesthesia, Cochrane Database of Systematic Reviews (1):Art. No.: CD008070, 2013.

Kopas M: A review of evidence-based practices for management of the second stage of labor, Journal of Midwifery & Women's Health 59(3):264–276, 2014.

Lai M-L, Lin K-C, Li HY, et al: Effects of delayed pushing during the second stage of labor on postpartum fatigue and birth outcomes in nulliparous women, The Journal of Nursing Research: JNR 17(1):62–71, 2009.

Lamont T, Dougall A, Johnson S, et al: Reducing the risk of retained swabs after vaginal birth: summary of a safety report from the National Patient Safety Agency, British Medical Journal 341:c3679, 2010.

Laughon SK, Berghella V, Reddy UM, et al: Neonatal and maternal outcomes with prolonged second stage, Obstetrics and Gynecology 124(1):57–67, 2014.

Lawrence A, Lewis L, Hofmeyr GJ, et al: Maternal positions and mobility during first stage labour, Cochrane Database of Systematic Reviews (10):Art. No.: CD003934, 2013.

Lemos A, Amorim M, de Andrade A, et al: Pushing/bearing down methods for the second stage of labour, Cochrane Database of Systematic Reviews (3):Art. No.: CD009124, 2017.

Long L: Redefining the second stage of labour could help to promote normal birth, British Journal of Midwifery 14(2):104–107, 2006.

Meyvis I, van Rompaey B, Goormans K, et al: Maternal position and other variables: effect on perineal outcomes in 557 births, Birth 39(2):115–120, 2011.

National Institute for Health and Care Excellence (NICE). Intrapartum care. Care of healthy women and their babies during childbirth clinical guideline 190, 2017. Online 20 February 2018. Available: www.nice.org.uk.

Nieuwenhuijze MJ, de Jonge A, Korstjens I, et al: Influence on birthing positions affects women's sense of control in second stage of labour, Midwifery 29(11):e107–e114, 2013.

Nkwabong E, Mballo JN, Dohbit JS: Risk factors for nuchal cord entanglement at delivery, International Journal of Gynaecology and Obstetrics: The Official Organ of the International Federation of Gynaecology and Obstetrics 141(1):108–112, 2018.

Osborne K, Hanson L: Directive versus supportive approaches used by midwives when providing care during the second stage of labor, Birth 20:142–147, 2012.

Pearson S: Warwick midwives are delivering women in upright positions, British Journal of Midwifery 20(7):522–523, 2012.

Priddis H, Dahlen H, Schmied V: What are the facilitators, inhibitors and implications of birth positioning? A review of the literature, Women and Birth: Journal of the Australian College of Midwives 25(3):100–106, 2012.

Prins M, Boxem J, Lucas C, et al: Effect of spontaneous pushing versus Valsalva pushing in the second stage of labour on mother and fetus: a systematic review of randomised trials, British Journal of Obstetrics and Gynaecology 118:662–670, 2011.

Queensland Health: Queensland clinical guidelines: normal birth, 2017. Online 20 February 2018. Available: www.health.qld.gov.au/__data/assets/pdf_file/0014/142007/g-normalbirth.pdf.

Ragnar I, Altman D, Tyden T, et al: Comparison of the maternal experience and duration of labour in two upright delivery positions—a randomised controlled trial, British Journal of Obstetrics and Gynaecology 113(2):165–170, 2006.

Raynor MD, Catling C: Myles survival guide to midwifery, 3rd ed., Elsevier, Philadelphia, 2017, p. 257.

Reed R: Supporting women's instinctive pushing behaviour during birth. Midwife Thinking (Blog), 2015. Available: https://midwifethinking.com/2015/09/09/supporting-womens-instinctive-pushing-behaviour-during-birth/.

Reed R, Barnes M, Allan J: Nuchal cords: sharing the evidence with parents, British Journal of Midwifery 17(2):106–109, 2009.

Royal Australian College of Obstetricians and Gynaecologists (RANZCOG): Instrumental vaginal birth, 2017a. Online 12 June 2018. Available: www.ranzcog.edu.au.

Royal Australian and New Zealand College of Obstetricians and Gynaecologists (RANZCOG): Intrapartum fetal surveillance clinical guideline—fourth edition 2019, 2019. Online 18 April 2021. Available: https://ranzcog.edu.au/RANZCOG_SITE/media/RANZCOG-MEDIA/Women%27s%20Health/Statement%20and%20guidelines/Clinical-Obstetrics/IFS-Guideline-4thEdition-2019.pdf?ext=.pdf.

Royal Australian College of Obstetricians and Gynaecologists (RANZCOG): Provision of routine intrapartum care in the absence of pregnancy complications, 2017b. Online: 3 February 2018. Available: www.ranzcog.edu.au.

Royal College of Midwives (RCM): Evidence-based guidelines for midwifery-led care in labour second stage of labour, Royal College of Midwives, London, 2012.

Russell JGB: Moulding of the pelvic outlet, Journal of Obstetrics and Gynaecology 76:817–820, 1969.

Rustamova S, Predanic M, Sumersille M, et al: Changes in symphysis pubis width during labor, Journal of Perinatal Medicine 37:370–373, 2009.

Sahai-Srivastava S, Amezcua L: Compressive neuropathies complicating normal childbirth: case report and literature review, Birth 34(2):173–175, 2007.

Sanderson TA: The movements of the maternal pelvis: a review, MIDIRS Midwifery Digest 22(3):319–326, 2012.

Sutton J: Birth without active pushing. In Wickham S, editor: Midwifery Best Practice, Elsevier Science, Edinburgh, 2003, pp. 90–92.

Yildirim G, Beji NK: Effects of pushing techniques in birth on mother and fetus: a randomized study, Birth 35(1):25–30, 2008.

CHAPTER 40

CARE OF THE PERINEUM BEFORE AND DURING BIRTH

Learning outcomes

Having read this chapter, the reader should be able to:

- discuss the evidence and opinions surrounding the management of the perineum during the second stage of labour
- discuss the impact of evidence around perineal massage and warm compresses
- discuss the differences between hands-off and hands-on techniques during birth
- describe how to infiltrate the perineum and perform an episiotomy
- discuss the role and responsibility of the midwife when performing an episiotomy
- list the factors that should be included with record keeping of episiotomies.

INTRODUCTION

In Australia, less than one-quarter (23%) of women have an intact perineum after giving birth vaginally. Of the remainder, 22% experience a first-degree tear or grazes and 30% sustain a second-degree laceration. A third- or fourth-degree injury occurs in 3% of women having a vaginal birth, 23% have an episiotomy (Australian Institute of Health and Welfare [AIHW] 2020). Spontaneous perineal injury statistics are not available for New Zealand; however, the episiotomy rate at 16% is slightly lower than that in Australia (Ministry of Health 2020). Effective management of the perineum is a priority for midwives because of the short- and long-term effects, such as associated urinary and anal incontinence, sexual dysfunction and broader psychological and emotional wellbeing that perineal trauma has for the woman (Crookall et al 2018, Dahlen & Priddis 2018). Pain is not only unpleasant for the woman but affects her ability to function normally and care for her baby (Albers & Borders 2007, Way 2012). This chapter will review the current evidence and clinical skills utilised in the management of the perineum during the second stage of labour and will include discussions around maternal positioning as a way of protecting the perineum, perineal massage and warm compresses and the hands-on versus the hands-off approach to facilitating birth. The chapter concludes with a discussion on episiotomies, including when and how to undertake an episiotomy.

MANAGEMENT OF THE PERINEUM

Sufficient time is helpful for the perineum to distend and stretch slowly during the second stage of labour. Moore and Moorhead (2013) suggest routine infiltration of the perineum is not evidence-based and may cause harm by increasing volume within the perineum, which can alter the elasticity of the perineal tissue, increasing the risk of spontaneous trauma. Importantly, a large number of women who prefer an elective caesarean section over a vaginal birth have previously been reported to make this decision due to fear of perineal damage (Premkumar 2005).

In 2018, Women's Healthcare Australasia (WHA) introduced a collaborative project that was proposed to reduce by 20% the number of women harmed by third- and fourth-degree perineal tears within the year. Known as the Perineal Bundle (see WHA 2018b), it is similar in nature to the Obstetric Anal Sphincter Injuries intervention introduced in the United Kingdom (UK) and both have caused controversy, predominantly because of the lack of evidence underpinning some bundle interventions, and because of the invasive and potentially psychologically traumatising nature of one in particular: a routine digital rectal examination for all women whose baby is born vaginally. A critique of the WHA perineal bundle by Australian midwife academic Dr Rachel Reed (see Reed 2018) and WHA's response (see WHA 2018a), as well as a critique of the UK intervention (see Thornton & Dahlen 2020), provide useful reading in relation to this topic.

RISK FACTORS FOR PERINEAL TRAUMA

Primiparous women and those who have an operative vaginal birth are at greater risk of **perineal trauma** (Dahlen et al 2013). A number of other factors, including maternal nutritional status, body mass, parity, history of prior trauma, ethnicity, older age, abnormal collagen synthesis, baby's birth weight, fetal sex (male), fetal malposition and malpresentation have been suggested as potential contributors to perineal trauma (Dahlen & Priddis 2018). Maternal comfort and perineal trauma during birth are also influenced by second stage management, including providing the woman with continuous support, maternal position, style of pushing, techniques to relax the perineum, immersion in water, epidurals (due to being associated with an increased risk of instrumental birth), episiotomy, hand manoeuvres and vacuum versus forceps birth (Aasheim et al 2011, Dahlen et al 2013, Dahlen & Priddis 2018). Giving birth at home or in a birth centre is also associated with a reduction in perineal trauma (Edqvist et al 2016), whereas attendance by an obstetrician is associated with higher instances of perineal trauma (Dahlen & Priddis 2018).

Maternal position

Meyvis and colleagues (2011) compared lithotomy with the left lateral position and found perineal damage increased with the use of the lithotomy position. Gupta and colleagues (2012) suggest an upright position or use of the birthing stool are associated with fewer episiotomies, but an increased risk of second-degree tears occurring. However, Albers and Borders (2007) found upright and lateral birth positions were associated with fewer perineal tears. When using a semisitting position during the expulsive phase, Da Silva and colleagues (2012) found an increased risk of second-degree tears and episiotomy compared to women who adopted a lateral, squatting or all-fours position. Soong and Barnes (2005) found a significant increase in perineal trauma in women adopting the semirecumbent position compared with the all-fours position. These effects were more noticeable with women undergoing their first vaginal birth and where the baby's birth weight was in excess of 3500 g. Women with epidural anaesthesia are more likely to adopt a horizontal position; for these women, Soong and Barnes (2005) found suturing was more likely to be required when injury occurred in a semirecumbent rather than a lateral position. Nicholl and Cattell (2006) agree, suggesting if a horizontal position is used for birth, a lateral position is preferable, as it results in a greater likelihood of an intact perineum and less risk of fourth-degree tears. De Jonge and colleagues (2010) compared sitting, semisitting and recumbent positions and found similar rates of intact perineums, but more perineal tears with the sitting group and more labial tears with the semisitting group. Gottvall and colleagues (2007) found there was a greater risk of third- and fourth-degree tears when women were in lithotomy (regardless of mode of birth) or squatting.

Blood loss may increase in the presence of perineal tears or episiotomy, but there is little evidence to suggest blood loss increases with one or more particular positions. Gupta and colleagues (2012) did find a blood loss > 500 mL occurred in association with an upright birthing position, but also noted the blood loss was collected in a receptacle; thus it could be measured rather than inaccurately estimated, and there were no differences in the rate of blood transfusions required.

Perineal massage

There has been extensive coverage in research literature about the effectiveness of perineal massage, both antenatal and intrapartum, for reducing perineal trauma over the last two decades. Essentially, the evidence is conflicting and many of the studies are small. Focusing on perineal massage during labour, a range of studies reported between 2001 and 2020 from a number of different practice contexts indicate that the intervention was associated with lower episiotomy rates and usually a lower incidence of spontaneous tears (Akhlaghi et al 2019, Arafah et al 2017, Aquino et al 2018). However, studies by Shahoei and colleagues (2017) and Oglak and Obut (2020) found the opposite in relation to the latter. Differently to all other published studies on the topic, Stamp and colleagues (2001) found that the rates of intact perineums, first- and second-degree tears and episiotomies were similar in the massage and the control groups in their study of 1340 women. With regard to antenatal perineal massage, Beckmann and Stock (2013) suggest women who perform antenatal perineal massage have a lower risk of perineal trauma primarily through a reduced risk of episiotomy; however, Seehusen and Raleigh (2014) suggest this is only for women who had not had a vaginal birth previously. Antenatal perineal stretching using a massage or stretching device (such as Epi-No) is not supported by evidence (Dahlen & Priddis 2018).

Warm compresses

Moore and Moorhead (2013) suggest women may find it beneficial to have their perineum soaked with warm or cool water during the second stage. Aasheim

2. What is the value of warm compresses during labour and how are these applied?
3. Describe the issues around the use of hands-on and hands-off approaches.
4. Describe how to infiltrate the perineum and perform an episiotomy.
5. Summarise the role and responsibilities of the midwife in relation to perineal care and intervention when providing complete care during the second stage of labour.

References

Aasheim V, Nilsen AB, Lukasse M, et al: Perineal techniques during the second stage of labour for reducing perineal trauma, Cochrane Database of Systematic Reviews (12):CD006672, 2011. Online 24 June 2018. Available: www.cochrane.org/CD006672/PREG_perineal-techniques-during-second-stage-labour-reducing-perineal-trauma.

Akhlaghi F, Sabeti Baygi Z, Miri M, Najaf Najafi M: Effect of perineal massage on the rate of episiotomy, Journal of Family & Reproductive Health September, 13(3): 160–166, 2019.

Albers LL, Borders N: Minimizing genital tract trauma and related pain following spontaneous vaginal birth, Journal of Midwifery and Women's Health 52(3):246–255, 2007.

Aquino CI, Guida M, Saccone G, et al: Perineal massage during labor: a systematic review and meta-analysis of randomized controlled trials, The Journal of Maternal-Fetal & Neonatal Medicine 33(6):1051–1063, 2018. Available: http://doi.org/10.1080/14767058.2018.1512574.

Arafah S, Lotisna D, Tiro E: Perineal massage during second stage of labor to the perineal laceration degree in primigravida, Majalah obstetri dan ginekologi Indonesia 218–221, 2017.

Australian Institute of Health and Welfare (AIHW): Australia's mothers and babies: 2018 in brief, 2020. Available: www.aihw.gov.au/getmedia/aa54e74a-bda7-4497-93ce-e0010cb66231/aihw-per-108.pdf.aspx?inline=true.

Australian Institute of Health and Welfare (AIHW): Australia's mothers and babies 2019 – web report, 2021. Online 11 October 2021. Available: www.aihw.gov.au/getmedia/bba093ef-a623-4cfd-818b-1bb5af9f0d20/Australia-s-mothers-and-babies.pdf.aspx?inline=true.

Beckmann MM, Stock OM: Antenatal perineal massage for reducing perineal trauma, Cochrane Database of Systematic Reviews (4):Art. No.: CD005123, 2013.

Crookall R, Fowler G, Wood C, Slade P: A systematic mixed studies review of women's experiences of perineal trauma sustained during childbirth, Journal of Advanced Nursing 74(9), 2038–2052, 2018.

Dahlen H, Priddis H: Perineal care and repair. In Pairman S, Tracy S, Dahlen HG, Dixon, L: Midwifery preparation for practice, 4th ed., Elsevier, Sydney, 2018.

Dahlen H, Priddis H, Schmied V, et al: Trends and risk factors for severe perineal trauma during childbirth in New South Wales between 2000 and 2008: a population-based data study, BMJ Open 3(5):e002824, 2013.

Da Silva FMB, de Oliveira SMJV, Bick D, et al: Risk factors for birth-related perineal trauma: a cross-sectional study in a birth centre, Journal of Clinical Nursing 21: 2209–2218, 2012.

De Jonge A, van Diem MT, Scheepers PLH, et al: Risk of perineal damage is not a reason to discourage a sitting position: a secondary analysis, International Journal of Clinical Practice 64(5):611–618, 2010.

Doğan B, Gün İ, Özdamar Ö, et al: Long-term impacts of vaginal birth with mediolateral episiotomy on sexual and pelvic dysfunction and perineal pain, The Journal of Maternal-Fetal & Neonatal Medicine 4, 457–460, 2017. http://doi.org/10.1080/14767058.2016.1174998.

Edqvist M, Blix E, Hegaard HK, et al: Perineal injuries and birth positions among 2992 women with a low risk pregnancy who opted for a homebirth, BMC Pregnancy and Childbirth 16(1):196, 2016.

Eogan M, Daly L, O'Connell P, et al: Does the angle of episiotomy affect the incidence of anal sphincter injury? British Journal of Obstetrics and Gynaecology 113: 190–194, 2006.

Gottvall K, Allebeck P, Ekeus C: Risk factors for anal sphincter tears: the importance of maternal position at birth, British Journal of Obstetrics and Gynaecology 114:1266–1272, 2007.

Gupta JK, Hofmeyr GJ, Shehmar M: Position in the second stage of labour for women without epidural anaesthesia, Cochrane Database of Systematic Reviews (5):Art No.: CD002006, 2012.

Homer C, Wilson A: Perineal Tears: A literature review. 2018. https://www.safetyandquality.gov.au/sites/default/files/migrated/D19-2045-Perineal-tears-lit-review-including-Commission-cover-for-external-publications_Jan-2019.pdf

Howie L, Rankin J: Pain relief in labour. In Rankin J, editor: Physiology in childbearing with anatomy and related biosciences, 4th ed., Edinburgh, 2017, Elsevier.

Johnson R, Taylor W: Skills for midwifery practice, 4th ed., London, 2016, Elsevier.

Lappen JR, Gossett DR: Changes in episiotomy practice: evidence-based medicine in action, Expert Review of Obstetrics & Gynecology 5(3):301a, 2010.

Magoga G, Saccone G, Al-Kouatly HB, et al: Warm perineal compresses during the second stage of labor for reducing perineal trauma: a meta-analysis, European Journal of Obstetrics & Gynecology and Reproductive Biology 240:93–98, 2019.

Meyvis I, van Rompaey B, Goormans K, et al: Maternal position and other variables: effect on perineal outcomes in 557 births, Birth 39(2):115–120, 2011.

Ministry of Health: Report on Maternity web tool, 15 September 2020. Online 14 February 2021. Available: www.health.govt.nz/publication/report-maternity-web-tool.

Moore E, Moorhead C: Promoting normality in the management of the puerperium during the second stage of labour, British Journal of Midwifery 21(9):616–620, 2013.

Nicholl MC, Cattell MA: Getting evidence into obstetric and midwifery practice: reducing perineal trauma, Australian Health Review 30(4):462–467, 2006.

O'Connell HE, Sanjeevan KV, Hutson JM. Anatomy of the clitoris, The Journal of Urology Oct;174(4 Pt 1):1189–1195, 2005. Available: http://doi.org/10.1097/01.ju.0000173639.38898.cd.

Oglak SC, Obut M: Effectiveness of perineal massage in the second stage of labor in preventing perineal trauma, Gynecology Obstetrics & Reproductive Medicine: GORM 26(2):1–93, 2020.

Premkumar G: Perineal trauma: reducing associated postnatal maternal morbidity, Midwives 8(1):30–32, 2005.

Reed R: Perineal 'bundles' and midwifery, Midwife Thinking, 2018. Online 28 July 2018. Available: https://midwifethinking.com/2018/05/09/the-perineal-bundle-and-midwifery/.

Royal Australian College of Obstetricians and Gynaecologists (RANZCOG): Provision of routine intrapartum care in the absence of pregnancy complications, 2017. Online 3 February 2018. Available: www.ranzcog.edu.au/.

Seehusen S, Raleigh M: Antenatal perineal massage to prevent birth trauma, American Family Physician 89(5):335–356, 2014.

Shahoei R, Zaheri F, Nasab LH, Ranaei F: The effect of perineal massage during the second stage of birth on nulliparous women perineal: A randomization clinical trial, Electronic physician 9(10):5588–5595, 2017.

Soong B, Barnes M: Maternal position at midwife-attended birth and perineal trauma: is there an association? Birth 32(3):164–169, 2005.

Stamp G, Kruzins G, Crowther C: Perineal massage in labour and prevention of perineal trauma: randomised controlled trial, BMJ, May, 322(7297):1277–1280, 2001.

Thornton J, Dahlen H: The UK Obstetric Anal Sphincter Injury (OASI) *Care Bundle*: A critical review, Midwifery, November, 90, 102801, 2020.

Way S: A qualitative study exploring women's personal experiences of their perineum after childbirth: expectations, reality and returning to normality, Midwifery 28(5):e712–e719, 2012.

Williams A: Third-degree perineal tears: risk factors and outcome after primary repair, Journal of Obstetrics and Gynaecology 23(6):611–614, 2003.

Women's Healthcare Australasia (WHA): Response to Rachel Reed 'The perineal bundle midwifery', 2018a. Online 28 July 2018. Available: https://women.wcha.asn.au/response-rachel-reed-perineal-bundle-midwifery.

Women's Healthcare Australasia (WHA): The how to guide: WHA CEC Perineal Protection Bundle©, 2019. Available: https://women.wcha.asn.au/sites/default/files/docs/wha_national_collaborative_how_to_guide_21.1.20.pdf.

Women's Healthcare Australasia (WHA): WHA National Collaborative, 2018b. Online 28 July 2018. Available: https://women.wcha.asn.au/wha-national-collaborative.

CHAPTER 41
ASSISTED AND OPERATIVE BIRTH

Learning outcomes

Having read this chapter, the reader should be able to:

- discuss conditions required to safely undertake an assisted birth
- identify the contraindications and indications for assisted birth
- discuss preoperative and intraoperative care prior to elective and emergency caesarean section (CS)
- identify the classifications of CS
- discuss recovery and post-CS care
- summarise the midwife's responsibilities in the scenario.

INTRODUCTION

While most babies are born via spontaneous vaginal birth there are times when the need arises to expedite the birth of the baby using forceps, a vacuum extraction or an emergency caesarean section (CS) as a result of maternal or fetal compromise. Birth by elective CS due to clinical indications or maternal choice, or a combination of both, also occurs. While the midwife does not perform these skills, they are required to assist in these instances and to provide the woman with support, information and reassurance before, during and after the birth of her baby. This chapter discusses assisted birth, including the reasons for forceps use or vacuum extraction; the indications and contraindications to this method of birth are considered, and the conditions under which an assisted birth can be undertaken safely are listed along with the possible complications associated with each method of assisted birth, before a brief discussion on rotational assisted birth. The skill of providing woman-centered care during a vacuum extraction is outlined. The chapter concludes with a discussion around CS, care prior to elective (or planned) and emergency CS, intraoperative care and postoperative recovery care after a CS birth.

ASSISTED BIRTH

Where there is a need to expedite birth for the benefit of mother or baby, **assisted birth** (also known as instrumental birth)—the use of either forceps or vacuum (Fig 41.1)—may be considered, providing there has been consideration for the clinical situation being appropriate, and the woman has provided informed consent. The goal for an assisted birth is to mimic a spontaneous vaginal birth, with minimal maternal and neonatal morbidity (RCOG 2011).

Forceps

The use of forceps requires significant experience by the operator, but can effect a rapid birth of the fetus in cases of fetal distress, and can be useful for the after-coming head in breech presentations and for fetal rotation.

A variety of types of forceps are available for use. The type of forceps chosen depends on the classification given according to the station of the vertex and whether rotation is required. The classifications (in brief), according to RANZCOG (2020, p. 8), include the following.

- Outlet
  - Fetal scalp visible without separating the labia
  - Fetal skull has reached the pelvic floor

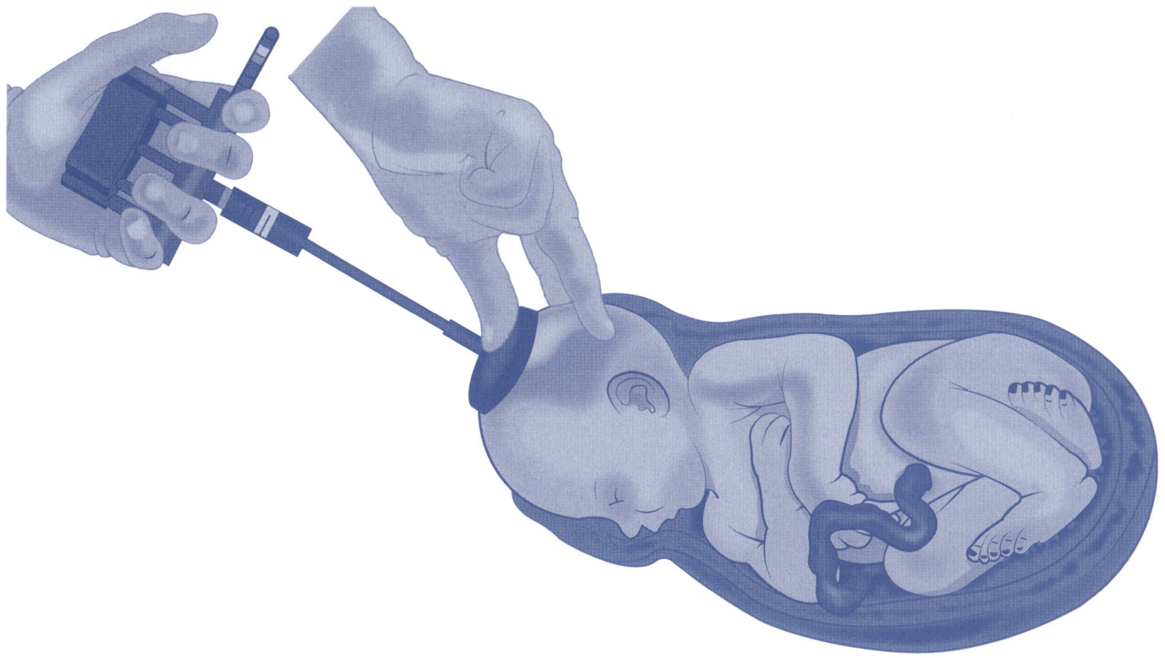

FIGURE 41.1 **Birth by vacuum extraction.**

  - Sagittal suture is in the antero-posterior diameter or right or left occiput anterior or posterior position (rotation does not exceed 45°)
  - Fetal head is at or on the perineum
- Low
  - Leading point of the skull (not caput) is at station plus 2 cm or more and not on the pelvic floor.
  - Two subdivisions:
    - rotation of 45° or less from the occipito-anterior position
    - rotation of more than 45° including the occipito-posterior position
- Mid
  - Fetal head is no more than ⅕ palpable per abdomen
  - Leading point of the skull is above station plus 2 cm but not above the ischial spines
  - Two subdivisions:
    - rotation of 45° or less from the occipito-anterior position
    - rotation of more than 45° including the occipito-posterior position
- High
  - Instrumental vaginal birth is not recommended in this situation where the head is ⅖ or more palpable abdominally and the presenting part is above the level of the ischial spines (except for a second twin).

Wrigley forceps are considered suitable for outlet classifications, whereas Neville-Barnes, Piper and Lauffe, and Simpson are suitable for low classifications. Kielland forceps are suitable for use in mid classifications where rotation is required (SA Maternal and Neonatal Clinical Network 2013). See Figure 41.2 for diagrams of Simpson, Wrigley and Kielland forceps.

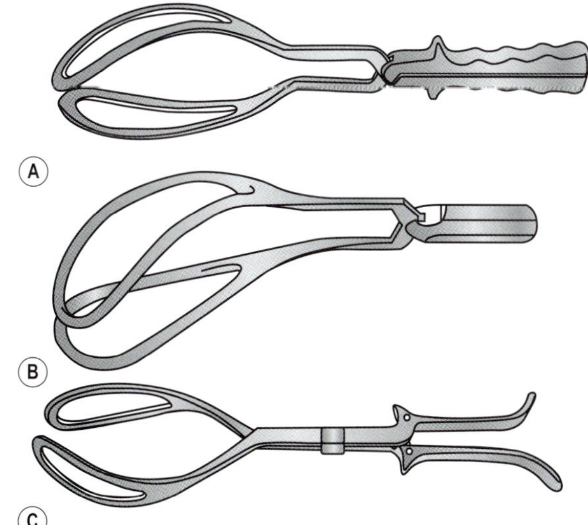

FIGURE 41.2 **A, Simpson, B, Wrigley and C, Kielland obstetric forceps.**

Vacuum extraction

There are two different types of vacuum extractor cups: synthetic and metal. Synthetic cups are either soft or rigid and suitable for straightforward deliveries, where there is no significant **caput** on the presenting part. Synthetic cups have a higher failure rate than metal cups but are associated with fewer neonatal scalp injuries (SA Maternal and Neonatal Clinical Network 2013). Metal cups are preferred for use in occipito-posterior and difficult occipito-anterior positions (O'Mahony et al 2010).

Indications for, and contraindications to, assisted birth

The decision to perform an assisted delivery depends on clinical circumstances, ensuring a balance between the potential risks of not expediting the birth of the fetus and the additional risks associated with performing a CS in the second stage of labour in the first instance. RANZCOG (2020, p. 6) suggests that there are few absolute indications for assisted birth, as follows:

- suspected or anticipated **fetal compromise**
- delay in the second stage
  - increased chance of fetal compromise with prolonged active pushing
  - maternal exhaustion
  - increased risk of pelvic floor injury, including anal sphincter dysfunction
- maternal effort is contraindicated
  - for example, in cases of maternal cerebral aneurysm, severe hypertension or cardiac failure.

Relative contraindications to assisted birth include fetal bleeding disorders (e.g. alloimmune thrombocytopenia) and fetal predisposition to fracture (e.g. osteogenesis imperfecta). Assisted birth using a vacuum should not be attempted in the case of face presentation or at gestations under 34 weeks, and should be used with caution between 34 and 36 weeks (RANZCOG 2020).

The decision for vacuum extraction or forceps

It is recognised that there is a place for both forceps and **vacuum extraction** in clinical practice. Largely, the choice of instrument relies on operator skill and choice, clinical circumstances and instrument availability (O'Mahony et al 2010). Forceps are less likely to result in neonatal morbidities, such as neonatal jaundice, subgaleal and retinal haemorrhage and cephalhaematoma, than vacuum extraction, but vacuum extraction is associated with less maternal pain 24 hours after birth and less serious maternal injury with less use of regional and general anaesthesia than forceps. Forceps use is, however, more likely to result in a successful assisted vaginal birth, and is suitable for assisted vaginal births where the baby is less than 36 weeks' gestation (RANZCOG 2015a, 2015b, RCOG 2011, SA Maternal and Neonatal Clinical Network 2013). The use of forceps was found in a Cochrane review to lead to fewer cases of shoulder dystocia, but a higher incidence of incontinence, third- or fourth-degree tears and any other type of vaginal trauma (RANZCOG 2020).

Conditions required for safe assisted birth

In order to ensure the optimal safety of both mother and baby during an assisted birth, the following conditions need to be met:

- the operator is experienced
- informed consent has been obtained
- the cervix is fully dilated
- the presenting part is engaged
- assessment of maternal pelvis is adequate
- membranes are ruptured
- adequate maternal analgesia has been provided
- the woman's bladder is emptied
- necessary support personnel and equipment are available and present in the room
- the operator is willing to abandon the procedure if necessary (Nielsen et al 2017).

Rotational assisted birth

In some cases rotation of the fetal head is required to move the vertex into an occiput anterior position, which is more favourable for descent. Manual rotation can occur alone or in conjunction with forceps or vacuum extraction, with success rates of 89–76% reported in two retrospective trials (Le Ray et al 2007, Shaffer et al 2006). In situations where the woman is a primipara, there is failure to progress or the cervix is not fully dilated prior to attempting a manual rotation, success is less likely; however, when successful, CS rates are significantly lower (Le Ray et al 2007, Shaffer et al 2006). Complication rates associated with manual rotation appear to be low, but it should be noted that limited data is available (RANZCOG 2020).

Possible complications of assisted birth

In addition to those complications listed in the previous section for aiding in making the decision between forceps or vacuum, there is a risk of postpartum haemorrhage for the mother, facial nerve palsy or corneal abrasion, the complications associated with shoulder dystocia and (rarely) cervical spine injury for the infant (RANZCOG 2020).

It is important to note that women commonly find assisted birth more traumatic than a spontaneous vaginal birth and this needs to be taken into consideration during birth and postnatally. Adequate time should be provided for debriefing and for the woman and/or her partner to ask any questions, and then again during any subsequent pregnancies to ensure she feels well informed and supported, and to minimise emotional trauma.

Caesarean section following attempted assisted birth

A **caesarean section (CS)** performed in the second stage of labour carries a greater risk of maternal morbidity, including haemorrhage and blood transfusion, bladder trauma, tears in relation to the uterine incision, and a potential for requiring intensive care. (Allen et al 2005, Pergialiotis et al 2014, RANZCOG 2020, Selo-Ojeme et al 2008). There is also an increased risk of subsequent pregnancies associated with repeat CS and uterine scar rupture in labour (RANZCOG 2020, Silver et al 2006).

SKILL 41.1 Assisting with a vacuum extraction

When assisting an obstetrician with a vacuum extraction, the midwife needs to ensure she supports the woman during the process and continues women-centred care. The midwife can do this by following this procedure.

1. Confirm the woman's identity if she is not known to the person who will be performing the procedure.
2. Provide continuous labour support.
3. Ensure the woman is given an opportunity to ask questions, and ensure she has given informed consent.
4. Ensure the woman is aware of what to expect at each stage of the process and what she may feel; guide her through each stage so she is aware of what is happening and what to expect.
5. Encourage the woman to push with each contraction to promote her being active in the birth process, except when contraindicated.
6. Provide verbal reassurance that she is part of the process with her pushing efforts.
7. Following the birth of the baby, ensure the woman is given ample opportunity to talk about the birth, debriefing with her why the vacuum extraction was indicated, answering any questions she may have, providing her with clarification and support, and discussing future labour and birth with her. Aim to resolve or talk through any negative feelings. Ensure support people who were present during the birth are available at this time and have the opportunity to debrief as well.
8. Discuss any side effects from the vacuum on the baby such as caput succedaneum or cephalohaematoma, providing them with reassurance that if either is present they should subside over the next 3–5 days.
9. Discuss signs and signs and symptoms of complications, including hyperbilirubinaemia, cerebral irritation (vomiting, neck and spin rigidity, and high-pitched cry) and infection, and what to do if they notice any of these.
10. Discuss possible difficulties with feeding, including the baby being sleepy; reassure the parents that this can be normal after a difficult birth, and provide them with management strategies for this.
11. Discuss perineal care with the woman, ensuring she is aware of any trauma she may have sustained and how to care for it (Chapter 45).
12. Ensure the woman is followed up with a physiotherapist to discuss pelvic floor rehabilitation.

OPERATIVE BIRTH

Midwives care for and support women who give birth by CS. The caesarean birth rate in Australia has increased from 30% in 2005 to 35% in 2018, with 20% of women requiring an assisted birth in 2018 (AIHW 2020). In New Zealand, 9% of births were instrumentally assisted and 27.2% of women gave birth by CS in 2018 (Ministry of Health 2020). The midwife has a significant role in caring safely for the woman, who may be feeling very anxious about the CS procedure and her baby's wellbeing before, during and after the birth. As for any birth setting, care includes that of the woman's partner or support person, who may also feel very anxious.

Reducing caesarean section rates

No surgery is without risks. The woman's early parenting skills and attachment with her baby can be affected by the postnatal complications of pain and immobility associated with CS (National Childbirth Trust 2011). Thromboembolism, infection and haemorrhage all feature as significant causes of maternal death (for which the risks are increased after CS) (Knight et al 2014). Neonatal respiratory morbidity, including transient tachypnoea of the newborn, pulmonary hypertension and surfactant deficiency, has been demonstrated to be associated with caesarean sections performed prior to labour (as in elective CS)—with a two- to three-fold increase in risk (Hansen et al 2007, Kolås et al 2006). Additionally, the infant is at risk of other injury, including lacerations and less effective temperature control. For the mother, a uterine scar can affect future pregnancies (e.g. they confer increased risks of uterine rupture and placenta praevia) (NICE 2021). These issues are just a snapshot; the decision for CS should be made with a consultant obstetrician and a clear clinical reason should be documented (NICE 2021). Attempting to reduce CS rates helps to reduce potential risks to both mother and baby, but additionally, aids in reducing the financial and resource demands on the maternity services.

Several non-clinical interventions have been recommended by the World Health Organization (WHO 2018) as having a positive influence on reducing CS rates, including a recommendation that women are cared for primarily by midwives with 24-hour obstetrician back-up. Further, in the face of year-on-year rises in CS numbers without any significant differences in population characteristics, the most recent 'Mothers, Babies and Children' report by Victoria's Consultative Council on Obstetric and Paediatric Mortality and Morbidity calls for maternity services to:

> develop and implement a formal time out process prior to every instrumental birth and emergency caesarean section, whether in a birth room or in the operating theatre, to improve situational awareness and decision making about whether it is the right mode of birth, in the right location, with the right instrument(s), and the right clinical team in attendance.
>
> Consultative Council on Obstetric and Paediatric Mortality and Morbidity (2021)

Categorising caesarean sections

In Australia and New Zealand, there is a four-grade classification system for use when determining the urgency of a CS (Table 41.1) RANZCOG (2019) and advises that each individual case should be managed according to the available clinical evidence of urgency, but recommends there be no specific time interval attached to each of the various categories. This may, however, be influenced by the judicial opinion that supports an optimal decision-to-delivery interval of 30 minutes in Australia and New Zealand, and RANZCOG acknowledges that this may influence professional practice. It should be noted that the clinical situation may change at any time and this may lead to greater urgency and therefore a change in category. All maternity services providing birth care should be equipped and staffed to promptly perform a CS within these guidelines.

TABLE 41.1 DETERMINING URGENCY FOR CAESAREAN SECTION

RANZCOG category	Level of urgency
Category 1	Urgent threat to the life or health of a woman or fetus
Category 2	Maternal or fetal compromise, but not immediately life threatening
Category 3	Needing earlier than planned delivery, but without current evident maternal or fetal compromise
Category 4	At a time acceptable to both the woman and the caesarean section team, understanding that this can be affected by a number of factors

Source: Royal Australian and New Zealand College of Obstetricians and Gynaecologists (RANZCOG): Categorisation of urgency for caesarean section, 2015a. Online 22 June 2018. Available: www.ranzcog.edu.au/.

Indications for caesarean sections

Reasons cited in the Australian clinical coding system for performing a CS (AIHW 2015) include:

- fetal compromise
- suspected fetal macrosomia
- malpresentation
- lack of progress; less than or equal to 3 cm cervical dilatation
- lack of progress in the first stage; greater than 3 cm to less than 10 cm cervical dilatation
- lack of progress in the second stage
- placenta praevia
- placental abruption
- vasa praevia
- antepartum/intrapartum haemorrhage
- multiple pregnancy
- unsuccessful attempt at assisted delivery
- cord prolapse
- previous adverse perinatal outcome
- previous CS
- previous severe perineal trauma
- previous shoulder dystocia
- other obstetric, medical, surgical, psychological indications
- maternal choice in the absence of any obstetric, medical, surgical, psychological indications.

Wherever possible, planned CS is undertaken after 39 weeks gestation (RANZCOG 2018). Good preparation for surgery, whether urgent or completed at leisure, aims primarily to facilitate uneventful surgery and smooth postoperative recovery.

PREPARATION FOR SURGERY

Given that around one-third of births are by CS in Australia (AIHW 2021), and one-quarter in New Zealand (Ministry of Health 2020), maternity services should aim to adopt a family-centred approach for all women scheduled for a CS, rather than the traditional procedure-centred approach, to help promote caesarean birth as a special and unique birth event rather than a surgical procedure (Bayes et al 2012).

Women will need to know what to bring to the hospital, what to expect throughout the process, fasting and arrival information and also the practicalities of aftercare once she returns home (e.g. no heavy lifting, driving, wound care). If the woman is on any regular medications she should be advised to keep taking her prescribed medications with a small amount of clear fluid, provided they are not contraindicated (Crenshaw

& Winslow 2006). Consideration needs to be given to providing an appropriate management plan for women on anticoagulation therapy to manage their dosages prior to surgery to reduce the risk of excessive bleeding; this should be done in consultation with her treating haematologist or obstetrician.

On the day of surgery, normal theatre preparation is required, including, but not limited to, being fasted, having had a shower (as a minimal requirement for skin preparation), noting that anything more is largely inconclusive at reducing postoperative wound infections, removal of any prostheses, changing into theatre attire without any underwear and not using any deodorant or talcum powder, as these may both be flammable. The woman should be advised not to wear make-up on the day of surgery and have nail polish removed to allow staff to recognise any cyanosis.

Hair removal from the wound site remains controversial; it is considered that if the hair is interfering with the wound or adhesive dressing then it should be removed. Shaving causes micro-abrasions on the skin that microorganisms can then colonise; shaving should be avoided (Jose & Dignon 2013). Better methods for hair removal are disposable head electric clippers or depilatory creams.

An indwelling catheter is used to prevent any trauma or over-distension to the bladder during surgery and is sometimes inserted prior to transfer to theatre, or at the time of surgery, where possible in accordance with the woman's wishes. It remains indwelling until the woman is mobile post-surgery.

Preparation for emergency surgery should include all of the above, but is often carried out much more quickly. If a general anaesthetic is being considered and the time since the woman last ate or drank something is possibly not sufficient, there are higher intraoperative and postoperative risks from emergency surgery.

Consultation with obstetrician and anaesthetist

Each woman should be seen by a registrar or obstetrician to have a detailed discussion of the risks and benefits of a CS in her individual circumstances and the decision made to proceed with CS delivery made in conjunction with her. The woman can be asked to sign a consent form at this point for a planned surgery. Should the surgery need to be carried out in a hurry to expedite the birth of the baby, the time allowed for the discussion of the CS may be much shorter and the midwife caring for the woman should ensure the woman is supported in making her decision, in either situation, whatever her decision may be (Charles 2013). The midwife caring for the woman having to undergo a medically necessary CS, whether planned or emergency, should acknowledge the woman's loss of her childbirth expectations, and assist her to recapture her losses to the greatest degree possible (Bayes et al 2012).

The woman will see an anaesthetist prior to surgery to assess her health, the reason for surgery and the suitability of the chosen anaesthetic (AAGBI & OAA 2005, American Society of Anesthesiologists 2007).The majority of caesarean sections should be performed under regional anaesthesia (spinal or epidural), as the risks are smaller than with a general anaesthetic (NICE 2021, SA Maternal and Neonatal Clinical Network 2014).

Prior to CS, blood group and save (or hold), along with a full blood count, must be taken to confirm haemoglobin level. Cross-matching should occur if heavy blood loss is anticipated, as in the case of placenta praevia or placenta creta, and blood transfusion services should be readily available. A baseline antenatal assessment and vital signs observation should also be on a Maternity Early Warning Score (MEWS) chart, in preparation for postoperative assessment and comparison. Allergies (e.g. to latex, antibiotics) should be carefully documented and the whole team made fully aware of them.

With the increasing popularity of establishing the baby's microbiome through vaginal seeding, both midwives and obstetricians should keep abreast with research relating to the practice, so they are able to answer questions and assist women wishing to undertake vaginal seeding following CS (Lee et al 2017).

INTRAOPERATIVE CARE

Care in the operating theatre is specialised, requiring cooperative teamwork between all the professional groups involved and ensuring the procedure is woman-centred (Yentis et al 2014). Theatre care is very detailed; some general principles are summarised below, but the reader is encouraged to consider other literary sources. The following general principles should be upheld in theatre.

- The most important person present is the woman. Her dignity and safety should be maintained, whether she is awake or anaesthetised and her preferences should be accommodated wherever possible, including immediate skin-to-skin contact with her infant, early breastfeeding and delayed cord clamping.
- Her safety is paramount, whether that relates to her internal safety or her external safety.
  - Internal safety
    - The theatre table should have a tilt of 15° to avoid aortocaval compression (NICE 2021).
    - Theatre is a sterile environment in which strict surgical asepsis is maintained. Asepsis (ANTT) is maintained throughout to reduce the risk of infection. Everyone in the theatre environment needs to be cautious to maintain the integrity of the sterile field and entering and exiting the theatre should be minimised (NICE 2013).

- External safety
  - Care of the immobile or unconscious woman: safety upon the operating table, care of numb limbs and pressure areas.

The operating theatre should also be appropriately stocked with all necessary and thoroughly checked equipment, including drugs and anaesthetic gases, anaesthetic machine, monitors, resuscitation equipment, IV fluids and infant Resuscitaire®, misoprostol and tamponade balloon, among other items (RANZCOG 2015a, WHO 2009).

Specific guidance is given within NICE guidelines (NICE 2021) as to the surgical techniques that reduce pain, haemorrhage and infection. These include issues such as transverse abdominal incision using the Joel Cohen incision (Mathai & Hofmeyr 2007)—a straight skin incision undertaken 3 cm above the symphysis pubis, blunt incision of the uterus and other layers (using scissors, not a knife, to extend if required), avoiding forceps, use of IV oxytocin (5 IU) and controlled cord traction for placental delivery (Anorlu et al 2008), uterine suturing in two layers within the abdomen, non-suturing of the visceral or parietal peritoneum or subcutaneous tissue (unless > 2 cm) and avoidance of superficial or routine wound drains (Gates & Anderson 2005). There is insufficient evidence to suggest that one type of skin closure is recommended over another.

The placenta and membranes are examined by the midwife, as for any other birth (Chapter 43). Cord blood is taken if the woman is Rh-negative and an umbilical artery and venous pH should be performed if there was fetal compromise.

Maternal-assisted caesarean section

Increasingly, maternity services are accommodating some women's wish to be an active part of her baby's birth in what is known as a maternal-assisted caesarean. This involves the woman actively lifting her baby through the surgical incision made into her abdomen, and requires her to perform a surgical scrub handwash and don a sterile gown and sterile gloves in advance of the procedure and to have undertaken preparatory meetings with clinicians in pregnancy. Women's experiences of maternal-assisted CS have yet to be reported in the research literature; anecdotally, though, they appear to imbue women with feelings of having some control over the birth process and to have bonding time sooner than they would in a 'usual' CS (Hill 2016).

POSTOPERATIVE CARE AND OBSERVATIONS

Regardless of anaesthetic type used for the CS, postoperative care following CS includes correct positioning, care of numb limbs and pressure areas, pain levels, administering analgesia if required or requested, education around patient-controlled analgesia if being used, care of IV infusion/blood transfusion/uterotonics and fluid balance, return of sensation following regional anaesthesia and appropriate thromboprophylaxis measures. The midwife caring for the woman post-CS should ensure the woman is supported in having time with her baby, including opportunities for skin-to-skin contact and feeding, and support and assistance to attend to baby cares such as nappy changes.

All vital sign observations, including level of consciousness and airway maintenance, respirations, temperature, blood pressure and heart rate, should be completed at regular short intervals initially and recorded on a MEWS chart. The timings are dictated by clinical condition and locally agreed policy, but are often at 5-minute intervals initially.

Vital signs should be inclusive of lochia (while keeping track of estimated blood loss in order to identify postpartum haemorrhage), urine output and wound assessment, inclusive of any drains which may have been placed. Further information is provided in Chapter 47.

THE BABY

A CS is a surgical procedure which adds an extra dimension as care of the newborn needs to be taken into consideration as well. Resuscitation equipment and personnel should be on hand if there has been a general anaesthetic or fetal compromise and the infant should have identification bands applied as soon as practical, and their body temperature monitored and maintained. When appropriate, delayed cord clamping can be considered, should informed maternal consent be obtained (Chapter 43).

The baby is cared for accordingly, noting that babies born in the operating theatre:

- are often cooler
- need to be fed as soon as possible
- may have had skin-to-skin care with birthing partner but needs skin-to-skin care with the mother
- should be labelled before leaving the area
- are more likely to experience respiratory distress.

ONGOING CARE

Psychologically, there is relief and enjoyment of the new baby, but it may be tinged by pain, immobility, distress (if rapid emergency or major complications were present) and frustration that progress appears slow. In the days following the surgery, the woman will appreciate sensitive and individualised midwifery care and should have the opportunity to review her care and future pregnancies with her obstetric team.

Postoperative care, while individualised, will include attention to hygiene and oral care, thromboembolic prophylaxis (Chapter 47), vital sign observations, pressure area care, urinary output and effective analgesia. Effective and regular pain relief is essential to the woman's recovery.

The woman may eat or drink as she wishes (NICE 2021). IV infusion is discontinued when appropriate—usually when the woman is tolerating fluids, although the cannula may be left in situ until the woman is mobile (often the following day but it will require flushing to maintain patency). The woman's postoperative haemoglobin levels should be checked prior to removal of her IV cannula, to ensure she does not require a blood transfusion. Once the woman is mobile, her urinary catheter can be removed; this should be at least 12 hours after the last regional analgesia dose. Early mobilisation is encouraged and naturally the woman will require support and care with her baby, particularly to establish breastfeeding. While this is often a motivating factor for the woman after CS, the midwife should ensure that the woman is having sufficient rest and is not over-tired.

The midwife should be sensitive to the woman's emotional state, noting that she has undergone two significant life experiences—having a baby and major surgery. Standard postnatal assessment is a part of each day's care in conjunction with specific postoperative needs.

Debriefing is recommended prior to leaving hospital, particularly in cases where the CS was an emergency or unplanned, so there can be discussion with the woman about why the CS took place and the implications for future childbearing (Baxter 2007).

Discharge from hospital will depend on the woman's progress and social support; it may be from 24 hours onwards. Post-surgery advice includes pain management, importance of rest and nutrition, what to do should complications arise and avoidance of lifting. Gould (2007) advises the amount lifted in the first 6 weeks should be no more than the weight of the baby, no driving in the first 6 weeks, effective contraception and attendance for assessment (often with the woman's general practitioner) at the end of the puerperium.

Role and responsibilities of the midwife

These can be summarised as:

- evidence-based practice throughout
- recognising deviations from normal and referring on when indicated
- assistance during assisted birth
- education, explanation, advocacy and support for the woman
- preoperative care to reduce intraoperative and postoperative complications
- skilled care within theatre and recovery for both mother and baby
- comprehensive postoperative care
- effective multidisciplinary teamwork and recognition of limitations where appropriate
- contemporaneous record keeping.

SUMMARY

- Birth can be expedited for maternal or fetal reasons or a combination of both, through the use of forceps and vacuum extraction assisted births.
- There are a number of different forceps and vacuum types, and the choice of which to use largely revolves around operator skill and choice, clinical circumstances and instrument availability.
- Theatre care is detailed and specialised; women undergoing a CS birth have increased risk factors associated with the changes of pregnancy, including aspiration, aortocaval occlusion and thromboembolism.
- Preoperative preparation should include consent, identity, care of the gastrointestinal and urinary tracts, skin preparation, removal of prostheses, thromboprophylaxis and psychological support; good preoperative care can reduce the intraoperative and postoperative risks.
- Intraoperative care considers the woman to be the highest priority for maintaining her internal and external safety; this comprises many aspects of care.
- Postoperative care focuses on vital sign observations, airway and consciousness, pain relief, assessment of wound and haemorrhage, care of infusions, bladder care, adaptation to parenthood and feeding and psychological support.
- There is the added dimension of the care requirements for the baby when a CS is performed.

Self-assessment exercises

The answers to the following questions may be found in the text.

1. List indications for assisted birth.
2. List the types of instruments used in assisted birth and the situations in which each may be used.
3. Discuss the indications and contraindications for assisted birth.
4. Discuss the requirements and rationale for preoperative preparation prior to emergency CS. Compare and contrast this with preparation for elective surgery.
5. Summarise the general principles of conduct and care in the theatre environment.
6. Discuss the midwife's role and responsibilities to the woman before, during and following CS.

References

Allen VM, O'Connell CM, Baskett TF: Maternal and perinatal morbidity of caesarean delivery at full cervical dilatation compared with caesarean delivery in the first stage of labour, BJOG: An International Journal of Obstetrics and Gynaecology 112(7):986–990, 2005.

American Society of Anesthesiologists: Practice guidelines for obstetric anesthesia, Anesthesiology 106:843–863, 2007.

Anorlu RI, Maholwana B, Hofmeyr GJ: Methods of delivering the placenta at caesarean section, Cochrane Database of Systematic Review (3):Art. No.: CD004737, 2008.

Association of Anaesthetists of Great Britain and Ireland and Obstetric Anaesthetists' Association (AAGBI & OAA): OAA/AAGBI guidelines for obstetric anaesthetic services, 2nd ed., London, 2005, AAGBI and OAA.

Australian Institute of Health and Welfare (AIHW): Australia's mothers and babies 2018 in brief, 2020. Online 18 April 2021. Available: www.aihw.gov.au/getmedia/aa54e74a-bda7-4497-93ce-e0010cb66231/aihw-per-108.pdf.aspx?inline=true.

Australian Institute of Health and Welfare (AIHW): Australia's Mothers and Babies 2019, 2021. Online 16 August 2021. Available: www.aihw.gov.au/reports/mothers-babies/australias-mothers-babies/contents/summary.

Australian Institute of Health and Welfare (AIHW): National Maternity Data Development Project: Research brief No. 5, 2015. Online 18 April 2021. Available: www.aihw.gov.au/getmedia/9e151b70-412a-4267-8ffc-b69fae2f474c/brief_5_per-79.pdf.aspx.

Baxter J: Do women understand the reasons given for their caesarean sections? British Journal of Midwifery 15(9):536–538, 2007.

Bayes S, Fenwick J, Hauck Y: Becoming redundant: Australian women's experiences of pregnancy after being unexpectedly scheduled for a medically necessary term elective cesarean section, International Journal of Childbirth 2(2):73–84, 2012.

Charles C: Caesarean section. In Chapman V, Charles C, editors: The midwife's labour and birth handbook, 3rd ed., Chichester, 2013, Wiley Blackwell, pp 179–192.

Crenshaw JT, Winslow EH: Actual versus instructed fasting times and associated discomforts in women having scheduled caesarean birth, Journal of Obstetric, Gynecologic, and Neonatal Nursing 35(2):257–264, 2006.

Consultative Council on Obstetric and Paediatric Mortality and Morbidity: Victoria's mothers, babies and children 2019, Victoria, 2021, Victorian Government. Online 18 April 2021. Available: www.bettersafercare.vic.gov.au/sites/default/files/2021-01/CCOPMM%20Mothers%20babies%20children%202019%20FINAL.pdf.

Gates S, Anderson ER: Wound drainage for caesarean section, Cochrane Database of Systematic Review (1): Art. No.: CD004549, 2005.

Gould D: Caesarean section, surgical site infection and wound management, Nursing Standard 21(32):57–66, 2007.

Hansen AK, Wisborg K, Uldbjerg N, et al: Elective caesarean section and respiratory morbidity in the term and near term neonate, Acta Obstetricia et Gynaecologica Scandinavica 86(4):389–394, 2007.

Hill K: Maternal-assisted caesarean: Mother helps deliver her baby boy Arlo, ABC News. 2016. Online 18 April 2021. Available: www.abc.net.au/news/2016-08-23/maternal-assisted-caesarean-mother-helps-delivery-baby-boy/7776654.

Jose B, Dignon A: Is there a relationship between preoperative shaving (hair removal) and surgical site infection? Journal of Perioperative Practice 23(1):23–25, 2013.

Knight M, Nair M, Shah A, et al: Maternal mortality and morbidity in the UK 2009–12: surveillance and epidemiology, Chapter 2. In Knight M, Kenyon S, Brocklehurst P, et al, eds: Saving lives, improving mothers' care—lessons learned to inform future maternity care from the UK and Ireland Confidential Enquiries into Maternal Deaths and Morbidity 2009–2012, Oxford, 2014, National Perinatal Epidemiology Unit.

Kolås T, Saugstad OD, Daltveit AK, et al: Planned caesarean versus planned vaginal delivery at term: comparison of newborn infant outcomes, American Journal of Obstetrics and Gynecology 195(6):1538–1543, 2006.

Lee L, Garland SM, Giles ML, Daley, A: Manipulating the baby biome: what are the issues?, Australia and New Zealand Journal of Obstetrics and Gynaecology 57(2):232–234, 2017.

Le Ray C, Serres P, Schmitz T, et al: Manual rotation in occiput posterior or transverse positions: risk factors and consequences on the cesarean delivery rate, Obstetrics and Gynaecology 110(4):873–879, 2007.

Mathai M, Hofmeyr GJ: Abdominal surgical incisions for caesarean section, Cochrane Database of Systematic Review (1):Art. No.: CD004453, 2007.

Ministry of Health: New Zealand Maternity Clinical Indicators 2018, 2020. Online 16 August 2021. Available: www.health.govt.nz/publication/new-zealand-maternity-clinical-indicators-2018.

Ministry of Health: Report on maternity 2018, 2020. Online 18 April 2021. Available: www.health.govt.nz/publication/report-maternity-web-tool.

National Childbirth Trust (NCT): Briefing for journalists: caesarean birth, 2011. NCT, London. Online 22 June 2018. Available: www.nct.org.uk/sites/default/files/related_documents/B3%20Caesarean%20Birth%20briefing%202011.pdf.

National Institute for Health and Clinical Excellence (NICE): Caesarean Section: NICE Clinical Guideline NG192, 2021. NICE, London. Online 18 April 2021. Available: www.nice.org.uk/guidance/ng192/resources/caesarean-birth-pdf-66142078788805.

National Institute for Health and Clinical Excellence (NICE): Surgical site infection NICE Quality Standard 49, 2013. NICE, London. Online 22 June 2018. Available: www.nice.org.uk/Guidance/QS49.

Nielsen PE, Deering SH, Galan HL: Operative vaginal delivery. In Gabbe SG, et al, eds: Obstetrics: normal and problem pregnancies, 7th ed., Philadelphia, 2017, Elsevier, pp 289–307.

O'Mahony F, Hofmeyr GJ, Menon V: Choice of instruments for assisted vaginal delivery, Cochrane Database of Systematic Review (11):Art. No.: CD005455, 2010.

Pergialiotis V, Vlachos DG, Rodolakis A, et al: First versus second stage C/S maternal and neonatal morbidity: a systematic review and meta-analysis, European Journal of Obstetrics and Gynaecology and Reproductive Biology 175:15–24, 2014.

Royal Australian and New Zealand College of Obstetricians and Gynaecologists (RANZCOG): Categorisation of urgency for caesarean section (C-Obs 14), 2019. Online 16 August 2021. Available: https://ranzcog.edu.au/RANZCOG_SITE/media/RANZCOG-MEDIA/Women%27s%20Health/Statement%20and%20guidelines/Clinical-Obstetrics/Categorisation-of-urgency-for-caesarean-section-(C-Obs-14).pdf?ext=.pdf

Royal Australian and New Zealand College of Obstetricians and Gynaecologists (RANZCOG): Categorisation of urgency for caesarean section, 2015a. Online 22 June 2018. Available: www.ranzcog.edu.au/.

Royal Australian and New Zealand College of Obstetricians and Gynaecologists (RANZCOG): Instrumental vaginal birth, 2020. Online 18 May 2021. Available: https://ranzcog.edu.au/RANZCOG_SITE/media/RANZCOG-MEDIA/Women%27s%20Health/Statement%20and%20guidelines/Clinical-Obstetrics/Instrumental-vaginal-birth-(C-Obs-16)-Review-March-2020.pdf?ext5.pdf.

Royal Australian and New Zealand College of Obstetricians and Gynaecologists (RANZCOG): Prevention, detection, and management of subgaleal haemorrhage in the newborn, 2015b. Online 22 June 2018. Available: www.ranzcog.edu.au/.

Royal Australian and New Zealand College of Obstetricians and Gynaecologists (RANZCOG): Timing of elective caesarean section at term (C-Obs 23), 2018. Online 16 August 2021. Available: https://ranzcog.edu.au/RANZCOG_SITE/media/RANZCOG-MEDIA/Women%27s%20Health/Statement%20and%20guidelines/Clinical-Obstetrics/Timing-of-elective-caesarean-section-(C-Obs-23)-March18.pdf?ext=.pdf.

Royal College of Obstetricians and Gynaecologists (RCOG): Operative vaginal delivery: Green-top guideline no. 26, 2011. Online 22 June 2018. Available: www.rcog.org.uk/.

SA Maternal and Neonatal Clinical Network: Clinical guideline: operative vaginal deliveries, 2013. Online 22 June 2018. Available: www.sahealth.sa.gov.au/.

SA Maternal and Neonatal Clinical Network: Clinical guideline: South Australian perinatal practice guidelines—caesarean section, 2014. Online 22 June 2018. Available: www.sahealth.sa.gov.au/.

Selo-Ojeme D, Sathiyathasan S, Fayyaz M: Caesarean delivery at full cervical dilatation versus caesarean delivery in the first stage of labour: comparison of maternal and perinatal morbidity, Archives of Gynaecology and Obstetrics 278(3):245–249, 2008.

Shaffer BL, Cheng YW, Vargas JE, et al: Manual rotation of the fetal occiput: predictors of success and delivery, American Journal of Obstetrics and Gynaecology 194(5):e7–e9, 2006.

Silver RM, Landon MB, Rouse DJ, et al: Maternal morbidity associated with multiple repeat cesarean deliveries, Obstetrics and Gynaecology 107(6):1226–1232, 2006.

Yentis S, Clyburn P, On behalf of the MBRRACE-UK Anaesthetic Chapter Writing Group, et al: Lessons for anaesthesia, Chapter 6. In Knight M, Kenyon S, Brocklehurst P, et al, eds: Saving Lives, Improving Mothers' Care—Lessons Learned to Inform Future Maternity Care from the UK and Ireland Confidential Enquiries into Maternal Deaths and Morbidity 2009–2012, Oxford, 2014, National Perinatal Epidemiology Unit.

World Health Organization (WHO): WHO recommendations—non-clinical interventions to reduce unnecessary caesarean sections, 2018. Online 18 April 2021. Available: http://apps.who.int/iris/bitstream/handle/10665/275377/9789241550338-eng.pdf?ua=1.

World Health Organization (WHO): WHO Surgical Safety Checklist, 2009. Online 22 June 2018. Available: www.nrls.npsa.nhs.uk/resources/?entryid45=59860.

CHAPTER 42
MATERNAL AND NEWBORN RESUSCITATION

Learning outcomes

Having read this chapter, the reader should be able to:

- anticipate and recognise maternal collapse
- discuss the modifications necessary for resuscitation of a pregnant woman
- recognise the importance of prompt, effective cardiac compressions
- demonstrate maternal resuscitation on a manikin
- recognise a neonate who requires resuscitation
- discuss the different ways of maintaining an open airway for the neonate during resuscitation
- discuss the rationale for using air to begin the resuscitation and when to increase the percentage of oxygen used
- describe when and how cardiac compressions are given to a neonate
- describe the equipment for both maternal and newborn resuscitation and how it is used
- discuss in detail the role and responsibilities of the midwife prior to, during and following a neonatal resuscitation
- demonstrate/simulate a neonatal resuscitation using a manikin, discussing how effective resuscitation is achieved.

The first half of this chapter focuses on maternal collapse and resuscitation, along with basic life support techniques, while the second half discusses newborn resuscitation, principles and management. While maternal collapse is a rare event associated with increased morbidity and mortality for the woman and her baby, the frequency of cardiac arrest in pregnancy is increasing (Edwards 2017). The increase in maternal collapse leading to cardiac arrest can be attributed to changes in demographics, including increased maternal age, increased maternal body mass index (BMI), increased incidence of birth by caesarean section and the increase in the incidence of preexisting co-morbidities (Government of South Australia 2017). Edwards (2017) suggests that cardiac arrest has an incidence of 1:20,000 to 1:30,000 during pregnancy internationally. There are two 'patients' involved in the resuscitation of a pregnant woman, effective resuscitation of the woman is the best way to optimise fetal survival (Jeejeebhoy & Windrim 2014).

MATERNAL COLLAPSE AND RESUSCITATION

Dohi et al (2017) state that in the event of maternal cardiac arrest, cardiopulmonary resuscitation should be commenced within 4 minutes to maximise the survival of both mother and fetus. If resuscitation has not been successful within 4 minutes then the baby's birth should be expedited (Zelop et al 2018).

Cardiac arrest occurs when the heart stops contracting effectively due to either an arrhythmia (e.g. ventricular fibrillation) or complete asystole. As a result, breathing will stop, although agonal breathing may be seen before cessation of respiration.

Physiological changes that occur during pregnancy can present challenges in the event of the requirement for cardiopulmonary resuscitation (Jeejeebhoy & Windram 2014). Adequate ventilation during a cardiac arrest can be compromised due to several physiological factors, including the upward displacement of the abdominal organs and the enlarged uterus. The decrease in pulmonary function and the increase in oxygen consumption demands can cause the pregnant woman to become hypoxic at a more rapid rate.

The midwife rarely undertakes maternal **cardiopulmonary resuscitation (CPR)**; thus, it is vital that the midwife undertakes regular training and practice to ensure she can do this effectively and efficiently when the need arises, and can modify the CPR to accommodate the particular needs of the collapsed pregnant woman.

Anticipation of collapse

The majority of pregnant women are healthy and at low risk of cardiac arrest, but there is the potential for complications from childbearing that may be life-threatening. It may be possible to anticipate collapse and prevent it from occurring. These include haemorrhage, cardiovascular conditions, hypertension, fever/sepsis, accidents, drugs, embolism and metabolic abnormalities (Zelop et al 2018).

Equipment

In the hospital environment, resuscitation equipment, including a defibrillator, should be readily available and are usually kept together in a resuscitation trolley which can be taken to the place where resuscitation is occurring. Midwives attending homebirths usually have equipment available for providing oxygen and ventilation breaths; the paramedic crew will bring other equipment as needed (e.g. a defibrillator). Equipment should be checked regularly to ensure it is working effectively, and drugs checked frequently to ensure they are within their use-by date.

Deteriorating patient

When the woman is an inpatient, utilising early warning systems, including rapid detection and response charts, can assist early identification of deterioration in the woman's condition. This enables the escalation process to be implemented by incorporating senior medical staff to assist in the timely response and management of the deteriorating patient, optimising outcome (Government of South Australia 2017).

Initial assessment

Collapse may be witnessed or unwitnessed. With an unwitnessed collapse, resuscitation may be less successful because of the delay in commencing cardiac compressions. The woman may be seen to look unwell (e.g. pale, cyanosed and clammy), and appear to be unmoving. It is important to ensure it is safe to approach the collapsed woman. A quick visual assessment of the area around the woman should be undertaken for hazards, such as a wet floor or dangling wires.

Assessing responsiveness

The midwife should initially determine if the woman is conscious or unconscious. This can be achieved by verbal and tactile stimulation.

Calling for help

If there is no response, help should be sought immediately. In a hospital setting this can be through use of the emergency buzzer or calling for help. It is important to call for the resuscitation team if the hospital has one, using the standard emergency number for the facility.

Airway

Opening the airway may be all that is needed to enable the woman to resume breathing. Check for obstruction in the mouth. The woman should then be turned onto her back and her airway opened using a head tilt and chin lift, so that her head is slightly extended. This is achieved by placing a hand on the woman's forehead and gently tilting her head back, then using fingertips under her chin to tilt her chin upwards.

Breathing

No more than 10 seconds should be taken to assess if the woman is breathing. The midwife does this by bringing her head close to the woman's face and chest, looking for chest rise, listening for breath sounds and feeling for breath on her cheeks. When no breathing is noted, cardiac arrest is assumed as the cause and CPR commenced immediately.

Circulation

High quality cardiopulmonary resuscitation is associated with increased chances of survival and involves the synchronisation of certain factors, including the correct compression depth, correct rate, correct positioning of the hands and complete chest recoil (Contri et al 2017). Cardiac compressions increase the chance of survival by maintaining the blood flow, and therefore the oxygen supply, to the heart, lungs and brain (Pendick 2015). This is achieved only if there is adequate perfusion of the coronary arteries to oxygenate the myocardium, and of the brain for a neurologically intact survival (Cunningham et al 2012). With each compression, coronary perfusion pressure gradually increases. Cunningham et al (2012) suggest it takes 40–45 seconds of continuous compressions to achieve the optimal perfusion pressure. Each time compressions are interrupted there is a rapid decrease in aortic relaxation (diastolic) pressure, which reduces both coronary and cerebral perfusion pressures; thus it is important to minimise interruptions to cardiac compressions (Beesems et al 2013).

The hand position when performing cardiac compressions is the same for both pregnant and non-pregnant individuals. This can be achieved by placing the heel of one hand in the centre of the chest, which positions the hand over the lower half of the sternum (Fig 42.1) (Bennett et al 2016). In the past, a higher placement of the hand on the sternum for cardiac compressions in a pregnant patient was recommended. However, most recent literature, guidelines and data do not support this recommendation (Kikuchi & Deering 2018).

With arms locked to make full use of upper body weight (Lewinsohn et al 2012), the hands compress the sternum 5–6 cm (2 inches) or at least one-third of the anteroposterior diameter. The extended arms should be vertical, at a 90° angle to the chest. Lee and colleagues (2012) caution that resuscitation on the bed makes this difficult unless the height of the bed matches the height of the person undertaking compressions. This reduces rescuer fatigue due to improved posture and produces more effective compressions (Lee et al 2012). Lewinsohn and colleagues (2012) advise the bed height should be at mid-thigh level to generate more effective intrathoracic pressure during compression and to reduce fatigue.

The Australian and New Zealand Committee on Resuscitation (ANZCOR n.d.) recommend that the compression rate for uninterrupted, continuous cardiac compressions should be 100–120 compressions per minute (almost two compressions per second). Some evidence highlights that compressions less than 100 or greater than 140 compressions per minute are linked with lower survival rates (ANZCOR n.d.). Following each compression, it is important to allow the chest to recoil to its precompression state to allow the heart's chambers to refill with blood between compressions (Contri et al 2017).

Defibrillation

An **automated external defibrillator (AED)** can be used by anyone regardless of whether or not they have any resuscitation training or experience. The machine should be turned on as soon as it arrives so that it can go through its self-checking program. When connected, the AED will give voice and visual prompts which are easy to follow. The AED has two electrode pads that are placed on the skin (ensuring first that the skin is dried) of the collapsed woman while compressions are happening—the right pad is placed to the right of her sternum below her clavicle. The left pad is placed laterally in the left mid-axillary line, clear of any breast tissue. When the machine is operational, it will analyse the heart rhythm and ascertain whether the rhythm is a shockable or a non-shockable cardiac rhythm. Shockable rhythms include ventricular fibrillation (VF) and pulseless ventricular tachycardia (VT).

An analysis of the heart rhythm is undertaken, but if there is too much movement this may not be possible; thus the AED may instruct the resuscitators to stand clear when it is analysing. The person undertaking cardiac compressions can maintain their position with hands poised just above the chest, so that when the command is given to recommence CPR this is undertaken quickly, minimising the interruption to compressions (Bennett et al 2016). If no shock has been given, the AED will continue to analyse until a shockable rhythm is detected or the AED is turned off. If a shock is to be administered, a warning noise will sound and all personnel should stand clear of the woman (and bed if she is on one). The risk of someone

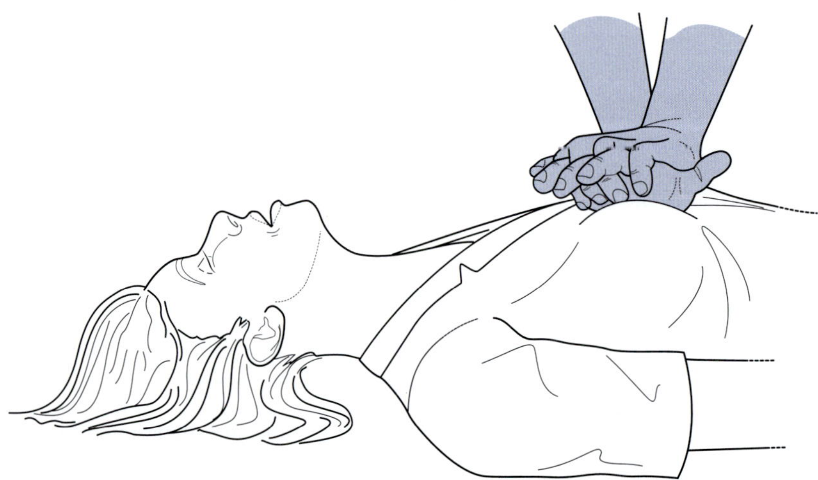

FIGURE 42.1 **Cardiac compression.**
Source: Adapted with kind permission from Peattie PI, Walker S: Understanding nursing care, 4th ed., Churchill Livingstone, Edinburgh, 1995.

else receiving an accidental shock if they are touching the woman or the bed that she is on is negligible. The person undertaking compressions is the last to stand clear and following a quick check to ensure everyone is clear, the shock button is pressed, delivering an electrical current to the woman's heart to depolarise cardiac muscle cells, disrupting abnormal cardiac rhythms and re-establishing sinus rhythm (Pourmand et al 2018). Defibrillation within 3–5 minutes of cardiac arrest can contribute to rates of survival between 50% and 70% (Ducloy-Bouthers et al 2016).

Pregnancy is not a contraindication to using the AED or receiving a shock and therefore concerns for fetal safety should not delay initiation of defibrillation (Kikuchi & Deering 2018). Kikuchi and Deering (2018) highlight that it is safe to use defibrillation at any gestation of pregnancy as a minimal amount of energy is transferred to the fetus. Defibrillation should not be delayed to remove fetal monitors as it is unlikely that defibrillation would cause arcing of fetal monitors. Studies show that modifications in the energy of the shock are not indicated (Kikuchi & Deering 2018).

Ventilation breaths

Compressions can be combined with ventilation breaths at a rate of 30 compressions to two breaths for an adult (Australian Resuscitation Council [ARC] 2021, New Zealand Resuscitation Council [NZRC] 2021). Ventilation breaths for basic life support can be undertaken using a facemask connected to a bag–valve–mask (BVM) system (e.g. Ambu bag), a pocket mask or mouth-to-mouth (Fig 42.2). When using a facemask for ventilation breaths, it is important to use the correct size (small, medium or large). Bosson and Gordon (2018) suggest that where the correct size is not available, a seal will be easier to achieve with a mask that is too big than one that is too small. Ideally the mask should not extend over the end of the woman's chin or into her eye sockets. It has a deformable rim that will fit snugly around the woman's nose and mouth when even pressure is applied and an airtight seal formed. It is important to hold the mask in place by placing slight pressure on the firm surface of the mask, as pressure on the rim may cause it to lose the seal. The woman's head should be slightly extended. It can be harder to achieve a good seal when there is a lack of teeth, BMI is above 26, age over 55 years, and there is a history of snoring (Bosson & Gordon 2018). Bosson and Gordon (2018) suggest that the mandible should be lifted to the mask rather than the mask pushed down onto the face.

There are several ways to hold the facemask in place using one or two hands. A common method is the E–C technique where the non-dominant hand is used by creating a C-shape with the thumb and index finger and placing them on the upper and lower part of the mask's firm surface (Fig 42.2). Gentle downward pressure is applied to create an airtight seal. The remaining three fingers are placed around the mandible in an E-shape to lift the chin up towards the mask.

If there is another person available to compress the bag, then two hands can be used to hold the mask in place with a double jaw thrust. Two opposing semicircles are made using the thumb and index finger of each hand and placed on either side of the facemask. The remaining three fingers of each hand are placed under the mandible and behind the angle of the jaw to pull the chin forwards.

A third technique is to place the length of the thumbs along the sides of the facemask to hold it in place using the remaining fingers under the mandible to pull

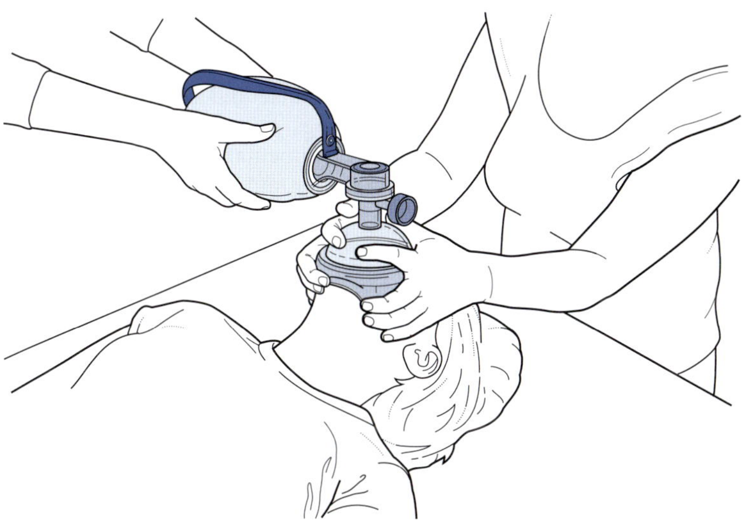

FIGURE 42.2 **Bag–valve–mask ventilation using two resuscitators.**
Source: Johnson R, Taylor W: Skills for midwifery practice, 4th ed., Elsevier, London, 2016.

the chin forwards. Care should be taken whichever technique is used to ensure the fingers under the mandible are only applying pressure on bone and not the soft tissue of the neck, as this may result in swelling and airway occlusion.

If a pocket mask is available, it should be placed over the woman's nose and mouth and her airway opened using a chin tilt. The mask should be held on the firm surface to prevent the rim from deforming. The midwife blows through the opening on the pocket mask using a normal expiratory breath as the chest rises. This is repeated once. If there is no chest movement noted, the head and mask position should be checked and corrected, and the two breaths re-attempted after the next set of compressions.

Mouth-to-mouth resuscitation can be undertaken if the midwife is willing to do so; however, it is acceptable to continue with compressions until suitable equipment arrives for ventilation, as there is a risk of coming into contact with body fluids. Patterson (2017) suggests the risk of disease transmission is extremely low.

In situations where ventilation breaths are not attempted, it is helpful to place an oxygen mask on the woman's face connected to 100% oxygen as this may facilitate the passive exchange of oxygen during compressions.

Currently, the recommendation is for 100% oxygen to be used with cardiac compressions (Bowden & Smith 2017). ANZCOR (n.d.) agree that the highest possible inspired oxygen concentration should be used on all patients while performing CPR and that oxygen should never be withheld due to fear of possible adverse effects.

The bag should be slowly compressed for one second for each ventilation, then released to refill while the operator observes for chest rise and fall. It may be difficult to see chest rise with pregnant women, particularly during the third trimester. Lateral chest and/or breast movement may be noted as an indication of lung inflation.

Considerations for the pregnant woman

Although the principles of resuscitation are the same as for any adult, the physiological changes occurring during pregnancy can influence resuscitation outcomes. The most important consideration is that of the gravid uterus and the compression effect it has on the inferior vena cava when the woman is lying in the supine position. However, there is limited research determining the optimum position for the pregnant woman when receiving CPR. Studies elucidate that importance be placed on the quality of the chest compressions rather than the positioning of the woman during CPR to maximise both maternal and fetal outcomes (ANZCOR 2011). ANZCOR (2011) suggest that once CPR has been initiated, and if significant resources are available, then either a wedge, rolled towel, pillow or cushion be placed under the woman's right hip to enable a 15–30° tilt of the woman's hips. This assists the gravid uterus, especially if the fundal height is over the level of the umbilicus, to avoid pressure on the major blood vessels of the abdomen. However, it is vital to ensure the shoulders are left flat to maximise the effectiveness of the cardiac compressions.

Airway management may be more difficult in the pregnant woman due to a higher oxygen requirement, the risk of hypoxemia and physical changes, including oedema and weight gain (Bennett et al 2016). Intubation may prove more difficult in the pregnant woman as the elevation in oestrogen levels promote vascularity, increasing the risk of bleeding and making the visualisation of the landmarks in the airway used to assist intubation more difficult (Jeejeebhoy & Windrim 2014).

In the event that there is no response within 4 minutes of the commencement of CPR then a perimortem caesarean section (CS) should be undertaken. This should be achieved within 5 minutes of the collapse and is undertaken in the place where the woman has collapsed (Government of South Australia 2017). Delivering the baby gives the woman a greater chance of surviving (depending on the reason for the cardiac arrest) as it reduces oxygen consumption, improves venous return and cardiac output and makes ventilation easier. All maternity units should have a pre-prepared perimortem CS kit available including a surgical scalpel, Mayo scissors and forceps (Government of South Australia 2017).

Additional measures

When the resuscitation team arrive, one of them will take overall control of the resuscitation to ensure the resuscitation is progressing as it should. A clear, concise, verbal handover of the history, treatment and response to-date should be given to the team. However, the obstetrician or midwife present will need to guide them on the particular adaptations necessary for the pregnant woman. While compression, ventilation breaths and use of the AED continue, other personnel can site two wide-bore gauge intravenous cannulae and commence fluid boluses or administer drugs as requested and maintain contemporaneous documentation. At this point the midwife also has an important role in supporting the family, setting up the Resuscitaire®, calling the paediatrician and assisting with resuscitating the baby if it is delivered.

Stopping resuscitation

The resuscitation will stop when there is return of spontaneous circulation, the people undertaking CPR are too exhausted to continue, or a senior team member makes the decision to stop. Because the collapse is usually unexpected, if the woman cannot be resuscitated the case will be referred to the coroner. It is important that any pieces of equipment inserted during the resuscitation remain in situ (e.g. airways, endotracheal tubes, cannulae), as these will be reviewed by the pathologist as part of the postmortem examination.

When the woman survives, post-resuscitation care will usually be provided in the intensive care unit following time in the operating theatre if a CS was performed. Debriefing for the woman, her family and staff involved is essential. Midwives can be a valuable support for other midwives involved in any maternal resuscitation, but particularly so when it is unsuccessful; this is a devastating event for the family and all involved in the care and resuscitation of the woman.

SKILL 42.1 Maternal resuscitation

1. Recognise the arrest and assess the situation for any potential dangers.
2. Assess the woman's level of responsiveness.
3. If the woman is unresponsive, call for emergency assistance.
4. Turn the woman on her back and tilt her head so that it is slightly extended.
5. Ensure the airway is open, using chin support.
6. Assess breathing, taking no more than 10 seconds.
7. If the woman is not breathing, commence cardiac compression at a rate of 100–120 beats per minute (bpm).
8. After every 30 cardiac compressions, undertake two ventilation breaths where possible, and maintain the rate at 30:2.
9. Apply AED electrodes and follow voice commands of the AED device.
10. Continue with resuscitation until spontaneous respiration or movement is seen, or until told to stop by the senior person present (or if too exhausted to continue and there is no one to take over from you).
11. If after 4 minutes there is minimal success, preparation should begin for CS (if pregnant) and the baby delivered within the next minute.
12. Participate within the multidisciplinary team and undertake other roles as needed; for example, intravenous cannulation, drug and fluid administration, support of family, assisting with neonatal resuscitation.
13. Maintain detailed records of all actions taken.
14. Fully debrief following the resuscitation.

NEWBORN RESUSCITATION

Approximately 3% of babies born at term will require assistance to transition to extrauterine life (Barber & Wyckoff 2006, Ersdal et al 2012, Perlman & Risser 1995). The aim of neonatal resuscitation is to restore tissue oxygen delivery before irreversible damage occurs, which may affect long-term neurodevelopment and increase the mortality rate (Harach 2013). Most neonates who require support require non-invasive assistance only to initiate spontaneous ventilation, and only very few are born truly lifeless and need intubation (2%) and/or cardiac compressions (0.1%) (ANZCOR n.d.). Prompt initiation of resuscitation is critical (Amin et al 2013) and the quality of care provided during the first few minutes after birth has a significant effect on long-term health (Rovamo et al 2013). Niermeyer and Clarke (2011) suggest that with each minute resuscitation is delayed, the time to the first gasp increases by about 2 minutes and the onset of spontaneous breathing can be delayed beyond 4 minutes. It is therefore vital that the midwife is able to anticipate and recognise the baby that requires resuscitative assistance at birth and provide this efficiently and competently to reduce morbidity and mortality associated with birth asphyxia. This section provides an overview of principles and processes for supporting the compromised or collapsed neonate, however the reader is advised to maintain neonatal resuscitation competence through regular accredited training and update courses and simulated practice.

The International Liaison Committee on Resuscitation (ILCOR) is a multinational group with representation from eight international resuscitation councils: the American Heart Association, the European Resuscitation Council, the Heart and Stroke Foundation of Canada, the Resuscitation Council of Asia, the Resuscitation Council of South Africa, the ANZCOR (comprising the Australian Resuscitation Council and the New Zealand Resuscitation Council: Whakahauora Aotearoa) and the InterAmerican Heart Foundation. ILCOR members review and debate the evidence on neonatal resuscitation and their recommendations are produced as guidelines by resuscitation councils; across the world. There may be subtle differences between guidelines adopted by different resuscitation councils; therefore, the midwife who intends to work in different countries is advised to review the resuscitation council guidelines of each before practising there.

At birth there are a number of adaptations the baby has to make to successfully transition from intrauterine to extrauterine life. The airways of the lungs are fluid-filled prior to birth and must quickly change to being air-filled for effective ventilation to occur. The alveoli in the lungs expand and maintain this expansion with the assistance of surfactant. A functional residual capacity (FRC) is created following the first few breaths. Pulmonary blood flow dramatically increases, which assists in the reversal of blood flow through the ductus arteriosus and the closure of the foramen ovale. Negative pressures as high as –80 cm H_2O can be generated by the baby with the first breaths, with lower pressures required for subsequent breaths. Lung expansion occurs in conjunction with an increase in the alveolar oxygen tension, which results in decreased pulmonary vascular resistance and increased pulmonary blood flow. Oxygen saturation levels increase slowly over the first 5–10 minutes. There is a significant difference in pre- and post-ductal oxygen saturation levels during the first 15 minutes of life. At this point, Beşkardeş and colleagues (2012) suggest it is possible the transfer of blood from right to left along the ductus arteriosus has stopped, increasing saturation levels in the extremities.

Babies who cannot produce adequate alveolar expansion develop respiratory failure and the change in pulmonary vascular resistance does not occur, resulting in persistent pulmonary hypertension, decreased pulmonary blood flow and hypoxaemia.

Very preterm babies can quickly succumb to surfactant deficiency preventing the alveoli from maintaining their expansion. They also may have weaker lung muscles, underdeveloped airway protective reflexes and a reduced drive to breathe. Post-mature babies may pass meconium into the amniotic fluid, which can be inhaled before or during labour, causing inflammation of the lungs and airway obstruction.

Pathophysiology of asphyxia

Asphyxia refers to inadequate tissue perfusion that does not meet the metabolic demands of the tissues for oxygen and removal of waste (Niermeyer & Clarke 2011), resulting in increasing hypoxia, hypercapnia and acidosis. This will cause a change in metabolism from aerobic to anaerobic, creating a metabolic acidosis, initially buffered by bicarbonate. As the bicarbonate is depleted, acidosis worsens. The initial response to asphyxia is an increased heart rate followed by decreased cardiac output and peripheral vasoconstriction in an attempt to maintain the blood pressure so that perfusion of the vital organs occurs. As acidosis worsens, cardiac failure can ensue with a decrease in heart rate and blood pressure.

Which newborns might need resuscitation?

There may be known maternal, fetal or intrapartum factors that increase the likelihood of the need for neonatal resuscitation. These include:

- maternal disease (e.g. pre-eclampsia)
- maternal infection (e.g. chorioamnionitis)
- maternal substance abuse
- fetal abnormality (e.g. diaphragmatic hernia)
- intrauterine growth restriction
- ante- or intrapartum haemorrhage
- prolonged rupture of membranes
- malposition or malpresentation (e.g. breech)
- abnormalities of the fetal heart rate indicative of fetal compromise
- induction and augmentation of labour
- preterm labour
- significant meconium within the amniotic fluid
- heavy maternal sedation
- prolonged labour
- instrumental and operative delivery
- obstetric emergency (e.g. cord prolapse, shoulder dystocia).

However, there will always be the unexpected situation that reminds the midwife of the importance of ensuring resuscitation equipment is available for every birth, highlighting the requirement that all midwives are trained in and practise neonatal resuscitation on at least a yearly basis so there is at least one person at the birth who is trained in newborn life support (Kattwinkel et al 2010, Richmond & Wyllie 2010). Ideally, two midwives are present at each birth, allowing one to attend to the immediate needs of the baby and the other to call for emergency assistance. In the hospital environment this may be through the use of the emergency bell or emergency phone number, while in the community the paramedic service should be accessed by ringing 000 in Australia, and 111 in New Zealand.

Training in neonatal resuscitation should occur in the environment and with the equipment the midwife uses in their work. Multidisciplinary training is ideal as good teamwork behaviours are correlated with higher quality of care during resuscitation (Sawyer et al 2013). Cusack and Fawke (2012) suggest significant decay in psychomotor skills occurs as soon as 3 months following training in resuscitation and advise refresher training and assessment should ideally occur 6 months after attending a resuscitation course to increase retention of knowledge and psychomotor skills.

Equipment

The majority of newborns that require assistance to transition to extrauterine life need minimal support, for which only a small amount of equipment is necessary. In the hospital or birth centre environment it is likely that a standard resuscitation platform (most commonly, a Resuscitaire®), with additional equipment, is available. The neonatal Resuscitaire® is equipped with a flat surface at optimal working height, good heat and light sources, an oxygen source (via either a cylinder or connection to piped oxygen), equipment for ventilation such as a NeoPuff/self-inflating bag and the ability to blend air and oxygen, and a clock. The neonatal Resuscitaire® can be switched on in preparation for the birth so the environment is pre-warmed, regardless of whether or not the need for resuscitation is anticipated. All of the equipment should be checked to ensure everything that may be required is available and working correctly, and the clock should be started when the baby is born. Most 'all-in-one' resuscitation surfaces are height-adjustable and on wheels, so they can be placed close to the newborn's mother to allow resuscitation to occur at the bedside with an unclamped umbilical cord; the newborn then has the benefit of delayed cord clamping (see Chapter 43).

In the home environment, the equipment for resuscitation should be laid out ready next to a flat surface and away from draughts. A supply of warm towels should be made available. This area may be close to the woman so that if resuscitation is required it can be undertaken with the cord still attached and unclamped.

The requirements for each aspect of resuscitation are listed in Box 42.1.

Principles of neonatal resuscitation

The following principles are underpinned by the Australia New Zealand Committee for Resuscitation Neonatal Resuscitation guidelines (ANZCOR, n.d.). These apply predominantly to term babies. For considerations specific to preterm and very preterm neonates, the reader is directed to consult a specialist neonatal care text.

Environment

Babies are born wet and into a cooler environment, which means heat loss can occur quickly. It is important to dry the newborn as soon as possible; this action provides stimulation and encourages spontaneous breathing. The newborn must be cared for away from drafts to help them maintain a temperature of 36.5°C to 37.5°C: on the mother's chest with both covered by a warm, dry towel or blanket, and then moved to a flat resuscitation surface with radiant heat if additional support is necessary.

Umbilical cord clamping

Delaying the clamping of the umbilical cord appears to be beneficial for term and preterm neonates in the short and long term (Polglase & Stark 2018), although it does increase the likelihood of the neonate needing phototherapy for jaundice (Mercer et al 2017). In preterm newborns, the benefits remain, but there is seemingly no increased risk of needing phototherapy

Box 42.1 Recommended equipment and drugs for resuscitation

General

- Firm, horizontal, padded resuscitation surface
- Overhead warmer
- Light for the area
- Clock with timer in seconds
- Warmed towels or similar covering
- Polythene bag or sheet, big enough for a baby less than 1500 g birthweight
- Stethoscope, neonatal size preferred
- Pulse oximeter plus neonatal probe

Equipment for airway management

- Suction apparatus and suction catheters (6F, 8F and either 10F or 12F)
- Oropharyngeal airways (sizes 0 and 00)
- Intubation equipment:
  - Laryngoscopes with infant blades (00, 0, 1)
  - Spare bulbs and batteries
  - Endotracheal tubes (sizes 2.5, 3, 3.5, and 4 mm ID, uncuffed, no eye)
  - Endotracheal stylet or introducer
  - Supplies for fixing endotracheal tubes (e.g. scissors, tape)
- End-tidal carbon dioxide detector (to confirm intubation)
- Meconium suction device (to apply suction directly to endotracheal tube)
- Magill forceps, neonatal size (optional)
- Laryngeal mask airway, size 1

Equipment for supporting breathing

- Facemasks (range of sizes suitable for premature and term infants)
- Positive pressure ventilation device, either:
  - T-piece device, or;
  - Flow-inflating bag with a pressure safety valve and manometer; and
  - Self-inflating bag (approximately 240 mL) with a removable oxygen reservoir
- Medical gases:
  - Source of medical oxygen (reticulated and/or cylinder, allowing flow rate of up to 10 L/min) with flow meter and tubing
  - Source of medical air plus air/oxygen blender
- Feeding tubes for gastric decompression (e.g. size 6F & 8F)

Equipment for supporting the circulation

- Umbilical venous catheter (UVC) kit (including UVC size 5F)
- Peripheral IV cannulation kit
- Skin preparation solution suitable for newborn skin
- Tapes/devices to secure UVC/IV cannula
- Syringes and needles (assorted sizes)
- Intraosseous needles

Drugs and fluids

- Adrenaline (epinephrine): 1 : 10 000 concentration (0.1 mg/mL)
- Volume expanders
- Normal saline
- Blood suitable for emergency neonatal transfusion needs to be readily available for a profoundly anaemic baby

Documentation

- Resuscitation record sheet

Source: Source: Australia and New Zealand Committee on Resuscitation (ANZCOR): All neonatal guidelines (Section 13.4), n.d. Online 18 April 2021. Available: https://resus.org.au/guidelines/.

(Wyllie et al 2015). ANZCOR thus suggest delaying cord clamping for preterm neonates that don't require immediate resuscitation, however, they caution that resuscitation measures should take priority, and the cord should be clamped and cut to facilitate these if necessary. On the basis of little evidence to recommend it, ANZCOR recommend against umbilical cord milking in any situation (n.d.).

Assessing the neonate

The need to begin neonatal resuscitation is established immediately following birth, and if it is necessary to commence resuscitation, the need to continue with it is continually assessed throughout. The first assessment focuses on three aspects: tone and response to stimulation; breathing, and heart rate. Other assessments to be considered are colour, pulse oximetry and umbilical artery cord blood gases.

Tone and response to stimulation

The majority of neonates will require no assistance: they usually begin moving, breathing spontaneously and maintaining a heart rate of > 100 bpm soon after birth. Those whose responses are absent or weak should be dried briskly but gently with a soft warm towel to stimulate breathing, while active resuscitation is likely to be needed by the neonate who is not responsive.

Breathing

Eighty-five per cent of babies born near or at term begin spontaneously breathing within 30 seconds of being born. Ninety-five per cent do so within 45 seconds (Ersdal et al 2014). If the neonate has a good tone and is maintaining a heart rate of 100 bpm or greater, immediate respiratory support may not be necessary. Persistent recession, retraction or drawing in of the lower rib cage and sternum, or persistent grunting on expiration, indicate that **continuous positive airway pressure (CPAP)** or **intermittent positive airway pressure (IPPV)** would be beneficial. The neonate who exhibits persistent apnoea, is hypotonic, and is bradycardic (HR < 100 bpm) is at risk of serious compromise and IPPV is required urgently.

Heart rate

Soon after birth, the heart rate of most well and healthy newborns is around 130 bpm, although the normal range is 110–160 bpm. A neonatal heart rate of < 100 bpm is a cause for concern. An increasing heart rate is the best sign that the neonate's condition is improving, while a decreasing one is an indicator of deterioration. CPAP or assisted ventilation is advised if the neonate's heart rate falls to and remains below 100 bpm at any time after about 2 minutes of age.

Colour

Well and healthy neonates often appear blue at birth, but become pink when regular respirations ensue. Acrocyanosis (blueish hands and feet) can remain for several months. If the neonate does not 'pink up', oxygen saturation levels should be checked. Cyanosis is suspected if the gums and mucous membranes appear blueish. The neonate who remains pallid, even despite ventilation, may be acidotic, hypotensive secondary to poor cardiac output and/or hypovolaemia, or severely anaemic.

Pulse oximetry

Pulse oximetry is recommended if it is anticipated that resuscitation will be necessary, when CPAP or IPPV has been commenced, when the neonate is cyanotic, and/or if the neonate is receiving supplemental oxygen.

Umbilical artery cord blood gases

Wherever possible, umbilical artery cord gases should be obtained and measured in neonates who undergo resuscitation, as they will help provide an understanding of whether cerebral palsy was the consequence of an intrapartum event (MacLennan 1999).

Airway management and mask ventilation

If the baby cannot maintain her/his own airway and respirations, assistance must be given. According to ANZCOR (n.d.), successful neonatal resuscitation depends on effective ventilation. The following guidance is drawn directly from that disseminated by the ANZCOR member organisations, the Australian and the New Zealand Resuscitation Councils, on their respective websites (see Resources at the end of the chapter).

Positioning and the airway

Where resuscitation is necessary, the neonate should be laid supine, and his/her head in a neutral or slightly extended position (Fig 42.3). Where moulding has occurred during birth and has not reduced by the time resuscitation is required, the placement of a 2 cm thick bolster (e.g. a folded blanket or towel) should be placed beneath the neonate's shoulders to optimise the effectiveness of resuscitative measures.

If the newborn is making an effort to breathe, but not doing so effectively and the heart rate remains

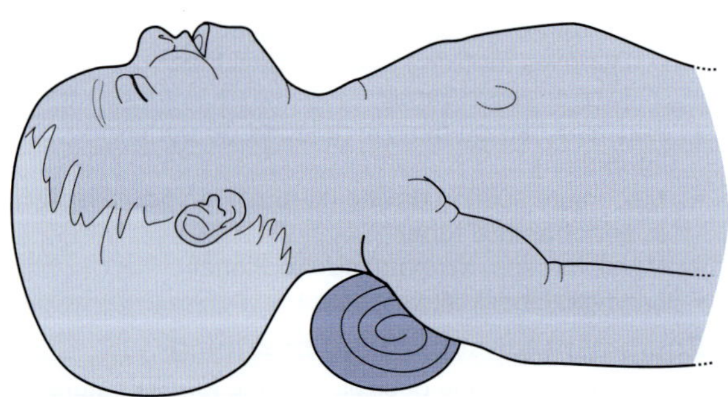

FIGURE 42.3 **Neutral position.**
Source: Johnson R, Taylor W: Skills for midwifery practice, 4th ed., Elsevier, London, 2016.

below 100 bpm, obstruction of the airway may have occurred. In this case, measures to improve the patency of the airway should be considered. These may include supporting the neonate's lower jaw, maintaining an open mouth or suctioning of the upper airways. Oral or pharyngeal suction should not be routinely performed, although it may be required to clear meconium, blood clots, tenacious mucous or vernix. For neonates born through meconium-stained liquor, routine endotracheal suction is no longer recommended on the basis that it has not been found to reliably prevent meconium aspiration syndrome. If meconium needs to be removed because it is obstructing the airway, the procedure should be performed briefly and with great care to prevent soft tissue damage and bradycardia.

Positive pressure ventilation

If drying and stimulation is ineffective in establishing adequate respirations (that is, the heart rate is not maintained at 100 bpm), either CPAP or intermittent positive pressure ventilation (IPPV) will be required. In a breathing neonate, CPAP may be commenced to augment her/his own efforts. In the non-breathing neonate, IPPV is necessary. Either a T-piece device (preferred by ANZCOR), a self-inflating bag or a flow-inflating bag may be used to ventilate neonates via a facemask, a laryngeal mask or an endotracheal tube, where this equipment is not available, ANZCOR (n.d.) recommend mouth-to-mouth-and-nose ventilation. The infant's face should first be cleaned of maternal blood and other fluids to decrease the risk of infection to the resuscitator. The mask should then be placed over the infant's mouth and nose, and tiny puffs should be delivered at a rate of 40–60 breaths per minute to cause the infant's chest to rise and fall slightly. This intervention is continued until the neonate's respiration improves. Laryngeal mask application and tracheal intubation is outside the scope of the midwife's role, and is thus not covered in this chapter.

When using a facemask, the correct size must be selected to ensure it effects a seal around the mouth and nose, and the head and jaw position must be correct (see above)(Fig 42.4). A rolling motion should be used to apply the facemask, starting from the chin and moving towards the nose bridge. A suitable grip should be used to hold the facemask in place and prevent the escape of air/oxygen (Figs 42.5 and 42.6). Effective ventilation clears lung liquid, establishes lung aeration and enables gas exchange. Initial pressures for term infants and preterm infants are suggested to be 30 cm, 20–25 cm H_2O. Where **positive end expiratory pressure (PEEP)** can be delivered, the initial setting is recommended to be 5 cm H_2O. Pressures should be increased or reduced according

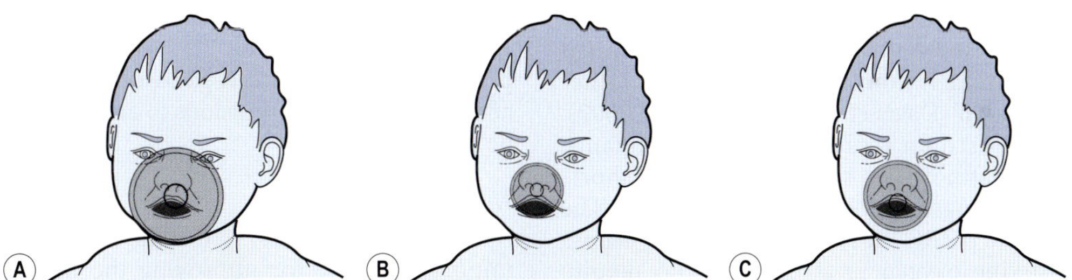

FIGURE 42.4 **Correct positioning of the facemask. A, Facemask too large. B, Facemask too small. C, Facemask correct size.**
Source: Johnson R, Taylor W: Skills for midwifery practice, 4th ed., Elsevier, London, 2016.

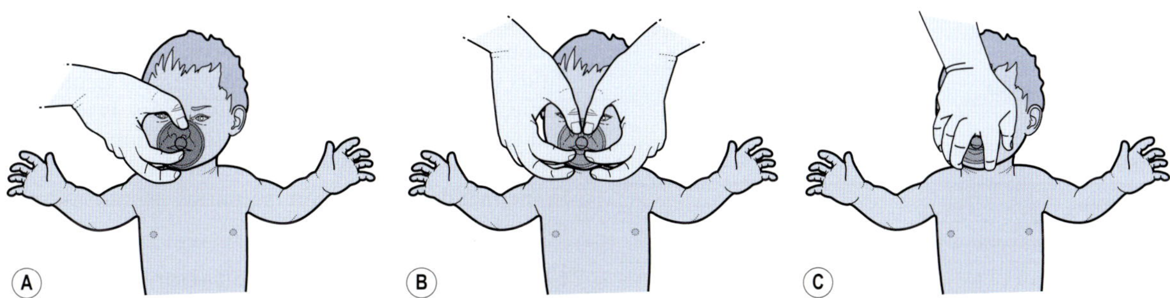

FIGURE 42.5 **Three ways of holding the facemask in position. A, Two-point top hold. B, Two-handed hold. C, Spider hold.**
Source: Johnson R, Taylor W: Skills for midwifery practice, 4th ed., Elsevier, London, 2016.

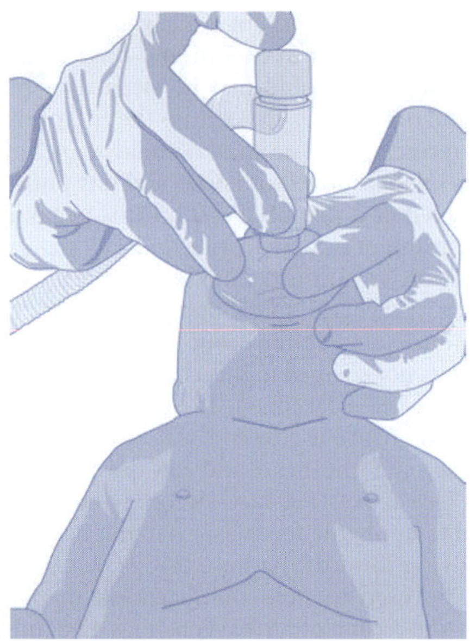

FIGURE 42.6 **Administering positive pressure ventilation via facemask.**
Source: Australia and New Zealand Committee on Resuscitation (ANZCOR): All neonatal guidelines (Section 13.4), n.d., p. 3. Online 18 April 2021. Available: https://resus.org.au/guidelines/.

to the response. For infants that have not made any respiratory effort, the first few inflations may need to be higher. Increased survival has been demonstrated when resuscitation is commenced with 21% rather than 100% oxygen (Davis et al 2004, Rabi et al 2007). Where IPPV is used for resuscitation of term infants, 100% oxygen has not been shown to have any short-term benefits (Saugstad 1998, Vento et al 2001). The ARC (2021) and NZRC (2021) assert that the purpose of administering oxygen to all infants who require it is to achieve a saturation level that resembles that

TABLE 42.1 TARGET SATURATIONS—OXYGEN

Time from birth	Target saturations for newborn infants during resuscitation
1 minute	60–70
2 minutes	65–85
3 minutes	70–90
4 minutes	75–90
5 minutes	80–90
10 minutes	85–90

Source: Australia and New Zealand Committee on Resuscitation (ANZCOR): All neonatal guidelines (Section 13.4), n.d., p. 6. Online 18 April 2021. Available: https://resus.org.au/guidelines/.

of a healthy term baby (see Table 42.1). Initially, air (21% oxygen) should be used, and the oxygen content increased as necessary to achieve that purpose.

Clinicians responsible for resuscitation should aim to assist the neonate to attain effective spontaneous breathing within one minute of birth. If this is not attained, or the neonate deteriorates, progress to the next step in the ANZCOR neonatal resuscitation algorithm (Fig 42.7).

Chest compressions

As noted earlier, a well and healthy newborn has a heart rate between 110 and 160 bpm once breathing has been established. Chest compressions are indicated when the heart rate is lower than 60 bpm despite the provision of adequate assisted ventilation for 30 seconds. Once it has been decided that cardiac compressions are necessary, venous access should be established and intravenous adrenaline should be administered. The correct location for the resuscitator to perform chest compressions is over the bottom third of the neonate's sternum, and each compression should depress the chest to one-third of his or her anterior–posterior chest diameter. The resuscitator places both thumbs, either superimposed or adjacent to one another, over the bottom third of the sternum (Fig 42.8). The remaining fingers are placed around the thorax and rest on the infant's back. The neonate can be positioned with his or her head either distal or proximal to the resuscitator (Figs 42.8 and 42.9). The ratio of inflations to chest compressions should be 3:1, with 90 compressions performed each minute. A pause of half a second is left after every three compressions to enable an inflation to be delivered.

Medications and fluids

As noted at the start of this section, the most important factor for improving the neonate's heart rate is adequate ventilation. If, despite competent resuscitation, a heart rate of less than 60 bpm persists, adrenaline (epinephrine) may be needed. Ideally, adrenaline (epinephrine) is given as close to the heart as possible, because part of its effect is by its action on the heart. If practical, it should be administered as a rapid bolus through an umbilical venous catheter. Intravascular crystalloid or colloid fluids will need to be considered when the neonate is suspected to have experienced blood loss, is in shock and is not responsive to other resuscitation methods. The administration of intravascular fluids and drugs in neonatal resuscitation scenarios is outside the midwife's scope of practice.

Discontinuation of resuscitation

Both the Australian and the New Zealand Resuscitation Councils agree that if a neonate's heartbeat cannot be detected after 10 minutes of competent resuscitation, both the likelihood of the neonate surviving, and

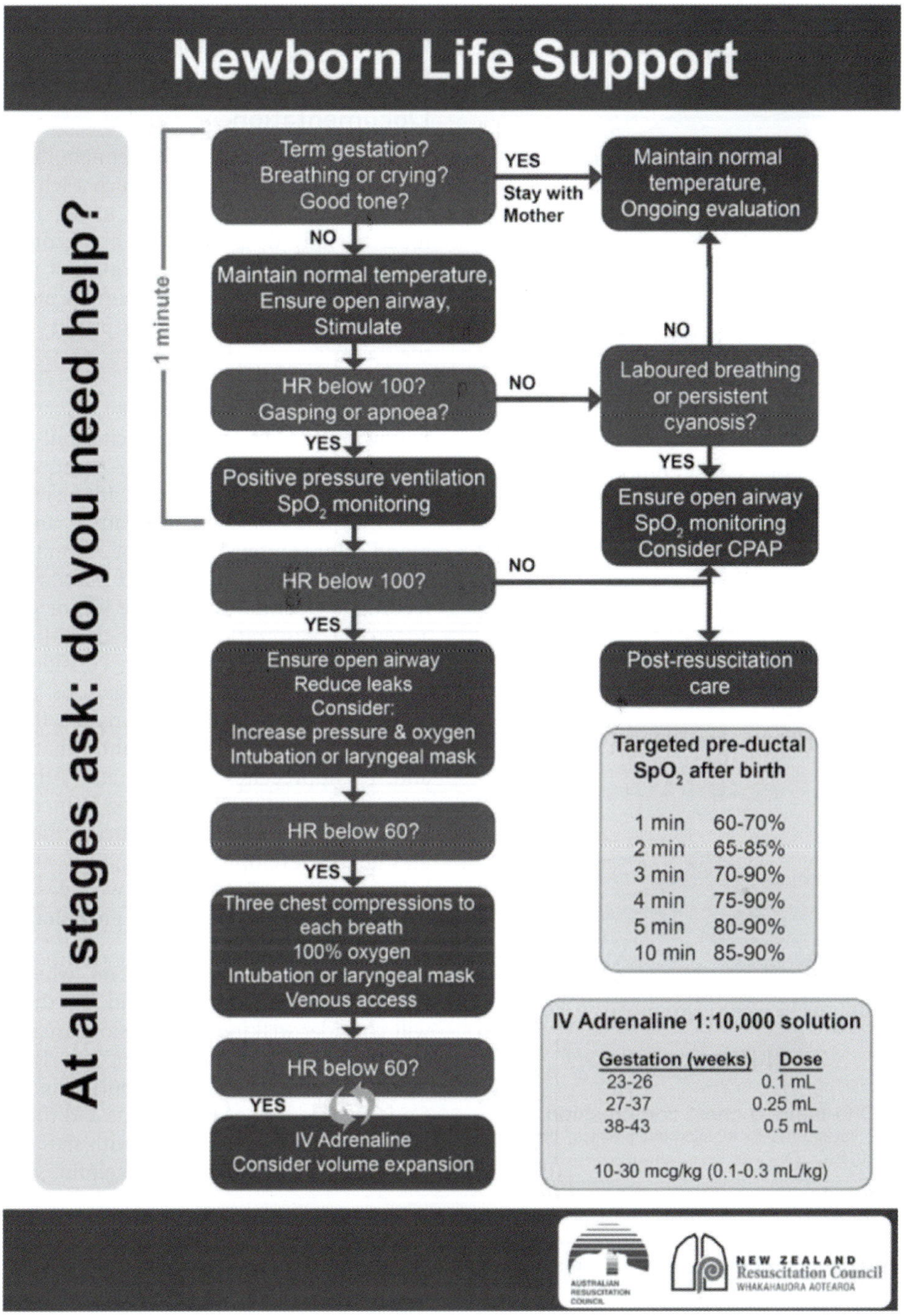

Newborn Life Support

At all stages ask: do you need help?

1 minute

Term gestation?
Breathing or crying?
Good tone?

YES — Stay with Mother → Maintain normal temperature, Ongoing evaluation

NO ↓

Maintain normal temperature,
Ensure open airway,
Stimulate

↓

HR below 100?
Gasping or apnoea?

NO → Laboured breathing or persistent cyanosis?
- NO → Maintain normal temperature, Ongoing evaluation
- YES ↓ Ensure open airway, SpO_2 monitoring, Consider CPAP

YES ↓

Positive pressure ventilation
SpO_2 monitoring

↓

HR below 100?

NO → Ensure open airway, SpO_2 monitoring, Consider CPAP / Post-resuscitation care

YES ↓

Ensure open airway
Reduce leaks
Consider:
Increase pressure & oxygen
Intubation or laryngeal mask

↓

HR below 60?

YES ↓

Three chest compressions to each breath
100% oxygen
Intubation or laryngeal mask
Venous access

↓

HR below 60?

YES ↓

IV Adrenaline
Consider volume expansion

Targeted pre-ductal SpO_2 after birth

1 min	60-70%
2 min	65-85%
3 min	70-90%
4 min	75-90%
5 min	80-90%
10 min	85-90%

IV Adrenaline 1:10,000 solution

Gestation (weeks)	Dose
23-26	0.1 mL
27-37	0.25 mL
38-43	0.5 mL

10-30 mcg/kg (0.1-0.3 mL/kg)

AUSTRALIAN RESUSCITATION COUNCIL

NEW ZEALAND Resuscitation Council WHAKAHAUORA AOTEAROA

FIGURE 42.7 **ANZCOR Neonatal resuscitation algorithm.**
Source: Australia and New Zealand Committee on Resuscitation (ANZCOR): All neonatal guidelines (Section 13.4), n.d., p. 7. Online 18 April 2021. Available: https://resus.org.au/guidelines/.

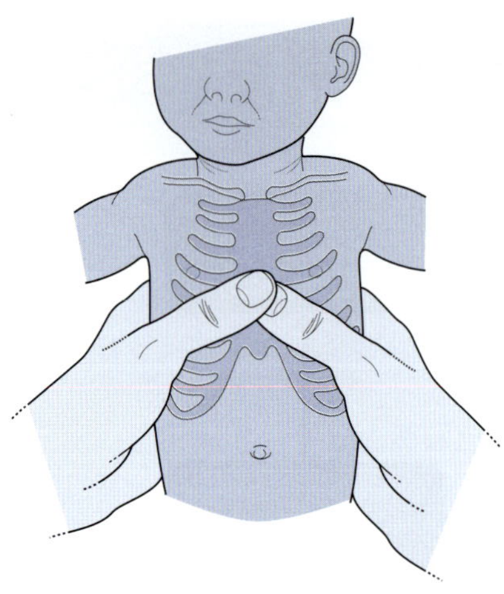

FIGURE 42.8 **Two-handed chest compression.**
Source: Johnson R, Taylor W: Skills for midwifery practice, 4th ed., Elsevier, London, 2016.

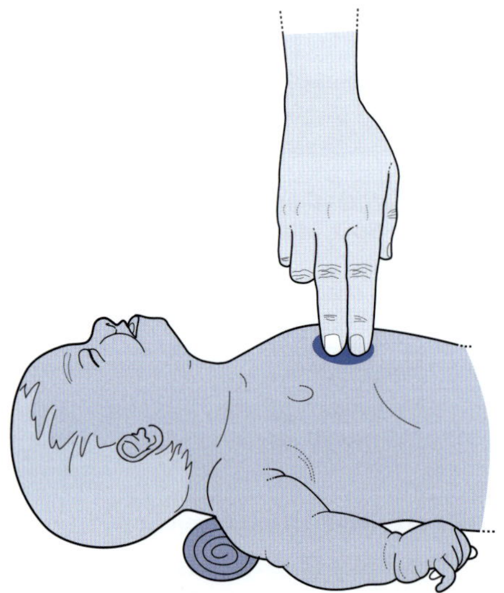

FIGURE 42.9 **One-handed chest compression.**
Source: Johnson R, Taylor W: Skills for midwifery practice, 4th ed., Elsevier, London, 2016.

the likely quality of his or her survival, deteriorate markedly. However, there are circumstances in which that timeframe may be extended (ANZCOR, n.d.).

Documentation

The observations made of the neonate, the interventions administered, the times at which each occurred, and the personnel present during neonatal resuscitation, must be fully documented. This record is made for clinical and medico–legal reasons, but it also provides the basis for the conversation with the neonate's parents that must occur to help them process and transition the event.

After the resuscitation

Following a successful resuscitation, the baby will either remain with his or her parents or, if unwell, will be moved to a neonatal intensive care setting. The neonate's body temperature and his or her blood glucose level must be monitored, because the baby may not be able to maintain these. Early feeding is essential due to the use of glucose during anaerobic respiration. As resuscitation may have been required due to sepsis, consideration should be given to whether investigations and antibiotic therapy are warranted. The parents will need support and information to understand what has occurred and to appreciate whether any further concerns exist. Therapeutic hypothermia is increasingly being recognised as helpful for reducing the risk of death and neuro-developmental disability at 18 months in babies $>$ 36 weeks gestation who develop moderate to severe **hypoxic ischaemic encephalopathy (HIE)** (Richmond & Wyllie 2010).

Local protocols will vary on when to halt the resuscitation if it is unsuccessful, but the paediatrician will consider making the decision usually when there has been no detectable heart rate for 10 minutes despite full resuscitation support (Finan et al 2011). Considerable care of the parents and the staff involved will be required. A debriefing with staff involved in the birth and resuscitation can be helpful.

SKILL 42.2 Neonatal resuscitation (Australia and New Zealand)

1. In hospital or birth centre settings: Check the neonatal Resuscitaire® is fully stocked and everything is in working order prior to the baby's birth; when birth is imminent, switch on the heater and light.
2. At home: Prepare the area and equipment for resuscitation, as outlined earlier in this section.
3. If possible, start the clock as soon as the baby is born.
4. Dry and stimulate the baby at birth and assess the need for resuscitation away from the woman.
5. When the need for resuscitation **away from the woman** is established, move the baby to the resuscitation area and turn on the clock (if not on), noting the time.
6. Dry and stimulate the baby thoroughly, remove the damp towel; wrap in a clean, warm towel, with the chest exposed.

SKILL 42.2 Neonatal resuscitation (Australia and New Zealand)—cont'd

7. Position the baby's head in the neutral position.
8. Assess breathing, tone and heart rate (and reassess every 30 seconds):
   - breathing spontaneously, heart rate > 100 bpm—keep the baby warm and return her/him to the woman for skin-to-skin contact
   - breathing irregularly with a heart rate > 100 bpm—provide tactile stimulation, keep the baby warm and the head in the neutral position; continue to assess tone, respiratory effort and heart rate, returning the neonate to her/his mother when breathing spontaneously and heart rate > 100 bpm
   - no respiratory effort, gasping evident, breathing remains irregular, or heart rate < 100 bpm—commence positive pressure ventilation.
9. Send out an emergency call for appropriate personnel (if an anticipated problem the paediatrician should already be present).
10. Ensure the baby's head is in the neutral position with an open airway.
11. Inflate the lungs at a rate of 40–60 breaths per minute, with air (21% oxygen), looking for chest movement. If no chest movement is seen, check the baby's head and mask position and repeat inflation.
12. Following 30 seconds of inflation breaths with concurrent chest movement, reassess the heart rate:
    - heart rate > 100 bpm—continue with ventilation breaths until spontaneous respiration occurs. Reassess breathing, heart rate and tone every 30 seconds.
    - heart rate < 60 bpm—commence chest compressions at a rate of three compressions to one ventilation breath and continue to reassess breathing, heart rate and tone every 30 seconds; when the heart rate is ≥ 60 bpm, stop chest compressions, but continue with ventilation breaths until spontaneous respiration occurs with the heart rate > 100 bpm.
13. Secure a neonatal oxygen saturation probe on the baby's right hand or wrist as soon as possible, then include saturation levels in the 30-second assessments:
    - if oxygen saturation levels are below the target level for the age of the baby, increase the amount of oxygen to the next level (e.g. from 21% to 30%)
    - once the oxygen saturation level is reached, begin to reduce the amount of oxygen given.
14. If the condition of the baby does not improve, the neonatologist will consider venous access, drugs and intravascular fluids.
15. Assist with preparing for transfer, if necessary.
16. Document all steps.
17. Discuss the resuscitation with the parents.

Role and responsibilities of the midwife

These can be summarised as follows.

Maternal collapse

- Keeping up-to-date with changes to the resuscitation guidelines
- Attending CPR updates on at least an annual basis
- Swift recognition and response in the event of collapse
- Undertaking CPR quickly and effectively, including cardiac compressions and ventilation breaths
- Attaching the AED leads as soon as possible and following the voice prompts of the AED device
- Recognising the need for and undertaking the adaptations necessary for resuscitating the pregnant woman
- Undertaking other aspects of care (e.g. intravenous cannulation, neonatal resuscitation, care of the family)
- Debriefing with appropriate members of the medical team
- Detailed contemporaneous records

Neonate resuscitation

- Ensuring knowledge around resuscitation and resuscitation guidelines is current
- Maintaining competent resuscitation skills, including correct use of equipment
- Anticipating the need for resuscitation and preparation of the environment and equipment
- Undertaking the assessment at birth and recognising the need for resuscitation
- Summoning appropriate medical/newborn life support (NLS) trained assistance, if not present
- Supporting and assisting others during the resuscitation
- Accurate contemporaneous record keeping
- Information for, and support of, the parents during and following the event
- Appropriate transfer of the care of the woman and baby

SUMMARY

Maternal collapse

- Maternal resuscitation is a rare occurrence; thus it is important that resuscitation skills are practised at least yearly.

- Calling for help is essential when a non-responsive person is found.
- If the person is not breathing or making gasping noises, cardiac arrest is assumed and compressions commenced.
- Cardiac compressions are the most important component of resuscitation and interruptions should be minimised.
- Cardiac compressions delivered at a rate of 100–120 per minute, at a depth of 5–6 cm, and with the chest allowed to recoil between compressions, are associated with an increased survival rate.
- A defibrillator should be attached and used early in the resuscitation, as this may increase the likelihood of survival.
- Adaptations are required when resuscitating a pregnant woman due to the physiological changes of pregnancy that make resuscitation more difficult: a wedge for displacement of the uterus and delivery of the baby at 5 minutes.

Neonate resuscitation

- The midwife has a responsible role in the recognition and management of neonatal resuscitation.
- Equipment should be accessible and the midwife should be familiar with its use.
- Appropriate help should be sought quickly.
- Management includes drying the baby and assessing tone, respiratory effort and heart rate.
- A neonatal oxygen saturation probe should be applied to the neonate as soon as possible.
- Resuscitation should begin in room air and the oxygen level increased according to the oxygen saturation level.
- Cardiac compressions using the two-handed technique are undertaken if the heart rate is below 60 bpm once the lungs have been oxygenated.
- Manoeuvres to open the airway and ventilate the lungs and chest compression should be undertaken efficiently when required.
- Routine oropharyngeal suctioning is not recommended.
- Drug and fluid therapy may be required when the response is poor.

Self-assessment exercises

The answers to the following questions may be found in the text.

1. What conditions may predispose the pregnant or postnatal woman to a cardiac arrest?
2. What actions would you take, in order, when finding a collapsed woman?
3. Describe how to perform effective cardiac compressions.
4. How can effective ventilation be achieved?
5. What adaptations may be needed for a woman being resuscitated at 38 weeks' gestation?
6. Summarise the role and responsibilities of the midwife when resuscitating a pregnant woman.
7. Identify five situations in which you would anticipate the need for neonatal resuscitation.
8. List the equipment required for neonatal resuscitation.
9. What would you assess in the baby at birth to determine if resuscitation is required?
10. How can the midwife ensure the baby's airway is patent?
11. What percentage of oxygen would you use to begin resuscitation?
12. When would you increase the amount of oxygen?
13. When would you undertake oropharyngeal suctioning?
14. When are chest compressions required and how are they undertaken?
15. Demonstrate/simulate a neonatal resuscitation, giving verbal explanations for the actions taken.

Resources

Australian Resuscitation Council (ARC): resus.org.au/.

Australian and New Zealand Committee on Resuscitation (ANZCOR) guidelines: https://resus.org.au/guidelines/ (Section 13) and www.nzrc.org.nz/assets/Guidelines/Neonatal-Resus/All-Neonatal-guidelines-June-2017.pdf.

International Liaison Committee on Resuscitation (ILCOR): www.ilcor.org/home/.

New Zealand Resuscitation Council: Whakahauora Aotearoa (NZRC): www.nzrc.org.nz/.

References

Amin HJ, Aziz K, Halamer LP, et al: Simulation-based learning combined with debriefing: trainers' satisfaction with a new approach to training the trainers to teach neonatal resuscitation, BMC Research Notes 6:251, 2013.

Australia and New Zealand Committee on Resuscitation (ANZCOR): All neonatal guidelines (Section 13), n.d. Online 18 April 2021. Available: https://resus.org.au/guidelines/.

Australia and New Zealand Committee on Resuscitation (ANZCOR): Resuscitation in special circumstances, 2011. Online 18 April 2021. Available: https://resus.org.au/guidelines/.

Australian Resuscitation Council (ARC): The ARC guidelines, 2021. Online 16 August 2021. Available: https://resus.org.au/guidelines/.

Barber CA, Wyckoff MH: Use and efficacy of endotracheal versus intravenous epinephrine during neonatal cardiopulmonary resuscitation in the delivery room, Pediatrics 118:1028–1034, 2006.

Beesems SG, Wijmans L, Tijssen JGP, et al: Duration of ventilations during cardiopulmonary resuscitation by lay rescuers and first responders: relationship between delivering cardiac compressions and outcomes, Circulation 127:1585–1590, 2013.

Bennett T-A, Katz VL, Zelop C: Cardiac arrest and resuscitation unique to pregnancy, Obstetric & Gynecology Clinics of North America 43:809–819, 2016.

Beşkardeş A, Salihoğlu Ö, Can E, et al: Oxygen saturation of healthy term neonates during the first 30 minutes of life, Pediatrics International 55:44–48, 2012.

Bosson N, Gordon PE: Bag-valve-mask ventilation, 2018. Online 26 July 2018. Available: https://emedicine.medscape.com/article/80184-technique#c2.

Bowden T, Smith D: An overview of adult cardiopulmonary resuscitation equipment, Nursing Standard 31(23): 54–63, 2017.

Contri E, Cornara S, Somaschini A, et al: Complete chest recoil during laypersons' CPR: is it a matter of weight? The American Journal of Emergency Medicine 35(9):1266–1268, 2017.

Cunningham LM, Mattu A, O'Connor RE, Brady, W: Cardiopulmonary resuscitation for cardiac arrest: the importance of uninterrupted cardiac compressions in cardiac arrest resuscitation, American Journal of Emergency Medicine 30:630–1638, 2012.

Cusack J, Fawke J: Neonatal resuscitation: are your trainees performing as you think they are? A retrospective assessment for neonatal medical trainees over an 8-year period, Archives of Disease in Childhood. Fetal and Neonatal Edition 97:F246–F248, 2012.

Davis PG, Tan A, O'Donnell CP, et al: Resuscitation of newborn infants with 100% oxygen or air: a systematic review and meta-analysis, Lancet 364:1329–1333, 2004.

Dohi S, Ichizuka K, Matsuoka R, et al: Coronary perfusion pressure and compression quality in maternal cardiopulmonary resuscitation in supine and left-lateral tilt positions: a prospective, crossover study using mannequins and swine models, European Journal of Obstetrics, Gynecology, and Reproductive Biology 216:98–103, 2017.

Ducloy-Bouthers A-S, Gonzalez-Estevez M, Constans B, et al: Cardiovascular emergencies and cardiac arrest in a pregnant woman, Anaesthesia Critical Care & Pain Medicine 35(Suppl 1):S43–S50, 2016.

Edwards M: Basic resuscitation, O&G Magazine 19(2):12–13, 2017.

Ersdal HL, Linde J, Mduma E, et al: Neonatal outcome following cord clamping after onset of spontaneous respiration, Pediatrics 134:265–272, 2014.

Ersdal HL, Mduma E, Svensen E, et al: Early initiation of basic resuscitation interventions including face mask ventilation may reduce birth asphyxia related mortality in low-income countries: a prospective descriptive observational study, Resuscitation 83:869–873, 2012.

Finan E, Aylward D, Aziz K: Neonatal resuscitation guidelines update: a case-based review, Paediatric Child Health 16(5):289–291, 2011.

Government of South Australia: Perinatal practice guideline: clinical guideline, 2017. Collapse (Maternal). SA Maternal, Neonatal & Gynaecology Clinical Community of Practice, 2017.

Harach T: Room air resuscitation and targeted oxygenation for infants at birth in the delivery room, Journal of Obstetric, Gynecologic, and Neonatal Nursing 42: 227–232, 2013.

Jeejeebhoy F, Windrim R: Management of cardiac arrest in pregnancy, Best Practice & Research Clinical Obstetrics and Gynaecology 28:607–618, 2014.

Kattwinkel J, Perlman JM, Aziz K, et al: Part 15: neonatal resuscitation: 2010 American heart association guidelines for cardiopulmonary resuscitation and emergency cardiovascular care, Circulation 122(Suppl):S909–S919, 2010.

Kikuchi J, Deering S: Cardiac arrest in pregnancy, Seminars in Perinatology 42:32–38, 2018.

Lee DH, Kim CW, Kim SG, et al: Use of step stool during resuscitation improved the quality of chest compressions in simulated resuscitation, Emergency Medicine Australasia 24:369–373, 2012.

Lewinsohn A, Sherren PB, Wijayatilake DS: The effects of bed height and time on the quality of cardiac compressions delivered during cardiopulmonary resuscitation: a randomised crossover simulation study, Emergency Medicine 29:660–663, 2012.

MacLennan A: A template for defining a causal relation between acute intrapartum events and cerebral palsy: international consensus statement, BMJ (Clinical Research Ed.) 319:1054–1059, 1999.

Mercer JS, Erickson-Owens DA, Collins J, et al: Effects of delayed cord clamping on residual placental blood volume, hemoglobin and bilirubin levels in term infants: a randomized controlled trial, Journal of Perinatology 37(3):260–264, 2017.

New Zealand Resuscitation Council (NZRC): Guidelines, 2021. Online 16 August 2021. Available: https://www.nzrc.org.nz/guidelines/.

Niermeyer S, Clarke SB: Delivery room care, Chapter 4. In Gardner SL, Carter BS, Enzman-Hines M, et al, eds: Merenstein & Gardner's handbook of neonatal intensive care, 7th ed., Mosby, St. Louis, 2011, pp. 52–77.

Patterson B: Fear of infection. The Journal of Emergency Dispatch, 2017. Online 26 July 2018. Available: https://iaedjournal.org/fear-of-infection/.

Pendick D: CPR during cardiac arrest: someone's life is in your hands. Harvard Health Publishing, Harvard Medical School, 2015.

Perlman JM, Risser R: Cardiopulmonary resuscitation in the delivery room: associated clinical events, Archives of Pediatrics & Adolescent Medicine 149:20–25, 1995.

Polglase GR, Stark M: Cord clamping in term and preterm infants: how should clinicians proceed? Evidence favours delayed cord clamping in most newborns, but further studies are needed, Medical Journal of Australia 208(8):330–331, 2018.

Pourmand A, Galvis J, Yamane D: The controversial role of dual sequential defibrillation in shockable cardiac arrest, The American Journal of Emergency Medicine 36(9):1674–1679, 2018. Online 26 July 2018. Available: www.ajemjournal.com/article/S0735-6757(18)30462-5/fulltext.

Rabi Y, Rabi D, Yee W: Room air resuscitation of the depressed newborn: a systematic review and meta-analysis, Resuscitation 72:353–363, 2007.

Richmond S, Wyllie J: European resuscitation council guideline for resuscitation 2010 section 7. Resuscitation of babies at birth, Resuscitation 81:1389–1399, 2010.

Rovamo LM, Mattila M-M, Andersson S, et al: Testing of midwife neonatal resuscitation skills with a simulator manikin in a low-risk delivery unit, Pediatrics International 55:465–471, 2013.

Saugstad OD: Resuscitation with room-air or oxygen supplementation, Clinics in Perinatology 25:741–756, xi, 1998.

Sawyer T, Laubach VA, Hudak J, et al: Improvements in teamwork during neonatal resuscitation after interprofessional team STEPPS training, Neonatal Network 32(1):26–33, 2013.

Vento M, Asensi M, Sastre J, et al: Resuscitation with room air instead of 100% oxygen prevents oxidative stress in moderately asphyxiated term neonates, Pediatrics 107:642–647, 2001.

Wyllie J, Perlman JM, Kattwinkel J, et al: Part 7: neonatal resuscitation: 2015 international consensus on cardiopulmonary resuscitation and emergency cardiovascular care science with treatment recommendations, Resuscitation 95:e169–e201, 2015.

Zelop CM, Einav S, Mhyre JM, Martin S: Cardiac arrest during pregnancy: ongoing clinical conundrum. American Journal of Obstetrics and Gynecology 219(1):52–61, 2018.

SECTION 11

MONITORING WELLBEING DURING AND AFTER THE THIRD STAGE

CHAPTER 43

PRINCIPLES OF INTRAPARTUM SKILLS: THIRD STAGE

Learning outcomes

Having read this chapter, the reader should be able to:

- recognise the importance of birthing the placenta for the health and wellbeing of the mother and neonate
- describe the physiology of the third stage of labour
- discuss the effects of delayed cord clamping and umbilical cord milking on the neonate
- discuss the different methods of managing the third stage
- discuss how blood loss is estimated
- describe the appearance and structure of the term placenta
- describe the examination of the placenta and the significance of the information obtained
- discuss how the midwife can obtain cord blood samples.

The midwife has a responsibility to ensure the placenta and membranes are born safely and completely following the birth of the neonate. This chapter focuses on management of the third stage of labour, estimation of blood loss, examination of the placenta, cord blood samples, cord blood banking and disposal of the placenta. The third stage is from the birth of the neonate to the complete expulsion of the placenta and membranes, involving: the separation, descent and expulsion of the placenta and membranes; monitoring of blood loss (see Chapter 44); and examination of the genital tract following birth (see Chapter 45).

PHYSIOLOGY OF THE THIRD STAGE OF LABOUR

During the third stage, rapid changes occur in maternal physiology involving a delicate and complex interaction of neurohormonal factors (Saxton et al 2014). The regulation of myometrial activity in the third stage is vital to reduce blood loss. The release of high levels of stress hormones can interfere with the ability of the uterus to contract by activating the fight or flight response, which directs blood away from the uterus and towards the heart, lung and muscles, disrupting oxytocin release (Saxton et al 2014). During the third stage, oxytocin release is enhanced when the neonate is skin-to-skin with their mother and this supports optimum uterine activity (Saxton et al 2014). Both health and attachment are optimised by early skin-to-skin and delayed cord clamping (Khyriem et al 2017).

Ultrasound measurements of myometrial thickness indicate that the uterus appears to prepare for the third stage by separating functionally into upper and lower segments, with the upper segment retracting and increasing in thickness while the lower segment relaxes and becomes thinner (Patwardhan et al 2015). Three phases of placental separation have been identified: latent, contraction/detachment and expulsion. The intrauterine volume reduces drastically (from 4 L pre-labour to 0.5 L) as the uterus becomes smaller following the birth of the neonate. Pressure within the uterus increases from 100 mmHg in the second stage to 140 mmHg in the third stage.

Phase 1: latent phase

The myometrium continues to contract and retract as in the first and second stages of labour, resulting in extensive thickening of most of the myometrium; the area of myometrium beneath the placental site does not thicken to the same degree.

Phase 2: contraction/detachment phase

The myometrium under the lower pole of the placenta begins to contract with a reduction in the surface area. Consequently, the shearing forces cause the placenta to separate from the spongy layer of the decidua. With the onset of placental detachment, the wave of separation passes upwards and the remaining placenta detaches, with the uppermost part of the placenta detaching last, leaving the maternal sinuses within the decidua exposed. The oblique muscle fibres surrounding the blood vessels contract to seal the torn ends of the maternal vessels to prevent haemorrhage.

Phase 3: expulsion phase

As the placenta descends into the lower uterine segment, the membranes (which had begun to detach from the uterine wall as the internal cervical os dilated) peel away from the walls of the uterus. With further contractions the placenta descends into the vagina, assisted by gravity, with the membranes following. Maternal effort will birth the placenta and membranes with the fetal surface appearing at the vulva, with the membranes behind containing any blood loss within them; this is often referred to as the 'Schultze' method of expulsion (Fig 43.1A). Sometimes the lower edge of the placenta will descend first, with the maternal surface appearing at the vulva and sliding out lengthways with the membranes (Fig 43.1B). This is a slower process, with increased blood loss as the mechanisms to control haemorrhage are less effective when the placenta is still partially attached. This has been referred to as the 'Matthews Duncan' method of expulsion.

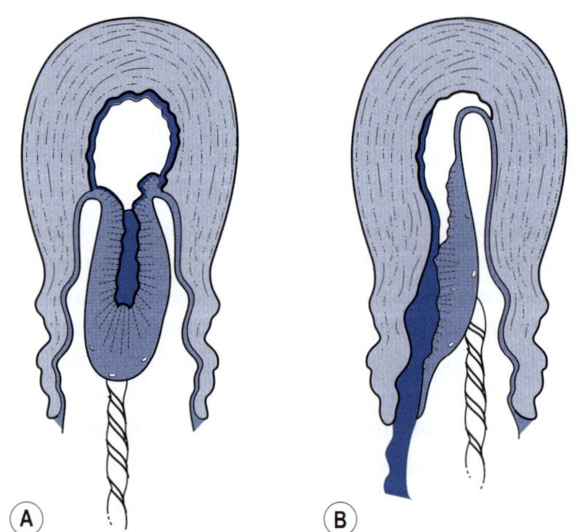

FIGURE 43.1 **Methods of placental expulsion. A, Schultze. B, Matthews Duncan.**
Source: Johnson R, Taylor W: Skills for midwifery practice, 4th ed., Elsevier, London, 2016.

The duration of the third stage varies according to the length of the latent phase. The time taken for the descent and birth of the placenta and membranes can vary and is influenced by factors such as posture and whether the third stage is managed actively or expectantly (Karim et al 2015). The actively managed third stage is completed in less than 30 minutes for 97% of women, with the remaining 3% of women taking up to 60 minutes with an average of 13.8 minutes (Shinar et al 2016).

In a normal third stage, dynamic and coordinated uterine action occurs as the myometrium of the upper uterine segment increases in thickness and the myometrium of the lower uterine segment decreases in thickness; these changes lead to birth of the placenta (Patwardhan et al 2015). However, according to Patwardhan and colleagues (2015), when women had postpartum haemorrhage (PPH), preterm birth or clinical chorioamnionitis the action of the uterine segment was less coordinated and followed a different pattern. The following additional differences were noted:

- PPH was associated with a thinner, lower uterine segment
- preterm birth was associated with a less clear differentiation between measurements of the upper and lower uterine segments
- chorioamnionitis was associated with lack of changes in the upper and lower uterine segment measurements
- a third stage lasting longer than 12 minutes was associated with significant differences in myometrium thickness and slower changes in thickness compared to women with an average third stage (Patwardhan et al 2015).

Despite varying patterns of uterine changes in the third stage, incremental thickening of the upper uterine segment and thinning of the lower uterine segment are required for spontaneous birth of the placenta (Patwardhan et al 2015).

SIGNS OF SEPARATION AND DESCENT

These are not absolute and may occur for other reasons.

- Bleeding, classed as a trickle of 30–60 mL of blood from the vagina; this could also be from a laceration or a partially separated placenta (although bleeding is often heavier).
- Cord lengthening may occur as the placenta descends, or from a coiled cord that is straightening out.
- A change in the shape and position of the uterus involves the uterus becoming globular, hard, high, mobile and ballottable. Before placental separation and descent into the lower uterine segment, the fundus is broad and palpable, usually below the umbilicus. With separation and descent, the fundus narrows and fundal height increases, usually above

the umbilicus (Fig 43.2). This can be assessed by gently palpating the fundus (it may provoke irregular contractions, which can interfere with placental separation and cause a partially separated placenta, resulting in excessive bleeding). The placenta may also appear as a bulge just above the symphysis pubis.
- The woman feels pressure or an urge to push as the placenta enters the vagina.

CORD CLAMPING

With the introduction of active management, the practice of immediate cord clamping following birth (within 30 seconds) became widespread. However, placental separation is reliant on the ability of the uterus to contract and retract. Early cord clamping prevents the transfer of blood to the neonate; this can prevent the placenta from reducing in size with the potential to inhibit contraction and retraction of the uterus, resulting in a slower separation process. This has two possible effects:

- delay in complete separation causes the torn maternal vessels to seal off more slowly, producing a retroplacental clot and increasing the risk of haemorrhage
- a retained placenta may occur if the cervix retracts before it is expelled, often necessitating a manual removal of the placenta and membranes under epidural, spinal or general anaesthetic.

Approximately 30% of fetal blood volume is within the placenta at any time; with immediate cord clamping, this blood remains within the placenta. When the cord is not clamped immediately, the process of placental separation is unaffected and the neonate receives the extra blood contained within the placenta. It has generally been accepted that blood flow via the umbilical arteries from neonate to placenta stops rapidly once the baby is born, whereas the umbilical vein remains open for longer, allowing blood from the placenta to flow to the newborn (Nandadasa et al 2020). According to Scheans (2013) the umbilical arteries close 20–25 seconds following birth, whereas the blood flow from the placenta to the neonate via the umbilical vein continues for up to 3 minutes. Newer research on the blood flow in the umbilical vessels immediately after birth using Doppler ultrasound has found blood flow in both the umbilical arteries and the umbilical vein continues for longer than previous information has indicated (Boere et al 2015). Placental transfusion appears to be complex, variable, influenced by multiple factors and unrelated to cessation of umbilical cord pulsations (Boere et al 2015). The first minute before cord clamping, when the neonate receives additional iron-rich blood, has been referred to as the 'iron minute' (McAdams 2014).

The cord clamp should be applied 3–4 cm from the abdominal wall. If the neonate is preterm the cord should be longer, as catheterisation of the umbilical vessels may be required; this is more successful with a longer cord. A clamp is usually applied to the maternal end of the cord and the section of cord between the two clamps cut. The woman's partner or a family member may wish to cut the cord; the midwife can direct them as to where to cut.

DELAYED CORD CLAMPING

Short-term benefits

Delayed cord clamping (DCC) is recommended for healthy preterm and term neonates (Kresch 2017,

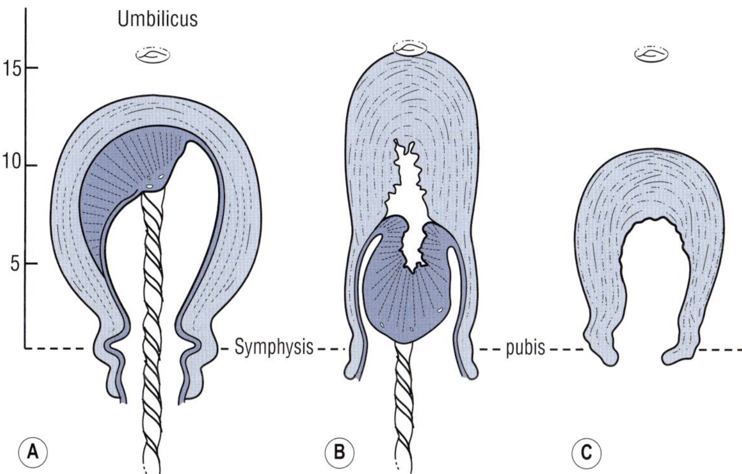

FIGURE 43.2 **A, Beginning of the third stage. B, Placenta in the lower segment. C, End of the third stage.**
Source: Johnson R, Taylor W: Skills for midwifery practice, 4th ed., Elsevier, London, 2016, p. 246.

National Institute for Health and Care Excellence [NICE] 2017, Polglase & Stark 2018, Vatansever et al 2018). Clamping the cord before respirations are established decreases cardiac ventricular output, compromises organ perfusion (Kresch 2017) and leads to hypovolaemia and hypoxia with oxygen saturation reduced by 20% (Yigit et al 2019). The Royal Australian and New Zealand College of Obstetricians and Gynaecologists (RANZCOG 2017) recognises the benefits of DCC for vigorous term infants (increased haematocrit and decreased iron deficiency) and vigorous preterm infants (decreased risk of requiring transfusion, infection, necrotising enterocolitis and intraventricular haemorrhage). The RANZCOG (2017) guideline on the provision of routine intrapartum care in the absence of pregnancy complications states: 'there should be no urgency to cut the umbilical cord and this can be done in an appropriate time frame'. The American College of Obstetricians and Gynaecologists (ACOG) recommend DCC for term and preterm infants (2020). In healthy full-term infants DCC for 5 minutes occurring during skin-to-skin on the maternal abdomen decreased residual placental blood volume and increased the infant's haematocrit and haemoglobin without any increase in jaundice (Mercer et al 2017).

Healthy term newborns with DCC ≥ 60 seconds had higher oxygen saturation and heart rate in the first 5 minutes following birth compared to infants undergoing immediate cord clamping (Padilla-Sánchez et al 2020). Benefits of DCC include improved cardiovascular and respiratory transition (Brodie 2018, Yigit 2019).

The Australian Placental Transfusion Study found infant mortality was lower in preterm infants who had the cord clamped after 60 seconds compared to infants receiving immediate cord clamping; however, the combined incidence of death or major morbidity at 36 weeks was not reduced (Tarnow-Mordi et al 2017). In the DCC group admission temperature was 0.1°C lower, the peak haematocrit was higher and fewer red cell transfusions were required (Tarnow-Mordi et al 2017). A systematic review found DCC reduced all-cause hospital mortality in preterm infants (Fogarty et al 2018). A meta-analysis found fewer transfusions for anaemia were required and less intraventricular haemorrhage and necrotising enterocolitis occurred (Rabe et al 2012). A review of results from multiple studies on DCC found that in term newborns blood pressure, blood volume, urine output and haemoglobin were higher with a lower incidence of iron deficiency and a minor increase in the requirement for phototherapy, with no change in the need to treat polycythaemia (Kresch 2017).

The most obvious benefit of DCC is increased blood volume, which assists with facilitating the pulmonary adaptation required at birth. DCC increases blood volume by 80–100 mL and iron levels are increased by 40–50 mg/kg (Buder 2015). According to Yigit and colleagues (2019) DCC increases blood volume by 10% for infants from 32–40 weeks gestation and by 15% for infants less than 30 weeks gestation.

In infants born between 32 and 34^{+6} weeks gestation, those with DCC showed an increased haematocrit and an improved respiratory transition at birth with no increase in hyperbilirubinaemia or the need for phototherapy (Chiruvolu et al 2018). When the cord is clamped immediately the newborn's venous return drops by 30–50%, which reduces cardiac output (Safarulla 2017). Following DCC, fewer infants are admitted to the neonatal intensive care unit (NICU) for respiratory support, suggesting DCC reduces resuscitation requirements by improving cardiopulmonary transition following birth (Chiruvolu et al 2018). DCC has been shown to improve preterm neonates' temperature, mean arterial blood pressure, haematocrit, blood volume, cardiac output and cerebral oxygenation, and decrease neonatal hypotension and intraventricular haemorrhage rates (Jelin et al 2016). A clinical trial on preterm neonates born by caesarean section found DCC decreased the incidence of intraventricular haemorrhage (IVH), periventricular leucomalacia (PVL) and seizures (Kazemi et al 2017). DCC improves cerebral oxygenation in infants less than 30 weeks gestation (Popat et al 2016). DCC increases birth weight by up to 2% (Buder 2015). In the context of red blood cell alloimmunisation, DCC improved the neonate's haemoglobin level and decreased the need for postnatal exchange transfusion (Garabedian et al 2016). In healthy pregnancy, normal birth inflammatory markers in neonatal serum were not altered by DCC (Daskalakis et al 2018).

One of the concerns preventing DCC is the need to resuscitate the neonate. To resolve this issue some companies have designed an adjustable-height table designed to facilitate resuscitation when the cord is intact (Malloy 2016). A small pilot study found that although providing assisted ventilation to preterm infants while they received DCC for 90 seconds can be challenging, it appears to be safe during both vaginal and caesarean births (Winter et al 2017). Caesarean births are associated with a reduced rate of DCC, both midwives and obstetricians may benefit from education on using DCC at operative births, including information indicating that maternal harm does not occur (Kuo et al 2018). Obstetricians may be concerned that DCC can delay hysterotomy closure and increase blood loss; however, DCC appears to cause minimal disruption during caesarean birth (Kuo et al 2018).

From the maternal perspective, DCC has been found to have no effect on the incidence of PPH or the need for maternal transfusion (Fogarty et al 2018). DCC made no significant difference to mean blood loss at birth or postnatal maternal haemoglobin levels (McDonald et al 2014). DCC does not increase risk of PPH for women with a vaginal birth (ACOG 2020, Brodie 2018) and appears to decrease blood loss at caesarean section

(Jenusaitis et al 2020). Research by Ruangkit and colleagues (2018) on multiple pregnancies found that DCC does not increase maternal blood loss, incidence of PPH or rates of maternal blood transfusion. A randomised controlled trial in Brazil found there was no statistically significant difference in mean blood loss, postpartum haematocrit or length of the third stage when the blood from the placenta was able to drain freely (Vasconcelos et al 2018). Following DCC, maternal haematological parameters, such as haemoglobin and haematocrit, did not decrease and the length of the third stage did not change significantly (De Paco et al 2016).

Cultural considerations may influence women's preferences. Australian Aboriginal women believe it is important to leave the cord intact until it stops pulsating because cutting the cord early affects activation of the *Miwi* (soul or spirit) print of the placenta. If, for medical reasons, the cord is clamped before it stops pulsating, a birthing ceremony and planting of the placenta in the Earth can mitigate these circumstances (Northern Sydney Local Health District [NSLHD] 2015).

Long-term benefits

A randomised controlled trial found DCC led to improved neurodevelopment, particularly in boys, who demonstrated better scores in fine motor and social domains at 4 years of age (Andersson et al 2015). Iron plays an important role in the rapid neurological development that occurs during the first 6 months of life (Bayer 2016). At 8 months, infants of mothers with anaemia had significantly less iron deficiency if they received DCC (Blouin et al 2013). According to Mercer and colleagues (2010), DCC seems to be a protective factor against motor disability at 7 months corrected age for very-low-birthweight infants (born at $24–31^{+6}$ weeks gestation). Long-term benefits include higher rates of stem cell transfer, lower occurrence of sepsis and reduced risk of iron deficiency (Brodie 2018).

Risks of DCC

Concern has been expressed that DCC may increase neonatal hypothermia and the extra blood may lead to polycythaemia and hyperbilirubinaemia (Bayer 2016, Tarnow-Mordi et al 2014). The incidence of polycythaemia and jaundice is increased with DCC; however, the incidence of partial exchange transfusion does not change (Fogarty et al 2018). Asymptomatic polycythaemia (haematocrit $> 65\%$) was more common in neonates who had DCC but was not associated with a significant difference in serum bilirubin levels or the need for phototherapy in the first 1–3 days (Scheans 2013). Term infants with DCC for 5 minutes did not have an increase in severe hyperbilirubinaemia, although more infants with DCC received phototherapy (Mercer et al 2017).

The infants of mothers with diabetes have an increased risk of polycythaemia associated with hyperbilirubinaemia. Concerns DCC may exacerbate the risk of jaundice in infants of mothers with diabetes have been investigated. Kotzen and colleagues (2021) found infants whose mothers had diabetes did not have an increased risk of phototherapy; therefore, DCC should not be withheld due to fears of increased jaundice. Infants with intrauterine growth restriction (IUGR) compensate for their decreased oxygen-carrying capacity by increasing haematocrit (Bayer 2016). A study evaluating DCC in neonates with IUGR found DCC had several benefits including improved systemic blood flow, haematocrit and serum ferritin levels without increasing the incidence of polycythaemia and phototherapy for hyperbilirubinaemia (Digal et al 2021). Newborns with congenital heart disease (CHD) require special consideration. Some infants with CHD benefit from DCC through higher blood volume, improved tissue oxygenation and decreased need for blood transfusions, whereas for other infants with CHD the increased haematocrit, blood viscosity and blood volume could be detrimental (Marzec et al 2020). RANZCOG (2017) indicate neonatal resuscitation must always be prioritised over DCC.

Duration of DCC

The optimal time for cord clamping has been debated. The appropriate time appears to be after the newborn has commenced breathing and can sustain their cardiac output (Hooper et al 2015). The prevailing view has been that when the infant is born the umbilical arteries constrict and prevent arterial flow from infant to placenta while blood flow through the vein continues until cord pulsation ceases, hence the directive to wait until cord pulsations cease before clamping the cord. However, Doppler ultrasound of the cord indicates umbilical blood flow is not related to cord pulsation (Boere et al 2015). Recommendations for cord clamping vary. ACOG (2020) recommends 30–60 seconds of DCC for vigorous term and preterm neonates, WHO (2014) suggests it should be for 30–120 seconds and Katheria and colleagues (2017) suggest 5 minutes.

Resuscitation and delayed cord clamping

A randomised controlled trial examined the differences between neonates at risk of resuscitation compared to cord clamping at 1 minute and 5 minutes (Katheria et al 2017). This trial found DCC for 5 minutes could be done safely while resuscitation was performed using a bedside resuscitation table; infants receiving 5 minutes of DCC had higher SpO_2 levels and a higher mean blood pressure compared with infants receiving 1 minute of DCC (Katheria et al 2017). An Australia feasibility study also indicates it is reasonable to resuscitate term and near-term infants at the bedside using baby-directed umbilical cord clamping, meaning the physiological readiness of the baby determines when DCC occurs (Blank et al 2018). Resuscitation and ventilation while the cord remains intact can occur when the infant has a congenital diaphragmatic hernia and results in higher Apgar scores and mean blood pressure with no increase in neonatal or maternal adverse events (Mur et al 2017).

POSITION OF THE NEONATE

Early studies recommended positioning the neonate 40 cm below the introitus for 30 seconds for maximal transfer of blood (Palethorpe et al 2010). When the newborn is skin-to-skin on the maternal abdomen during DCC, the transfusion of blood from the placenta is slower and 5 minutes may be required for infants to receive a full placental transfusion (Mercer et al 2017). No significant difference in mortality or serious morbidity has been demonstrated between neonates placed 5 cm or 20 cm below the mother's introitus or caesarean section incision (Fogarty et al 2018), indicating that placental transfusion will occur effectively if the baby is placed on the mother's chest while the cord drains. Gravity probably has little influence on placental transfusion.

MILKING THE CORD

DCC is now recommended for vigorous term and preterm infants due to the beneficial impact on survival and neurodevelopmental outcomes. In situations with no time for DCC, it was suggested milking the cord may offer some advantages and could be performed in approximately 20 seconds (Safarulla 2017). Early research showed promising benefits including: reduced rates of mortality, IVH and transfusion (Backes et al 2010); higher haemoglobin (Hb) and serum ferritin and relatively higher blood pressure during the first 48 hours (Upadhyay et al 2013); higher urine output levels within the first 24 hours, decreased need for volume expanders (Patel et al 2014) and improved cerebral perfusion (Takami et al 2012),

Tarnow-Mordi and colleagues (2014) suggest milking the umbilical cord disrupts the fetoplacental circulation and the transition of the cardiopulmonary and cerebral circulation. More recent studies indicate an association between umbilical cord milking and an increase in severe IVH (Kumbhat et al 2021), particularly for extremely preterm infants between 23 and 27 weeks gestation (Reister et al 2019). It now appears DCC is of more benefit to preterm infants and milking the umbilical cord should be avoided (Steinhorn 2021).

MANAGEMENT OF THE THIRD STAGE

Considerable variations in the management of the third stage exist internationally and within countries. However, all women require sensitive care and the opportunity to bond with their baby without separation or disruption (NICE 2017). Midwives should be competent with both expectant (physiological, conservative, passive) and active management and discuss the benefits and risks of each with women antenatally. The RANZCOG (2017) guideline on the provision of routine intrapartum care in the absence of pregnancy complications recommends active management of the third stage using oxytocics and assisted expulsion of the placenta for all women. Most of the studies on management of the third stage have focused on births occurring in hospitals. In this setting high numbers of women are induced or augmented and the normal physiological process is disrupted. In this situation saturation of the oxytocin receptors may occur.

Holistic psychophysiological care during the third stage has been described by Fahy and colleagues (2010) as involving: immediate skin-to-skin contact; gentle support focused on the mother–neonate dyad, which enables women to feel safe and secure; and unobtrusive observation of placental separation without interference. In clinical settings, the natural physiology of the third stage is frequently disrupted due to clinical practice and guidelines designed to decrease the length of the third stage and reduce PPH. In practice, mixed management is often used with a combination of active and expectant management. Mixed management may include administration of prophylactic uterotonic, clamping the cord after pulsation ceases and then controlled cord traction (CCT) (Begley et al 2019).

PHYSIOLOGICAL THIRD STAGE OF LABOUR

Physiological third stage refers to spontaneous birth of the placenta without interference and is also known as expectant management. Women who have experienced a physiological labour and birth can choose a physiological third stage for birthing their placenta (New Zealand College of Midwives [NZCOM] 2013). The process of placental separation depends on a finely tuned balance of hormonal, physiological, psychological and neurological interactions (Buckley 2009). If any of these processes have been disturbed by interventions, such as induction, augmentation, epidural or narcotic analgesia, safety can be compromised (NZCOM 2013). In Australia and New Zealand, the use of oxytocin to induce or augment labour is common, with over one-third of labours (34%) induced in Australia (AIHW 2021). In New Zealand in 2019 the overall rate of induction for all births was 35.8%; nulliparae had the highest rate of induction (46.9%), followed by multiparae with no previous caesarean section (39.8%) and multiparae with a previous caesarean section (9.9%) (Auckland District Health Board 2019).

A calm, warm, relaxed environment with skin-to-skin contact with the neonate reduces adrenaline levels that may interfere with oxytocin levels and the physiological process of uterine contraction and retraction, and thus placental separation and descent (Buckley 2009). Ideally, the woman can feel safe and be undisturbed; this lowers catecholamine levels and encourages oxytocin and prolactin release (Charles 2018).

With physiological third stage, the placenta is born by maternal effort assisted by gravity, skin-to-skin contact and the neonate suckling at the breast. There should be no intervention and no prophylactic administration of a uterotonic agent, and the uterus should not be palpated. The cord is not clamped and cut until pulsation has ceased. Physiological third stage is a hands-off approach which includes watching for signs of separation and descent, such as lengthening of the umbilical cord. A New Zealand study found low-risk women had a lower risk of blood loss > 1000 mL with physiological third stage when compared with active management (Davis et al 2012). In 2019, New Zealand data indicated 4.6% of *wāhine* (women) who birthed vaginally had their third stage managed physiologically. Paradoxically, these *wāhine* were less likely to have a PPH or to require blood transfusion postpartum.

Physiological third stage is possible following preterm birth if active full resuscitation of the neonate can be performed. In this situation, the cord can be left unclamped to facilitate drainage of blood from the placenta, helping to reduce its overall size. The blood drained from the placenta should not be included in the total estimate of blood loss following birth as it is placental not maternal blood.

A Cochrane review concluded it is uncertain if there is a difference between active and physiological management and incidence of severe PPH (> 1000 mL) (Begley et al 2019). Active management may increase blood loss in the early postpartum period when compared to a physiological third stage (Kashanian et al 2010). It is important to discuss options for the third stage with each woman, including the advantages and disadvantages of both active and physiological management (Begley et al 2019, Selfe & Walsh 2015). In practice, women often receive information with more emphasis on active management (Selfe & Walsh 2015). The woman needs to be aware of the risk of haemorrhage and the possibility of needing to change from physiological to active third stage and administer a uterotonic in the presence of haemorrhage. Women may feel they are not given adequate information from their health providers and need to undertake their own research (Reed et al 2019).

The duration of the third stage is often longer with a physiological third stage (Patwardhan et al 2015). In the absence of bleeding, it can last more than an hour without an increased risk of PPH (Dixon et al 2009). If the woman's condition remains stable, with no excessive bleeding, there is no cause for concern; breastfeeding can be initiated, with the added benefit of increased oxytocin release to promote uterine contraction. NZCOM (2013) recommends the woman should be encouraged to adopt an upright position to shorten the duration of the third stage. NICE (2014) suggests the placenta should be birthed within 1 hour and that management should change to active if this does not happen. Odent (1998) believes it is not necessary to 'manage' the third stage of labour.

During the physiological third stage, clamping and cutting the cord does not occur until after the cord has stopped pulsating. Some women request lotus birth (umbilical non-severance); in this case the cord is not clamped or cut and the placenta remains attached to the newborn until the cord shrivels and separates naturally. Usually the placenta is rinsed and patted dry within the first 24 hours and both sides of the placenta are salted before the placenta is wrapped in a clean cloth (Zinsser 2018). The woman may add essential oils (e.g. lavender) with or without powdered herbs (e.g. goldenseal). The neonate is fed, held and bathed as normal and wrapped in loose clothes. If the placenta is not kept dry it may develop a musky odour. By the sixth day the umbilical cord has generally separated from the placenta (Zinsser 2018). Applying human breast milk may be applied to the umbilical cord to reduce cord separation time (Kirk et al 2019). A case of idiopathic neonatal hepatitis associated with a lotus birth has been reported in Italy (Tricarico 2017). Cases of neonatal omphalitis possibly related to lotus births have also been reported (Steer-Massaro 2020).

Safer Care Victoria and the Royal Australian and New Zealand College of Obstetricians and Gynaecologists Victoria (2021) have developed a consensus statement on lotus birth indicating they do not recommend it due to a lack of empirical data. It would seem prudent to discuss the following with women: hygiene measures such as handwashing prior to touching the placenta or umbilical cord; monitoring the neonate for signs of infection; and seeking medical help if signs of infection are present (Steer-Massaro 2020).

RANZCOG (2017) does not recommend physiological management on the basis of evidence associated with an increase in the incidence of PPH and the need for blood transfusion when compared with active management.

SKILL 43.1 Physiological third stage

1. The principles of standard precautions (Chapter 1) and aseptic non-touch technique (ANTT) (Chapter 2) are followed to reduce the risk of infection.
2. Note the time of birth of the neonate.
3. Keep the neonate covered on the woman's abdomen, skin-to-skin.

Continued

SKILL 43.1 Physiological third stage—cont'd

4. Maintain a safe, warm and private environment, unobtrusively observe normal physiology and take steps to reduce any anxiety in the woman (Schorn 2020).
5. The woman's bladder should remain empty.
6. Encourage the woman to adopt an upright position.
7. Observe the general condition of the woman throughout, particularly blood loss per vaginam, colour, respirations (NICE 2014) and discomfort (Schorn 2020).
8. Do not touch the cord, allowing it to stop pulsating naturally.
9. Encourage neonate-led breastfeeding.
10. Do not palpate the uterus unless blood loss becomes excessive.
11. Place a suitable receptacle under or next to the woman when she is ready to birth the placenta.
12. Observe for signs of placental separation and descent (small fresh blood loss, cord lengthening, fundus becoming smaller and more globular).
13. When the woman has the urge to push, encourage her to birth the placenta by her own efforts.
14. Note the time the placenta and membranes are expelled.
15. The cord can be clamped and cut when it has stopped pulsating, unless the woman has requested a lotus birth.
16. Assess the condition of the woman, noting the tone of the uterus (should be firm and central), amount of blood loss, pulse and blood pressure following completion of the third stage; the condition of the genital tract should also be determined, with suturing undertaken when appropriate.
17. Assist the woman into a comfortable position, removing any soiled linen; enable the woman and newborn to stay together (with her partner or labour supporter), ensuring the call bell is close at hand.
18. Examine the placenta and record total blood loss.
19. Dispose of the placenta and equipment correctly (if the woman is taking the placenta home, it should be double wrapped and placed in a suitable container).
20. Document findings and act accordingly.

ACTIVE MANAGEMENT OF THE THIRD STAGE OF LABOUR

Traditionally, the strict definition of active management includes a prophylactic uterotonic drug, early cord clamping and CCT (NICE 2014, Westhoff et al 2013). However, early cord clamping is no longer considered best practice. NICE (2014) now discusses active management as:

- routine use of uterotonics
- deferred clamping and cutting of the cord
- CCT after signs of placental separation.

Active management of third-stage labour (AMTSL), including the use of uterotonics such as oxytocin to reduce the risk of PPH, is recommended for all women (RANZCOG 2017, WHO 2012). Assisted birth of the placenta using CCT is optional according to WHO (2012). Women who receive prophylactic oxytocin have a lower risk of blood loss ≥ 500 mL, but their risk of PPH ≤ 1000 mL and the need for blood transfusion or additional treatment with uterotonics is not altered (Erickson et al 2017). In New Zealand, 2019 data indicates studies calculating blood loss by weight indicate 500 mL may be normal and well tolerated by women with a healthy physiological increase in blood volume (Erickson et al 2017). According to Erickson and colleagues, routine use of uterotonics may pathologise normal blood loss and lead to a loss of awareness about normal physiological postpartum blood loss. Prophylactic oxytocin may have an adverse effect related to the potential for exogenous oxytocin to desensitise and down-regulate oxytocin receptor function. Women whose labour is induced or augmented with oxytocin have an increased risk of PPH (Erickson et al 2017).

A Cochrane review found the admission of neonates to special care and the incidence of jaundice requiring treatment did not differ between active and expectant management of the third stage (Begley et al 2019). Active management may reduce the risk of PPH > 1000 mL at the time of birth; however, it is unclear if it reduces the incidence of PPH > 1000 mL and the incidence of maternal Hb < 9 g/dL in the 24 to 72 hours following birth (Begley et al 2019). When birth of the placenta does not occur after 30–60 minutes, the risk of haemorrhage is increased. It is important women are advised of the risks and benefits of both active and expectant third-stage management, preferably during the antenatal period so they can make an informed choice (Begley et al 2019).

Uterine massage

Uterine massage involves placing a hand on the lower abdomen to stimulate uterine contraction through the use of repetitive massaging or squeezing movements. Hofmeyr and colleagues (2013) do not support the routine use of uterine massage following birth of the placenta, suggesting that if a uterotonic has been administered the potential for further benefit is limited. The evidence as to whether uterine massage should be undertaken routinely when there is an increased risk of PPH and no uterotonics available is inconclusive (Hofmeyr et al 2013). The use of uterine massage is not recommended by WHO (2012) when oxytocin has been administered as there is insufficient evidence to support its use as part of routine PPH prevention. Although uterine massage did not reduce the amount of blood lost during the first 2 hours following the birth, it did increase the number of therapeutic uterotonics administered (Chen et al 2013).

Controlled cord traction

Traditionally **controlled cord traction (CTT)** has been a component of active management. A comparison between CCT immediately after birth with a contraction and awaiting signs of spontaneous separation and descent assisted by maternal effort found no significant effect on the incidence of PPH, duration of the third stage or the need for manual removal of the placenta, with women experiencing less pain, discomfort, anxiety and fatigue (Deneux-Tharaux et al 2013). DCC is facilitated when CCT is avoided. CCT has little effect on the incidence and severity of PPH (Culliney & Williams 2016, Deneux-Tharaux et al 2013, Hofmeyr et al 2015). CCT does not decrease the rate of PPH greater than 1000 mL and results in a minimal increase in the rate of manual removal of the placenta (Hofmeyr et al 2015), with 161 CCT required to avoid one manual removal of the placenta (Culliney & Williams 2016). The risk of cord rupture is increased to 1 in 23 and, rarely, uterine inversion may occur. CCT does not alter the risk of blood transfusion, severe morbidity or mortality, operative procedures or the use of additional uterotonics (Culliney & Williams 2016). The focus should be on the uterotonic component of active management with CCT optional unless Syntometrine (oxytocin and ergometrine) or ergometrine have been administered (NZCOM 2013). Omitting CCT from the active management package has been recommended by Hofmeyr and colleagues (2015). CCT can cause shreds of placental membrane to be retained in utero, increasing the incidence of a woman returning to hospital with bleeding (Begley et al 2019). According to the New Zealand College of Midwives, CCT should not be used if a uterotonic drug has not been given and if there are no signs of placental separation (NZCOM 2013).

EXAMINATION OF THE GENITAL TRACT

The midwife should examine the woman's genital tract following birth to ascertain the degree of trauma and whether suturing is indicated. Examination of the genital tract following birth of the placenta is described in Chapter 45.

SKILL 43.2 Active management of the third stage

1. The principles of standard precautions (Chapter 1) and ANTT (Chapter 2) are followed to reduce the risk of infection.
2. Avoid taking third-stage oxytocics into the birth room until active second stage has commenced and do not draw up until birth is imminent.
3. Following birth of the anterior shoulder or neonate, an intravenous or intramuscular uterotonic drug is administered.
4. Clamp and cut the cord within 5 minutes unless contraindicated, ensuring both ends are secure and placing the maternal end in a sterile receiver, positioned close to the vulva.
5. Place a sterile towel over the woman's abdomen and place the non-dominant hand over the fundus and await a contraction, keeping the hand still, during which time signs of placental separation and descent may be seen.
6. Birth of the placenta and membranes.
   - Either encourage the woman to birth the placenta through her own effort

   OR
   - controlled cord traction (CCT) (only used when a uterotonic has been given, the uterus is contracted and signs of separation and descent have been seen): place the non-dominant hand above the symphysis pubis, with the thumb and fingers stretched across the abdomen and palm facing inwards to push the uterus upwards (there is no evidence this reduces the risk of uterine inversion, but it may act as a counter-pressure and the movement of the placenta may be felt)
   - using the dominant hand, grasp the cord and apply steady downward traction
   - CCT is accomplished more easily by keeping the hand applying traction close to the vulva; the grip should be secured by placing the artery forceps on the cord close to the vulva, then as the cord lengthens, the clamp should be moved up to remain near the vulva—alternatively, wrap the cord around the fingers of the dominant hand, moving them nearer to the vulva as necessary
   - if the uterus relaxes or resistance is felt, stop, relieve the pressure from the dominant then the non-dominant hand and wait for 1 minute before attempting again, ensuring the uterus is contracted
   - when the placenta appears at the vulva, traction should be applied in an upward direction to follow the curve of the birth canal

Continued

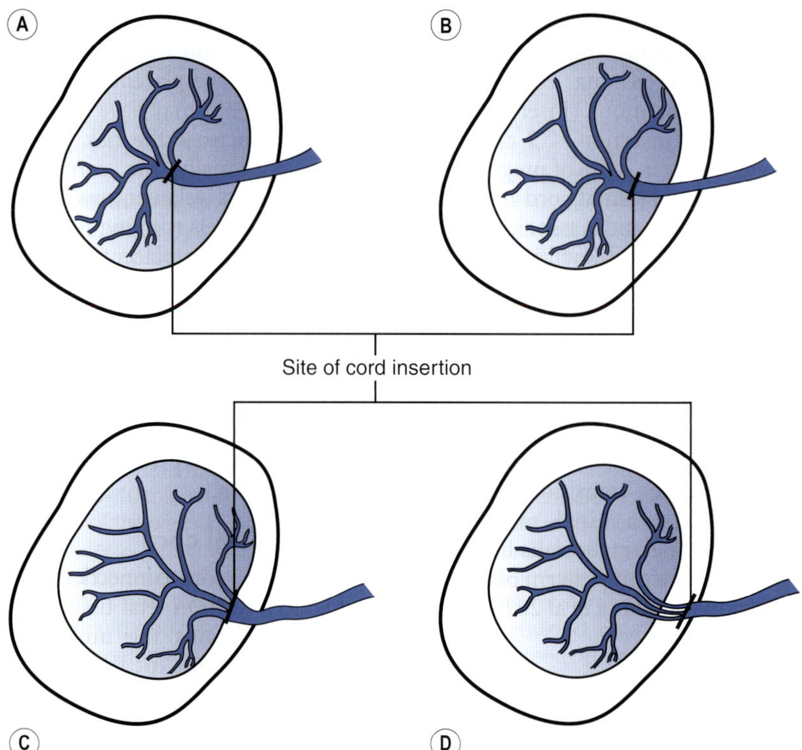

FIGURE 43.4 **Cord insertions. A, Central. B, Eccentric. C, Battledore. D, Velamentous.**
Source: Johnson R, Taylor W: Skills for midwifery practice, 4th ed., Elsevier, London, 2016, p. 261.

through the pelvis, which can lead to an abnormal fetal heart rate pattern. Long cords are associated with knots in the cord, fetal entanglement and cord prolapse (Khong 2015). Conditions associated with larger uterine size (e.g. multiparity and higher maternal age) are related to long cords (Khong 2015). There is a risk of a long cord wrapping around the fetus or becoming knotted, resulting in occlusion of the vessels. A true knot occurs in 0.1–2.1% of cords and there is also an increased risk of cord presentation and prolapse, particularly if the presenting part is poorly applied to the cervix (e.g. with a malposition or malpresentation).

The cord is 1–2 cm wide; a thicker cord is associated with diabetes, macrosomia and hydrops (Khong 2015), whereas a thinner cord is associated with IUGR (Baergen 2011). In women with diabetes the umbilical cord has thickened vessel walls (Koskinen et al 2015). The cord is twisted in a spiral with one coil every 5 cm, which protects the vessels from pressure and provides an enhanced capacity to withstand kinking, compression and torsion. False knots may be noted in the cord and can occur when the blood vessels are longer than the cord, forming a loop in the Wharton's jelly.

The fetal membranes

Two membranes surround the fetus and form the amniotic sac: the amnion and chorion. The amnion and chorion are generally fused by 16 weeks gestation (Gerson et al 2019). When examining the placenta they can be separated by stripping one from the other. The amnion covers the cord and fetal surface of the placenta and is the inner lining of the amniotic sac; it is smooth, tough and translucent. The chorion begins at the placental edge, extends around the decidua and is thick, friable and opaque. Following expulsion of the placenta, the membranes will have a hole in them through which the neonate has been born. They should be carefully examined, as a piece of membrane may be retained in utero and is likely to give the appearance of ragged membranes. Even a small fragment of retained membrane can result in uterine atony and PPH. Both ragged and incomplete membranes are associated with an increased risk of primary PPH (Keating et al 2018). Retained membranes provide a site for microorganisms to grow, predisposing the woman to infection. Pieces of membrane may be found in clots passed postpartum, hence the need to examine postpartum clots for the presence of membranes, particularly when the membranes are ragged.

Maternal surface of the placenta

The maternal side is composed of 15–20 **cotyledons** (divided by septa), which have arisen from two or more main stem villi and their branches. Fibrin deposition can occur around the villi during the second and third trimesters, resulting in isolated villi infarction. While this is usually insignificant, an excessive number of infarctions can affect the exchange of nutrients and waste products between the fetal and maternal circulation, resulting in IUGR. Lime salt deposition can result in small areas of calcification appearing on the surface, giving the surface a gritty feel; these are insignificant. If a cotyledon is separated from the other cotyledons, it will be seen in the membranes connected to the main part of the placenta by blood vessels—this is a 'succenturiate' lobe (Fig 43.5). It is important to examine the membranes for unexplained holes or blood vessels that do not connect to anything, as it is possible the succenturiate lobe has been retained in utero and can predispose to uterine atony, haemorrhage and infection. While the surface has a dark red appearance, it may appear paler if DCC or fetal haemorrhage has occurred.

SKILL 43.3 Examination of the placenta

1. Explain the procedure to the parents and ascertain if they wish to observe the examination.
2. Gather equipment:
   - non-sterile gloves and apron
   - disposable protective cover
   - disposal bag for placenta
   - placenta
   - equipment for cord blood sampling if indicated.
3. Perform hand hygiene and apply apron and gloves.
4. Place the disposable protective cover onto a firm surface.
5. Lay the placenta onto the cover with the fetal surface uppermost. Note the size, shape, smell and colour.
6. Inspect the cord, noting the length, insertion point and presence of knots.
7. Count the number of vessels in the cut end of the cord.
8. If cord blood is required and has not yet been obtained, the samples should be taken now (see below).
9. Observe and feel the fetal surface for irregularities.
10. Taking hold of the cord with the non-dominant hand, lift the placenta from the surface and examine the hole in the membranes, looking to see if the membranes appear complete or ragged; then re-place it onto the surface.
11. Spread the membranes outwards, looking for extra vessel or lobes, or unexplained holes.
12. Separate the amnion and chorion, pulling the amnion back over the base of the umbilical cord.
13. Turn the placenta over so the maternal side is uppermost.
14. Examine the cotyledons, ensuring all are present, noting the size and amount of areas of infarction or blood clots.
15. Weigh or swab the placenta, if indicated (see Chapter 12).
16. If the placenta is being disposed of by the hospital, dispose of it according to the hospital protocol.
17. If the placenta is being taken home by the parents, securely wrap it in two plastic bags or place in an appropriate container and seal, then give it to the parents.
18. Remove gloves and apron.
19. Perform hand hygiene.
20. Discuss the findings with the parents.
21. Document findings and act accordingly.

Source: Johnson R, Taylor W: Skills for midwifery practice, 4th ed., Elsevier, London, 2016.

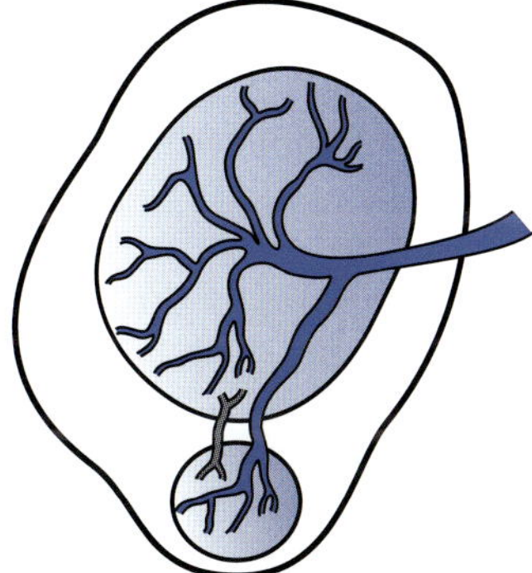

FIGURE 43.5 **Succenturiate lobe.**
Source: Johnson R, Taylor W: Skills for midwifery practice, 4th ed., Elsevier, London, 2016, p. 262.

CORD BLOOD SAMPLES

The midwife may be required to obtain cord blood when the mother is Rh-negative to ascertain the neonate's blood group and Rh-factor and determine if the mother requires anti-D administration. Cord blood may also be collected for blood gas analysis, or as part of the postmortem assessment following stillbirth. The sample should be undertaken as soon as possible after birth and before the blood has clotted. Blood can be obtained from one of the cord blood vessels or from a vessel on the fetal surface of the placenta. When a mother is Rh-negative, cord blood is collected in an EDTA tube; this can be done by draining the cut end of the cord into the barrel of a 20 mL syringe and funnelling the blood directly into the EDTA tube by placing the end of the syringe in the EDTA tube. To prevent contamination with maternal blood, the site of sampling should be wiped with a gauze swab before the sample is obtained.

For blood gas analysis, paired samples of arterial and venous blood are taken from the cord vessels and should be collected within 1 hour of clamping the cord. The **arterial sample** reflects the neonatal status, while the venous sample reflects the maternal acid–base status and placental function. If only one sample can be obtained for an umbilical cord blood gas, an arterial sample is preferable. Umbilical cord gases assist in determining the neonate's metabolic condition at birth. The acid–base status measures placental aerobic and anaerobic metabolism, reflecting the fetal exposure and response to intrauterine intrapartum hypoxia (Simhan 2020). The main cause of respiratory or metabolic acidaemia in the fetus is uteroplacental hypoperfusion. Only a minority of neonates with a low Apgar score are acidotic at birth and depression at birth may be related to something other than prolonged intrauterine hypoxia (Simhan 2020). Approximately 13% of neonates with low Apgar scores have severe metabolic acidosis and 50% have a normal pH (Wong & MacLennan 2011).

Metabolism and gaseous exchange can continue within the cord and placenta following birth, leading to different results depending on how long it takes to obtain the samples. When a cord blood gas analysis is required, a 10–20 cm segment of cord should be double-clamped as soon as possible after birth. A delay in cord clamping may affect the results; however, maternal requests for DCC are a consideration. The **cord blood gases** are collected in heparinised syringes from both vessels. The artery should be sampled first as the thicker vein provides support for the thinner arteries. To obtain the sample the cord is held by the non-dominant hand. The needle is held in the dominant hand and inserted slowly into the vessel following a 45° angle with the bevel of the needle pointing down to reduce the risk of puncturing the posterior vessel wall. When the sample is obtained, the air bubbles should be expelled by gently rolling the syringe between the fingers, as air bubbles can interfere with the results. The syringe is capped and labelled as arterial, and the second venous sample obtained in the same way and labelled as venous. Although cord blood samples remain stable at room temperature for 60 minutes, samples should be taken to the laboratory as soon as possible. Results should be documented and the neonatologist notified if health results are abnormal.

Umbilical cord blood banking

Umbilical cord blood contains stem cells which can be used to treat blood and immune system disorders. Cord blood is collected by inserting a needle into the umbilical cord and draining the blood from the placenta into a collection bag, which is later frozen. It is generally not possible to have DCC if cord blood is being collected for storage (RANZCOG 2020), although some companies indicate they can allow less than 60 seconds of DCC. In Australia, cord blood can be donated to a public cord blood bank or stored in a private cord bank for personal use and will attract a storage fee. In New Zealand cord blood storage only occurs through private cord blood banks.

DISPOSING OF THE PLACENTA

The majority of women leave the placenta for the hospital to dispose of, usually by incineration (local policy should be followed). The placenta and/or cord are collected in some maternity units and frozen for research purposes. Histological investigation may be required in certain situations (e.g. multiple births, preterm births, stillbirths, suspected infection).

Placentophagy—ingestion of the placenta—is undertaken by some women. This may be by ingesting the raw or cooked placenta or liquidising it to drink. More women have been using encapsulation of the placenta, which is usually cooked by steaming then slicing, dehydrating, grinding and placing it into capsules for easy consumption. The placenta is ingested for its mood-enhancing and unspecified health benefits (Selander et al 2013). A Cochrane review found there to be no benefits from placentophagy as the nutrients and hormones remaining following placental encapsulation are minimal (Farr et al 2018). The Centers for Disease Control and Prevention has recommended avoiding placental capsules as in one case a newborn developed group B streptococcus sepsis after maternal ingestion of contaminated placenta capsules (Farr et al 2018).

For Australian Aboriginal women, the placenta is important for the infant's spiritual journey, as every placenta has a unique *Miwi* (spirit or soul) print that contains instructions for their life journey (Northern Sydney Local Health District [NSLHD] 2015). The placenta is planted in *Nungeena-tya* (mother earth), near a tree of significance (NSLHD 2015) on family ground (Nappaljari Jones, n.d.). In Māori culture, the placenta is known as *whenua*, which also means land, and it is considered *tapu* (sacred). Traditionally, the placenta is buried in tribal lands to link the newborn to the earth and to symbolise being part of a collective tribal nation (Te Ahukaramū Charles Royal 2007). The midwife should ascertain the wishes of the woman regarding the placenta.

Role and responsibilities of the midwife

These can be summarised as:

- undertaking the procedures correctly and following evidence-based and/or best practice guidelines
- maintaining competency with both active and expectant management of labour
- recognising deviations from normal, taking actions and instigating referral

- taking appropriate action to prevent and reduce the complications arising from postpartum haemorrhage
- undertaking the examination of the placenta correctly
- recognising the normal, identifying deviations and instigating referral
- obtaining cord blood when required
- appropriate use of personal protective equipment (PPE)
- appropriate record keeping.

SUMMARY

- The third stage of labour is concerned with the expulsion of the placenta and membranes and the control of haemorrhage.
- During this stage, the woman is at increased risk of morbidity and mortality from haemorrhage.
- The placenta and membranes may be birthed expectantly (by the woman) or actively (facilitated by the midwife).
- Delayed cord clamping (DCC) confers many benefits for the neonate and does not appear to compromise the woman.
- Active management decreases the length of the third stage of labour and blood loss, but is associated with increased side effects from the uterotonic drugs and retained placenta.
- Cord clamping is optional with active management, but the cord should be cut within 5 minutes.
- Estimation of blood loss is often inaccurate and underassessed; as the blood loss increases, inaccuracy also increases.
- All swabs used should be double-counted at the end of labour care, to ensure none is retained within the woman, and documented.
- The placenta has fetal and maternal components; both sides should be examined carefully.
- Examination of the placenta should be undertaken to ensure it is complete; retained products predispose to PPH and infection.
- Deviations from normal can indicate underlying problems for the neonate (e.g. infection, congenital abnormality).
- PPE should always be used when handling and disposing of the placenta.
- Cord blood gases provide an assessment of the acid–base status of the neonate at birth.
- Women vary in how they want to dispose of their placenta and the woman's wishes should be established and facilitated.

Self-assessment exercises

The answers to the following questions may be found in the text.

1. Describe how the placenta separates and descends.
2. What are the advantages for the neonate of DCC?
3. What is the midwife's role when the third stage is physiological?
4. How and when is CCT used?
5. Why is it important to double-count the number of swabs at the end of labour care?
6. Describe the general appearance of the term placenta.
7. What are the differences between the fetal and maternal placental surfaces?
8. Describe the procedure for examining the placenta.
9. How would the midwife obtain cord blood for blood gas analysis?
10. What is a lotus birth?

References

American College of Obstetricians and Gynecologists (ACOG): Delayed cord clamping after birth, Committee opinion no. 814, 2020. Online 18 April 2021. Available: www.acog.org/-/media/project/acog/acogorg/clinical/files/committee-opinion/articles/2020/12/delayed-umbilical-cord-clamping-after-birth.pdf.

Andersson O, Lindquist B, Lindgren M, et al: Effect of delayed cord clamping on neurodevelopment at 4 years of age: a randomized clinical trial, JAMA Pediatrics 169(7):631–638, 2015.

Auckland District Health Board: National Women's Health Pūrongo Haumanu ā tau annual clinical report, 2019. Online 18 April 2021. Available: https://www.nationalwomenshealth.adhb.govt.nz/healthprofessionals/annual-clinical-report/national-womens-annual-clinical-report/.

Australian Institute of Health and Welfare (AIHW): Australia's mothers and babies. Cat. no. PER 101. AIHW, Canberra, 2021. Online 13 August 2021. Available: www.aihw.gov.au/reports/mothers-babies/australias-mothers-babies.

Backes CH, Rivera BK, Haque U, et al: Placental transfusion strategies in very preterm neonates, Obstetrics and Gynecology 124(1):47–56, 2010.

Baergen RN: Ch. 3. Manual of pathology of the human placenta, 2nd ed., Springer, New York, 2011, pp. 23–42.

Bayer K: Delayed umbilical cord clamping in the 21st century: indications for practice, Advances in Neonatal Care 16(1):68–73, 2016.

Begley CM, Gyte GML, Devane D, et al: Active versus expectant management for women in the third stage of labour, Cochrane Database System Reviews (3):Art. No.:CD007412, 2019.

Blank D, Badurdeen S, Omar F Kamlin C, et al: Baby-directed umbilical cord clamping: a feasibility study, Resuscitation 131, 1–7, 2018.

Blouin B, Penny ME, Maheu-Giroux M, et al: Timing of umbilical cord-clamping and infant anaemia: the role of maternal anaemia, Paediatrics and International Child Health 33(2):79–85, 2013.

Boere I, Roest A, Wallace E, et al: Umbilical blood flow patterns directly after birth before delayed cord clamping, Archives of Disease in Childhood, Fetal and Neonatal Edition 100(2), F121–F125, 2015.

Brodie K: Delayed cord clamping. Women and Birth: Journal of the Australian College of Midwives 31, S2–S2, 2018.

Buckley S: Gentle birth, gentle mothering, Celestial Arts, Berkeley, 2009.

Buder A: Implementation of delayed cord clamping in the active management of the third stage of labour, MIDIRS Midwifery Digest 25(2):211–217, 2015.

Charles, C. Labour and normal birth. Chapter 1. In: Chapman V, Charles C, editors, The midwife's labour and birth handbook, John Wiley & Sons, 2018.

Chen M, Chang Q, Duan T, et al: Uterine massage to reduce blood loss after vaginal delivery: a randomized controlled trial, Obstetrics and Gynecology 122(2):290–295, 2013.

Chiruvolu A, Huanying Q, Nguyen ET, et al: The effect of delayed cord clamping on moderate and early late-preterm infants, American Journal of Perinatology 35(3):288–291, 2018.

Culliney EM, Williams PM: Controlled cord traction during the third stage of labor, American Family Physician 93(5):350B–351B, 2016.

Daskalakis G, Papapanagiotou A, Siristatidis C, et al: The influence of delayed cord clamping and cord milking on inflammatory cytokines in umbilical vein and neonatal circulation, Acta Obstetricia et Gynecologica Scandinavica 97(5):624–628, 2018.

Davis D, Baddock S, Pairman S, et al: Risk of severe postpartum hemorrhage in low-risk childbearing women in New Zealand: exploring the effect of place of birth and comparing third stage management of labor, Birth: Issues in Perinatal Care 39(2):98–105, 2012.

De Paco C, Herrera J, Garcia C, et al: Effects of delayed cord clamping on the third stage of labour, maternal haematological parameters and acid-base status in fetuses at term, European Journal of Obstetrics, Gynecology & Reproductive Biology 207:153–156, 2016.

Deneux-Tharaux C, Sentilhes L, Maillard F, et al: Effect of routine controlled cord traction as part of the active management of the third stage of labour on postpartum haemorrhage: multicenter randomized controlled trial (TRACOR), British Medical Journal 346:F1541, 2013.

Digal K, Singh P, Srivastava Y, et al: Effects of delayed cord clamping in intrauterine growth-restricted neonates: a randomized controlled trial. European Journal of Pediatrics Jun;180(6):1701–1710, 2021.

Dixon L, Fletcher L, Tracy S, et al: Midwives care during the third stage of labour: an analysis of the New Zealand College of Midwives Midwifery Database 2004–2008, New Zealand College of Midwives 41:20–25, 2009.

Dunn AD, Ngu S, Lederman S, et al: The relationship between birth and placental weights changes with placental size, Early Human Development 111:56–59, 2017.

Ebbing C, Kiserud T, Johnsen SL, et al: Third stage of labor risks in velamentous and marginal cord insertion: a population-based study, Acta Obstetricia et Gynecologica Scandinavica 94(8):878–883, 2015.

Erickson EN, Lee CS, Emeis CL: Role of prophylactic oxytocin in the third stage of labor: physiologic versus pharmacologically influenced labor and birth, Journal of Midwifery & Women's Health 62(4):418–424, 2017.

Fahy K, Hastie C, Bisits A, et al: Holistic physiological care compared with active management of the third stage of labour for women at low risk of postpartum haemorrhage: a cohort study, Women and Birth: Journal of the Australian College of Midwives 23(4):146–152, 2010.

Farr A, Chervenak FA, McCullough LB, et al: Human placentophagy: a review, American Journal of Obstetrics & Gynecology 218(4):401.e1–401.e11, 2018.

Fogarty M, Osborn DA, Askie L, et al: Delayed vs early umbilical cord clamping for preterm infants: a systematic review and meta-analysis, American Journal of Obstetrics & Gynecology 218(1):1–18, 2018.

Garabedian C, Rakza T, Drumez E, et al: Benefits of delayed cord clamping in red blood cell alloimmunization, Pediatrics 137(3):29, 2016.

Gerson K, Modest A, Hecht J, Young B: Persistent amnion-chorion membrane separation, The Journal of Obstetrics and Gynaecology Research 45(2):352–357, 2019.

Gibbins KJ, Silver RM, Pinar H, et al: Stillbirth, hypertensive disorders of pregnancy and placental pathology, Placenta 43:61–68, 2016.

Hayward CE, Lean S, Sibley CP, et al: Placental adaptation: what can we learn from birthweight: placental weight ratio? Frontiers in Physiology 7:28, 2016.

Hilde G, Eskild A, Owe KM, et al: Exercise in pregnancy: an association with placental weight? American Journal of Obstetrics and Gynecology 216(2):168e1–168e9, 2017.

Hofmeyr GJ, Abdel-Aleem H, Abdel-Aleem A: Uterine massage for preventing postpartum haemorrhage, Cochrane Database System Review (7):Art. No.:CD006431, 2013.

Hofmeyr GJ, Mshweshwe NT, Gülmezoglu AM: Controlled cord traction for the third stage of labour, Cochrane Database System Reviews (1):Art. No.:CD008020, 2015.

Hooper SB, Polglase GR, te Pas AB: A physiological approach to the timing of umbilical cord clamping at birth, Archives of Disease in Childhood—Fetal and Neonatal Edition, July, 100(4):F355–F360, 2015. PMID: 25540147. Available: http://doi.org/10.1136/archdischild-2013-305703.

Ismail KI, Hannigan A, O'Donoghue K, et al: Abnormal placental cord insertion and adverse pregnancy outcomes: a systematic review and meta-analysis, Systematic Reviews 6:242), 2017. Online 22 April 2021. Available: https://systematicreviewsjournal.biomedcentral.com/track/pdf/10.1186/s13643-017-0641-1.

Jauniaux E, Moffett A, Burton GJ: Placental implantation disorders, Obstetrics and Gynecology Clinics of North America, March 47(1):117–132, 2020.

Jelin AC, Zlatnik MG, Kuppermann M, et al: Clamp late and maintain perfusion (CLAMP) policy: delayed cord clamping in preterm infants, Journal of Maternal–Fetal & Neonatal Medicine 29(11):1705–1709, 2016.

Jenusaitis L, Keplinger KB, Dean K, et al: Impact of a delayed cord clamping protocol on maternal and neonatal outcomes in patients undergoing term cesarean section, The Journal of Maternal–Fetal & Neonatal Medicine, 1–7, 2020.

Karim R, Pervaiz F, Muhammad MF: Comparison of active versus expectant management of third stage of labour, Journal of Postgraduate Medical Institute 29(1): 14–17, 2015.

Kashanian M, Fekrat M, Masoomi Z, et al: Comparison of active and expectant management on the duration of the third stage of labour and the amount of blood loss during the third and fourth stages of labour: a randomised controlled trial, Midwifery 26(2): 241–245, 2010.

Katheria AC, Brown MK, Faksh A, et al: Delayed cord clamping in newborns born at term at risk for resuscitation: a feasibility randomized clinical trial, Journal of Pediatrics 187:313–317, 2017.

Kazemi MV, Akbarianrad Z, Zahedpasha Y, et al: Effects of delayed cord clamping on intraventricular hemorrhage in preterm infants, Iranian Journal of Pediatrics 27(5):1–4, 2017.

Keating J, Barnett M, Watkins V, Gwini S: The association between ragged or incomplete membranes and postpartum haemorrhage: a retrospective cohort study, Australian and New Zealand Journal of Obstetrics and Gynaecology, 58(6):612–619, 2018.

Khong TY: The placenta and umbilical cord. In Khong TY, Malcomson DG, eds: Keeling's Fetal and Neonatal Pathology, 5th ed., Springer, 2015.

Khyriem B, Venkadalakshmi V, Rana AK: A pilot study to assess the current practices of immediate newborn care for term newborns in relation to early skin-to-skin contact and delayed cord clamping among health personnel of Labour Room, Nursing & Midwifery Research Journal 13(3):97–103, 2017.

Kirk AP, Yang J, Sim WC, et al: Systematic review of the effect of topical application of human breast milk on early umbilical cord separation. Journal of Obstetric, Gynecologic & Neonatal Nursing 48(2):121–130, 2019.

Koskinen A, Lehtoranta L, Laiho A, et al: Maternal diabetes induces changes in the umbilical cord gene expression, Placenta 36(7):767–774, 2015.

Kotzen M, Dhudasia M, Mukhopadhyay S, et al: 898 Delayed cord clamping does not increase need for phototherapy in infants of women with diabetes, American Journal of Obstetrics and Gynecology 224(2):S557–S557, 2021.

Kresch MJ: Management of the third stage of labor: how delayed umbilical cord clamping can affect neonatal outcome, American Journal of Perinatology 34(14): 1375–1381, 2017.

Kumbhat N, Eggleston B, Davis A, et al: Umbilical cord milking vs delayed cord clamping and associations with in-hospital outcomes among extremely premature infants, The Journal of Pediatrics May;232:87-94.e4, 2021.

Kuo K, Gokhale P, Hackney DN, et al: Maternal outcomes following the initiation of an institutional delayed cord clamping protocol: an observational case-control study, Journal of Maternal–Fetal & Neonatal Medicine 31(2):197–201, 2018.

Larsen S, Bjelland EK, Haavaldsen C, et al: Placental weight in pregnancies with high or low hemoglobin concentrations, European Journal of Obstetrics, Gynecology & Reproductive Biology 206:48–52, 2016.

Malloy ME: Delayed cord clamping requires a new table for stressed newborns, Midwifery Today 117:59–62, 2016.

Marzec L, Zettler E, Cua C, et al: Timing of umbilical cord clamping among infants with congenital heart disease, Progress in Pediatric Cardiology December, 59, 2020.

McAdams RM: Time to implement delayed cord clamping, Obstetrics & Gynecology 123(3):549–552, 2014.

McDonald SJ, Middleton P, Dowswell T, et al: Effect of timing of umbilical cord clamping of term infants on maternal and neonatal outcomes, Cochrane Database System Reviews (7):Art. No.:CD004074, 2014.

Mehta S, Khoury J, Miodovnik M, et al: Placental weight in pregnant women with type 1 diabetes mellitus: the association with fetal growth, American Journal of Perinatology 33(13):1255–1261, 2016.

Mercer JS, Erickson-Owens DA, Collins J, et al: Effects of delayed cord clamping on residual placental blood volume, hemoglobin and bilirubin levels in term infants: a randomized controlled trial, Journal of Perinatology 37(3):260–264, 2017.

Mercer JS, Vohr BR, Erickson-Owens DA, et al: Seven-month developmental outcomes of very low birthweight infants enrolled in a randomized controlled trial of delayed versus immediate cord clamping, Journal of Perinatology 30(1):11–16, 2010.

Mur S, Storme L, Lefebvre C, et al: Feasibility and safety of intact cord resuscitation in newborn infants with congenital diaphragmatic hernia (CDH), Resuscitation 12020–12025, 2017.

Nandadasa S, Szafron J, Pathak V, et al: Vascular dimorphism ensured by regulated proteoglycan dynamics favors rapid umbilical artery closure at birth, eLife, September 10(9), 2020.

Nappaljari Jones J: Birthing: Aboriginal women. Journal of Indigenous Policy 13:103–109, n.d. Online 22 April 2021. www.austlii.edu.au/au/journals/JlIndigP/2012/8.pdf.

National Institute for Health and Care Excellence (NICE): CG190 Intrapartum care: care of healthy women and their neonates during childbirth, NICE, London, 2014. Online 22 April 2021. Available: www.nice.org.uk/guidance/cg190.

National Institute for Health and Care Excellence (NICE): Quality statement 6: Delayed cord clamping, 2017. Online 22 April 2021. Available: www.nice.org.uk/guidance/qs105/chapter/Quality-statement-6-Delayed-cord-clamping.

New Zealand College of Midwives (NZCOM): Consensus statement: facilitating the birth of the placenta, 2013. Online 18 April 2021. Available: www.midwife.org.nz/wp-content/uploads/2019/05/Facilitating-the-Birth-of-the-Placenta.pdf.

Northern Sydney Local Health District (NSLHD): First Australian birthing practices in Gaimariagal Country: a guide for mothers and families, NSLHD, Sydney, 2015. Online 27 August 2021. Available: httpswww.nslhd.

health.nsw.gov.au/aboriginal_health/Documents/A%20guide%20for%20mothers%20and%20families,%20first%20Australian%20birthing%20practices%20in%20Gaimariagal%20Country.pdf.

Odent M: Don't manage the third stage of labour! Practising Midwife 11(9):31–33, 1998.

Padilla-Sánchez C, Baixauli-Alacreu S, Cañada-Martínez A, et al: Delayed vs immediate cord clamping changes oxygen saturation and heart rate patterns in the first minutes after birth, The Journal of Pediatrics 227: 149-156.e1, 2020

Palethorpe RJ, Farrar D, Duley L: Alternative positions for the neonate at birth before clamping the umbilical cord, Cochrane Database System Reviews (10):Art. No.: CD007555, 2010.

Patel S, Clark EAS, Rodriguez CE, et al: Effect of umbilical cord milking on morbidity and survival in extremely low gestational age neonates, American Journal of Obstetrics & Gynecology 211(519):e1–e7, 2014.

Patwardhan M, Hernandez-Andrade E, Ahn H: Dynamic changes in the myometrium during the third stage of labor, evaluated using two-dimensional ultrasound, in women with normal and abnormal third stage of labor and in women with obstetric complications, Gynecologic & Obstetric Investigation 80(1):26–37, 2015.

Polglase GR, Stark M: Cord clamping in term and preterm infants: how should clinicians proceed? Evidence favours delayed cord clamping in most newborns, but further studies are needed, Medical Journal of Australia 208(8):330–331, 2018.

Popat H, Robledo KP, Sebastian L, et al: Effect of delayed cord clamping on systemic blood flow: a randomized controlled trial, Journal of Pediatrics 178:81–86, 2016.

Rabe H, Diaz-Rossello JL, Duley L, et al: Effect of timing of umbilical cord clamping and other strategies to influence placental transfusion at preterm birth on maternal and infant outcomes, Cochrane Database System Reviews (8):Art. No.:CD003248, 2012.

Reed R, Gabriel L, Kearney L: Birthing the placenta: women's decisions and experiences, BMC Pregnancy and Childbirth 19(1):140–140, 2019.

Reister K, Reister F, Essers J et al: Association of umbilical cord milking vs delayed umbilical cord clamping with death or severe intraventricular hemorrhage among preterm infants, JAMA: the Journal of the American Medical Association 322.19, 2019.

Richardson BS, Ruttinger S, Brown HK, et al: Maternal body mass index impacts fetal-placental size at birth and umbilical cord oxygen values with implications for regulatory mechanisms, Early Human Development 112:42–47, 2017.

Royal Australian and New Zealand College of Obstetricians and Gynaecologists (RANZCOG): Altruistic and directed umbilical cord banking for families at risk, 2020. Online 22 April 2021. Available: ranzcog.edu.au/RANZCOG_SITE/media/RANZCOG-MEDIA/Women%27s%20Health/Statement%20and%20guidelines/Clinical-Obstetrics/Umbilical-cord-blood-banking-(C-Obs-18)-Review-July-2020.pdf?ext=.pdf.

Royal Australian and New Zealand College of Obstetricians and Gynaecologists (RANZCOG): Provision of routine intrapartum care in the absence of pregnancy complications, 2017. Online 22 April 2021. Available: www.ranzcog.edu.au/RANZCOG_SITE/media/RANZCOG-MEDIA/Women%27s%20Health/Statement%20and%20guidelines/Clinical-Obstetrics/Provision-of-routine-intrapartum-care-in-the-absence-of-pregnancy-complications-(C-Obs-31)review-July-2017.pdf?ext=.pdf.

Ruangkit C, Leon M, Hassen K, et al: Maternal bleeding complications following early versus delayed umbilical cord clamping in multiple pregnancies, BMC Pregnancy and Childbirth 18:131, 2018.

Safarulla A: A review of benefits of cord milking over delayed cord clamping in the preterm infant and future directions of research, Journal of Maternal–Fetal & Neonatal Medicine 30(24):2966–2973, 2017.

Safer Care Victoria and the Royal Australian and New Zealand College of Obstetricians and Gynaecologists Victoria: Consensus statement, 2021. Online 25 April 2021. Available: www.bettersafercare.vic.gov.au/clinical-guidance/maternity/vaginal-seeding-and-lotus-births-consensus-statement.

Saxton A, Fahy K, Skinner V, et al: Effects of immediate skin-to-skin contact and breastfeeding after birth on postpartum haemorrhage (PPH) rates: a cohort study, Women and Birth: Journal of the Australian College of Midwives 26:S16–S17, 2014.

Scheans P: Delayed cord clamping: a collaborative practice to improve outcomes, Neonatal Network 32(5):369–373, 2013.

Schorn M: Management terminology during the third stage of labor, Journal of Midwifery & Women's Health 65(3):301–305, 2020.

Selander J, Cantor A, Young SM, et al: Human maternal placentophagy: a survey of self-reported motivations and experiences associated with placenta consumption, Ecology of Food and Nutrition 52:93–115, 2013.

Selfe K, Walsh DJ: The third stage of labour: are low-risk women really offered an informed choice? MIDIRS Midwifery Digest 25(1):66–72, 2015.

Shinar S, Shenhav M, Maslovitz S, et al: Distribution of third-stage length and risk factors for its prolongation, American Journal of Perinatology 33(10):1023–2028, 2016.

Simhan HN: Umbilical cord blood acid-base analysis at delivery. In Lockwood CJ, Barss VA, editors: UpToDate, 2020. Online 25 April 2021. Available: www.uptodate.com.

Stanek J: Placental pathology varies in hypertensive conditions of pregnancy, Virchows Archiv 472(3): 415–423, 2018.

Steer-Massaro C: Neonatal omphalitis after lotus birth, Journal of Midwifery & Women's Health 65(2):271–275, 2020.

Steinhorn, RH: Umbilical cord milking should be avoided in preterm infants. Journal of Pediatrics, May, 232: 1–3, 2021.

Takami T, Suganami Y, Sunohara D, et al: Umbilical cord milking stabilizes cerebral oxygenation and perfusion in infants born before 29 weeks of gestation, Journal of Pediatrics 161:742–747, 2012.

Tarnow-Mordi W, Morris J, Kirby A, et al: Delayed versus immediate cord clamping in preterm infants, New England Journal of Medicine 377(25):2445–2455, 2017.

Tarnow-Mordi WO, Duley L, Field D, et al: Timing of cord clamping in very preterm infants: more evidence is needed, American Journal of Obstetrics & Gynecology 211:118–123, 2014.

Te Ahukaramū Charles Royal: Papatūānuku—the land—Whenua—the placenta, Te Ara—the Encyclopedia of New Zealand, 2007. Online 27 August 2021. Available: www.TeAra.govt.nz/en/papatuanuku-the-land/page-4.

Tricarico A: Lotus birth associated with idiopathic neonatal hepatitis, Paediatric Neonatology 58(3):281–282, 2017.

Upadhyay A, Gothwal S, Parihar R, et al: Effect of umbilical cord milking in term and near term infants: randomized controlled trial, American Journal of Obstetrics & Gynecology 208:120e1–120e6, 2013.

Vasconcelos FB, Katz L, Coutinho I, et al: Placental cord drainage in the third stage of labor: randomized clinical trial, PLoS ONE 13(5):1–10, 2018.

Vatansever B, Demirel G, Ciler Eren E, et al: Is early cord clamping, delayed cord clamping or cord milking best? Journal of Maternal–Fetal & Neonatal Medicine 31(7):877–880, 2018.

Westhoff G, Cotter AM, Tolosa JE: Prophylactic oxytocin for the third stage of labour to prevent postpartum haemorrhage, Cochrane Database System Reviews (10):Art. No.: CD001808, 2013.

Winter J, Kattwinkel J, Wilson S, et al: Ventilation of preterm infants during delayed cord clamping (ventfirst): a pilot study of feasibility and safety, American Journal of Perinatology 34(2):111–116, 2017.

Wong L, Maclennan AH: Gathering the evidence: cord gases and placental histology for births with low Apgar scores, Australia NZ Journal of Obstetrics and Gynaecology 51:17–21, 2011.

World Health Organization (WHO): WHO recommendations for the prevention and treatment of postpartum haemorrhage, 2012. Online 22 April 2021. Available: apps.who.int/iris/bitstream/handle/10665/75411/9789241548502_eng.pdf;jsessionid=935F15DF8E55616AEDF74B831244959A?sequence=1.

World Health Organization (WHO): Guideline: Delayed umbilical cord clamping for improved maternal and infant health and nutrition outcomes, 2014. Online 22 April 2021. apps.who.int/iris/bitstream/handle/10665/148793/9789241508209_eng.pdf?sequence=1.

Yamamoto Y, Aoki S, Oba MS, et al: Relationship between short umbilical cord length and adverse pregnancy outcomes. Fetal and Pediatric Pathology 35(2):81–87, 2016.

Yigit B, Tutsak E, Yıldırım C, et al: Transitional fetal hemodynamics and gas exchange in premature postpartum adaptation: immediate vs. delayed cord clamping. Maternal Health, Neonatology and Perinatology 5(1):5–5, 2019.

Zinsser LA: Lotus birth, a holistic approach on physiological cord clamping, Women and Birth: Journal of the Australian College of Midwives 31(2):e73–e76, 2018.

CHAPTER 44
POSTPARTUM HAEMORRHAGE

Learning outcomes

Having read this chapter, the reader should be able to:

- define postpartum haemorrhage
- discuss the risk factors for postpartum haemorrhage
- describe how blood loss is estimated
- list how uterotonics are used for postpartum haemorrhage management
- describe emergency management of post-partum haemorrhage
- summarise the role and responsibilities of the midwife.

Globally, **postpartum haemorrhage (PPH)** is the leading cause of maternal mortality, accounting for over one-quarter of maternal deaths (Say et al 2014), with one woman dying from PPH about every 4 minutes (Sebghati & Chandraharan 2017). In Australia, obstetric haemorrhage was responsible for 15 maternal deaths between 2009–2018, with one direct maternal death occurring in 2018 (Australian Institute of Health and Welfare [AIHW] 2020). In New Zealand there were four direct maternal deaths from obstetric haemorrhage between 2006–2018 (Perinatal & Maternal Mortality Review Committee 2021). Australian Indigenous women continue to have a higher incidence of adverse outcomes (AIHW 2021). Māori women also have a higher incidence of adverse outcomes (Health Quality & Safety Commission New Zealand [HQSC] 2021). New Zealand's Severe Acute Maternal Morbidity (SAMM) audit found delay or failure to recognise deterioration occurred with major PPH (HQSC 2017). New Zealand has developed a *National Consensus Guideline for the Treatment of Postpartum Haemorrhage* (Ministry of Health 2013). **Obstetric haemorrhage** relates to bleeding from the uterus, usually the placental site, and is used in reporting to distinguish mortality and morbidity from non-obstetric haemorrhage, such as intracerebral haemorrhage.

PPH is excessive blood loss from the genital tract after the infant is born and during the 6 weeks postpartum. The traditional definition of PPH is blood loss of 500 mL or more during the puerperium, with severe or major PPH defined as blood loss of 1000 mL or more (Royal Australian And New Zealand College of Obstetricians and Gynaecologists [RANZCOG] 2017a). In addition, major PPH can be classified into moderate if between 1001–2000 mL and severe if > 2000 mL (Dey & Weeks 2020). PPH definitions differ depending on the mode of birth, with loss of 500 mL or more after vaginal birth and loss of 1000 mL or more after caesarean section considered as a PPH. Further classification is related to timing of the haemorrhage, with primary PPH occurring within 24 hours of birth and secondary PPH occurring between 24 hours and 6 weeks postpartum (RANZCOG 2017a). The American College of Obstetricians and Gynecologists (ACOG 2017, p. 923) have updated their definition of maternal haemorrhage to: 'a cumulative blood loss of greater than or equal to 1000 mL or blood loss accompanied by signs or symptoms of hypovolaemia within 24 hours after the birth process'. Most definitions of PPH discuss the importance of recognising signs of haemodynamic instability (RANZCOG 2017b, Sebghati & Chandraharan 2017). It is essential that the response to PPH considers blood loss as a proportion of circulating blood volume in relation to a woman's body weight (Tuffnell & Knight 2020). Smaller women may tolerate less blood loss (see Table 44.1).

PPH can cause serious morbidity including multi-organ failure, multiple blood transfusions, damage

TABLE 44.1 ESTIMATED BLOOD VOLUMES AND BLOOD LOSS IN RELATION TO BODY WEIGHT

Weight	Total blood volume*	Moderate haemorrhage 15% blood volume loss	Severe haemorrhage 30% blood volume loss	Life-threatening haemorrhage 40% blood volume loss
50 kg	5000	750	1500	2000
60 kg	6000	900	1800	2400
70 kg	7000	1050	2100	2800
80 kg	8000	1200	2400	3200
90 kg	9000	1350	2700	3600
100 kg	10000	1500	3000	4000

*Based on 100 mL/kg blood volume in pregnancy; may over-estimate blood volume in obese women (Lemmens et al 2006).
Source: Lemmens HJ et al: Estimating blood volume in obese and morbidly obese patients, Obesity Surgery 16(6):773–776, 2006. Tuffnell D, Knight M on behalf of the MBRRACE-UK haemorrhage and AFE chapter-writing group: Chapter 7, Lessons for care of women with haemorrhage or amniotic fluid embolism. In Knight M, Bunch K, Tuffnell D, et al, eds, on behalf of MBRRACE-UK. Saving lives, improving mothers' care—lessons learned to inform maternity care from the UK and Ireland Confidential Enquiries into Maternal Deaths and Morbidity 2016–18, National Perinatal Epidemiology Unit, University of Oxford, Oxford, 2020, pp. 58–63.

to pelvic organs, hysterectomy, loss of fertility and psychological trauma (Sebghati & Chandraharan 2017). PPH can result in anaemia and fatigue, making it more difficult for mothers to care for their infant (AIHW 2016). Significant haemorrhage also increases the risk of venous thromboembolism (VTE) (Kennedy & McMurtry Baird 2017).

The national Australian incidence of PPH is between 5% and 15% of births (Keating et al 2018). However, the incidence of PPH appears to be increasing substantially in Australia and other developed countries (Flood et al 2018a, 2018b, Kearney et al 2018, Nathan 2019). Due to inconsistent definitions and reporting variations within Australia, it is difficult to provide current national estimates of PPH (Flood et al 2018a, 2018b). A study in Queensland using gravimetric assessment of blood loss found a 28.1% rate of PPH of > 500 mL in women who had a vaginal birth (Kearney et al 2018). A Victorian study found 21.8% of women experienced a primary PPH between 2009 and 2013 (Flood et al 2019). The lowest incidence of primary PPH occurred in women with an unassisted vaginal birth and the highest incidence in women with an unplanned caesarean section (Flood et al 2019). In 2020 in New Zealand, primary PPH ≥ 500 mL occurred in 39.1% of births and primary PPH of ≥ 1000 mL occurred in 12.2% of births (Auckland District Health Board 2020).

PHYSIOLOGY OF POSTPARTUM HAEMORRHAGE

Third stage

For the majority of women, the **third stage of labour** occurs with no adverse outcomes. However, vigilance is important as it is during the third stage that PPH is most likely to occur. The placental circulation is approximately 750 mL/min at term (RANZCOG 2017a); therefore, bleeding from the placental site can be profuse and rapid. Control of bleeding is achieved in three ways.

1. The middle oblique fibres of the uterus contract, constricting and kinking the blood vessels passing through them. Blood flow slows down and stops, allowing time for clot formation at the placental site.
2. The uterine walls become in apposition to each other, exerting pressure on the placental site.
3. The coagulation process begins to work at the placental site, within the sinuses and torn vessels. The damaged tissues release thrombokinase, which converts prothrombin to thrombin. Then thrombin combines with fibrinogen to form fibrin, which forms a clot by combining with platelets. Vitamin K, calcium and the other clotting factors are required for this process to happen efficiently.

RISK FACTORS FOR PPH

Identified risk factors

The majority of women who develop PPH have no identifiable risk factors (Dey & Weeks 2020). Identified risk factors include induction of labour, caesarean section, fetal macrosomia, retained placenta and prolonged third stage (Finlayson et al 2021). **Abnormally adherent placentation** is an increasing cause of PPH and reflects the increased incidence of caesarean section (Goh & Zalud 2016, Jauniaux et al 2019). Disorders of placental implantation (placenta praevia, placenta accreta spectrum) and velamentous cord insertion are mostly iatrogenic with > 90% occurring as a result of caesarean section and in vitro fertilisation (Jauniaux et al 2019). Risks factors for placenta accreta include increased maternal age, previous caesarean section, placenta praevia and multiple birth (Farquhar et al 2017). The incidence of placenta praevia is now 1 in 200 pregnancies with approximately 4.1% of women with one previous caesarean section diagnosed antenatally (Jauniaux et al 2019). **Placenta accreta** spectrum occurs in approximately 1 in 533 pregnancies (Goh & Zalud 2016). **Placenta praevia** is a major risk factor with a 45.5% risk of PPH ≥ 1000 mL.

Active management of third stage is recommended for women with risk factors for PPH (RANZCOG 2017a). The **four Ts**—tone, trauma, tissue and thrombin—are commonly cited as the underlying reasons for PPH. **Uterine atony** is the cause of over 60% (Nyfløt et al 2017) to 90% of PPH (Say et al 2014), making atony the most common cause (Dey & Weeks 2020). It is important to note in the case of uterine atony the extent of blood loss may not be visible because the dilated uterus has poor tone and can conceal a significant amount of blood (Belfort 2021). The following is a list of risk factors (adapted from RANZCOG 2017a).

Tone

- Prolonged labour, particularly second stage
- Prolonged third stage
- Induction of labour
- Anaemia and high parity
- Oxytocin withdrawal
- Uterine over-distention: multiple pregnancy, polyhydramnios, macrosomia
- Obesity (body mass index [BMI] > 35)
- Previous PPH
- Asian ethnicity
- Age (> 40 years, nulliparous)
- Medications promoting atonia, such as magnesium sulfate

Trauma

- Elective or emergency caesarean section
- Uterine rupture
- Cervical, vaginal or perineal tear
- Episiotomy
- Instrumental birth
- Large for gestational age (LGA) baby

Tissue

- Retained products of conception: placenta, membranes
- Placenta praevia, placenta accreta
- Uterine inversion

Thrombin

- Bleeding disorders such as von Willebrand's disease
- Thrombocytopenia
- Disseminated intravascular coagulation (DIC)
- Severe pre-eclampsia, sepsis, fetal death in utero (FDIU), amniotic fluid embolism
- Unsuspected or proven placental abruption
- Pyrexia in labour
- Massive PPH from any cause results in coagulopathy.

Unclassified

- Anaemia (< 9 g/dL) will exacerbate the response to haemorrhage

RISK FACTORS FOR SEVERE PPH

A PPH > 1500 mL occurred in 1.4% of births in a Victorian study; the risk factors for PPH > 1500 mL identified by Davey and colleagues (2020) included:

- multiple pregnancy
- older maternal age
- overweight/obesity
- first births
- placental complications
- macrosomia
- instrumental vaginal birth
- third- and fourth-degree perineal laceration
- in-labour caesarean section
- birth outside 37–41 weeks gestation
- 12- to 24-hour labour
- use of oxytocin infusion in labour.

In this study PPH > 1500 mL occurred in 0.7% of women with no identified risk factors (Davey et al 2020). A cohort-based study found women with a previous caesarean section, women with an induced or augmented labour, and women who gave birth to a baby with a birth weight > 4000 g had increased risk of severe PPH (Graugaard & Maimburg 2021).

RISK MITIGATION STRATEGIES

Caesarean section increases the risk of PPH; therefore, avoiding unnecessary caesarean sections has the potential to decrease the incidence of PPH (Hofmeyr & Qureshi 2016). Uterine hyperstimulation following induction of labour has occurred in women who died from PPH. During labour induction or augmentation, attention must be given to avoidance of uterine hyperstimulation and uterine tachysystole (Knight et al 2014). Oxytocin for induction of labour should be used for the shortest time and at the lowest effective dose as the risk of severe PPH is increased with longer duration of oxytocin infusion, possibly due to desensitisation of oxytocin receptors (Page et al 2017). Examination of the rates of PPH in women with an induction who had cessation of intravenous oxytocin at 15, 30 or 60 minutes after birth found no statistically significant differences (Lewis et al 2020). The risk of PPH in Australia is increased with induction or augmentation of labour, possibly due to uterine desensitisation and downregulation of oxytocin receptors (Springhall et al 2017). The rate of PPH was 34% in women who were augmented, 26% for women who were induced and 19.3% for women who had a spontaneous birth (Springhall et al 2017). In contrast, an Australian study using retrospective data found nulliparity, induction of labour and augmentation were not associated with PPH (Kearney et al 2018). This study found high neonatal body weight, perineal injury, labour complications and the baby being separated from their mother during the first hour following birth were factors associated with PPH (Kearney et al 2018). Induction or augmentation of labour should not occur without women being fully informed about their options and the risks and benefits of these interventions. The International Confederation of Midwives (ICM) statement related to caring for women during the COVID-19 pandemic indicates routine interventions such as induction of labour increase the risk of complications, length of hospital stay and possible exposure to COVID-19 (ICM 2020).

Significant risk factors, such as previous PPH and placenta accreta, should be flagged in the woman's health record. Women with abnormal placentation, such as placenta accreta or **placenta percreta**, require multidisciplinary planning including blood group, antibody testing and cross-match, availability of blood products and care by staff with resuscitation and intensive care skills. Maternal haemoglobin screening for anaemia and correction of iron-deficiency anaemia improves women's tolerance to blood loss; therefore, haemoglobin should be optimised during pregnancy. Women with blood disorders require specialist care and a birth plan regarding appropriate care during labour, birth and the postpartum period to provide a guide for all staff. Women may benefit from prophylactic intravenous (IV) access as it may be difficult to cannulate in the setting of haemorrhage and hypovolaemia.

Every facility benefits from a PPH protocol and a PPH kit containing appropriate rapidly accessible resources (Belfort 2021). Interdisciplinary high-quality simulation exercises help staff be well prepared and identify any gaps in protocol, staff, equipment and knowledge (Davis 2018). Checklists can be utilised effectively in the emergency management of PPH and assist with communication, coordination and ensuring critical tasks are completed (Elmezzi & Deering 2019).

Women who are Jehovah's Witnesses should discuss their preferences and acceptance of blood derivatives (such as cryoprecipitate), techniques (such as intraoperative cell salvage) and the use of erythropoiesis-stimulating agents and pharmacological drugs (such as tranexamic acid and intravenous iron transfusion). If a woman has declined blood products, this should be documented in her health record.

MANAGEMENT OF THIRD STAGE

Active management of third stage with uterotonics and controlled cord traction (CCT) is recommended to prevent PPH (RANZCOG 2017a, World Health Organization [WHO] 2012). According to RANZCOG (2017a), the risk of PPH is reduced by approximately 50% with use of prophylactic oxytocin. For vaginal birth, oxytocin 10 international units (IU) is given intramuscularly (IM). For caesarean section births, oxytocin 5 IU is given IV over 1 to 2 minutes. Variations in local protocols may occur and these should be followed. Active management includes CCT and is performed by a trained midwife or obstetrician following administration of uterotonics (see Chapter 43). If excessive bleeding occurs with a physiological third stage, uterotonics are recommended. Interestingly, data from the National Women's Health Annual Report (Auckland District Health Board 2020) shows women who had a physiological third stage following a vaginal birth were less likely to have a PPH or to require blood transfusion postpartum. Delayed cord clamping (DCC) does not increase the risk of PPH and is recommended.

UTEROTONIC DRUGS

Uterotonic drugs are used prophylactically for women at increased risk for PPH and during a PPH to stimulate the uterus to contract. They primarily consist of oxytocin (Syntocinon), and ergometrine, or a combination of the two (Syntometrine). A list of the various uterotonic drugs is presented in Table 44.2.

Oxytocin

Oxytocin is a cyclic 9-aminoacid peptide secreted by the posterior lobe of the pituitary gland. It is released into the systemic circulation during labour and breastfeeding. Syntocinon is the synthetic form of oxytocin. Oxytocin binds with oxytocin receptors within the uterus, triggering calcium release from intracellular stores, which leads to rhythmic contraction of smooth muscle, primarily of the upper segment of the uterus, mimicking the body's own actions. Oxytocin also has a weak antidiuretic activity and water intoxication can occur with repeated administration in large volumes of electrolyte-free solutions (Therapeutic Goods Administration [TGA] 2020a).

Oxytocin appears to be the most effective first-line treatment of PPH (Parry Smith et al 2020). The usual dose of Syntocinon is 5 or 10 IU. When administered intravenously (IV), oxytocin takes effect within 60 seconds; with IM use, it takes around 2–4 minutes to take effect, with the response lasting 30–60 minutes (TGA 2020a). Infusions containing Syntocinon are diluted in an isotonic electrolyte solution (e.g. 0.9% normal saline). IV infusions containing Syntocinon must be administered using a mechanical infusion pump.

Side effects

Syntocinon has a direct relaxing effect on vascular smooth muscle. A rapid IV bolus injection of oxytocin can cause acute short-lasting hypotension accompanied with flushing, reflex tachycardia and electrocardiograph

TABLE 44.2 UTEROTONICS FOR PREVENTION AND TREATMENT OF PRIMARY PPH

Drug	Dose and route	Side effects	Contraindications
Syntocinon (synthetic oxytocin)	Before birth of placenta: 5 IU slow IV injection (1–2 minutes) OR 5–10 IU by IM injection	Nausea, vomiting Water intoxication Transient vasodilation with undiluted IV doses	Hypersensitivity to oxytocin
	After completion of third stage 40 IU Syntocinon in 1 L warmed Hartmann's or normal saline solution over 4 hours		Do not give IV Syntocinon in a 5% dextrose solution
Syntometrine (ergometrine maleate 500 microgram/mL)	IM Syntometrine 1 mL after birth of placenta or to treat PPH Repeat after more than 2 hours Total dose should not be > 3 mL in 24 hours	Nausea, vomiting, uterine hypertonicity, abdominal pain, headache, dizziness, skin rashes, hypertension, bradycardia, cardiac arrhythmia, chest pain Anaphylactic reaction	Possible retained placenta Hypertension, eclampsia, pre-eclampsia, diastolic bp > 90 mmHg Severe or persistent sepsis Impaired hepatic or renal function
Ergometrine maleate (500 microgram/mL)	Ergometrine 250 microgram IMI OR 250 microgram IV over 1 minute or diluted to 5 mL with normal saline 0.9%	Nausea, vomiting, abdominal pain, headache dizziness, rash, peripheral vasoconstriction, hypertension, cardiac arrhythmias, chest pain, anaphylactic reaction	Must not be added to IV fluids containing any other medications
15-methyl-PGF2α (Carboprost 250 microgram/mL): Only available in Australia using the Special Access Scheme	IM injection of 250 microgram (0.25 mg) repeated at 15-minute intervals to a maximum cumulative dose of 2.0 mg **Must not be given IV**	Pulmonary hypertension, bronchospasm, pulmonary oedema, acute hypertension, usually transient, abdominal cramps, diarrhoea and vomiting	Cardiac and pulmonary disease, pulmonary hypertension, reactive airway disease, history of asthma
Tranexamic acid (100 mg/mL)	1 g IV over 10 minutes. Rapid injection can cause dizziness and/or hypertension hypersensitivity	Nausea, vomiting, dizziness, anxiety, blurred vision, chest pain, confusion, cough, tachycardia	History of thrombosis, active deep vein thrombosis (DVT), acquired defective colour vision, hypersensitivity

Sources: NSW Government: Postpartum haemorrhage (PPH), NSW Health guideline summary, July 2021. Online 5 September 2021. Available: www1.health.nsw.gov.au/pds/ActivePDSDocuments/GL2021_010.pdf; Royal Australian and New Zealand College of Obstetricians and Gynaecologists (RANZCOG): Management of post-partum haemorrhage (PPH), 2017a. Online 6 September 2021. Available: www.ranzcog.edu.au/RANZCOG_SITE/media/RANZCOG-MEDIA/Women%27s%20Health/Statement%20and%20guidelines/Clinical-Obstetrics/Management-of-Postpartum-Haemorrhage-(C-Obs-43)-Review-July-2017.pdf?ext=.pdf; Therapeutic Goods Administration (TGA): Cytotec® (misoprostol). Australian product information, 2019b. Online 6 September 2021. Available: www.ebs.tga.gov.au/ebs/picmi/picmirepository.nsf/pdf?OpenAgent&id=CP-2010-PI-05416-3; Therapeutic Goods Administration (TGA): DBL™ ergometrine injection (ergometrine maleate). Australian product information, 2020b. Online 6 September 2021. Available: www.ebs.tga.gov.au/ebs/picmi/picmirepository.nsf/pdf?OpenAgent&id=CP-2018-PI-01920-1; Therapeutic Goods Administration (TGA): Syntocinon® (oxytocin injection). Australian product information, 2020a. Online 6 September 2021. Available: www.ebs.tga.gov.au/ebs/picmi/picmirepository.nsf/pdf?OpenAgent&id=CP-2018-PI-02394-1; Therapeutic Goods Administration (TGA): Syntometrine® (oxytocin/ergometrine maleate). Full product information, 2019a. Online 6 September 2018. Available: www.ebs.tga.gov.au/ebs/picmi/picmirepository.nsf/pdf?OpenAgent&id=CP-2014-PI-02336-1; Therapeutic Goods Administration (TGA): Tranexamic-AFT (tranexamic acid). Australian product information, 2019c. Online 6 September 2018. Available: www.ebs.tga.gov.au/ebs/picmi/picmirepository.nsf/pdf?OpenAgent&id=CP-2015-PI-02748-1.

changes. These rapid haemodynamic changes may result in myocardial ischaemia, particularly in women with preexisting cardiovascular disease. Therefore, Syntocinon is used with caution for women with cardiovascular conditions and long QT syndrome (TGA 2020a). Common side effects include headache, tachycardia, bradycardia, nausea and vomiting (TGA 2020a). The plasma half-life of Syntocinon ranges from 3 to 20 minutes.

Syntocinon is usually stored at temperatures of 2–8°C. However, where this is not possible it can be stored at 30°C for 3 months.

Ergometrine

Ergometrine is an amine ergot alkaloid that stimulates contraction of uterine and vascular smooth muscle, as well as the cervix. Ergometrine causes sustained tonic uterine contractions of both the upper and lower uterine segments. Ergometrine also causes vasoconstriction via several pathways, including stimulation of alpha-adrenergic and serotonin receptors (TGA 2020b). With doses around 200 micrograms, the uterine contraction is intense and usually followed by periods of relaxation; however, with larger doses the contraction is sustained and forceful with little or no period of relaxation (TGA 2020b). As the amplitude and frequency of uterine contraction and tone are increased by ergometrine, uterine blood flow reduces, promoting haemostasis. Constriction of vascular smooth muscle can result in an increase in both venous and arterial blood pressure and thus should not be routinely administered to women with hypertension, eclampsia or severe cardiac disease (Sebghati & Chandraharan 2017).

Ergometrine is contraindicated for retained placenta and severe or persistent sepsis (TGA 2020b).

Intravenous ergometrine takes effect within 1 minute, with the effects lasting for 45 minutes (TGA 2020b). The use of IV ergometrine is only recommended for severe uterine bleeding or a life-threatening emergency. IV ergometrine must be administered slowly, at least over 1 minute and preferably diluted to 5 mL with sodium chloride 0.9% to reduce the risk of serious adverse effects occurring. Ergometrine is rapidly absorbed after IM injection with uterine contractions occurring within 2–5 minutes and persisting for 3 hours or more (TGA 2020b). A Cochrane review found a lack of evidence for the effectiveness of ergometrine as a first-line treatment for PPH (Parry Smith et al 2020).

Side effects

Side effects are mainly related to the effects of smooth muscle contraction and include tinnitus, headache, transient chest pain and palpitations, cramp-like pains in the back and legs, nausea and vomiting, a sharp rise in blood pressure and a decreased prolactin level (if multiple doses are given). Ergometrine should be stored at temperatures of 2–8°C and protected from light. The usual dose is 250–500 micrograms.

Syntometrine

This is composed of ergometrine 500 micrograms and oxytocin 5 IU in 1 mL (TGA 2019a). It combines the effects of the two drugs but it also combines the side effects of the two drugs (nausea, vomiting, abdominal pain, headache, dizziness, rash and hypertension). Syntometrine begins to work after 2.5 minutes and its effect lasts for several hours, so it has the advantage of working faster than ergometrine alone and lasts longer than oxytocin alone. It is particularly useful when IV administration of a uterotonic is not possible.

An Australian study found minimal difference between the rates of PPH with treatment with oxytocin alone compared to Syntometrine (Springhall et al 2017). Syntometrine appears to reduce the need for additional uterotonics but made no difference to measured blood loss when compared with oxytocin; however, Syntometrine increased maternal side effects and reduced mothers' ability to bond with their baby in the first 2 hours following birth (van der Nelson et al 2021). A Cochrane review found a lack of evidence for the effectiveness of Syntometrine as a first-line treatment for PPH (Parry Smith et al 2020).

Side effects

Side effects include a significant increase in the incidence of diastolic hypertension, vomiting and nausea when Syntometrine is used compared with oxytocin. McDonald and colleagues (2004) suggest the advantages of reducing the risk of blood loss of 500–1000 mL should be measured against the risk of side effects occurring when deciding whether to use Syntocinon or Syntometrine. Westhoff and colleagues (2013) found oxytocin at either 5 or 10 IU was superior to ergometrine for preventing PPH > 500 mL, with less side effects such as nausea and vomiting, and did not find any improvement when they were added together.

Route and dose

Oladapo and colleagues (2012) found no evidence to recommend the use of IM over IV Syntocinon and vice versa for a vaginal birth in relation to the benefits, risks and side effects. WHO (2012) advises using 10 IU, IV or IM, whereas the National Institute for Health and Care Excellence (NICE 2014) suggests 10 IU given IM.

Traditionally, the uterotonic had been administered with the birth of the anterior shoulder. However, if the drug is administered at this time it has implications for DCC because it means a second person who is qualified to administer an injection has to be present (Soltani et al 2011). According to Soltani et al (2011), administering oxytocin (mainly IV) at the delivery of the anterior shoulder or after delivery of the placenta did not significantly influence the major clinical outcomes such as PPH or the duration of the third stage. NICE (2014) recommends the uterotonic be administered as the anterior shoulder is delivered or immediately after the birth of the baby, but before the cord is clamped (before 5 minutes). NSW Health recommends Syntocinon before delivery of the placenta (NSW Government 2021). The New Zealand College of Midwives (NZCOM 2013) recommends the uterotonic should be given after the cord has been clamped and cut.

15-methyl-PGF$_{2}\alpha$ (Carboprost)

Carboprost is a smooth muscle stimulant used to treat PPH due to uterine atony. Carboprost is only licensed for IM injection, but is used off-label as an intramyometrial injection by obstetricians. Carboprost must not be given intravenously as it can cause bronchospasm, hypertension, vomiting or anaphylaxis. It must be kept refrigerated between 2°C and 8°C as it is light- and heat-sensitive. A Cochrane review of evidence on the effectiveness of Carboprost for treatment of PPH was lacking (Parry Smith et al 2020).

Tranexamic acid

Tranexamic acid is a haemostatic agent and antifibrinolytic that acts on the process of coagulation by stabilising clots and preventing the breakdown of fibrin. In women with PPH, tranexamic acid reduces morbidity with no adverse effects (Brenner et al 2018). Once excess bleeding is recognised, tranexamic acid should be given as soon as possible, preferably within 3 hours (Brenner et al 2019, Sudhof et al 2019) The WOMAN (World Maternal Antifibrinolytic) Trial found IV administration of tranexamic acid reduced blood loss after vaginal birth and caesarean section (Shakur et al 2018). Tranexamic acid is effective in arresting bleeding that is not related to uterine atony (Dey & Weeks 2020).

Misoprostol

Misoprostol is a synthetic prostaglandin E_1 analogue (TGA 2019b). It inhibits gastric acid secretion and has mucosal cytoprotective properties. Misoprostol causes uterine contractions and is contraindicated in pregnancy. Misoprostol is less effective for treating PPH than oxytocin and tends to be used in low-resource settings where oxytocin is not available (Dey & Weeks 2020). Misoprostol used in combination with oxytocin has more side effects and probably does not improve effectiveness outcomes; however, it may possibly reduce the need for blood transfusion and reduce additional blood loss ≥ 1000 mL (Parry Smith et al 2020). Misoprostol is excreted in breast milk and may lead to diarrhoea in breastfeeding infants (TGA 2019b).

ESTIMATION OF BLOOD LOSS

It is essential to monitor blood loss at birth and in the early postpartum period. An estimated blood loss (EBL) figure is required for all births. It is essential to recognise excessive blood loss promptly as a delay in recognition of excessive blood loss can have serious consequences (Belfort 2021). Blood loss is generally underestimated (Flood et al 2018a, 2018b) and is notoriously inaccurate. Student midwives underestimate blood loss more frequently than midwives, indicating the need for supervision of students regarding accuracy (Pranal et al 2018). Underestimating blood loss will artificially 'lower' PPH rates and estimates of measures taken to prevent PPH (Sloan et al 2010). Blood loss is often visually estimated; calibrated drapes can be used and blood-soaked materials weighed. A Cochrane review on methods for blood loss estimation after vaginal birth found insufficient evidence to support one specific method (Diaz et al 2018).

Begley and colleagues (2015) suggest healthy women with a normal pregnancy haemoglobin level can tolerate a blood loss of 600–750 mL, (routine blood donation is approximately 470 mL); however, the effect of blood loss will vary considerably depending on the woman's general health state, current haemoglobin value, coagulation status and the speed of blood loss. In a cohort of healthy women in Japan who had midwifery care for physiological birth without intervention, the average blood loss at 2 hours after birth was 608 mL; 32% of women had blood loss between 500 and 999 mL, which was well tolerated (Oishi et al 2017). Blood loss of 500 mL may represent normal postpartum blood loss and identifying this as a PPH may be pathologising normal blood loss (Erickson et al 2017).

Bose and colleagues (2006) found there was significant underestimation for large floor spillages, large gauze swabs and where blood loss was over the bed and onto the floor. They developed guidelines to assist with the visual estimation of blood loss, which include looking at saturated gauze swabs (small 10 × 10 cm = 60 mL, medium 30 × 30 cm = 140 mL, large 45 × 45 cm = 350 mL), saturated sanitary pads (100 mL), floor spillages (50 cm diameter = 500 mL, 75 cm = 1000 mL, 100 cm = 1500 mL), and whether the bleeding with a PPH is restricted to the bed (unlikely to exceed 1000 mL) or spills over the bed and onto the floor (likely to exceed 1000 mL) (Bose et al 2006).

Weighing pads, swabs and drapes improves the accuracy of blood loss estimation (RANZCOG 2017a). Estimation of blood loss during and after the third stage includes blood loss on disposable sheets, linen and within containers. It is important to retrieve as much blood from the sheets as possible into a container for measurement. Obvious blood loss can be measured in a jug, but when the blood has seeped onto the sheets it becomes harder to estimate blood loss; in this case linens should be weighed for greater accuracy. Estimated blood loss was improved by use of drapes with calibrated markings placed under the woman to 'catch' the blood (Toledo et al 2007). Gravimetric measurement (weighing of blood-soaked pads, linen etc.) of postpartum blood loss is considered more accurate than visual estimation. A study comparing gravimetric measurement and visual estimation of blood loss found the estimated blood loss was on average 78% of the measured value with 76% of estimates within 100 mL of the measured value (Kearney et al 2018).

Recognition of blood loss appears to be a dynamic process which includes the rapidity and force of blood loss, the condition of the woman and estimation of blood loss (Hancock et al 2015). Women are 'acutely aware' of their level of blood loss and should be encouraged to notify the midwife if they are concerned about it (Hancock et al 2015, p. 8). The measured and estimated amount of blood loss should be documented and prompt action taken if this is excessive or the woman is compromised.

VIGILANT ASSESSMENT

Accurate assessment of blood loss and observation of a woman's vital signs and condition are essential to prevent and manage PPH. The midwife must act on vital signs outside the normal parameters using the **Modified Early Obstetric Warning System (MEOWS)** or the early warning system in use locally. The effect of blood loss is cumulative and calculation of ongoing blood loss is necessary. Women who died from haemorrhage in the United Kingdom did not have ongoing blood loss calculated and staff relied on a single point-of-care haemoglobin test, which gave false reassurance (Knight & Paterson-Brown 2017). Transfusion is recommended with a haemoglobin level of 70–80 g/L; however, haemoconcentration in the early stages of PPH means results should be interpreted with caution (Collis & Guasch 2017). The majority of women with life-threatening PPH had tachycardia and agitation, but were not hypotensive until they were seriously compromised. Of note, hypotension is a very late sign of haemorrhage (Tuffnell & Knight 2020). Tachycardia is often the first sign of reduced blood volume.

Midwives must be aware of the signs of PPH, which may include:

- increase in visible blood loss (blood loss may be concealed)
- tachycardia with heart rate ≥ 110 beats per minute
- downward blood pressure trend (> 15% drop)
- hypotension and/or collapse
- pallor
- agitation/restlessness
- drowsiness, altered level of consciousness
- poor uterine tone
- oliguria
- oxygen saturation less than 95%.

PRIMARY POSTPARTUM HAEMORRHAGE

Primary PPH is an acute emergency with the potential for serious consequences. Emergency management is required and the situation may deteriorate rapidly. Significant blood loss must be detected early before irreversible collapse and coagulopathy occur (Dilby 2018). Midwives must recognise and take action when abnormal blood loss is suspected in order to prevent serious consequences. Midwifery, medical and ancillary staffing needs to be adequate for monitoring women carefully and for emergencies such as PPH. Table 44.3 lists some of the signs and symptoms of shock in primary PPH.

Prompt action is required to avoid cardiovascular collapse; women may not exhibit cardiovascular signs of shock until they have lost 30–50% of their circulating blood volume (Collis & Guasch 2017). Prior haemoglobin and the size of the woman should be considered when assessing PPH as blood volume is approximately 100 mL/kg at term; therefore, a 70 kg woman would have a blood volume of around 7000 mL while a 50 kg woman's blood volume would be around 5000 mL (RANZCOG 2017a).

The goals of PPH treatment defined by Belfort (2021) are to:

- restore/maintain adequate circulatory volume to prevent organ hypoperfusion
- restore/maintain adequate tissue oxygenation
- reverse/prevent coagulopathy
- eliminate cause of PPH.

Obstetric management of PPH may include bimanual compression of the uterus (Hofmeyr et al 2016); uterine balloon tamponade; thromboelastography; tranexamic acid (Dilby 2018); haemostatic compression sutures (e.g. B-Lynch suture); and artery occlusion and aortic compression (Dey & Weeks 2020). Thromboelastography tests clotting factors and fibrinogen concentrations to determine if plasma transfusion is indicated (Collis & Guasch 2017). Early thromboelastography provides rapid results in the context of PPH and can analyse clotting time, clot firmness, rate of clot growth and lysis, as well as platelet count, activated partial thromboplastin

TABLE 44.3 SIGNS AND SYMPTOMS OF SHOCK IN PRIMARY PPH

Blood loss	Blood pressure (systolic)	Signs and symptoms	Degree of shock
500–1000 mL (10–15% of blood volume)	Normal	Palpitations, dizziness, tachycardia	Compensation
1000–1500 mL (15–25% of blood volume)	Sight decrease (80–90 mmHg)	Mild anxiety, weakness, sweating, tachycardia	Mild
1500–2000 mL (25–35% of total blood volume)	Marked decrease (70–80 mmHg)	Restlessness, anxiety, confusion, pallor, oliguria	Moderate
2000–3000 mL (35–45% of total blood volume)	Profound decrease (50–70 mmHg)	Confusion, lethargy, collapse, air hunger, anuria	Severe

Source: Adapted from National Blood Authority: Patient Blood Management Guidelines Module 1: Table 3.1, Canberra, 2011. Online 17 April 2021. Available: www.blood.gov.au/pbm-module-1; NSW Government: Postpartum haemorrhage (PPH), NSW Health guideline summary, July 2021. Online 5 September 2021. Available: www1.health.nsw.gov.au/pds/ActivePDSDocuments/GL2021_010.pdf.

time, prothrombin time, fibrinogen, antithrombin and D-dimer (Karlsson et al 2014). Laboratory testing should also include potassium and calcium levels (Dilby 2018).

Responding to a PPH requires a multidisciplinary team to work together efficiently (Collis & Guasch 2017, RANZCOG 2017a) and to communicate effectively (Cooper et al 2019). Four Rs have been described by ACOG (2017) as necessary for the management of PPH; the final step involves systems-based quality improvement:

- Readiness
- Recognition
- Response
- Reporting.

SKILL 44.1 Management of primary postpartum haemorrhage

Note that the steps may not be carried out in the order below as context may vary and evidence-based management changes rapidly. This skill is a guide and local algorithms/flowcharts should be followed.

1. Call for help; activate a call for the medical emergency team (obstetrician, anaesthetist, registrar, midwives, haematologist, resuscitation team, radiologist may be required).
2. Assess airway and breathing and administer high-flow oxygen (10–15 L/min), regardless of oxygen saturation.
3. Commence resuscitation, if indicated.
4. Insert wide-bore IV cannula; two IV cannulas are optimal.
5. Send blood for a full blood count, coagulation profile, crossmatch (if not done), chemistry profile, blood gas. (Do not wait for results before treating.)
6. Commence rapid infusion of fluids (preferably warmed).
7. Restore oxygen-carrying capacity by transfusing group-specific blood or O Rh(D)-negative blood; commence with two units of red blood cells.
8. Monitor vital signs, including pulse, oxygen saturation and blood pressure (every 5–10 minutes). Monitor temperature and respiratory rate.
9. Continue to evaluate bleeding and level of consciousness/shock.
10. Allocate a team member to record vital signs, fluids, drugs and events.
11. Allocate someone to care for the neonate, partner and family.
12. Call an anaesthetist if the woman's airway is compromised.
13. Urgently order blood and fresh frozen plasma—initiate massive transfusion protocol, if indicated.
14. Keep the woman warm and in a flat position; avoid hypothermia.
15. Insert an indwelling catheter (IDC) if one is not already in place and monitor urine output.
16. Identify the cause of bleeding.
17. Treat uterine atony with uterine massage and expel uterine clots (treat all PPH as atony until proven otherwise).
    - Commence uterotonic medication in steps following local protocol; usually 5 IU oxytocin (Syntocinon) by slow IV bolus or IM injection.
    - Commence 40 units of oxytocin as an IV infusion in 500 mL or 1000 mL over 4 hours.
    - Ergometrine 250 micrograms can be given IV or by IM injection. If IV, it must be given by slow IV bolus (over at least 1 minute), or diluted to a volume of 5 mL with sodium chloride injection 0.9%.
    - Misoprostol (800–1000 micrograms) can be given per rectum,
    - Prostaglandin and prostaglandin analogues may be given (contraindicated if the patient has a history of asthma).
    - IM injection of 15-methyl-PGF$_2\alpha$ (Carboprost): IM injection of 250 micrograms repeated at 15-minute intervals to a maximum cumulative dose of 2 mg (eight doses) (or 500 micrograms intramyometrial).
    - Tranexamic acid 1 g IV is given over 10 minutes; early administration is preferred.
18. Retained placenta or retained products of conception: proceed to theatre for manual removal/evacuation of uterus.
19. Assess for uterine rupture or inversion, haematoma, amniotic fluid embolism.
20. Evaluate for vaginal or cervical tears and uterine rupture.
21. Repair genital tract injury.
22. Conduct point-of-care testing for platelets and clotting factors, if available.
23. Carry out emergency measures such as: bimanual compression of the uterus; uterine tamponade (e.g. Bakri balloon); haemostatic suturing (e.g. B-Lynch suture); bilateral ligation of uterine arteries or internal iliac arteries; selective arterial embolisation; and hysterectomy may be considered.
24. Continue monitoring for the next 24–48 hours.
25. Transfer to intensive care, high dependency or tertiary unit as required.
26. Postpartum VTE prophylaxis and treatment of anaemia may be required.

A PPH is a traumatic experience for a woman, her partner and family, and the health practitioners involved in her care. An opportunity to evaluate, review, discuss and debrief should be made available.

SECONDARY POSTPARTUM HAEMORRHAGE

Secondary PPH is associated with endometritis and/or retained products of conception. Conservative management with antibiotics and sometimes uterotonics is generally successful; if excessive bleeding is present, surgical evacuation of retained products may be considered (RANZCOG 2017a).

Role and responsibilities of the midwife

These can be summarised as:

- early recognition of risk factors
- assessment and recognition of PPH
- regular training and simulation to maintain skill and competence
- estimation and monitoring of blood loss
- assessment of vital signs and clinical deterioration
- competence in emergency management of PPH
- assessment of vital signs and clinical deterioration
- correct documentation.

SUMMARY

- PPH can result in severe morbidity and mortality.
- Estimation of blood loss is important and is often underestimated.
- Competent emergency management of primary PPH is essential.
- Morbidity and mortality are decreased by a timely and coordinated team response.

Self-assessment exercises

The answers to the following questions may be found in the text.

1. Discuss the signs and symptoms of PPH.
2. Describe the major risk factors for PPH.
3. Discuss the types of uterotonics available and their use.
4. Explain why the rate of PPH is increasing.
5. How is primary PPH managed?
6. Summarise the role and responsibilities of the midwife when she recognises a PPH.

References

American College of Obstetricians and Gynecologists (ACOG): Postpartum hemorrhage: Practice Bulletin no. 183, 2017. Online 17 April 2021. Available: www.acog.org/clinical/clinical-guidance/practice-bulletin/articles/2017/10/postpartum-hemorrhage.

Auckland District Health Board: National women's health annual clinical report, 2020. Online 5 September 2021. Available: www.nationalwomenshealth.adhb.govt.nz/assets/Womens-health/Documents/ACR/2020-Annual-Clinical-Report.pdf.

Australian Institute of Health and Welfare (AIHW): Australia's mothers and babies, Cat. no. PER 101, AIHW, Canberra, 2021. Online 6 September 2021. Available: www.aihw.gov.au/reports/mothers-babies/australias-mothers-babies.

Australian Institute of Health and Welfare (AIHW): Maternal deaths in Australia 2018, Cat. no. PER 99, AIHW, Canberra, 14 December 2020. Online 17 April 2021. Available: www.aihw.gov.au/reports/mothers-babies/maternal-deaths-in-australia.

Australian Institute of Health and Welfare (AIHW): National maternity data development project: primary postpartum haemorrhage, Research brief no. 8, Cat. No. PER 82, AIHW, Canberra, 2016.

Begley CM, Gyte GML, Devane D, et al: Active versus expectant management for women in the third stage of labour, Cochrane Database of Systematic Reviews (3):Art. No.:CD007412, 2015.

Belfort M: Overview of postpartum hemorrhage. In Lockwood CJ, Barss VA, eds, UpToDate, 2021. Online 18 April 2020. Available: www.uptodate.com/contents/overview-of-postpartum-hemorrhage.

Bose P, Regan F, Paterson-Brown S: Improving the accuracy of estimated blood loss at obstetric haemorrhage using clinical reconstructions, British Journal of Obstetrics and Gynaecology 113(8):919–924, 2006.

Brenner A, Ker K, Shakur-Still H, Roberts I: Tranexamic acid for post-partum haemorrhage: What, who and when, Best Practice & Research Clinical Obstetrics & Gynaecology 61:66–74, 2019.

Brenner A, Shakur-Still H, Chaudhri R, et al: The impact of early outcome events on the effect of tranexamic acid in post-partum haemorrhage: an exploratory subgroup analysis of the WOMAN trial, BMC Pregnancy and Childbirth 18(1):215–215, 2018.

Collis R, Guasch E: Managing major obstetric haemorrhage: pharmacotherapy and transfusion, Best Practice & Research Clinical Anaesthesiology 31(1):107–124, 2017.

Cooper N, O'Brien S, Siassakos D: Training health workers to prevent and manage post-partum haemorrhage (PPH), Best Practice & Research Clinical Obstetrics & Gynaecology 61:121–129, 2019.

Davey M, Flood M, Pollock W, et al: Risk factors for severe postpartum haemorrhage: A population-based retrospective cohort study, Australian & New Zealand Journal of Obstetrics & Gynaecology 60(4):522–532, 2020.

Davis A: Inspiring change: an interprofessional simulation for managing postpartum hemorrhage, Nursing 48(5):17–20, 2018.

Dey T, Weeks A: Identification, prevention and management of post-partum haemorrhage, Obstetrics, Gynaecology and Reproductive Medicine 30(8):231–241, 2020.

Diaz V, Abalos E, Carroli G, Diaz V: Methods for blood loss estimation after vaginal birth, Cochrane Library 2018(9):CD010980–CD010980, 2018.

Dilby GA: How to prepare for postpartum hemorrhage, Contemporary OB/GYN 63(3):22–31, 2018.

Elmezzi K, Deering, S: Checklists in emergencies, Seminars in Perinatology Feb;43(1):18–21, 2019.

Erickson EN, Lee CS, Emeis CL: Role of prophylactic oxytocin in the third stage of labor: physiologic versus pharmacologically influenced labor and birth, Journal of Midwifery & Women's Health 62(4):418–424, 2017.

Farquhar C, Li Z, Lensen S, et al: Incidence, risk factors and perinatal outcomes for placenta accreta in Australia and New Zealand: a case–control study, BMJ Open 7(10):e017713–e017713, 2017.

Finlayson K, Vogel J, Althabe F, et al: Healthcare providers experiences of using uterine balloon tamponade (UBT) devices for the treatment of post-partum haemorrhage: A meta-synthesis of qualitative studies, PloS One 16(3):e0248656–e0248656, 2021.

Flood M, McDonald S, Pollock W, et al: Incidence, trends and severity of primary postpartum haemorrhage in Australia: a population-based study using Victorian Perinatal Data Collection data for 764,244 births, Australian & New Zealand Journal of Obstetrics & Gynaecology 59(2):228–234, 2019.

Flood M, Pollock W, McDonald SJ, et al: Accuracy of postpartum haemorrhage data in the 2011 Victorian Perinatal Data Collection: results of a validation study, The Australian and New Zealand Journal of Obstetrics & Gynaecology 58(2):210–216, 2018a.

Flood MM, Pollock WE, McDonald SJ, et al: Monitoring postpartum haemorrhage in Australia: opportunities to improve reporting, Women and Birth: Journal of the Australian College of Midwives 31(2):89–95, 2018b.

Goh WA, Zalud I: Placenta accreta: diagnosis, management and the molecular biology of the morbidly adherent placenta, Journal of Maternal–Fetal and Neonatal Medicine 29(11):1795–1800, 2016.

Graugaard H, Maimburg R: Is the increase in postpartum hemorrhage after vaginal birth because of altered clinical practice? A register-based cohort study. Birth 10 March 2021.

Hancock A, Weeks AD, Lavender DT: Is accurate and reliable blood loss estimation the 'crucial step' in early detection of postpartum haemorrhage? An integrative review of the literature, BMC Pregnancy and Childbirth 15(1):1–9, 2015.

Health Quality and Safety Commission New Zealand (HQSC): Fourteenth annual report of the Perinatal and Maternal Mortality Review Committee: Reporting mortality and morbidity 2018, Wellington, February 2021. Online 17 April 2021. Available: www.hqsc.govt.nz/assets/PMMRC/Publications/14thPMMRCreport/report-pmmrc-14th.pdf.

Hofmeyr GJ, Qureshi Z: Preventing deaths due to haemorrhage, Best Practice & Research. Clinical Obstetrics and Gynaecology 36:68–82, 2016.

International Confederation of Midwives (ICM): Women's rights in childbirth must be upheld during the coronavirus pandemic, 2020. Online 5 September 2021. Available: www.internationalmidwives.org/assets/files/news-files/2020/03/icm-statement_upholding-womens-rights-during-covid19-5e83ae2ebfe59.pdf.

Jauniaux E, Grønbeck L, Bunce C, et al: Epidemiology of placenta previa accreta: a systematic review and meta-analysis, BMJ Open 9(11):e031193–e031193, 2019.

Karlsson O, Jeppsson A, Hellgren M: Major obstetric haemorrhage: monitoring with thromboelastography, laboratory analyses or both? International Journal of Obstetric Anesthesia 23(1):10–17, 2014.

Kearney L, Kynn M, Reed R, et al: Identifying the risk: a prospective cohort study examining postpartum haemorrhage in a regional Australian health service, BMC Pregnancy and Childbirth 18(1):214–214, 2018.

Keating J, Barnett M, Watkins V, Gwini S: The association between ragged or incomplete membranes and postpartum haemorrhage: a retrospective cohort study, Australian & New Zealand Journal of Obstetrics & Gynaecology 58(6):612–619, 2018.

Kennedy BB, McMurtry Baird S: Collaborative strategies for management of obstetric hemorrhage, Critical Care Nursing Clinics of North America 29(3):315–330, 2017.

Knight M, Kenyon S, Brocklehurst P, et al, eds: Chapter 8. In Saving lives, improving mothers' care—lessons learned to inform future maternity care from the UK and Ireland confidential enquiries into maternal deaths and morbidity 2009–12, National Perinatal Epidemiology Unit, University of Oxford, Oxford, 2014.

Knight M, Paterson-Brown S, on behalf of the Haemorrhage and AFE Chapter-Writing Group: Messages for care of women with haemorrhage or amniotic fluid embolism. In Knight M, Nair M, Tuffnell D, et al, eds: On behalf of MBRRACE-UK. Saving lives, improving mothers' care—lessons learned to inform maternity care from the UK and Ireland confidential enquiries into maternal deaths and morbidity 2013–15, National Perinatal Epidemiology Unit, University of Oxford, Oxford, 2017, pp. 74–81.

Lewis L, Doherty D, Conwell M, et al: Spontaneous vaginal birth following induction with intravenous oxytocin: Three oxytocic regimes to minimise blood loss post birth. Women and Birth: Journal of the Australian College of Midwives May;34(3):e322–e329, 2020.

McDonald SJ, Abbott JM, Higgins SP: Prophylactic ergometrine-oxytocin versus oxytocin for the third stage of labour, Cochrane Database of Systematic Reviews (1):CD000201, 2004.

Ministry of Health: National consensus guideline for treatment of postpartum haemorrhage, Ministry of Health, Wellington, 2013. Online 17 April 2021. Available: www.health.govt.nz/system/files/documents/publications/national-consensus-guideline-for-treatment-of-postpartum-haemorrhage-nov13-v2_0.pdf.

Nathan LM: An overview of obstetric hemorrhage, Seminars in Perinatology 43:2–4, 2019.

National Institute for Health and Care Excellence (NICE): CG190 Intrapartum care: care of healthy women and their neonates during childbirth, NICE, London, 2014. Online 17 April 2021. Available online: www.nice.org.uk.

New Zealand College of Midwives (NZCOM): Consensus statement: facilitating the birth of the placenta, 2013. Online 17 April 2021. Available: www.midwife.org.nz/midwives/professional-practice/consensus-statements/

NSW Government: Postpartum haemorrhage (PPH), NSW Health guideline summary, July 2021. Online

5 September 2021. Available: www1.health.nsw.gov.au/pds/ActivePDSDocuments/GL2021_010.pdf.

Nyfløt LT, Stray-Pedersen B, Forsén L, et al: Duration of labor and the risk of severe postpartum hemorrhage: a case-control study, PLoS ONE 12(4):1–10, 2017.

Oishi T, Tamura T, Yamamoto U: Outcomes of blood loss post physiological birth with physiological management in the third stage of labour at a maternity home in Japan, New Zealand College of Midwives Journal 53:23–29, 2017.

Oladapo OT, Okusanya BO, Abalose E: Intramuscular versus intravenous prophylactic oxytocin for the third stage of labour, Cochrane Database of Systematic Reviews (2): Art. No.: CD009332, 2012.

Page K, McCool WF, Guidera M: Examination of the pharmacology of oxytocin and clinical guidelines for use in labor, Journal of Midwifery & Women's Health 62(4):425–433, 2017.

Parry Smith W, Papadopoulou A, Thomas E, et al: Uterotonic agents for first-line treatment of postpartum haemorrhage: a network meta-analysis, Cochrane Library, Nov 24;11(11):CD012754, 2020.

Perinatal & Maternal Mortality Review Committee. Fourteenth Annual Report of the Perinatal & Maternal Mortality Review Committee, 2021. Online 5 September 2021. Available: www.hqsc.govt.nz/assets/PMMRC/Publications/14thPMMRCreport/Maternal_mortality.pdf.

Pranal M, Guttmann A, Ouchchane L, et al: Do estimates of blood loss differ between student midwives and midwives? A multicenter cross-sectional study, Midwifery 59:17–22, 2018.

Royal Australian And New Zealand College of Obstetricians and Gynaecologists (RANZCOG): Management of post-partum haemorrhage (PPH), 2017a. Online 17 April 2021. Available: www.ranzcog.edu.au/RANZCOG_SITE/media/RANZCOG-MEDIA/Women%27s%20Health/Statement%20and%20guidelines/Clinical-Obstetrics/Management-of-Postpartum-Haemorrhage-(C-Obs-43)-Review-July-2017.pdf?ext=.pdf.

Royal Australian And New Zealand College of Obstetricians and Gynaecologists (RANZCOG): Provision of routine intrapartum care in the absence of pregnancy complications, 2017b. Online 17 April 2021. Available: ranzcog.edu.au/statements-guidelines.

Say L, Chou D, Gemmill A, et al: Global causes of maternal death: a WHO systematic analysis, The Lancet, Global health, 2(6):e323–e333, 2014.

Sebghati M, Chandraharan E: An update on the risk factors for and management of obstetric haemorrhage, Women's Health 13(2):34–40, 2017.

Shakur-Still H, Roberts I, Fawole B, et al: Effect of tranexamic acid on coagulation and fibrinolysis in women with postpartum haemorrhage (WOMAN-ETAC): a single-centre, randomised, double-blind, placebo-controlled trial, Wellcome Open Research 3:100, 2018.

Sloan NL, Durocher J, Aldrich T, et al: What measured blood loss tells us about postpartum bleeding: a systematic review, British Journal of Obstetrics and Gynaecology 117(7):788–800, 2010.

Soltani H, Poulose TA, Hutchon DR: Placental cord drainage after vaginal delivery as part of the management of the third stage of labour, Cochrane Database of Systematic Reviews (9):Art. No.: CD004665, 2011.

Springhall E, Wallace EM, Stewart L, et al: Customised management of the third stage of labour, Australian and New Zealand Journal of Obstetrics and Gynaecology 57(3):302–307, 2017.

Sudhof LS et al, Tranexamic acid in the routine treatment of post-partum hemorrhage in the United States: a cost-effectiveness analysis, American Journal of Obstetrics and Gynecology Sep;221(3):275.e1–275.e12, 2019.

Therapeutic Goods Administration (TGA): Cytotec® (misoprostol). Australian product information, 2019b. Online 6 September 2021. Available: www.ebs.tga.gov.au/ebs/picmi/picmirepository.nsf/pdf?OpenAgent&id=CP-2010-PI-05416-3.

Therapeutic Goods Administration (TGA): DBL™ ergometrine injection (ergometrine maleate). Australian product information, 2020b. Online 6 September 2021. Available: www.ebs.tga.gov.au/ebs/picmi/picmirepository.nsf/pdf?OpenAgent&id=CP-2018-PI-01920-1.

Therapeutic Goods Administration (TGA): Syntocinon® (oxytocin injection). Australian product information, 2020a. Online 6 September 2021. Available: www.ebs.tga.gov.au/ebs/picmi/picmirepository.nsf/pdf?OpenAgent&id=CP-2018-PI-02394-1.

Therapeutic Goods Administration (TGA): Syntometrine® (oxytocin/ergometrine maleate). Full product information, 2019a. Online 6 September 2018. Available: www.ebs.tga.gov.au/ebs/picmi/picmirepository.nsf/pdf?OpenAgent&id=CP-2014-PI-02336-1.

Toledo P, McCarthy RJ, Hewlett BJ, et al: The accuracy of blood loss estimation after simulated vaginal delivery, Anesthesia and Analgesia 105(6):1736–1740, 2007.

Tuffnell D, Knight M on behalf of the MBRRACE-UK haemorrhage and AFE chapter-writing group: Chapter 7, Lessons for care of women with haemorrhage or amniotic fluid embolism. In Knight M, Bunch K, Tuffnell D, et al, eds, on behalf of MBRRACE-UK. Saving lives, improving mothers' care—lessons learned to inform maternity care from the UK and Ireland Confidential Enquiries into Maternal Deaths and Morbidity 2016–18, National Perinatal Epidemiology Unit, University of Oxford, Oxford, 2020, pp. 58–63.

van der Nelson H, O'Brien S, Burnard S et al: Intramuscular oxytocin versus Syntometrine® versus carbetocin for prevention of primary postpartum haemorrhage after vaginal birth: a randomised double-blinded clinical trial of effectiveness, side effects and quality of life, BJOG: an International Journal of Obstetrics and Gynaecology Jun;128(7):1236–1246, 2021.

Westhoff G, Cotter AM, Tolosa JE: Prophylactic oxytocin for the third stage of labour to prevent postpartum haemorrhage, Cochrane Database of Systematic Reviews (10):Art. No.: CD001808, 2013.

World Health Organization (WHO): WHO recommendations for the prevention and treatment of postpartum haemorrhage, 2012. Online 17 April 2021. Available: www.who.int/reproductivehealth/publications/maternal_perinatal_health/9789241548502/en/.

CHAPTER 45

EXAMINATION AND REPAIR OF THE GENITAL TRACT FOLLOWING BIRTH

Learning outcomes

Having read this chapter, the reader should be able to:

- state the aims of perineal repair
- describe the four degrees of perineal trauma
- discuss the role and responsibilities of the midwife when undertaking perineal repair
- discuss the current evidence for the choice of materials and techniques used
- describe how to infiltrate the perineum
- demonstrate tying a knot, continuous non-locked and subcuticular sutures
- list the factors that should be included with record keeping.

INTRODUCTION

Approximately 75% of women who have a vaginal birth in Australia experience some degree of perineal trauma (AIHW 2020); comprehensive data is not available about perineal state for women in New Zealand. Steen and Roberts (2011) suggest a second-degree tear is the most common spontaneous perineal injury during childbirth. Recognising the degree of perineal trauma and undertaking the repair are important skills for the midwife. Chapter 40 covers the skill of inspection of the perineum immediately post-birth. Perineal trauma and repair are associated with both short- and long-term problems (Beckman & Stock 2013). This chapter reviews the anatomy of the pelvic floor, the damage that may occur during childbirth, the significance of correct repair, the evidence around perineal suturing, and the materials and techniques used. While care of the perineum postnatally is an important aspect of postnatal care, it is not covered within this chapter.

THE PELVIC FLOOR

Within the pelvis two layers of muscles in a hammock-shaped arrangement provide support to the pelvic organs and prevent them from prolapsing; the urethra, vagina and anal canal pass through them (Fig 45.1). The pelvic floor is an important component in the correct functioning of the vagina, bladder, uterus and rectum; a damaged or weakened pelvic floor may cause long-term urinary, faecal and sexual morbidity. The deep muscles provide strength to the pelvic floor and are made up of three muscles—the pubococcygeus, iliococcygeus and ischiococcygeus—collectively referred to as the levator ani muscles. The superficial muscles consist of the ischiocavernosus, bulbocavernosus and transverse perineal muscles. The perineal body is a triangular-shaped structure situated between the vagina and rectum, with its apex pointing upwards. It is composed of two superficial muscles (bulbocavernosus and transverse perineal) and one deep muscle (pubococcygeus). As the presenting part descends during the second stage of labour, it flattens and displaces, but can be damaged spontaneously during the birth of the baby or via an episiotomy. It has also been recognised in recent years that the anatomy of the clitoris extends much further than previously thought (Blechner 2017), and so it may also be implicated in any damage sustained to genitalia while giving birth.

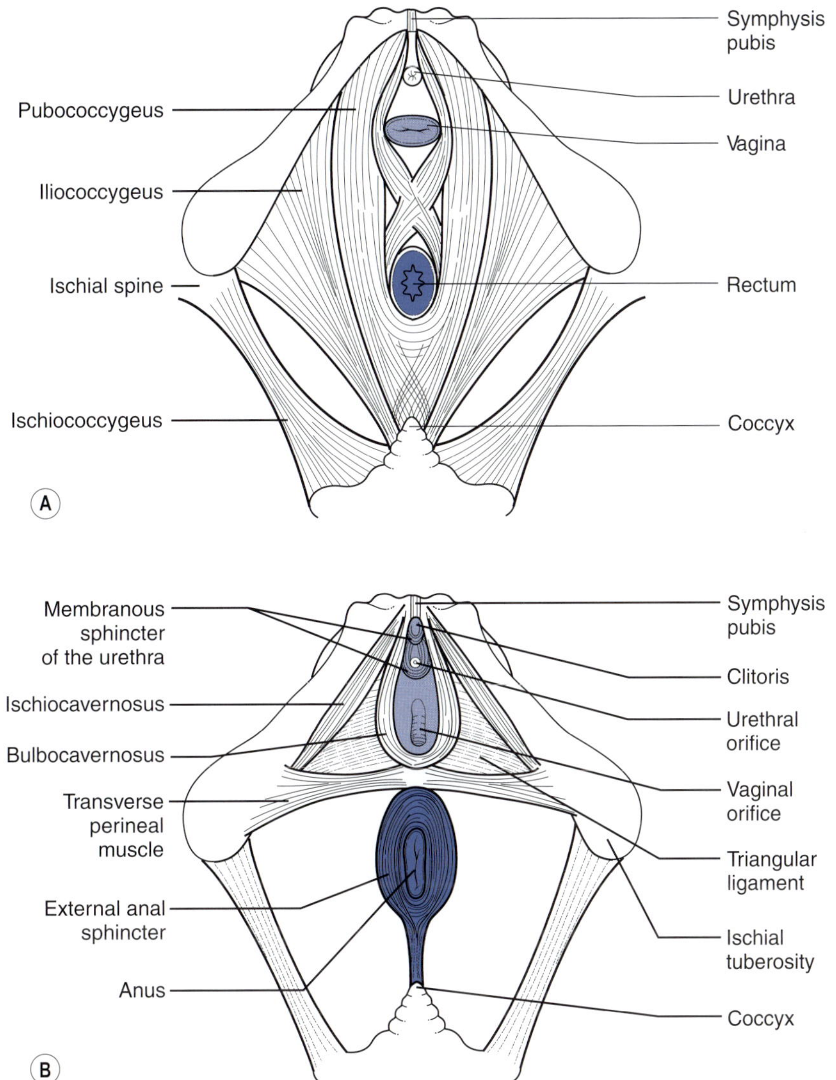

FIGURE 45.1 **A, Deep muscle layer of the pelvic floor. B, Superficial muscle layer of the pelvic floor.**
Source: Johnson R, Taylor W: Skills for midwifery practice, 4th ed., Elsevier, London, 2016.

AIMS OF PERINEAL REPAIR

The aim or repairing the perineum is to realign the tissues in their correct anatomical position, promote healing by primary intention, and prevent haemorrhage by sealing bleeding vessels and reducing the dead space into which bleeding can occur, causing a haematoma. Ultimately the aim is to restore the integrity of the woman's pelvic floor and normal physiological and sexual function as far as possible; however, damage to the dorsal nerve of the clitoris during childbirth may result in an extended period of reduced sensation, while its complete dissection is only reparable with surgery (Turin & Placik 2020).

PERINEAL DAMAGE

The degree of perineal trauma is classified according to the structures involved and does not include any reference to the depth or size of the injury. Classification of perineal tears in clinical guidance related to perineal injury (see RANZCOG 2015, for example) generally takes the form described by Sultan in 1999. The specifications for each perineal tear 'type' are as follows.

- First-degree tear: Injury to perineal skin and/or vaginal mucosa.
- Second-degree tear: Injury to perineum involving perineal muscles but not involving the anal sphincter.

- Third-degree tear: Injury to perineum involving the anal sphincter complex.
  - Grade 3a tear: Less than 50% of external anal sphincter (EAS) thickness torn.
  - Grade 3b tear: More than 50% of EAS thickness torn.
  - Grade 3c tear: Both EAS and internal anal sphincter (IAS) torn.
- Fourth-degree tear: Injury to perineum involving the anal sphincter complex (EAS and IAS) and anorectal mucosa (Sultan 1999).

Anterior perineal injury may also occur and involves injury to the labia, anterior vagina, urethra or clitoris. Concern around repair of labial grazes is largely related to achieving haemostasis, bilateral tears (where there is a risk of them adhering to one another when healing) or in situations where they are deep or do not oppose well (Dahlen & Priddis 2018). If the woman declines suturing of bilateral labial tears, she should be advised about the risks and encouraged to part her labia daily to reduce the likelihood of fusion.

The genital tract should be independently examined by two midwives as soon as possible post-birth to assess the extent of perineal (and other) trauma and decide whether it requires repair, by whom, in which environment and using which materials.

In 2018, Women's Healthcare Australasia, in collaboration with the Australian Clinical Excellence Commission and New South Wales Health, implemented a set of interventions known as the WHA CEC Perineal Protection Bundle. These interventions were 'aimed at reducing by 20% the number of women harmed by third- and fourth-degree perineal tears by the end of that year' (WHA 2018b). They were introduced into 28 Australian maternity services; however, this caused controversy. A critique of the Bundle by Australian midwife academic Dr Rachel Reed (see Reed 2018), updated in 2020, and WHA's response to Dr Reed's article (see WHA 2018a) provide useful reading in relation to this topic.

The importance of genital tract repair being performed by either a skilled midwife or obstetrician, using the best techniques and suture materials, has been emphasised by Kettle and colleagues (2012) as resulting in the least amount of short- and long-term morbidity for the woman. Notably, extensive trauma, such as third- and fourth-degree tears, will require suturing by a senior obstetrician, often in the operating theatre under general or regional anaesthesia. Accurate diagnosis and repair of obstetric anal sphincter injury is of utmost importance, and primary repair by an experienced obstetrician using the correct technique in the correct setting (usually the operating theatre), is associated with improved outcomes and reduced faecal incontinence rates (Preston & Fowler 2016). Suturing by a genitourinary specialist may be indicated if the urethra has been damaged.

Suturing is the most common method of perineal repair; however, there is increasing interest in the use of tissue adhesives. Currently, adhesive is used widely in other areas, such as paediatric and ophthalmic surgery. Initially it was thought the perineum would be an unsuitable site for adhesive use due to the amount of moisture in the area. However, Mota and colleagues (2009) found the use of adhesive for skin closure shortened the time taken to close the skin layer and a similar rate of complications and pain compared with subcuticular suturing. Feigenberg and colleagues (2014) report cosmetic and functional results equal to traditional suturing with surgical glue for first-degree tears..

TO SUTURE, OR NOT TO SUTURE?

Being able to identify the difference between a simple, small and well-apposed tear that is not bleeding, and a larger, ragged poorly apposed and bleeding second-degree tear is largely dependent on the experience of the midwife making the decision to suture or not (Dahlen & Priddis 2018). Importantly, as mentioned earlier, the decision to suture labial grazes is largely related to achieving haemostasis, when the graze is deep or poorly apposed, or when there is a risk of the labia adhering during the healing process if, bilateral labial grazes are present (Dahlen & Priddis 2018). The risk of fusion and the importance of daily cleansing and parting of the labia is an important part of education for women who decline suturing of bilateral labial tears. However, Elharmeel and colleagues (2011) suggest that small tears can heal well without being sutured and short-term outcomes are similar to sutured tears. Long-term outcomes were not evaluated in the studies they reviewed and the sample sizes were small. They conclude there is insufficient evidence to recommend whether suturing or non-suturing is best practice and propose that women should be offered information and informed choice around perineal suturing until conclusive studies are available. As noted earlier, surgical glue may be considered for these injuries (Feigenberg et al 2014). The Royal College of Midwives (RCM) (2008) suggests there appears to be neither benefit nor disadvantage in relation to suturing or not suturing the skin. Viswanathan and colleagues (2005) advise it is preferable to leave both the superficial vaginal and perineal skin unsutured. In a large randomised controlled trial (RCT) comparing two-stage repairs where the skin was left unsutured and three-stage repairs, where the skin was sutured, women who had resumed intercourse at 3 months post-birth and had a two-stage repair reported significantly less dyspareunia than those who had a three-stage repair (Gordon et al 1998). Additionally, fewer women reported that their perineum felt different from before birth at the 1-year mark (Gordon et al 1998).

When discussing with the woman whether or not to suture, the midwife should include the rationale for suturing, with the advantages and disadvantages, to allow the woman to make a more informed choice. The advantages of suturing include quicker initial healing of the tissues with better wound alignment compared with not suturing (Langley et al 2006, Leeman et al 2007) and reduced urinary problems (Metcalfe et al 2006). However, suturing can be a painful procedure, may require the use of lithotomy position, which can be difficult for some women (e.g. those with pelvic girdle pain) and may result in increased use of analgesia (Langley et al 2006, Leeman 2007). Metcalfe and colleagues (2006) found reported levels of perineal pain were similar between sutured and unsutured women.

Choice of suture material

Historically, both non-dissolvable and dissolvable sutures have been used to repair perineal trauma, with dissolvable sutures more popular in recent years. Kettle and colleagues (2010) suggest the ideal suture material causes minimal tissue reaction, is able to hold the tissues in apposition during the healing process and is absorbed once healing has occurred. While the sutures remain in the tissues, the body views them as foreign material, which may cause a significant inflammatory response. If microorganisms colonise the implanted sutures or knots it can be difficult to eradicate any resulting infection that may predispose the area to abscess formation and wound dehiscence (Kettle et al 2010).

Synthetic sutures include polyglycolic acid (e.g. Dexon), polyglactin 910 (e.g. Vicryl and Vicryl Rapide) and Biosyn. The polyglycolic acid suture is made of 100% glycolide and is converted into a braided suture material. It is designed to maintain wound support for up to 30 days and be completely absorbed by 120 days (Kettle et al 2010). Polyglactin 910 is a copolymer of glycolide (90%) and lactide (10%), which is derived from glycolic and lactic acids. They are also braided and coated with a copolymer of lactide, glycolide and calcium stearate to reduce bacterial adherence and tissue drag (Kettle et al 2010). They are absorbed more rapidly, by 90 days. Vicryl Rapide has the same chemical composition as polyglactin 910, but is irradiated during the sterilisation process, creating a faster absorption rate of 42 days while providing wound support for 14 days (Kettle et al 2010). Biosyn is a newer monofilament product composed of glycolide (60%), trimethylene carbonate (26%), and dioxanone (14%). It provides wound support for up to 21 days and is fully absorbed between 90 and 110 days (Kettle et al 2010). This suture has less tissue drag and less tissue reactivity and promotes better wound healing (Kettle et al 2010).

So which is the best type of suture to use for perineal repair? In the most recently published Cochrane systematic review on the topic, Kettle and colleagues (2010) reported that catgut increases short-term pain and wound dehiscence with an increased need to re-suture compared to synthetic sutures, and also that there is an increased need to remove synthetic sutures. For synthetic sutures, Kettle and colleagues (2010) suggest there is little difference between polyglactin 910 and Vicryl Rapide. Fewer sutures required removal in the first 3 months with Vicryl Rapide use, but there was a slightly increased risk of superficial partial skin dehiscence causing the skin edges to gape (Kettle et al 2010).

Wound dehiscence is associated with infection and provides a potential route for systemic infection with increased risk for septic shock. Infection causes the edges of the wound to become softened, which can lead to the suture cutting out of the tissue and causing the wound to break down (Kettle et al 2010).

Overall, the fast-absorbing polyglactin sutures are currently considered to be the suture material of choice as they are associated with less perineal pain, a reduced need for analgesia, less uterine cramping at 24–48 hours and at 6–8 weeks, a significant reduction in the need for suture removal, fewer healing problems in the short term, and earlier resumption of sexual activity (Greenberg et al 2004, Leroux & Bujold 2006, Viswanathan et al 2005). Size 2/0 sutures are recommended for perineal tissue.

Needles

Parantainen and colleagues (2011) suggest the use of blunt needles will noticeably reduce the risk of exposure to blood and body fluids by reducing the risk of needlestick injuries and also the risk of glove perforation by 54% compared to using sharp needles. The American College of Surgeons also support the use of blunt-ended needles when suturing muscle to reduce the risk of needlestick injury (ACS 2016). However, Wilson and colleagues (2008) found no difference in the rate of surgical glove perforation between blunt and sharp needles during perineal repair, but reported that the use of blunt needles increased the difficulty of perineal repair. Blunt needles do not penetrate the skin as easily as sharp needles and are better suited for subcutaneous wound closure (Parantainen et al 2011).

PRINCIPLES OF PERINEAL SUTURING

It is important that the midwife encourages the woman to maintain skin-to-skin contact with her newborn(s) and breastfeed as she feels comfortable throughout the process of checking her perineum following childbirth. The midwife should ensure the woman is supported in doing so, and attempt to facilitate this bonding as much as able in the early postnatal period, including while repair is carried out. Additionally, optimal perineal repair incorporates all of the principles listed below and on the following pages.

Effective analgesia for the woman

Pain during suturing can be greater than midwives realise for women who do not have regional analgesia (Sanders et al 2002); thus it is important to ensure effective analgesia. Where an epidural has been used effectively during labour, the infusion should be maintained if it is providing effective anaesthesia. If this does not achieve effective anaesthesia or regional analgesia has not been used, the perineum should be infiltrated using 20 mL 1% lignocaine or equivalent (NICE 2017). Nitrous oxide is a satisfactory and effective alternative to the use of lignocaine (Berlit et al 2013). Consideration needs to be given during the procedure as 16% of women report severe perineal pain during repairs (Sanders et al 2002); these women may require multiple forms of analgesia. Following repair, a non-steroidal rectal suppository (e.g. diclofenac 100 mg) is recommended, provided it is not contraindicated, as it is associated with reduced pain during the first 24 hours following the repair and less analgesia used within the first 48 hours (Hedayati et al 2003, Kenyon & Ford 2004, NICE 2017).

Asepsis and standard precautions

The midwife should use a sterile suturing pack and appropriate personal protective equipment (PPE); for example, sterile gloves, full body gown, apron and any other necessary items for infection control as indicated by local protocols. An aseptic non-touch technique (ANTT) should be used, with a critical aseptic field. Research into suitable fluids for perineal swabbing remains limited, but water is widely used.

Swabs and sharps

All swabs and sharps opened should be counted and recorded and the count repeated after the repair is completed with an entry in the woman's notes to record that both counts are correct.

Alignment of the tissues to encourage granulation and healing by primary intention

Familiarity with the pelvic floor anatomy can assist with alignment of the tissues; the distinction in colour between the tissues may be helpful. For assessment and repair, it is essential to have a good light source and access to the perineum. Occasionally, further examination with the woman in lithotomy may indicate the tear is more extensive than originally thought. Decisions should be reviewed and, if necessary, an obstetrician called. While the lithotomy position is still widely used in hospitals, its use is not always essential.

The woman must be comfortable and able to open her legs sufficiently. However, care must be taken to ensure the woman's legs are not abducted excessively. Resting her legs against the lithotomy poles may be more comfortable. With proper tissue alignment, the process of wound healing begins; sutures that are too tight or too loose may hamper this process. Tissues with a good blood supply heal rapidly. If there is tension at the wound edges, the tissue can become devascularised (Kettle et al 2010), disrupting the healing process.

Cessation of haemorrhage

This must be achieved in each part of the repair, otherwise haemorrhage can continue between the layers, resulting in a haematoma or postpartum haemorrhage. When a bleeding vessel is located, it should be tied off.

Reduction of any dead space

If bleeding occurs into areas of dead space a haematoma can result; thus it is important to bring the tissues into apposition to reduce this risk.

Minimal amount of suture material

Foreign material in tissue can cause an inflammatory reaction, which will impair healing and increase the risk of infection. Fewer knots and less suture material minimise this risk and result in improved healing.

Infiltration of perineum for repair

Anaesthetic, usually 20 mL 1% lignocaine, is administered using ANTT and is infiltrated into the four aspects of the tear, along the left- and right-hand sides of the vaginal wall and perineum. The tissue is held with tissue forceps while the needle is inserted at point A along to point B (Fig 45.2) and the plunger withdrawn to ensure the needle has not punctured a blood vessel. If blood is seen in the syringe, withdraw the needle and recommence the procedure using a new

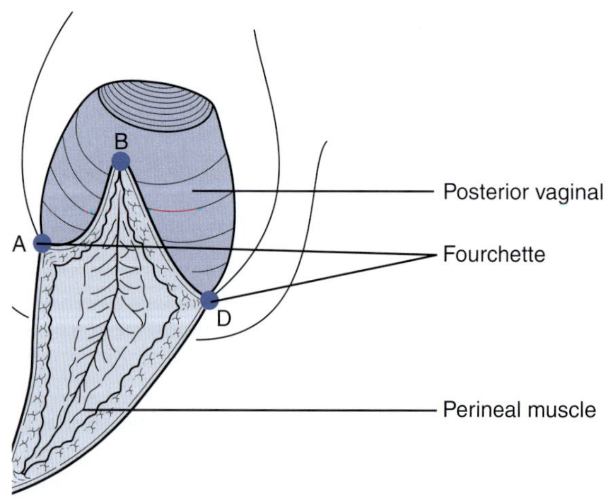

FIGURE 45.2 **Infiltration prior to suturing.**
Source: Johnson R, Taylor W: Skills for midwifery practice, 4th ed., Elsevier, London, 2016.

needle, syringe and solution (aspiration is repeated each time the position of the needle is changed). If no blood is seen, the needle is slowly withdrawn as the anaesthetic is injected along line B to A, the needle is reversed rather than removed and inserted to point C and the line C to A is infiltrated. The needle is withdrawn and inserted into point D and the process repeated B to D, C to D. Sufficient time should be allowed for the anaesthetic to work prior to commencing suturing.

Using a needle holder

The needle holder appears very similar in appearance to artery forceps; however, the grooves are designed to retain a better grip on the needle. The suture is positioned in the packet so that as the packet is torn at the right-hand side, the needle is exposed in the correct position to attach it to the needle holder without having to remove the suture from the packet. The suture is attached to the needle, the needle being appropriately shaped to reduce tissue trauma and also levelled off approximately one-third of the way along the needle to allow the needle holder to grasp it securely. The needle holder should be placed on the last third of the needle (the part closest to the thread) at right angles to the curve of the needle.

The needle holder is held by the shank with the wrist curved backwards; then the needle is inserted into the tissue. The wrist is then turned forwards to guide both the direction and depth of the needle through the tissue. The free end of the needle is secured using tissue forceps while the needle holder is removed from the needle and then re-clamped on the end of the needle protruding through the tissue. With the palm facing down, the needle is pulled completely through the tissue using a flicking movement of the wrist along the curve of the needle.

TECHNIQUE

Perineal repair is usually undertaken in three stages:

1. posterior vaginal wall
2. perineal muscle layer
3. perineal skin.

The use of a loose continuous suture is currently recommended for all three layers, as it results in less short-term pain than interrupted or locked sutures (Kettle et al 2012). In the past, a continuous locked suture was used to repair the vaginal wall, as it was thought it would prevent shortening of the vagina by avoiding concertinaing of the vaginal wall if the continuous non-locked suture were pulled too tight; however, there is a lack of good quality evidence to support this (Kettle et al 2012). Furthermore, Kettle and colleagues (2012) caution that if stitches that are too tight the distribution of tissue oedema can be restricted, resulting in increased pain; the use of a loose continuous suture enables the tension to be transferred throughout the length of the whole stitch, thereby reducing pain. Oedema can apply excessive pressure on the wound edges and capillaries, resulting in ischaemia. Consequently the wound edges necrose, resulting in a nidus for infection.

Suturing techniques

The basic suturing techniques described are for a right-handed midwife; a left-handed person will need to adapt these principles. If there is any possible exposure to the needle, tissue forceps rather than fingers should be used to hold the tissue.

Tying a knot

The knot is tied three times, to the right with two throws, to the left (one throw) and back to the right (one throw), so that it will not slip and will lie flat.

1. The needle is inserted through the tissue from the woman's left to her right side so that it is protruding through the right side (Fig 45.3A).
2. The needle holder is removed from the needle and placed on the opposite end of the needle and the needle and thread pulled through, leaving 6–8 cm of thread on the left side (Fig 45.3B).
3. Holding the needle holder in the right hand parallel to the maternal tissue, the thread is grasped on the right side between the thumb and index finger of the left hand and passed twice around the needle holder (Fig 45.3C).
4. Keeping the loops on the needle holder, open the needle holder and use it to grasp the free short end of the thread and draw/pull it through the loops (Fig 45.3D).
5. The two ends of the knot should be pulled at a 180° angle to each other to tighten the knot; encourage it to stay as flat as possible and prevent the thread pulling through to a sliding hitch (Fig 45.3E).
6. Repeat from Fig 45.3C to Fig 45.3E, but pass the thread around the needle holder in the opposite direction once.
7. Repeat again, passing the thread over the needle holder once it is in the original direction.
8. The knot ends should be cut short if this is the final knot, or just the free end if suturing is to continue.
9. If the thread is kinked or not tightened enough, the security of the knot is reduced due to breakage or slippage. Using a needle holder rather than fingers to tie the knot is usually more economical on the amount of suture thread used.

Continuous non-locked suture

A **continuous non-locked suture** is recommended for use on the posterior vaginal wall and perineal muscles. The apex of the tear is located and visualised to ensure the tear is repaired completely—inserting a lubricated tampon may assist by minimising lochial blood loss.

1. The first stitch enters the tissue above the apex and a knot tied to anchor it and the short end cut.
2. The next stitch is placed below and parallel to the first one, entering on the woman's left side. The left hand applies slight tension to the thread

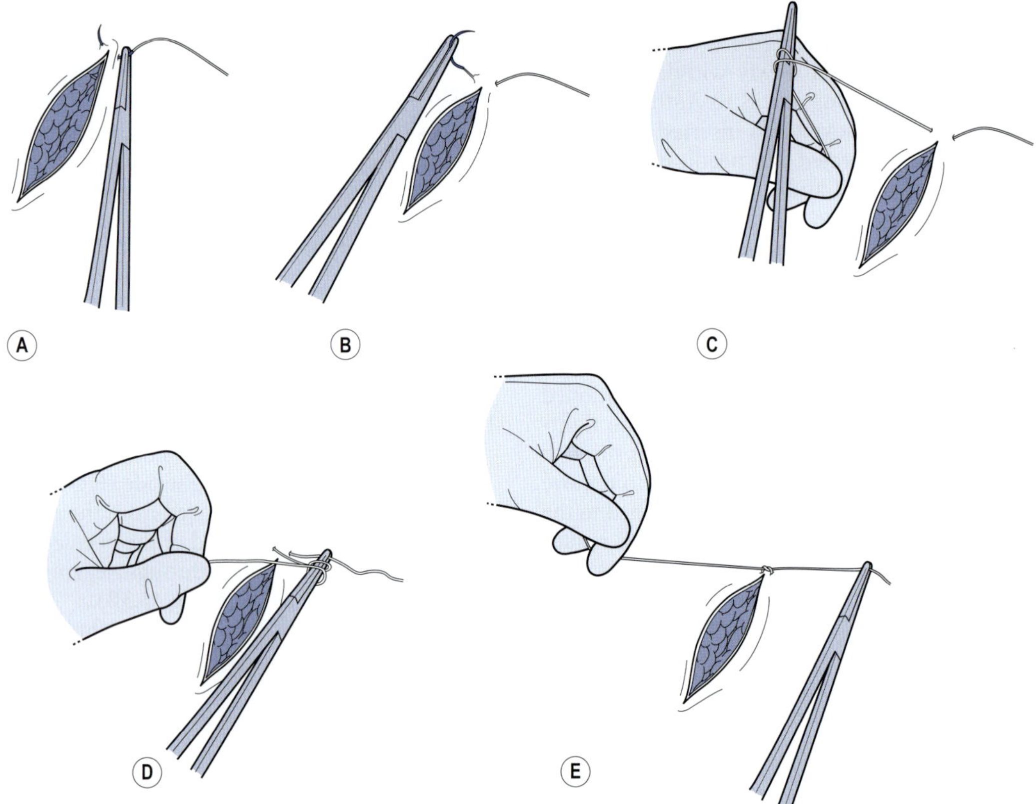

FIGURE 45.3 **A, B, C, D, E, Instrument-tied knot: consisting of three throws to 'lock' and prevent slippage.**
Source: Johnson R, Taylor W: Skills for midwifery practice, 4th ed., Elsevier, London, 2016.

so the needle emerges below and to the far side of the thread that is held (Fig 45.4). The needle should enter and exit at a 90° angle and traverse a vertically semicircular course to follow the curve of the needle. It is important to visualise the needle at the trough of the wound to ensure the dead space will be closed and prevent the suture from going through the rectal mucosa. If the wound is not deep, it may be possible to enter and exit in one movement, but if it is deep, the sides may need two separate actions. The thread is pulled completely through both sides of the wound.

3. Suturing is continued at approximately 1 cm intervals down the vaginal wall to the fourchette and, if required, along the perineal muscle layer taking the same size 'bites' from each side of the wound, ensuring the sutures are not pulled too tight.
4. If the skin does not require suturing, the suture is tied and a loop is retained to act as the short end.
5. The knot is then tied in the same way; it may be buried for comfort. Burying a knot is achieved by cutting the short end then passing the needle under the suture line to take the knot into the tissue. The long end is then cut (Fig 45.5).

Subcuticular suture to perineal skin

A **subcuticular suture** is one that is just beneath the skin surface. If the perineal muscles have not been sutured or there is no thread to continue with, a new stitch is begun at the anal end with a knot tied beneath the skin. The needle is inserted deeply on the left-hand side of the tear, emerging (still on the left) superficially just below the skin and a knot tied. The needle is then reversed on the needle holder (so the point of the needle emerges in front of the needle holder). The needle is inserted superficially beneath the skin on the right-hand side of the tear, opposite the knot on the left. The needle emerges superficially (still on the right) at approximately the length of the needle and the thread pulled through. The next bite is taken along the left side of the incision, entering opposite where the last suture emerged on the right (Fig 45.6). It is important the bites are parallel to the skin surface, at the same depth and length to prevent an uneven vertical overlap. The process is repeated until the fourchette is reached. A loop is retained with the last suture to tie off a knot, which is then buried. Both ends are cut. There should not be any suture material apparent on the outside of the perineum.

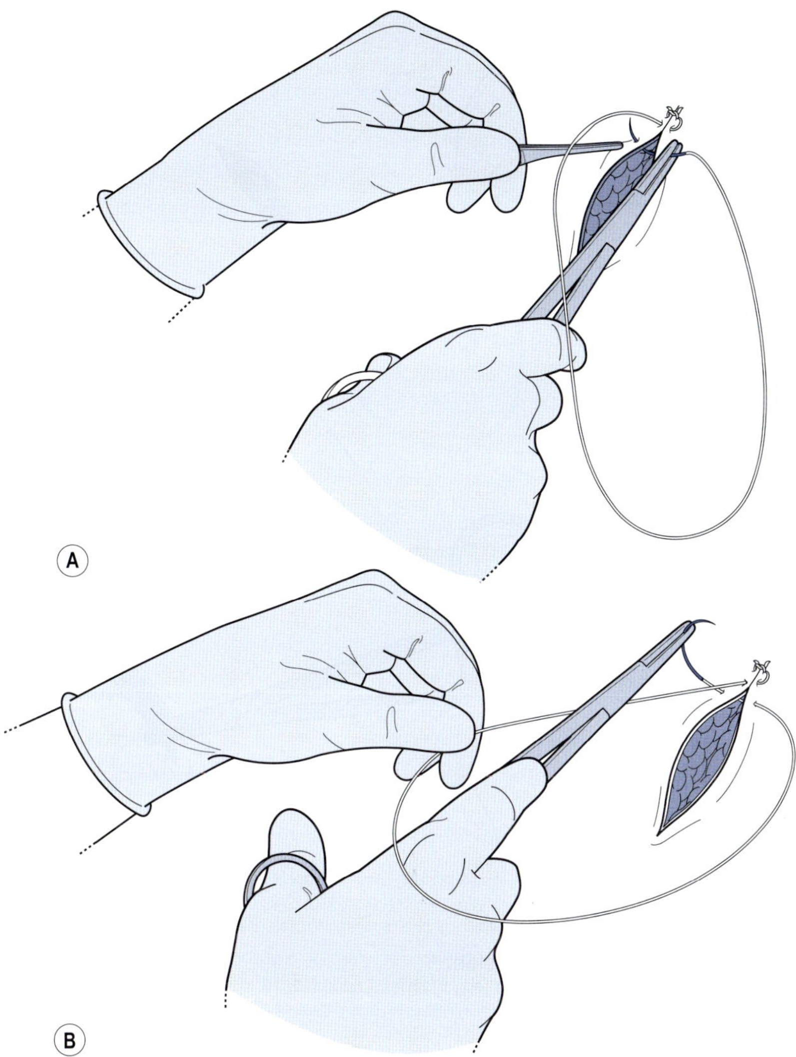

FIGURE 45.4 **A, B, Continuous non-locked suture.**
Source: Johnson R, Taylor W: Skills for midwifery practice, 4th ed., Elsevier, London, 2016.

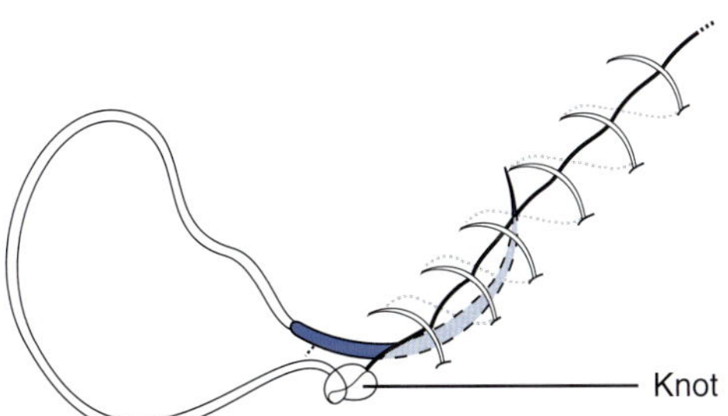

FIGURE 45.5 **Burying a knot.**
Source: Johnson R, Taylor W: Skills for midwifery practice, 4th ed., Elsevier, London, 2016.

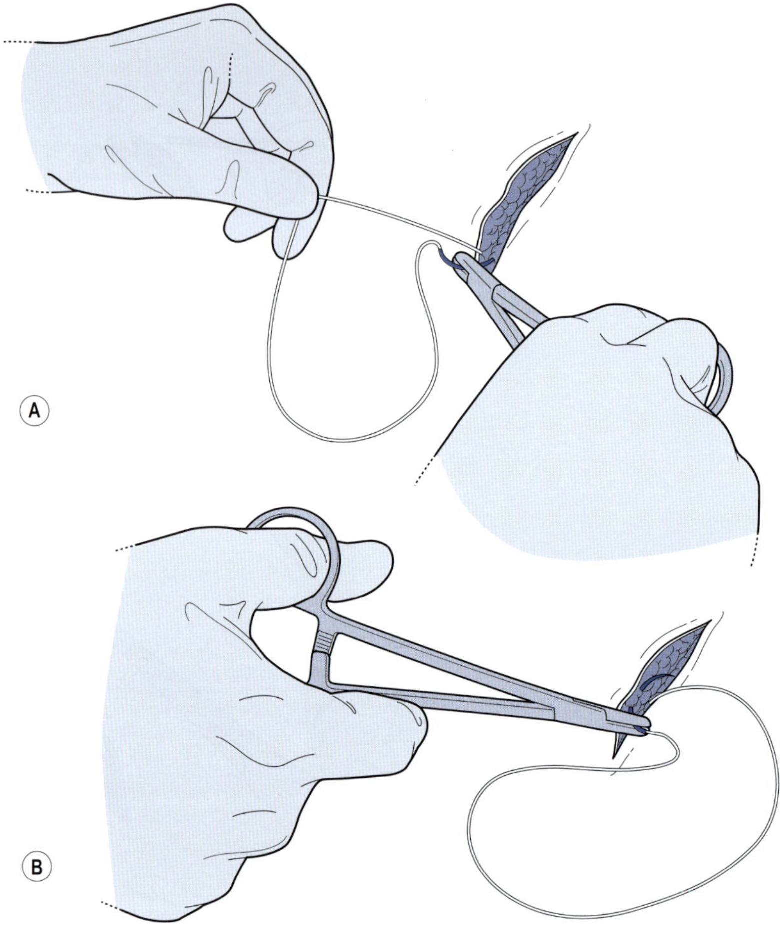

FIGURE 45.6 **A, B, Subcuticular suture to the skin.**
Source: Johnson R, Taylor W: Skills for midwifery practice, 4th ed., Elsevier, London, 2016.

SKILL 45.1 Perineal repair

1. Ensure operator is directly supervised by an expert or is competent in repair techniques.
2. Ensure adherence to local workplace policies and procedures.
3. Gain informed consent.
4. Collect equipment and place on a cleaned dressings trolley or suitable cleaned working surface:
   - sterile repair pack (with sterile gown)
   - water/lotion/locally approved skin cleanser
   - plastic apron
   - sterile gloves
   - sterile sutures
   - 20 mL lignocaine with sterile needle (21-g green) and syringe
   - lubricant—sterile, single-use
   - diclofenac suppository (if not contraindicated)
   - alcohol-based hand rub
   - sharps bin.
5. Assist the woman into a suitable position and keep her covered. A stool should be available for the midwife to sit on and the light positioned appropriately.
6. With clean hands, open the outer covering of the repair pack (an assistant can do this).
7. Put on apron, wash and dry hands.
8. Open the pack.
9. Using ANTT, open and place on sterile field other items required (e.g. sutures, swabs, needle, syringe, gloves, gown, diclofenac suppository) and add lotion and lubricant to bowl/gallipots (this can be done by an assistant, if present).
10. If using lignocaine, open the ampoule and place within easy reach on a clean surface unless an assistant is present to open and hold the ampoule.
11. Uncover the woman as necessary.
12. Perform hand hygiene.

SKILL 45.1 Perineal repair—cont'd

13. Put on the gown and gloves.
14. Check and count the swabs, needles and instruments.
15. Arrange the trolley in a way that suits.
16. Draw up the anaesthetic using ANTT—if no assistant is present, the ampoule can be held using a swab to maintain sterility.
17. Cleanse the vulva using ANTT, working from top to bottom, using each swab only once.
18. Establish a sterile field beneath the woman's buttocks, over her legs and abdomen using the sterile towels and fenestrated drape.
19. If required, infiltrate the perineum as described above; time is given for anaesthesia to be achieved.
20. Re-examine the genital tract to establish the extent of the trauma and realign the tissues; refer if necessary.
21. Insert a lubricated vaginal tampon to absorb the lochial loss, so visibility while suturing is good; attach the tail to the sterile drapes using artery forceps.
22. Locate the apex, insert the first suture just above it, and anchor with a knot.
23. Complete a continuous, loose, non-locked suture down the vaginal wall.
24. Locate the perineal muscles and suture with a continuous non-locked suture, securing with a buried knot if the skin is in good apposition (0.5 cm maximum gap). If necessary, the deep and superficial muscles can be sutured in two layers.
25. If the skin is not in good apposition, complete a subcuticular suture, beginning at the anal end and ending at the fourchette and burying the knot.
26. Examine the vagina and perineum to establish that the tissue is in good alignment and all bleeding has stopped.
27. Remove the tampon, examine the repair gently, and insert one lubricated finger into the anus to establish the sutures have not gone through the rectal mucosa. Administer rectal analgesia if not contraindicated.
28. Remove the drapes, assist the woman into a comfortable position, and cover her, placing a sanitary towel over the perineum. Advise her with regard to ongoing perineal care.
29. Count the swabs, instruments and needles and dispose of sharps correctly.
30. Dispose of the equipment, remove gloves and apron.
31. Wash and dry hands.
32. Document the repair and act accordingly.

RECORD KEEPING

The following should be included:

- information provided to the woman prior to the procedure and during the consent process
- time and date of the procedure
- nature and extent of the tear—a diagram can be helpful
- position of the woman (e.g. lithotomy)
- amount and type of anaesthetic drugs used (also documented on the medicine administration record)
- tampon inserted and removed
- suture material used
- order of repair
- techniques used at which area
- examinations *per vaginam* and *per rectum* following the repair
- swabs, needles and instrument counted and correct
- analgesia administered following procedure (also documented on the medicine administration record)
- legible signature and name of suturing midwife
- any specific aftercare instructions provided to the woman.

Role and responsibilities of the midwife

These are summarised as:

- regular training and assessment of competency for suturing
- regular review of evidence-based practice around suturing to ensure knowledge level is up-to-date
- appropriate assessment of the wound to establish who should suture, where, with which anaesthetic/analgesia and which material
- providing the woman with evidence-based information to allow her to make an informed decision regarding suturing
- use of appropriate materials, technique, asepsis and standard precautions
- education and support of the woman before, during and following the procedure
- contemporaneous records
- Follow-up with the woman at 6 weeks to ascertain how she is healing.

SUMMARY

- The repair is a sterile procedure using ANTT approach; the aims include alignment of the tissue, stemming haemorrhage and reducing dead space.

- When indicated, a perineal wound should be sutured using a rapidly absorbing polyglactin suture (e.g. Vicryl Rapide) with a loose, continuous, unlocked suture to the posterior vaginal wall and muscle layer, bringing the skin into good apposition.
- If skin closure is indicated, a continuous subcuticular technique should be used.
- To reduce the risk of short- and long-term morbidity for the woman, perineal repair should be undertaken by a skilled operator; thus it is important the midwife is trained appropriately, updated and able to acknowledge any limitations in her ability, referring as necessary.
- Evidence-based practice should be used with regard to the materials and techniques used.

Self-assessment exercises

The answers to the following questions may be found in the text.

1. How is perineal trauma currently classified?
2. List the aims of successful perineal repair.
3. When might a midwife ask a senior obstetrician to complete the suturing?
4. What is the current material of choice for perineal repair?
5. Describe how to successfully infiltrate the perineum prior to suturing.
6. Give a rationale for the techniques used when suturing the posterior vaginal wall and perineal muscles.
7. What technique should be used for suturing the perineal skin?
8. Summarise the role and responsibilities of the midwife in relation to perineal repair.
9. List all the aspects of the repair that should be documented.
10. Find some suitable suturing equipment and demonstrate tying a knot, continuous non-locked and subcuticular suturing.

References

American College of Surgeons (ACS). Revised statement on sharps injury, 2016. Online 11 June 2018. Available: www.facs.org/about-acs/statements/94-sharps-safety.

Australian Institute of Health and Welfare (AIHW). Australia's mothers and babies data visualisations 2018, 2020. Online 25 May 2020. Available: www.aihw.gov.au/reports/mothers-babies/australias-mothers-babies-data-visualisations/contents/summary.

Beckman MM, Stock OM: Antenatal perineal massage for reducing perineal trauma, Cochrane Database of Systematic Reviews (4):Art. No.: CD005123, 2013.

Berlit S, Tuschy B, Brade J, et al: Effectiveness of nitrous oxide for postpartum perineal repair: a randomised controlled trial, European Journal of Obstetrics and Gynecology and Reproductive Biology 170(2): 329–332, 2013.

Blechner MJ: The clitoris: anatomical and psychological issues, Studies in Gender and Sexuality 18(3):190–200, 2017.

Dahlen H, Priddis H: Perineal care and repair. In Pairman S, Pincombe J, Thorogood C, et al, eds: Midwifery: preparation for practice, 4th ed., Elsevier, Sydney, 2018.

Elharmeel SMA, Chaudhary Y, Tan S, et al: Surgical repair of spontaneous perineal tears that occur during childbirth versus no intervention, Cochrane Database of Systematic Reviews (8):Art. No.: CD008534, 2011.

Feigenberg T, Maor-Sagie E, Zivi E et al: Using adhesive glue to repair first degree perineal tears: a prospective randomized controlled trial, BioMed Research International, 2014, 526590. Available: https://doi.org/10.1155/2014/526590.

Gordon B, Mackrodt C, Fern E, et al: The Ipswich Childbirth Study: 1. A randomised evaluation of two stage postpartum perineal repair leaving the skin unsutured, BJOG: An International Journal of Obstetrics and Gynaecology 105(4):435–440, 1998.

Greenberg JA, Lieberman E, Cohen AP, et al: Randomized comparison of chromic versus fast absorbing polyglactin 910 for postpartum perineal repair, Obstetrics and Gynaecology 103(6):1308–1313, 2004.

Hedayati H, Parsons J, Crowther CA: Rectal analgesia for pain from perineal trauma following childbirth, Cochrane Database of Systematic Reviews (3):Art.No.: CD0003931, 2003.

Kenyon S, Ford F: How can we improve women's postbirth perineal health? MIDIRS Midwifery Digest 14(1): 7–12, 2004.

Kettle C, Dowswell T, Ismail KMK: Absorbable suture materials for repair of episiotomy and second-degree tears, Cochrane Database of Systematic Reviews (6):Art. No.: CD000006, 2010.

Kettle C, Dowswell T, Ismail KMK: Continuous and interrupted suturing techniques for repair of episiotomy or second-degree tears, Cochrane Database of Systematic Review (11):Art. No.: CD000947, 2012.

Langley V, Thoburn A, Shaw S, Barton, A: Second degree tears: to suture or not? A randomized controlled trial, British Journal of Midwifery 14(9):550–554, 2006.

Leeman LM, Rogers RG, Greulich B, Albers, L: Do un-sutured second-degree perineal lacerations affect postpartum functional outcomes?, Journal of the American Board of Family Medicine 20(5):451–457, 2007.

Leroux N, Bujold E: Impact of chromic catgut versus polyglactin 910 versus fast-absorbing polyglactin 910 sutures for perineal repair: a randomized controlled trial, American Journal of Obstetrics and Gynaecology 194(6):1585–1590, 2006.

Metcalfe A, Bick D, Tohill S, et al: A prospective cohort study of repair and non-repair of second-degree perineal trauma: results and issues for future research, Evidence Based Midwifery 4(2):60–64, 2006.

Mota R, Costa E, Amaral A, et al: Skin adhesive versus subcuticular suture for perineal skin repair after episiotomy—a randomized controlled trial, Acta Obstetrica et Gynecologica Scandinavia 88(6): 660–666, 2009.

National Institute for Health and Care Excellence (NICE). Intrapartum care. Care of healthy women and their babies during childbirth Clinical Guideline 190, 2017. Online 20 February 2018. Available: www.nice.org.uk.

Parantainen A, Verbek JH, Lavoie MC, et al: Blunt versus sharp suture needles for preventing percutaneous exposure incidents in surgical staff, Cochrane Database of Systematic Review (11):Art. No.: CD009170, 2011.

Preston HL, Fowler GE: Risk factors for and management of obstetric anal sphincter injury, Obstetrics, Gynaecology and Reproductive Medicine 26(11):65–71, 2016.

Reed R: The perineal bundle and midwifery. Midwife Thinking, 2018. Online 28 July 2018. Available: https://midwifethinking.com/2018/05/09/the-perineal-bundle-and-midwifery/.

Royal Australian and New Zealand College of Obstetricians and Gynaecologists (RANZCOG): The management of third- and fourth-degree perineal tears: Green-top Guideline No. 29, 2015. Available: https://ranzcog.edu.au/RANZCOG_SITE/media/RANZCOG-MEDIA/Women%27s%20Health/Statement%20and%20guidelines/Clinical-Obstetrics/RCOG-Management-of-Third-and-Fourth-Degrees-Perineal-Tears.pdf?ext=.pdf.

Royal College of Midwives (RCM). Suturing the perineum. Midwifery Practice Guidelines. Royal College of Midwives, London, 2008.

Sanders J, Campbell R, Peters T: Effectiveness of pain relief during perineal suturing, British Journal of Obstetrics and Gynaecology 109:1066–1068, 2002.

Steen M, Roberts T: The consequences of pregnancy and birth for the pelvic floor, British Journal of Midwifery 19(11):692–698, 2011.

Sultan AH: Obstetric perineal injury and anal incontinence, Clinical Risk 5:193–6, 1999.

Turin SY, Placik OJ: Commentary on: anatomical dissection of the dorsal nerve of the clitoris, Aesthetic Surgery Journal 40(5):548–550, 2020.

Viswanathan M, Hartmann K, Palmieri R, et al. The use of episiotomy in obstetrical care: a systematic review, 2005. Agency for Healthcare Research and Quality. Online 11 June 2018. Available: www.ncbi.nlm.nih.gov/books/NBK11967/.

Wilson LK, Sullivan S, Goodnight W, et al: The use of blunt needles does not reduce glove perforations during obstetrical laceration repair, American Journal of Obstetrics and Gynaecology 199(6):1097–6868, 2008.

Women's Healthcare Australasia: Response to Rachel Reed 'The perineal midwifery', 2018a. Online 28 July 2018. Available: https://women.wcha.asn.au/response-rachel-reed-perineal-bundle-midwifery.

Women's Hospitals Australasia: WHA National Collaborative, 2018b. Online 28 July 2018. Available: https://women.wcha.asn.au/collaborative/intervention-bundle.

PART 3

WORKING WITH THE WOMAN AND BABY AFTER BIRTH

SECTION 12

SKILLS FOR OPTIMISING THE WOMAN'S AND BABY'S PHYSIOLOGICAL WELLBEING

CHAPTER 46

PROMOTING PHYSIOLOGICAL STABILITY IN THE MOTHER–BABY DYAD IMMEDIATELY AFTER NORMAL TERM BIRTH

Learning outcomes

Having read this chapter, the reader should be able to:

- discuss the immediate physiological monitoring and care needs of a woman who has had a normal term birth
- summarise the midwife's responsibilities in this aspect of her/his roles.

When a woman has given birth normally at term, the midwife's role includes optimising the woman's physiological stability and promoting maternal–newborn attachment. This chapter considers the specific observations and care that must be undertaken in the first 2 hours after a normal term birth in a context of fostering the woman's connection with her baby.

FACILITATING PHYSIOLOGICAL STABILITY AFTER NORMAL OR INSTRUMENT-ASSISTED VAGINAL BIRTH AT TERM

In the first 2 hours after giving birth normally at term and in the hours and days that follow, women are at risk of a range of physiological complications, including (but not limited to):

- blood loss
- deep vein thrombosis (DVT)
- pulmonary embolus
- urine retention.

Further, if women have had instrumental assistance to give birth and/or have a perineal injury, they face the additional possibility of:

- perineal and/or genital pain
- perineal and/or genital wound infection

In all cases of vaginal birth, the woman is also vulnerable to urine retention.

Detection of these complications relies on timely observations being made of a number of physiological features. The woman's physiological condition should be closely monitored in the immediate postpartum period, and then regularly thereafter until she is physiologically stable. The accepted definition of the postnatal period, or 'puerperium', is the 6-week period following the birth of the placenta(e), during which the woman's body progressively returns to its pre-pregnant physiological state. This chapter is concerned with the immediate postpartum period, defined as the first 2 hours after completion of the third stage of labour and birth (Dixon 2013); however, this time is also

CHAPTER 47

CARING FOR A WOMAN AFTER A CAESAREAN SECTION

Learning outcomes

Having read this chapter, the reader should be able to:

- discuss the physiological monitoring needs of a woman who has had a caesarean section
- describe how maternal–newborn attachment between the mother–baby dyad might be facilitated following a caesarean section
- discuss post-caesarean section care
- summarise the midwife's responsibilities in these roles.

When a woman has a caesarean section, the midwife's role includes optimising the woman's physiological stability and promoting maternal–newborn attachment. Information about the rationale for caesarean section and the midwife's role during it is found in Chapter 41. This chapter considers the specific observations that must be made of the woman's condition in the hours and days after a caesarean section, the ways in which the midwife can support the establishment of the mother–baby relationship after operative birth, and the midwifery care women require postoperatively.

The information in this chapter pertains to women who have given birth by caesarean section under regional (usually combined spinal/epidural, or 'CSE') anaesthesia. In Australasia, 6% of women having a caesarean section do so under general anaesthetic (GA). For information and guidance on care specifically related to GA, the reader is recommended to consult a text on the topic and/or review their own organisation's postoperative care policy and guideline documents.

FACILITATING PHYSIOLOGICAL STABILITY AFTER CAESAREAN SECTION

Immediately post-caesarean section and in the hours and days that follow, women are at risk of a range of physiological complications including (but not limited to):

- blood loss
- effects of damage to organs near the operation site, including the bladder
- anaesthetic risks, such as low blood pressure, nausea and vomiting and post-dural puncture headache
- wound infection
- deep vein thrombosis (DVT)
- pulmonary embolus.

All these risks are increased if the woman is overweight (Royal Australian and New Zealand College of Obstetricians and Gynaecologists [RANZCOG] 2017).

Detection of these complications relies on timely observations being made of a number of physiological features. The woman's physiological condition should be assessed in the immediate postoperative period and regularly thereafter.

SUPPORTING THE ESTABLISHMENT OF THE MATERNAL–NEWBORN RELATIONSHIP

To optimise maternal–newborn attachment, the guidance for women who have had a caesarean section and have a well, healthy baby is the same as those for

SKILL 47.1 Monitoring the woman's physiological wellbeing after caesarean section

Immediately following the caesarean section and while the woman is in the operating theatre recovery area, the timings of observations are dictated by clinical condition and locally agreed policy, but are often made at 5-minute intervals initially. As time passes and observations remain within normal limits, the frequency of observations may be reduced to every 15 minutes, 30 minutes, etc. They should then be half-hourly for at least 2 hours and hourly thereafter until satisfactory (National Institute for Health Care Excellence [NICE] 2021). If the woman has given birth under GA, she should be continuously monitored one-to-one by a healthcare professional with airway management skills until she has regained airway control, is haemodynamically stable and is able to communicate (NICE 2021). Maternity service protocols will vary; however, the frequency of observations tends to lessen as time goes on, as long as they remain within normal parameters.

On collecting the woman from the recovery room, and at each assessment thereafter, the midwife should check:

- the wound drainage system, and record the amount and type of fluid (until removed): drains should be emptied at midnight and the volume recorded on the woman's fluid balance chart
- any intravenous infusion(s) and the IV access site, and check the IV fluid prescription (until discontinued): fluid intake and output should be carefully recorded on the woman's fluid balance chart
- the patient-controlled analgesia (PCA) or patient-controlled epidural analgesia (PCEA) pump (until discontinued), the woman's pain level, the level of sensory and motor block, and the prescription for further analgesia
- the epidural catheter site
- that appropriate venous thromboembolus prophylaxis is in place (graduated pressure stockings and/or a sequential compression device according to hospital policy, and anticoagulant medication) is in place
- that oxygen is prescribed and administered as necessary
- the patency of the urinary catheter, as well as the colour and amount of the woman's urine (until removed)
- that the wound dressing is intact and the wound is not oozing
- the amount of lochia
- that an oxytocic is prescribed, should it be required
- that breastfeeding has been initiated
- that all of the above is documented in the woman's clinical record.

women who have had a normal birth (see Chapter 46). According to NICE (2017):

> women should be encouraged to have skin-to-skin contact with their babies as soon as possible after birth; the baby should be dried and covered with a warm, dry blanket or towel while maintaining skin-to-skin contact with his/her mother; separation of a woman and her baby within the first hour of the birth for routine postnatal procedures, for example, weighing, measuring and bathing, should be avoided unless necessary or the woman requests it; initiation of breastfeeding should occur as soon as possible after the birth, within 1 hour if at all possible.

SKILL 47.2 Facilitating maternal–newborn attachment after caesarean section

RANZCOG (2016) advises that, assuming he or she does not need resuscitating, the baby born by caesarean section should:

- be placed skin-to-skin with his or her mother as soon as possible after the birth
- have warmed blankets placed over his or her back
- have a bonnet placed on his or her head.

WOUND CARE

Closure of the caesarean section wound aims to bring the skin edges in neat apposition so that healing may begin by first intention. Gurusamy and colleagues (2014) found little conclusive evidence as to the value of continuous or interrupted sutures in reducing surgical site infection (SSI). There was less wound breakdown when subcuticular suturing was used, but the quality of studies was limited and none of them were obstetric surgery. Wetter and colleagues (1991) and Johnson, Young and Reilly (2006) both recommend the use of subcuticular suturing, and Ward and colleagues (2008) found that wound infection was higher with staples than with a continuous suture. Olsen and colleagues (2008) agreed. Mangram and colleagues (1999) highlighted that a monofilament suture carried less infection risk than a multifilamented one. Reilly (2002) found that if sutures were left in place for longer than 10 days infection rates were greater. Gould (2007) recommends that for a transverse wound the sutures or staples can be removed after 4 or 5 days, once the new epithelium has become intact. The recommended length of time for removal from a vertical incision is 7 to 10 days. NICE (2011) indicates that superficial wound drains should be avoided for caesarean section wounds. If one is used, it should be removed as soon as drainage ceases, ideally the next day (Gould 2007).

Wound dressings

It is now well accepted that a moist wound environment promotes wound healing. There are various types of dressings available for a range of wound types. The wound dressing performs several important functions (adapted from Doran-Williams et al 2011).

- It protects the wound from injury, hypothermia and external infection (until natural healing has begun).
- It absorbs any wound secretions, maintaining the moisture balance.
- It minimises pain, odour and bleeding.

Generally, after caesarean section an absorbent non-adherent dressing is applied. This varies; however, it is often locally agreed on and can be based on cost as well as effectiveness. In the event of haemorrhage, a pressure dressing may be applied to aid haemostasis.

Postoperative wound care

Cleaning and dressing wounds

A carefully sutured incision that has achieved haemostasis will be sealed by fibrin within 24 hours (Reilly 2002). In relation to wound infection, NICE (2021) indicates that no type of wound dressing has been shown to be better than another at reducing the risk of wound infections, and that dressing removal can occur from 6 hours onwards because there is no difference in the risk of wound infection when dressings are removed 6 hours postoperatively compared with 24 hours postoperatively. The woman is encouraged to wear cotton underwear and loose clothing. The wound should be cleaned and dried daily. Suture or staple removal (if necessary) is undertaken from day 5 onwards. In instances where dressings need changing, aseptic non-touch technique (ANTT) should be used.

Caesarean section wounds—summary

For a woman with a lower segment caesarean section (LSCS) wound, the following principles are suggested at the time of writing, but the reader is encouraged to be aware of the emerging evidence.

- The theatre dressing can be removed after a minimum of 6 hours.
- The woman should shower daily, the wound being gently patted dry. A dry dressing can be applied to offer protection against clothing rubbing against the wound; otherwise, it may be left uncovered. The woman should wear cotton underwear and loose clothing.
- The wound should be assessed at every postoperative/postnatal assessment.
- Suture/staple removal is planned for the correct day, often day 5 onwards.
- If the wound is exuding fluid or shows any other signs of potential complications it should be swabbed (see Chapter 12 for technique), cleansed and re-dressed. Referral may be necessary for antibiotic therapy.
- If a wound requires cleansing and re-dressing, ANTT is used.

Longer-term care

Gould (2007) indicates that women need to be aware that wound healing involves several layers of tissue and that it takes time for the maturation phase to be completed (1–2 years). In both the short and the long term, women need to be aware of what constitutes impairment or complications of wound healing and so seek appropriate referral.

Aseptic wound dressing

Chapter 2 discusses the principles of asepsis which are then applied to each situation. In many instances caesarean section wounds do not require re-dressing, but for a wound that does, an ANTT approach should be used (Rowley et al 2010). Wounds that need an aseptic dressing usually require cleansing. This removes bacteria, exudate and debris, among other things. However, unnecessary cleaning may disturb the healing process. 0.9% sodium chloride (at room temperature) or warm tap water is used (Doran-Williams et al 2011). Sterile gauze, foam or a 10 mL syringe is used according to availability and suitability.

The question of when a wound dressing should be changed remains unanswered. It would appear sensible to make a daily *assessment,* but not to disturb the wound by cleaning or re-dressing it unless necessary.

SKILL 47.3 Aseptic dressing technique

1. Confirm the woman's identity, gain informed consent and establish that re-dressing is indicated.
2. Decontaminate hands and collect a clean-dressings trolley.
3. Put on non-sterile gloves and clean the trolley with the locally approved surface wipes. Remove gloves and wash and dry hands.
4. Gather and place the following equipment onto the lower shelf of the trolley:
   - alcohol-based hand rub and non-sterile gloves
   - apron
   - sachet of 0.9% sodium chloride at body temperature
   - sterile dressing pack (in date) (should contain disposable bag and suitable dressing)
   - 10 mL syringe.

SKILL 47.3 Aseptic dressing technique—cont'd

5. Position the woman appropriately, maintaining privacy and dignity.
6. Wash and dry hands and put on the apron.
7. Loosen the existing dressing, but keep the wound covered and decontaminate hands.
8. Open the outer layer of the pack, dropping the wrapped contents carefully onto the top shelf of the trolley.
9. Open the inner wrapper of the pack, touching only the edges of the paper; slide the other sterile items onto the sterile field and pour the saline into the gallipot, all with ANTT.
10. Loosen the existing dressing, place the disposable bag over the hand and remove the dressing (see Nicol and colleagues 2008).
11. Invert the bag, with the dressing inside, and attach it to the side of the trolley as a refuse bag.
12. Use alcohol-based hand rub and apply non-sterile gloves.
13. If appropriate, place a sterile field under the wound.
14. Assess the wound; if irrigation is indicated, draw up the saline in the syringe.
15. Cleanse the skin around the wound with gauze.
16. Then either (depending on local protocol):
    - clean the wound with gauze and gloved hands, ensuring that it is only the sterile gauze that touches the wound; use each swab to wipe once only, wiping from areas of discharge outwards, then discard the swab and repeat as necessary; OR
    - hold a piece of gauze at the dirtier end of the wound and irrigate with the syringe, from clean to dirty, catching the fluid in the gauze (this is the preferable method).
17. Dry the surrounding skin.
18. Apply and secure the replacement dressing.
19. Remove gloves and apron; wash and dry hands.
20. Ensure the woman is comfortable; discuss findings and ongoing care with her.
21. Dispose of equipment correctly and clean the trolley.
22. Return the trolley to the clean area.
23. Decontaminate hands.
24. Document findings, including the appearance of the wound and the future plan of care. Take action accordingly.

Removal of sutures or staples

The decision to remove sutures or staples is taken according to the assessment of how the wound is healing. Removal is often 4–5 days after the surgery. Sutures that are retained for too long increase the infection risk and delay wound healing. Suture removal is an aseptic procedure; a receptacle is required to place staples in so that they can be disposed of correctly in a sharps container. If the wound gapes after any of the sutures/staples have been removed, the midwife will refer the woman before removing them all, and may apply an adhesive suture and sterile dressing in the meantime. Obviously, only non-absorbable sutures need to be removed.

SKILL 47.4 Removal of sutures

The aim of correct suture removal is to ensure that no part of the external suture is taken through internally. It is an aseptic procedure for which a dressings trolley is prepared and used as mentioned previously, to which sterile scissors/stitch cutter or staple remover are added accordingly. Suture removal packs are sometimes available containing forceps; if unavailable, then individual sterile forceps are used.

1. Clean the wound as described in Skill 47.3.
2. Lift and hold the external part of the suture with forceps, using the non-dominant hand.
3. Cut beneath the knot as near to the skin as possible using scissors or stitch cutter in the dominant hand.
4. Remove the suture by pulling it gently through the skin.
5. This last principle applies whether the sutures are interrupted or subcuticular. Subcuticular suturing is sometimes held in place with a bead, the bead should be removed at the distal end of the wound so that on removal the suture is pulled from the end nearest to the midwife. The removal should be smooth; the woman may experience the pulling sensation rather than discomfort.

Source: Johnson R, Taylor W: Skills for midwifery practice, 4th ed., Elsevier, London, 2016.

SKILL 47.5 Removal of staples

1. Clean the wound as described in Skill 47.3.
2. Hold the staple remover as if it was a pair of scissors.
3. Insert the lower blade directly under the staple.
4. Squeeze the handles together; the staple will be lifted from the skin as it concertinas.

Continued

SKILL 47.5 Removal of staples—cont'd

5. Lift clear, place into sterile receptacle on the trolley and dispose of into a sharps box when finished completely.
6. The removing of sutures/staples must be recorded, including whether the removal was partial or complete. If some sutures/staples still need to be removed, a clear plan of care (including referral if needed) should be documented. Wound assessment should be completed; in some instances this is on a locally agreed wound chart.

Source: Johnson R, Taylor W: Skills for midwifery practice, 4th ed., Elsevier, London, 2016.

PROMOTION OF SKIN INTEGRITY

Restricted mobility is a given after a caesarean section and puts women at risk of a pressure injury occurring. This risk increases further if the woman is unwell. While the occurrence of pressure injuries within the maternity setting is low, they do occur and every patient is potentially at risk of developing a pressure injury if risk factors are present (Butcher 2004, McInnes and colleagues 2011, NICE 2014).

Thus it is important the midwife understands why pressure injuries occur and how they can be prevented. Pressure injuries are reportable in most health services as an untoward incident and an investigation is usually initiated to determine if there were any omissions in care that led to their development.

This section focuses on the principles of pressure area care, including a discussion of the aetiology and classification of pressure injuries. The factors that influence the development of pressure injuries are given, followed by a discussion of the assessment of skin integrity.

Pressure injuries

A **pressure injury** is a skin ulceration that forms due to localised tissue necrosis, commonly found on the parts of the body that have received unrelieved pressure. It has previously been referred to as a 'decubitus ulcer', 'pressure sore' or (less commonly) a 'bedsore'.

Common sites for pressure injury formation

Although pressure injuries can form on any part of the body, the most common sites are the sacrum, buttocks, trochanter and calcaneus (heels) (Bowen & Noble 2014b, McGinnis & Stubbs 2014) with toes, knees, ischial tuberosities, shoulders, elbows and ears also having the potential to be affected (Fig 47.1). Pressure may also occur from drainage tubes, indwelling catheters (against labia), nasogastric tubes (nasal passages), nasal oxygen cannulae and graduated compression stockings. Babies may also develop a pressure injury in the occipital region.

Effects of pressure

When sitting or lying, pressure is transferred from the external surface to the underlying bone via the different skin layers. This results in compression of the skin, subcutaneous fat, muscle and blood vessels. The pressure is directed downwards in an inverted cone shape and has a pressure gradient with the highest pressure at the apex. The pressure within these deep tissues is up to five times greater than within the epidermis (Dolan 2011). Consequently, the pressure within the blood vessels increases. Normal capillary pressure is 12–32 mmHg; when the pressure exceeds this, the blood vessel becomes distorted and occludes (Colwell 2015). Blood flow is reduced and ischaemic injury can occur. Additionally, the lymphatic supply can be occluded with accumulation of toxic substances that further increase cell damage (Hosking 2013).

For the majority of people, once the pressure is removed reactive hyperaemia occurs as blood flow begins again and reperfuses the area. The area then becomes red and warm with the redness lasting up to 50–75%, as long as the time the pressure prevented blood flow (deWit & O'Neill 2014). It can be difficult to detect hyperaemia in darkly pigmented skin. Bowen & Noble (2014b) advise touching the skin to detect warmth. If the redness resolves or the area blanches under fingertip pressure, it is unlikely damage has occurred to the underlying tissues. However, a cycle of ischaemia and tissue reperfusion during periods of prolonged pressure is thought to contribute to tissue damage (Hosking 2013).

If the pressure is not relieved, the risk of ischaemic injury increases, so that when the pressure is removed non-blanchable hyperaemia occurs. No blanching is seen with fingertip palpation; this is the first stage of skin injury and indicates deep tissue injury, although it may still be possible to reverse the damage at this stage (Colwell 2015). The cells rub together causing the cell membranes to rupture, releasing toxic intracellular material and normal skin colour is not restored. Damage can occur within 1–2 hours of continued pressure but generally is affected by the duration and amount of pressure, **skin integrity** and ability of supporting structures to redistribute pressure (Bowen & Noble 2014b, Colwell 2015). A deep pressure injury can arise when the lymphatic vessels and muscle fibres tear. In the healthy adult with full sensation, this will result in pain, causing the individual to move (Benbow 2008). Where sensation is impaired (e.g. epidural anaesthesia), the change of position does not occur spontaneously.

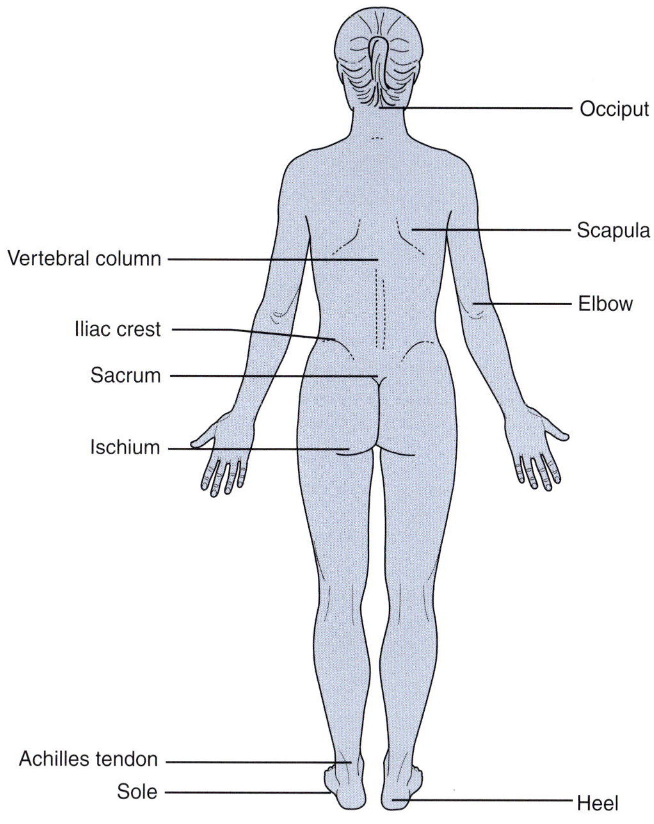

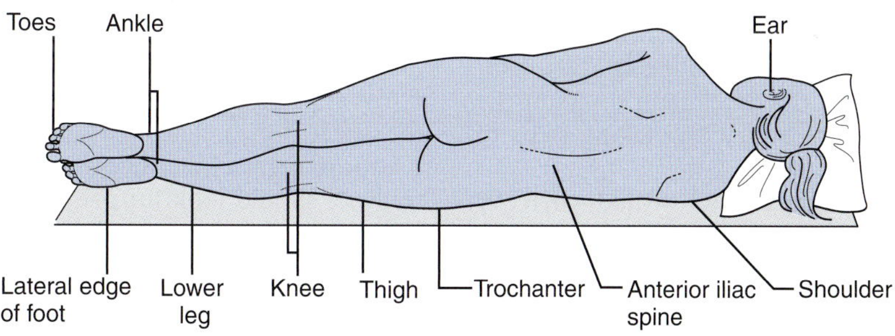

FIGURE 47.1 **Pressure area sites.**
Source: Johnson R, Taylor W: Skills for midwifery practice, 4th ed., Elsevier, London, 2016.

Shearing can compound the effects of pressure. A shearing force is the pressure exerted against the skin in a direction parallel to the body's surface, occurring when the body moves up or down the bed while in an upright position. As the layers of muscle and bone slide in the direction of the body movement, the skin and subcutaneous layers stick to the bed surface, causing the bone to slide down into the skin, with a force exerted onto the skin. This can happen if the woman is pulled up the bed rather than lifted. A shearing force results at the junction of the deep and superficial tissues. The microcirculation is compressed, stretched and damaged, causing microscopic haemorrhage and necrosis deep within the tissues. This is compounded by the decreased capillary blood flow, resulting from the external pressure against the skin. Eventually, a channel opens through the skin and the necrotic area drains through this (tunnelling). The areas commonly affected by shearing forces are the sacrum and coccygeus.

The skin can also be damaged by friction, but this is no longer considered a cause of pressure injuries. Friction is the mechanical force exerted when the skin is dragged across a coarse surface (e.g. bedding). Antokal and colleagues (2012) suggest that friction may cause mechanical damage to the superficial tissue cells, thus damage is due to excessive deformation rather than ischaemia. The epidermis is rubbed away, giving the appearance of a shallow abrasion injury, often on the elbows and heels. The effects of friction are exacerbated by moisture (as for shearing) (Benbow 2008).

Classification of pressure injuries

Pressure injuries are classified using the National Pressure Injury Advisory Panel (NPIAP) classification system. There are four stages of pressure injury that relate to the depth of tissue damage and involvement of associated structures, as well as a number of additional 'unstageable' injury classifications (Edsberg et al 2016).

- Stage I Pressure Injury: Non-blanchable erythema of intact skin
- Stage II Pressure Injury: Partial-thickness skin loss with exposed dermis
- Stage III Pressure Injury: Full-thickness skin loss
- Stage IV Pressure Injury: Full-thickness loss of skin and tissue

Factors influencing development

According to NICE (2015), all people are potentially at risk of developing a pressure injury but they are more likely to occur in people who are seriously ill, have a neurological condition, have impaired mobility, have poor posture or a deformity, have compromised skin or who are malnourished.

Pressure area care

This is undertaken to reduce the incidence of pressure injury formation. It involves undertaking an assessment of the risk of pressure injuries developing, assessing the skin for signs of pressure injury and taking steps to reduce the effects of pressure.

The ideal risk assessment tool would correctly identify those at risk of developing a pressure injury and those who are not at risk, and do so consistently with each successive assessment irrespective of who undertakes the assessment (Guy 2012). NPUAP/EPUAP/PPPIA (2014) advise that although there is no worldwide agreement as to the best approach for conducting a risk assessment, it should be one that is structured. There is a variety of structured risk assessment tools available for use in the clinical setting (e.g. the remodified Norton Scale, Braden Scale, RAPS scale), all of which have varying degrees of appropriateness for maternity environments; they are designed for nursing settings. However, of the tools available, Pancorbo-Hidalgo and colleagues (2006) found the Braden Scale offered the best balance between specificity and sensitivity and the best risk estimate for pressure injury formation, and concluded that both this scale and the Norton Scale were more accurate than nurses' judgment in predicting the risk of pressure injury formation. Previously, NICE's guidance on postnatal care (2015) has included a recommendation that a risk assessment be undertaken on all those in in-patient settings; however, Moore and Cowman (2014) suggest there is no reliable evidence to demonstrate that using these tools can reduce the incidence of pressure injuries. NPUAP/EPUAP/PPPIA (2014) caution that the risk assessment tool should not be used in isolation when assessing individual risk. Consequently, NICE (2021) no longer refers to pressure injury risk in its most recent Postnatal Care guidance.

Regardless of whether a risk assessment tool is used or not, it is important to identify individuals who at risk of developing pressure injuries by considering the woman's general medical condition, undertaking an assessment of her skin, mobility, moistness (including level of continence), nutrition and pain levels. For those identified as being at increased risk, appropriate interventions should be utilised.

Assessment of skin integrity

The midwife, using good (preferably natural) lighting, should inspect the skin and potential pressure injury sites. The frequency is determined by individual needs and influenced by the presence of risk factors. For those women who are willing and able, the midwife can show them how to inspect their own skin and that of their baby. The condition of the skin, particularly over the bony prominences (e.g. sacrum, heels, hips, ankles, elbows, occiput) should be assessed initially to determine whether it is intact, dry, oedematous, red, indurated or cracking. All skin folds on a bariatric woman should be examined, as pressure injuries can also arise from tissue pressure across the buttocks and other areas of high adipose tissue.

The presence of hyperaemia should be noted when it first appears and steps taken to minimise pressure on the affected area. The area should be rechecked after 1 hour to determine if hyperaemia is still present. The midwife should look for persistent erythema and the absence of blanching on fingertip pressure in lightly pigmented skin by depressing the skin firmly but gently with a clean fingertip. When the pressure is removed, the colour of the skin is noted. In darkly pigmented skin the colour should be observed; purplish/bluish discolouration that is darker than the surrounding skin is abnormal. The location, size and colour of the affected area should be recorded; Colwell (2015) recommends using a marker pen to outline the area to make re-assessment easier and more accurate. Photographs or tracings of the pressure injury with a ruler by the side of it may be required to enable accurate assessment of how the pressure injury is changing.

The skin is also assessed for other signs of potential damage, including:

- localised heat over the affected area; with further tissue damage this heat is replaced by coolness, a sign of tissue devitalisation
- localised oedema: the area will feel spongy and the skin may appear shiny and taut
- localised induration

- break in the skin integrity (e.g. blister, pimple).

Where signs of pressure injury formation are seen, it is important the midwife documents:

- the cause (if known)
- site/location
- dimension (measured with a ruler/tape measure)
- grade of pressure injury
- amount and type of exudate
- signs of local infection
- wound appearance
- presence of sinus tracts or tunnelling
- pain score
- description of surrounding skin and any odour emitted.

For women at risk of a pressure injury, or for those with a Stage 1 pressure injury, a plan should be developed and implemented to prevent any deterioration in the condition (e.g. using high-specification foam mattresses and pressure-relieving devices, positioning and repositioning regimen). It should be fully documented using the approved assessment tool.

Preventing the development of pressure injuries

The aim is to prevent the development of pressure injuries by:

- ensuring people admitted to hospital or a care home with nursing have a pressure injury risk assessment within 6 hours of admission (NICE 2015)
- regular assessment of the skin, noting the colour, integrity, presence of blanching, oedema, tissue consistency, pain or heat
- changing the woman's position if non-blanching erythema is noted and re-examining the skin at least 2-hourly until it has resolved (NICE 2014)
- relieving pressure by assisting the woman or baby to change position on a regular basis (Moore & Cowman 2012) (NICE [2014] advises this should be at least 6-hourly); a turning chart may be used to record the time of turning and the positions used
- ensuring there is no pressure from tubing (e.g. indwelling urethral catheters, drains)
- using high-specification foam mattresses with pressure-relieving properties for women and babies at elevated risk (McInnes et al 2011)
- raising the bedclothes from the body (e.g. bedding should be loosened at the end of the bed or left untucked, or using a bed cradle)
- placing a pillow between the knees of the woman when lying laterally to reduce the pressure from the top leg
- encouraging a 30–40° position when side-lying rather than 90° to distribute the pressure
- placing a foam cushion underneath the full length of the calves and flexing the knees 5–10° if elevating the heels; check regularly that the leg has not slipped off the pillow onto the bed as this will increase pressure on the heels (Clegg & Palfreyman 2014)
- removing all creases, crumbs, and so on from the bedding as these can exert unnecessary pressure
- increasing circulation by passive or active exercises (see pp. 473–474)
- ensuring the woman or the baby is adequately hydrated; a fluid balance chart may be required
- ensuring the diet is well balanced, referring to the dietician if there are any difficulties
- using appropriate equipment for manual handling to prevent shearing
- good hygiene, especially if incontinent or sweating profusely, using water-based and pH neutral cleansers after washing and drying the skin with a gentle patting motion
- using soft cotton bedding in preference to synthetic fibres
- using medical grade rather than synthetic sheepskin
- avoiding contact with plastic surfaces
- NOT using ring cushions, water-filled gloves or donut-shaped devices as they move the pressure to another body surface (Bowen & Noble 2014b, Hosking 2013)
- NOT massaging reddened skin; to restore the circulation to a deprived area, gently rub around the area using circular outward movements (deWit & O'Neill 2014).

If a pressure injury is found, it should be cleaned with tap water or normal saline and a suitable dressing applied to facilitate moist wound healing (Bowen & Noble 2014b). Areas with necrotic tissue may need debridement, as necrotic tissue is a barrier to tissue healing.

PREVENTION OF VENOUS THROMBOEMBOLISM

Restricted mobility can influence the development of a venous thromboembolism (VTE), which affects morbidity and mortality. From 2009 to 2018 in Australia VTE was the third equal-highest direct cause of maternal mortality, with one woman dying of this cause during this period (Australian Institute of Health and Welfare [AIHW] 2020). In New Zealand, six women died of VTE in the period 2006–2018 (Perinatal and Maternal Mortality Review Committee [PMMRC] 2021). This section focuses on the principles of VTE prevention, the physiological changes that occur during pregnancy, the risk factors that increase the likelihood of VTE developing and prophylactic measures that can be used: exercises, graduated compression stockings (GCS) and sequential compression devices.

Venous thromboembolism

A thrombosis (clot) forms in response to stasis of blood flow, altered coagulation status and/or damage to the blood vessel walls (known as Virchow's triad), all of which are present at some point during pregnancy, labour and the postnatal period. Pregnancy is a state of hypercoagulability; there is a progressive change in the balance between anticoagulant and prothrombotic factors, an increase in fibrin deposition and decreased fibrinolysis, which create a procoagulant state (Arya 2011, Blackburn 2013). Blood flow in the lower limbs is reduced by up to 50% and venous distension during pregnancy can result in vessel wall damage, with further trauma occurring at delivery (Arya 2011). The changes to the coagulation factors begin with conception and may not return to their prepregnancy levels until 8 weeks following delivery (James 2011). The clot that forms is referred to as a deep vein thrombosis (DVT). If a part of the DVT breaks away, it is carried in the circulation to the major organs where it may lodge in a smaller vein causing ischaemia and may be referred to as an embolism.

During pregnancy the risk of a DVT increases 4- to 6-fold (Arya 2011, RCOG 2015) with the risk of a pulmonary embolism being 1.3 per 1000 pregnancies (RCOG 2015). While DVTs are often symptomatic, Meyer (2010) suggests the rates of asymptomatic DVT following surgery range from 10% for minor surgery (e.g. repair of third-degree tear) to 10–40% for major surgery (e.g. caesarean section). It is more common for a DVT to form in the left leg during pregnancy because of the increased pressure from the gravid uterus on the left common iliac vein, but postnatally it can occur in either leg (Virkus et al 2013). Many antenatal VTEs occur during the first trimester (RCOG 2015), although Chan and colleagues (2012) consider the incidence does not vary much across the trimesters. The Royal College of Obstetricians and Gynaecologists (RCOG 2015) advises the first 3 weeks postpartum is the highest risk period for VTE and PE formation, with the risk increased 22-fold.

Complications of DVT

The most serious complication is death; 3.5% of women who develop a PE during pregnancy through to the puerperium will die (RCOG 2015). Approximately 89% of the women who died during 2006–2008 had risk factors, and care was substandard for 56% of women (Drife 2011). Thus, it is important to identify women who are at high risk of VTE and manage them appropriately. Post-thrombotic syndrome (PTS) is thought to occur in 20–50% of DVT events (Wik et al 2012). This develops from valve incompetence causing venous stasis, resulting in chronic swelling and discomfort in the affected limb, with some limbs becoming ulcerated (Roswell & Law 2011). The use of GCS worn for 2 years following the DVT can reduce the incidence of PTS by 50% (Wik et al 2012).

Risk factors

The most recent summary of risk factors for VTE are noted by the RCOG (2015) as follows.

Preexisting factors

- Previous venous thromboembolism
- Thrombophilia inherited (e.g. factor V Leiden) or acquired (e.g. persistent lupus anticoagulant)
- Medical comorbidities (e.g. sickle cell disease)
- Age > 35 years
- Obesity: BMI > 30
- Parity ≥ 3
- Smoking
- Gross varicose veins (symptomatic or above knee or with associated phlebitis, oedema/skin changes)
- Paraplegia

Obstetric factors

- Multiple pregnancy
- Assisted reproductive therapy
- Pre-eclampsia
- Caesarean section
- Prolonged labour
- Mid-cavity rotational operative delivery
- Postpartum haemorrhage (PPH) (> 1 L) requiring transfusion

New-onset/transient factors

- Surgical procedure in pregnancy or puerperium (e.g. evacuation of retained products of conception [ERPC], appendicectomy)

Potentially reversible factors

- Hyperemesis, dehydration
- Ovarian hyperstimulation syndrome
- Admission or immobility (≥ 3 days' bed rest) (e.g. symphysis pubis dysfunction restricting mobility)
- Systemic infection (requiring antibiotics or admission to hospital) (e.g. pyelonephritis, postpartum wound infection)
- Long-distance travel (> 4 hours)
- Additionally, Roswell & Law (2011) advise dehydration can also predispose women to VTE formation.

Risk assessment

The RCOG (2015) recommends that all women have a documented assessment of risk factors for VTE in early pregnancy or, if possible, before pregnancy. They advise the assessment should be repeated each time the woman is admitted to hospital or, if she develops other problems, in labour and following delivery, as her risk status may have changed (RCOG 2015). The Australian Commission on Safety and Quality in Health Care (ACSQHC) has produced a Clinical Care Standard for VTE prevention in Australian hospitals (ASCQHC 2020), and New Zealand has a national policy framework in place for the same purpose (Blumgart 2012). The risk assessment should identify women at increased risk of developing a VTE and the RCOG (2015) recommends prophylactic treatment based on the degree of risk. However, Bennett-Day (2011) argues the amount of high-grade evidence around the unique risk factors associated with VTE and the benefit of thromboprophylaxis is limited. Thus many women will be advised to have prophylactic treatment if they deliver in hospital, and Bennett-Day (2011) questions the value of this. The reader is advised to read her article for further detail.

Preventing VTE formation

While some factors (e.g. age) are unchangeable, other factors may be modifiable or preventable. For example, advice on smoking cessation and weight reduction can be given where appropriate. Dehydration should be prevented and immobilisation kept to a minimum. Encouraging women to remain active is important; however, for some women (e.g. those with severe pelvic girdle pain) postoperative immobility may be unavoidable; thus specific exercises, both passive and active, should be encouraged to assist with venous blood flow. An obstetric physiotherapist can assist with these, but the midwife is also in a good position to support and encourage these exercises.

EXERCISES

Both passive and active exercises can be undertaken and involve moving the muscles and joints through their normal range of motion to promote circulation. They also assist in maintaining and improving muscle tone and can prevent joint contracture developing with long-term immobility. Tritak (2015) advises that they can also prevent thrombophlebitis from developing and refers to them as 'anti-embolic' exercises, suggesting they should be undertaken each hour the woman is awake. Passive exercises are rarely needed and are undertaken when the woman cannot do them herself (e.g. if she is unconscious). Active exercises are undertaken by the woman until she is fully ambulatory.

- Ankle pumps: The woman should be sitting or lying comfortably with straight knees and alternate dorsiflexion and plantar flexion by flexing her feet towards her body then extending them towards the bed (Tritak 2015). This can be done at least 10 times (Fig 47.2).
- Foot circles: The woman should be sitting or lying comfortably with straight knees, then circle her ankles by moving her feet in a clockwise direction at least 10 times, then an anticlockwise direction for 10 times, keeping her hips and knees still (Fig 47.3).
- Leg tightening: The woman should sit or lie on the bed with straight legs and pull her toes towards her legs pressing the back of her knees down towards the bed, holding the position for 4 seconds, then relaxing. This should be repeated five times.

Deep breathing exercises

Venous return is improved with each deep breath taken, but additionally the secretions within the lungs can be removed preventing hypostatic pneumonia that can occur with decreased activity (deWit & O'Neill 2014). It is particularly useful following a GA.

Two to three deep breaths should be taken while sitting up; this can be repeated often. The expiration of each breath should be followed by a short forced expiration, referred to as 'huffing', to loosen secretions.

Anticoagulation

Following the risk assessment, women may be advised to commence low molecular weight heparin prophylactically (RCOG 2015). This is a subcutaneous injection that is administered once or sometimes twice

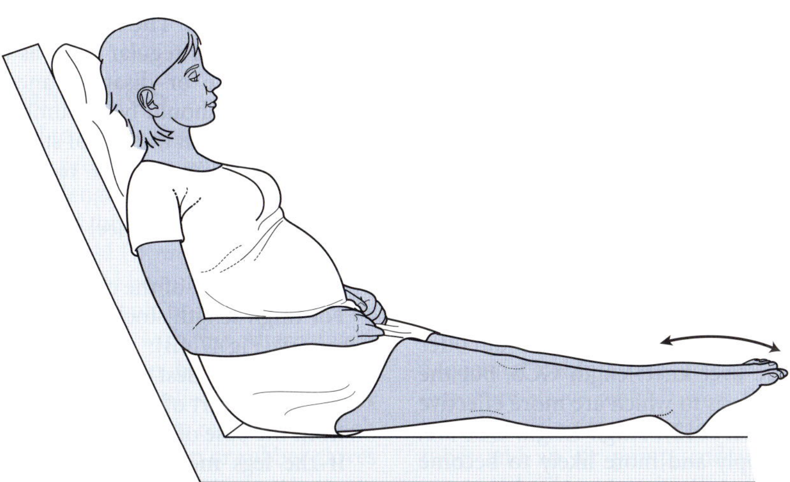

FIGURE 47.2 **Foot exercises—flexing the feet.**
Source: Johnson R, Taylor W: Skills for midwifery practice, 4th ed., Elsevier, London, 2016.

sequential SCDs can inflate legs together or separately, but are designed to move the pressure up the leg in increments (Hill 2014). Caprini (2010) recommends inflation pressures of 35–55 mmHg, with a compression cycle of 10–35 seconds and a deflation period of 1 minute to allow the leg/foot veins to refill with blood.

SCDs reduce VTE formation by enhancing blood flow in the lower limbs and stimulating the fibrinolytic system, which may help modulate hypercoagulability (Arabi et al 2013, Caprini 2010). They are often applied in the operating theatre, but can also be used for women at high risk of VTE formation who have an epidural during labour. It is recommended that SCDs are used for all women having a caesarean section, as this is the time when most emboli develop (Clarke 2015), and work by Arabi and others (2013) supports this: they found a higher reduction in the incidence of VTE when SCDs were used in critically ill patients compared with GCS. It is unclear for how long the SCDs should be worn, with recommendations varying from until 'fully ambulant' to 'discharge' (Brady et al 2015).

SKILL 47.7 Applying a sequential compression device (SCD)

1. Discuss the reason for applying the SCD and gain consent.
2. Gather and assemble equipment:
   - SCD insufflator with air hoses attached
   - adjustable Velcro compression stockings/ SCD sleeve.
3. Wash and dry hands.
4. Ensure privacy and ask the woman to lie down and remove any clothing around her legs.
5. Inspect the condition of the skin on the legs for a baseline and ensure the legs are dry.
6. Place the SCD sleeve under the woman's leg using the position indicated on the inner lining of the sleeve:
   - the back of the ankle should line up with the ankle position indicated
   - the back of the knee lines up with the popliteal opening.
7. Wrap the SCD sleeve around the woman's legs and secure with the Velcro fastening.
8. Check the SCD sleeve tightness by placing the pads of two fingertips side-by-side between the woman's leg (by her ankle) and the SCD sleeve.
9. Attach the SCD sleeve to the air insufflator and turn on the device.
10. Remain with the woman for one full cycle to ensure the sleeves are comfortable and working correctly.
11. Assist the woman into a comfortable position.
12. Wash and dry hands.
13. Document condition of skin, SCD applied and advice given to the woman.

Role and responsibilities of the midwife

These can be summarised as:

- providing comprehensive postoperative care
- applying evidence-based care
- undertaking all procedures correctly with ANTT approach when indicated
- being aware of how pressure injuries develop
- identifying women who are vulnerable to and at elevated risk of developing pressure injuries
- undertaking appropriate assessment of the skin to look for evidence of pressure damage
- assisting the woman with measures to reduce pressure injury formation
- up-to-date knowledge regarding the aetiology of VTE and risk factors pertinent to the pregnant woman
- undertaking a risk assessment at booking, at each hospital admission, including labour, following birth and if the clinical condition changes and referral as necessary
- ensuring the woman does not become dehydrated
- encouraging active exercises for women with reduced mobility
- undertaking competent clinical care, particularly in relation to anticoagulation prophylaxis, application of graduated compression stockings and SCDs
- educating the woman
- referring, if indicated
- undertaking contemporaneous record keeping.

SUMMARY

- Postoperative physiological care focuses on vital sign observations, pain relief, assessment of wound and haemorrhage, care of infusions, bladder care, prevention of VTE, maternal–newborn attachment and support of the initiation of breastfeeding.
- ANTT is required if a wound needs dressing or sutures/staples removing.
- Caesarean section wounds are often uncovered after a minimum of 6 hours; ongoing assessment of the wound should be undertaken at each consultation.
- Pressure injuries develop as a result of unrelieved pressure.
- The majority of pressure injuries are avoidable; the midwife needs to be aware of who is vulnerable or at elevated risk and able to assess the skin condition regularly.
- There are a number of measures that can be taken to reduce the likelihood of pressure injury formation; the midwife should be familiar with these.
- Thromboembolism remains a major cause of maternal mortality; pregnancy alone is a risk factor, other risks include previous VTE, reduced mobility, smoking and obesity.
- Gentle foot and leg exercises, deep breathing, anticoagulation prophylaxis, and the use of

graduated compression stockings or SCDs can all contribute to reducing the risk of VTE.
- Immobility and dehydration should be avoided whenever possible.
- Graduated compression stockings must be fitted and worn correctly to be effective.

Self-assessment exercises

The answers to the following questions may be found in the text.

1. Describe the care that the woman needs in the immediate and ongoing recovery period after a caesarean section under regional anaesthesia.
2. Describe the management of the wound following caesarean section.
3. Describe how to remove sutures correctly. Compare and contrast the removal of staples with sutures.
4. What complications are associated with wound healing?
5. How do pressure ulcers arise?
6. What factors predispose to pressure ulcer formation?
7. Describe the different stages of pressure ulcer formation and how these are recognised.
8. What is the midwife looking for when an assessment of the skin is undertaken?
9. How can the midwife provide pressure area care to reduce the risks of pressure ulcers forming?
10. Identify the women most at risk of VTE.
11. Why is pregnancy a time of increased risk for VTE formation?
12. What measures can be taken to promote venous circulation?
13. How would the midwife ensure that a knee-length graduated compression stocking is the correct size?
14. How would you fit a sequential compression device?
15. What are the role and responsibilities of the midwife in relation to the prevention of thromboembolism in a woman with restricted mobility?

References

Antokal S, Brienza D, Bryan N, et al: Friction induced skin injuries—are they pressure ulcers? A National Pressure Ulcer Advisory Panel White Paper, 2012. Online 23 March 2018. Available: www.npuap.org/resources/white-papers.

Arabi YM, Khedr M, Dara SI, et al: Use of intermittent pneumatic devices and not graduated compression stockings associated with lower incident of venous thromboembolism in critically ill patients: a multiple propensity scores adjusted analysis, Chest 144(1): 152–159, 2013.

Arya R: How I manage venous thromboembolism in pregnancy, British Journal of Haematology 153: 698–708, 2011.

Australian Commission on Safety and Quality in Health Care: Venous Thromboembolism Prevention Clinical Care Standard, ACSQHC Sydney, 2020. Online 22 September 2021. Available: www.safetyandquality.gov.au/sites/default/files/2020-01/venous_thromboembolism_prevention_clinical_care_standard_-_jan_2020_2.pdf.

Australian Institute of Health and Welfare (AIHW): Maternal deaths in Australia 2009–2018, Canberra, 2020. Online 27 August 2021. Available: www.aihw.gov.au/getmedia/64189da2-a826-4d42-ad23-1c36a50ac4ff/Maternal-deaths-in-Australia.pdf.aspx?inline=true.

Benbow M: Pressure ulcer prevention and pressure-relieving surfaces, British Journal of Nursing 17(13):830–835, 2008.

Bennett-Day S: Universal risk assessments to guide use of thromboprophylaxis, British Journal of Midwifery 19(2):778–785, 2011.

Blackburn S: Maternal, fetal and neonatal physiology: a clinical perspective, 4th ed., Saunders, St. Louis, 2013.

Blumgart A, editor: National Policy Framework: VTE prevention in adult hospitalised patients in NZ, Health Quality and Safety Commission, Wellington, 2012. Online 23 March 2018. Available: www.hqsc.govt.nz/assets/Other-Topics/QS-challenge-reports/VTE-Prevention-programme-National-Policy-Framework.pdf.

Bowen L, Noble D: Hygiene. In Dempsey J, Hillege S, Hill R, eds: Fundamentals of nursing and midwifery—2nd Australian and New Zealand ed., Lippincott Williams & Wilkins, Sydney, 2014a.

Bowen L, Noble D: Skin integrity and wound care. In Dempsey J, Hillege S, Hill R, eds: Fundamentals of nursing and midwifery—2nd Australian and New Zealand ed., Lippincott Williams & Wilkins, Sydney, 2014b.

Brady MA, Carroll AW, Cheang KI, et al: Sequential compression device compliance in postoperative obstetrics and gynecology patients, Obstetrics & Gynecology 125(1):19–25, 2015.

Butcher M: Risk of pressure damage for women using maternity services, Nursing Times 100(41):46–47, 2004.

Caprini JA: Mechanical methods for thrombosis prophylaxis, Clinical and Applied Thrombosis/Hemostasis 16(6): 668–673, 2010.

Chan N, Merriman E, Hyder S, et al: How do we manage venous thromboembolism in pregnancy? A retrospective review of the practice of diagnosing and managing pregnancy-related venous thromboembolism at two major hospitals in Australia and New Zealand, International Medical Journal 42(10):1104–1112, 2012.

Clarke SL: Peripartum venous thromboprophylaxis. Where do we go from here? Obstetrics & Gynecology 125(1): 16–18, 2015.

Clegg R, Palfreyman S: Elevation devices for the prevention of heel pressure ulcers: a review, British Journal of Nursing 23(20):S4–S11, 2014.

Colwell JC: Skin integrity and wound care. In Potter PA, Perry AG, Stockert PA, et al, eds: Essentials for nursing practice, 8th ed., Elsevier, St. Louis, 2015.

deWit S, O'Neill P: Fundamental concepts and skills for nursing, 4th ed., Elsevier, St. Louis, 2014.

Dolan S: Risk management. In Dougherty L, Lister SE, eds: Royal Marsden Hospital manual of clinical nursing procedures, 8th ed, Blackwell Publishing, Chichester, 2011.

Doran-Williams P, Jackson B, Tinne N: Wound management. In Doughty L, Lister S, eds: Royal Marsden Hospital manual of clinical nursing procedures, 8th ed., Wiley Blackwell, Chichester, 2011.

Drife J: Thrombosis and thromboembolism. In: Centre for Maternal and Child Enquiries (CMACE). Saving Mothers' Lives: reviewing maternal deaths to make motherhood safer: 2006–08. The eighth report on confidential enquiries into maternal deaths in the United Kingdom, British Journal of Obstetrics & Gynecology 118(Suppl 1):57–65, 2011.

Edsberg LE, Black JM, Goldberg M, et al: (2016). Revised national pressure ulcer advisory panel pressure injury staging system: revised pressure injury staging system, Journal of Wound, Ostomy, and Continence Nursing: official publication of The Wound, Ostomy and Continence Nurses Society 43(6):585-597. Available: https://doi.org/10.1097/WON.0000000000000281

Gould D: Caesarean section, surgical site infection and wound management, Nursing Standard 21(32):57–66, 2007.

Gurusamy K, Toon C, Allen V, Davidson, B: Continuous versus interrupted skin sutures for non-obstetric surgery, Cochrane Database of Systematic Reviews (2):Art.No. CD010365, 2014.

Guy H: Pressure ulcer risk assessment, Nursing Times 108(4):16–20, 2012.

Hill R: Perioperative care. In Dempsey J, Hillege S, Hill R, eds: Fundamentals of nursing and midwifery 2nd Australian and New Zealand ed., Lippincott, Williams & Wilkins, Sydney, 2014.

Hosking G: Skin integrity and wound care. In Koutoukidis G, Stainton K, Hughson J, eds: Tabbners' nursing care, 6th ed., Elsevier, Chatswood, 2013.

James A: Practice bulletin no. 123: thromboembolism in pregnancy, Obstetrics & Gynecology 118(3):718–729, 2011.

Johnson A, Young D, Reilly J: Caesarean section surgical site infection surveillance, Journal of Hospital Infection 64(1):30–35, 2006.

Mangram AJ, Horan TC, Pearson ML, et al: Guideline for prevention of surgical site infection, American Journal of Infection Control 27(2):97–134, 1999.

McGinnis E, Stubbs N: Pressure-relieving devices for treating heel pressure injuries, Cochrane Database of Systematic Reviews (2):Art. No.: CD005485, 2014.

McInnes E, Jammali-Blasi A, Bell-Syer SE, et al: Support surfaces for pressure ulcer prevention, Cochrane Database of Systematic Reviews (4):Art. No.: CD001735, 2011.

Meyer S: Leg compression and pharmacologic prophylaxis for venous thromboembolism prevention in high-risk patients, American Family Physician 81(3):284–285, 2010.

Miller JA: Use and wear of anti-embolism stockings: a clinical audit of surgical patients, International Wound Journal 8(10):74–83, 2011.

Milne J, Vowden P, Fumarola S, Leaper, D: Postoperative incision management, Wounds UK Suppl 8(4):1–4, 2012.

Moore ZEH, Cowman S: Risk assessment tools for the prevention of pressure ulcers, Cochrane Database of Systematic Reviews (2):Art. No.: CD006471, 2014.

Moore ZEH, Cowman S: Repositioning for treating pressure ulcers, Cochrane Database of Systematic Reviews (9):Art. No.: CD006898, 2012.

National Institute for Health and Care Excellence (NICE): CG179 Pressure ulcers: prevention and management of pressure ulcers, London, 2014. Online 23 Mar 2018. Available: www.nice.org.uk/guidance/cg179.

National Institute for Health and Care Excellence (NICE): CG190 Intrapartum care for healthy women and babies, London, 2017. Online 23 March 2018. Available: www.nice.org.uk/guidance/cg190/chapter/Recommendations#third-stage-of-labour.

National Institute for Health Care Excellence (NICE): Postnatal Care up to 8 weeks after birth: NICE Clinical Guideline 37, London, 2015, NICE. Available: www.nice.org.uk/guidance/cg37.

National Institute for Health and Clinical Excellence (NICE): NG192 Caesarean birth. NICE, London, 2021. Online 23 May 2021. Available: www.nice.org.uk/guidance/ng192/resources/caesarean-birth-pdf-66142078788805.

National Institute for Health and Care Excellence (NICE): Postnatal Care: NG194, London, 2021. Available: www.nice.org.uk/guidance/ng194/resources/postnatal-care-pdf-66142082148037

Nicol M, Bavin C, Cronin P, et al: Essential nursing skills, 3rd ed., Elsevier, Edinburgh, 2008.

Ohayon R, Rose R, Ebert K, et al: Incidence of incorrectly sized graduated compression stockings and lower leg irregularities in postoperative orthopedic patients, Medsurgical Nursing 22(6):370–374, 2013.

Olsen MA, Butler AM, Willers DM, et al: Risk factors for surgical site infection after low transverse cesarean section, Infection Control and Hospital Epidemiology 29(6):477–484, 2008.

Pancorbo-Hidalgo PL, Garcia-Fernandez FP, Lopez-Medina IM, et al: Risk assessment scales for pressure ulcer prevention: a systematic review, Journal of Advanced Nursing 54(1):94–110, 2006.

Perinatal and Maternal Mortality Review Committee (PMMRC): Fourteenth annual report of the perinatal and maternal mortality review committee, Te Pūrongo ā-Tau Tekau mā Whā o te Komiti Arotake Mate Pēpi, Mate Whaea Hoki: Reporting mortality 2006–2018, Health Quality and Safety Committee, Wellington, 2021. Online 23 May 2021. Available: www.hqsc.govt.nz/our-programmes/mrc/pmmrc/publications-and-resources/publication/4210/.

Royal Australian and New Zealand College of Obstetricians and Gynaecologists (RANZCOG): Management of obesity in pregnancy: C-Obs 49. RANZCOG, Melbourne, 2017. Online 3 June 2018. Available: www.ranzcog.

edu.au/RANZCOG_SITE/media/RANZCOG-MEDIA/Women%27s%20Health/Statement%20and%20guidelines/Clinical-Obstetrics/Management-of-obesity-(C-Obs-49)-Review-March-2017.pdf?ext=.pdf.

Royal Australian and New Zealand College of Obstetricians and Gynaecologists (RANZCOG): Caesarean section, RANZCOG, Melbourne, 2016. Online 23 March 2018. Available: www.ranzcog.edu.au/RANZCOG_SITE/media/RANZCOG-MEDIA/Women%27s%20Health/Patient%20information/Caesarean-section-pamphlet.pdf?ext=.pdf.

Reilly J: Evidence based surgical wound care on surgical wound infection, British Journal of Nursing 11(16):S4–S12, 2002.

Roswell H, Law C: Reducing patients' risk of venous thromboembolism, American Family Physician 81(3):284–285, 2011.

Rowley S, Clare S, Macqueen S, et al: ANTT v2: an updated practice framework for aseptic technique, British Journal of Nursing 19(5):S5–S11, 2010.

Royal College of Obstetricians and Gynaecologists (RCOG), 2015. Reducing the risk of venous thromboembolism during pregnancy and the puerperium. Green-Top Guideline No. 37a. Online 23 May 2021. Available: www.rcog.org.uk/en/guidelines-research-services/guidelines/gtg37a/.

Sajid MS, Desai M, Morris RW, et al: Knee length versus thigh length graduated compression stocking for prevention of deep vein thrombosis in postoperative surgical patients, Cochrane Database of Systematic Reviews (5):Art. No.: CD007162, 2012.

Tritak A: Immobility. In Potter PA, Perry AG, Stockert PA, Hall, A, eds: Essentials for nursing practice, 8th ed., Elsevier, St. Louis, 2015.

Virkus RA, Løkkegaard ECL, Lidegaard Ø, et al: Venous thromboembolism in pregnancy and the puerperal period: a study of 1210 events, Acta Obstetrica et Gynecologica Scandinavica 92(10):1135–1142, 2013.

Ward VP, Charlett A, Fagan J, et al: Enhanced surgical site infection surveillance following caesarean section: experience of a multicentre collaborative post-discharge system, Journal of Hospital Infection 70:166–173, 2008.

Wetter LA, Dinneen MD, Levitt MD, et al: Controlled trial of polyglycolic acid versus catgut and nylon for appendicectomy wound closure, British Journal of Surgery 78(8):985–987, 1991.

Wik HS, Jacobsen AF, Sandvik L, et al: Prevalence and predictors for post-thrombotic syndrome 3 to 16 years after pregnancy-related venous thrombosis: a population-based, cross-sectional, case-control survey, Journal of Thrombosis Haemostasis 10(5):840–847, 2012. Available: https://onlinelibrary.wiley.com/doi/10.1111/j.1538-7836.2012.04690.x

CHAPTER 48

CARING FOR THE BABY'S PHYSIOLOGICAL WELLBEING AFTER BIRTH

Learning outcomes

Having read this chapter, the reader should be able to:

- discuss how the Apgar score is undertaken and the significance of the scores
- describe the initial examination of the baby at birth, identifying how normality is confirmed
- describe the observations that should be made during the daily examination of the baby and identify how normal progress is recognised
- discuss the factors that contribute to developmental dysplasia of the hips (DDH)
- describe DDH and how it is classified
- describe the different tests that are used to assess for DDH
- discuss how DDH may be prevented once the baby is born
- discuss the midwife's role and responsibilities regarding assessment of the baby immediately following birth and during each daily examination of the baby.

Once the baby is born, the midwife's role and responsibilities extend to assessing and optimising the baby's wellbeing in the immediate postnatal period. This includes assessing the baby's condition at and soon after birth, detection and prevention of developmental dysplasia of the hips (DDH), and evaluating his or her adaptation to extrauterine life in the early days and weeks. This chapter considers the specific observations that must be made of the baby in these three aspects.

ASSESSING THE BABY AT BIRTH

There are two components to assessing the baby at birth: the Apgar score, which is undertaken to determine how well the baby is adjusting from intrauterine to extrauterine life, and the **top-to-toe physical examination** that looks to confirm normality and detect any deviations from this, so that referral can be made. These examinations are usually undertaken by the midwife as part of the care of the baby at birth (National Institute for Health and Care Excellence [NICE] 2014b), thus it is important the midwife is competent in both of these assessments and understands the significance of what is being assessed and the findings.

Although in some settings the midwife will undertake a more extensive examination, this is only undertaken if the midwife has had further training; therefore these aspects are not discussed within this chapter. Further, pulse oximetry screening is increasingly being introduced into immediate postnatal care of the newborn; however, at the time of writing this is not a universal inclusion in either Australia or New Zealand and therefore is not discussed herein. The reader is advised to check local policy.

The reader may wish to consider the information and skills that follow in the broader discussion of newborn health and wellbeing, and the influences upon it, that is found in Pairman, et al *Midwifery: Preparation for practice* (Chapter 29).

The Apgar score

The **Apgar score** was formulated by Dr Virginia Apgar in the 1950s as a way of assessing the baby's condition at birth and the need for resuscitation. Five interrelated variables, assessed at 1, 5 and 10 minutes (although these can be repeated at different timeframes), are based on what happens and can be seen if the baby does not breathe effectively at birth (Pinheiro 2009). Each of the five variables is given a score of 0, 1 or 2, with a total score out of 10 (Table 48.1). The variables are breathing, heart rate, colour, tone and reflex irritability. If the baby is not breathing there is less oxygen reaching cardiac tissue. This causes the heart rate to decrease which results in less oxygen reaching the tissues. This will affect the colour, muscle tone and reflex irritability. Thus a low score will indicate the need for resuscitation. As breathing occurs, the heart rate improves, resulting in the baby becoming pinker, with improved muscle tone and reflex irritability. A high score reflects a baby who does not need resuscitation and can reflect the baby who has made the adjustment well or has had a good response to resuscitative measures undertaken. However, it must be remembered that resuscitation should begin before 1 minute if indicated by the condition of the baby and an Apgar score calculated during resuscitation is not equivalent to that of a baby who is breathing spontaneously. There is no accepted standard for calculating Apgar scores for babies who are being resuscitated (Pinheiro 2009).

A low score at 1 minute does not correlate with future outcome, whereas at 5 minutes it is associated with neonatal mortality from 24 weeks' gestation, but there is conflicting evidence around neurological disability (Lee et al 2010, O'Donnell et al 2006, Pinheiro 2009). Iliodromiti and colleagues (2014) found an increased risk of infant death for babies who had a 5-minute Apgar score of 0–3. Dijxhoorn and colleagues (1986) suggest changes in the fetal heart rate do not compare well with Apgar scores at delivery, making it difficult to anticipate which babies will have a low score at birth. This may account for why some emergency caesarean sections undertaken because of serious concerns regarding the fetal heart rate deliver a baby with a total Apgar score of 9 or 10. Additionally, a persistently low Apgar score on its own should not be considered a specific indicator of intrapartum asphyxia. Salustiano and colleagues (2012) undertook a retrospective study to assess risk factors associated with an Apgar score < 7 at 5 minutes and found that while prolonged second stage of labour and repeated late decelerations on the cardiotocograph (CTG) were predictive, age, parity and breech birth were not. They also found these babies had an increased risk of respiratory distress, mechanical ventilation, admission to the neonatal intensive care unit, and a strong association with hypoxic–ischaemic encephalopathy (Salustiano et al 2012).

TABLE 48.1 THE APGAR SCORING SYSTEM: THE FIVE CLASSIFICATIONS USED AND THE CRITERIA FOR SCORING 0–2

Sign	0	1	2
Appearance (colour)	Blue, pale	Body pink, limbs blue	All pink
Pulse (heart rate)	Absent	< 100	> 100
Grimace (response to stimuli)	None	Grimace	Cry
Activity (muscle tone)	Limp	Some flexion of limbs	Active movements, limbs well flexed
Respiratory effort	None	Slow, irregular	Good, strong cry

Source: Johnson R, Taylor W: Skills for midwifery practice, 4th ed., Elsevier, London, 2016.

The Apgar score is vulnerable to bias, as it is a subjective score and is often undertaken retrospectively. McCarthy and colleagues (2013) found that babies being resuscitated were given an Apgar score at 1 minute, even though there was no documented evidence that the heart rate had been recorded, suggesting that the score does not accurately reflect the events occurring during resuscitation or when interventions are occurring. Ideally, Apgar scoring should be undertaken by someone other than the midwife in attendance at the birth, as the midwife can be distracted by what is happening to the mother and the baby. The retrospective scoring is often based on what happened to the baby; thus a baby who had no resuscitative measures will score high. In some situations the Apgar score is jointly assigned by all midwives and doctors present at delivery, but again is often retrospective and O'Donnell and colleagues (2006) caution that there is poor interobserver reliability even when undertaken independently.

There are a number of factors that can influence the score: the quality of lighting, for example, can affect the perception of the baby's colour, as can skin pigmentation and haemoglobin levels. Tone can be affected by gestational age, congenital abnormality and maternal drugs. Silverton (1993) advises that skin pigmentation in non-Caucasian babies usually develops from the fifth day of life, which can make these babies appear less well perfused. If the skin is darkly pigmented, colour can be assessed by observing the mucous membranes, palms of the hand, and soles of the feet: these should be pink. The preterm baby has an immature neurological system, resulting in poorer muscle tone and slower reflexes, as well as a bluish-red skin colour, which can lead to a low Apgar score, even though the baby requires no resuscitation.

Assessing the Apgar score

The five variables that are assessed in Apgar scoring have been used to develop the acronym 'Apgar', which stands for Appearance, Pulse, Grimace, Activity and Respiration (see Table 48.1). The assessor(s) should do the following.

- Observe the appearance: is the baby pink all over (score 2), is the body pink but the extremities blue (score 1) or is the baby pale or blue all over (score 0)?

- Assess the heart rate by palpating the umbilicus or placing two fingers across the chest over the apex, count the rate for 6 seconds, then multiply by 10. Determine whether the heart rate is < 100 (10 beats or more over the 6-second period) (score 2), > 100 (less than 10 beats in 6 seconds) (score 1) or absent (score 0). A baby who is pink, active and breathing is likely to have a heart rate < 100.
- The response of the baby to stimuli should be noted. Determine whether the baby cries in response to stimuli (score 2), whether it is trying to cry but is only able to grimace (score 1) or whether there is no response (score 0).
- Assess the degree of muscle tone by observing the amount of activity and degree of flexion of the limbs: are there active movements using well-flexed limbs (score 2), is there some flexion of the limbs (score 1) or is the baby limp (score 0)?
- Observe the respiratory effort made by the baby: is it good and strong (often seen in conjunction with a crying baby) (score 2), is respiration slow and irregular (score 1) or is there no respiratory effort (score 0)?

The scores are added and a total score is documented. Babies scoring above seven rarely need resuscitation.

SKILL 48.1 Apgar scoring

1. Ensure the lighting facilitates good visualisation of colour and there is access to the baby, which may involve uncovering the baby briefly.
2. Note the time of birth, wait 1 minute, then undertake the first assessment; the five variables should be assessed quickly and simultaneously, and the score totalled.
3. Act promptly and appropriately according to the score; for example, a baby scoring 0–3 requires immediate resuscitation (it may already have commenced if the baby is obviously compromised at birth).
4. Repeat at 5 minutes; the score should increase if previously 8 or below.
5. If resuscitation is still continuing, repeat again at 10 minutes and every 5 minutes thereafter until efforts cease.
6. Document findings and act accordingly.

Source: Johnson R, Taylor W: Skills for midwifery practice, 4th ed., Elsevier, London, 2016.

BIRTH EXAMINATION

The **initial birth examination** is a physical examination undertaken to confirm normality and detect deviations from normal. In New Zealand the newborn assessment is undertaken as part of primary maternity care by the midwife, who carries out In New Zealand, the newborn assessment is undertaken as part of primary maternity care by the midwife, who carries out examinations of the baby that are consistent with the requirements of the Well Child Tamariki Ora Schedule (Ministry of Health 2021). If any problems are detected the baby is referred to a paediatrician for further investigation. In Australia, the legal and professional responsibilities of midwives relating to neonatal assessment vary according to state and local protocols. However, generally a midwife will perform an initial general assessment soon after birth, after which a medical practitioner will perform a more detailed examination within the next 24 hours or before discharge from the maternity unit (Pairman et al 2018).

The initial assessment is usually undertaken within the first couple of hours of life, having given the baby time for skin-to-skin contact with his or her mother and to complete his first feed (NICE 2014a). The examination should be undertaken in a warm environment, free from draughts (to ensure the baby does not become cold), and with a good light source. This examination is likely to reveal obvious abnormalities, but others, some of which may not be apparent at birth, will be detected during the physical examination undertaken within the first 72 hours of birth (NICE 2014b). The examination must be performed by a health practitioner experienced in hip examination; this may be a midwife who has undertaken further training and assessment in the examination of the newborn, or a paediatrician. The midwife will develop their own systematic approach to examining the baby; however, the order is less important than ensuring the examination is thorough and complete.

SKILL 48.2 Birth examination

1. Discuss the procedure with the parents and gain their informed consent, requesting that one or both are present for the examination (if the mother is unable to move from the bed, the examination can take place at the bedside or on the bed).

SKILL 48.2 Birth examination—cont'd

2. Gather equipment:
   - thermometer suitable for use with a baby (pp. 47–48)
   - scales for weighing the baby
   - disposable tape measure
   - disposable sheet
   - non-sterile gloves
   - nappy.
3. Wash and dry hands and put on non-sterile gloves.
4. Place the baby on to the disposable sheet that has been placed on top of a firm, safe surface with good lighting.
5. Perform a full set of vital observations, taking care to check that the baby is warm enough by taking his or her temperature before beginning the procedure; to maintain the temperature only uncover the part of the baby being examined and re-cover the baby quickly.
6. Examine the baby systematically and thoroughly, noting the colour, tone and activity throughout the procedure.
7. Begin by examining the head, face and neck, then moving onto the clavicles, arms, hands, chest and abdomen. The genitalia are then examined, followed by the legs, feet, spine and buttocks. Reflexes can be assessed during the procedure (see later this chapter for more detail).
8. Measure the baby's weight, head circumference and length, and note if any urine and meconium are passed.
9. Place the baby skin-to-skin with his mother or dress him/her (the parents should be encouraged to do this).
10. Dispose of disposable sheet and gloves, wash and dry hands.
11. Discuss the findings with the parents during the procedure or at the end if they are not present.
12. Document findings and act accordingly.

Source: Johnson R, Taylor W: Skills for midwifery practice, 4th ed., Elsevier, London, 2016.

The head

The size of the head should be reviewed in relation to the rest of the baby; the head will appear large and out of proportion to the body and limbs in the preterm baby, where asymmetrical growth restriction has occurred and in cases of hydrocephaly, whereas one that appears too small is associated with microcephaly and fetal alcohol spectrum disorders. Look for signs of moulding and caput succedaneum, as these may result in the head appearing asymmetrical and will influence the measurement of the head circumference. The parents should be reassured that both the moulding and caput swelling will resolve spontaneously over the ensuing 48 hours and that the head will become more rounded. On rare occasions the swelling may be due to a subgaleal haemorrhage, especially if the birth was by vacuum extraction. The swelling will be present at birth, but may not pit on pressure and will increase in size as the condition of the baby deteriorates. Urgent paediatric referral is required in this case (Swanson et al 2011). Visible signs of trauma should be looked for, particularly if an amnihook, fetal scalp electrode, forceps or vacuum cup has been used, as should signs of bruising, which may increase the risk of physiological jaundice developing.

The suture lines and fontanelles should be palpated to assess their size and appearance. Widely spaced sutures may be indicative of a preterm baby, lack of moulding or hydrocephalus. Narrowly spaced sutures are usually a result of moulding. The triangular-shaped posterior fontanelle should feel small and often appears closed at birth due to moulding. The diamond-shaped anterior fontanelle should be palpated; Bailey (2014) advises it should measure 3–4 cm in length and 1.5–2 cm in width (this may vary with moulding). A large fontanelle may be due to prematurity, hypothyroidism or hydrocephalus; a small one is suggestive of microcephaly. If the fontanelle is raised/bulging, this may be due to raised intracranial pressure (from birth injury, bleeding, hydrocephalus), while a depressed fontanelle is suggestive of dehydration—rarely seen at birth. Occasionally a third fontanelle can be felt between the anterior and posterior fontanelles and is suggestive of trisomy 21.

Head circumference

The occipitofrontal circumference is used to measure the head circumference, which is the measurement around the occiput and forehead. However, due to the changes that can occur at birth from moulding, this measurement is likely to change over the next 48 hours. England (2014) suggests the normal measurement for a term baby is 32–36 cm, whereas Michaelides (2011) proposes it is 33–38 cm. Johnston and colleagues (2003) state it as 33–37 cm with the average cited as 35 cm, while Gardner and Hernandez (2011) advise it should be 32–38 cm.

Shape of the face

There should be a symmetrical shape to the face, so the size and position of the eyes, nose, mouth, chin and ears should be noted in relation to each other. Moderate facial asymmetry may be associated with prolonged second stage, forceps delivery, macrosomia and birth trauma; for example, facial (Bell's) palsy (Stellwagen et al 2008). If the face appears unusual in appearance, England (2014) recommends looking at the face of each parent before expressing concern.

Eyes

If the baby's eyes are closed, gently tip the baby backwards, then raise the baby slowly as this may encourage him or her to open the eyes. The eyes are examined to ensure two are present with an assessment of their size, shape, symmetry and any slanting (which may be normal). Widely spaced or narrowly spaced eyes are abnormal and may be indicative of an underlying syndrome. Epicanthic folds are normal in some ethnic groups (e.g. people of East, Southeast, Central and North Asian descent) and may occur in those of South Asian, Polynesian or Micronesian origin, but may also be associated with an underlying syndrome (e.g. trisomy 21). The cornea should be clear; if it is cloudy-looking it could be infection, trauma (from forceps), dystrophies, metabolic abnormality or congenital glaucoma. While the sclera should be clear, conjunctival haemorrhage can be present, usually acquired during the second stage of labour, and should be noted. The parents should be reassured that this is likely to resolve within a few days. Any profuse or purulent discharge should be noted and a swab taken; this is not normal and could be indicative of infection. On examination, the pupils should appear round and clear, occasionally a keyhole shape is present (coloboma), which could be indicative of an underlying retinal defect. They should constrict to light. White or grey cloudiness within the pupil could indicate congenital cataracts (an early red eye reflex examination is required). White speckles on the iris, Brushfield's spots, may be indicative of trisomy 21, but can also be a normal variant.

Nose

Observe the shape of the nose and width of the bridge, which should be greater than 2.5 cm in the term baby. Two patent nares should be present; if either or both are blocked it will affect the baby's ability to breathe as babies are initially nose breathers rather than being able to use the mouth and the nose. Gardner and Hernandez (2011) suggest patency can be assessed by closing the baby's mouth and obstructing one nostril and observing breathing from the other nostril, then repeating with the other side, or placing a stethoscope diaphragm under the nostrils and looking for bilateral 'fogging'. It is not unusual for the nose to be squashed at birth; if so, this should be noted, particularly if it is affecting the baby's ability to breathe. The nostrils should not flare; if they do, this is usually indicative of respiratory illness.

Mouth

The lips should be formed and symmetrical; asymmetry could be indicative of facial (Bell's) palsy. The size of the baby's mouth should be reviewed; a small mouth may be due to micrognathia, often associated with underlying abnormality. The area between the lips and the nose is then examined for the presence of a cleft lip. The inside of the mouth should be visualised using a good light source and is more easily achieved when the baby is crying or by pressing gently on the chin or the angle of the jaw to encourage the mouth to open. The palate is then observed for intactness, particularly at the junction of the hard and soft palates where a cleft palate may occur; the palate should be high and arched. Digital examination is only undertaken if a submucous cleft palate is suspected (Habel et al 2006). The presence of white spots on the gums or palate is usually due to epithelial (Epstein's) pearls, which are of no significance, or teeth, and are noted, as is the length of the frenulum to assess for tongue tie.

Ears

The ears are examined to ensure two are present, which should be fully formed and in the correct position. There should be enough cartilage in the ears of a term baby to allow them to spring back into position when moved forwards gently. The pinna should be well formed with defined curves in the upper part. Correct positioning of the ears is determined by tracing an imaginary line from the outer canthus of the eyes horizontally back to the ears, with the top of the pinna above this line. Low-set ears may be associated with an underlying chromosomal abnormality (e.g. trisomy 21), renal abnormality or a normal variation. Gardner and Hernandez (2011) advise the ears are positioned almost vertically and suggest it is abnormal if the angle is $> 10°$. The external auditory meatus should be examined to ensure patency. The presence of accessory skin tags or auricles should be noted and may be associated with renal abnormalities and hearing impairment (Roth et al 2008).

Neck

Babies generally have short necks, which should be examined for symmetry. The presence of swelling (e.g. cystic hygroma, sternomastoid tumour) can be detected by feeling all around the neck. The baby should be able to move his or her head to both sides well past the shoulder 100–110° from the midline and flex the head 50–60° laterally towards his or her ear. The head should also flex towards the chest so that it almost or does touch the chest and extend backwards so the back of the occiput reaches or is almost touching the back (Michaelides 2011). Limited lateral movement is associated with torticollis (Stellwagen et al 2008). Webbing is unusual and could be indicative of a chromosomal abnormality (e.g. Turner's syndrome); redundant skin folds at the back of the neck are suggestive of trisomy 21.

Clavicles

Feel along the clavicles using the index finger to ensure they are intact, particularly if there was a breech presentation that required manipulation or shoulder dystocia; both increase the risk of a fractured clavicle, resulting in little or no movement in the associated arm.

Arms

The arms should be the same length, confirmed by straightening them down the side of the body and comparing the two together. Both arms should be moving freely; spontaneous arm movements can usually be elicited by stroking the forearm or hand. Lack of movement may be associated with underlying trauma (e.g. fractures, nerve damage) or poor motor control associated with neurological impairment. The number of digits is then counted and examined for webbing between them; polydactyly and/or syndactyly is noted. The palm should be straightened and the number of palmar creases noted; a single crease may be associated with chromosomal abnormality (e.g. trisomy 21), but can also be a normal variant. The nails should be examined for the presence of paronychia and hangnails; hangnails may become infected or get caught on bedding, causing them to tear and bleed.

Chest

The chest is observed for a rounded shape and symmetry of movement with respiration; asymmetrical movement may be due to unilateral pneumothorax or phrenic nerve injury, particularly if there was a shoulder dystocia at birth. The respiratory rate can be counted if it appears abnormal and signs of respiratory distress (e.g. sternal recession, intercostal recession) reported to a paediatrician immediately. The nipples and areolae are well formed in the term baby and appear symmetrical on the chest wall but not widely spaced (this may be indicative of an underlying chromosomal abnormality). Any accessory nipples should be noted. The breasts may appear enlarged; this is normal and of little significance unless there are signs of infection.

Abdomen

Observe the abdomen, which should appear rounded and move in synchrony with the chest during respiration, inspecting the area to confirm it is intact and gently palpating to ensure there are no abnormal swellings. The abdomen usually protrudes slightly; a flat or sunken abdomen may be associated with decreased tone or diaphragmatic hernia (this is likely to cause respiratory difficulty, particularly when the baby is laid flat). Diastasis recti (separation of the rectus muscles) is common and may facilitate the presence of a midline hernia around the umbilicus, which should resolve spontaneously within 24 hours (Michaelides 2011). Midline defects (e.g. gastroschisis, exomphalos) require covering and urgent referral. The umbilical cord should be securely clamped and inspected to ensure there are no signs of haemorrhage.

Genitalia

With boys, the length and shape of the penis should be assessed—this is usually about 3 cm and straight—and the position of the urethral meatus confirmed (easier to see when the baby passes urine). England (2014) suggests an apparently short penis is common and usually due to the presence of suprapubic fat, which may reassure parents. The foreskin should not be retracted, as it is adherent to the glans penis and physically retracting it at this age can lead to phimosis. The scrotum is observed for symmetry, suggestive of two descended testicles and gently palpated to feel for both testicles, Michaelides (2011) advises they are 1.5–2 cm long and feel similar to a pea. England (2014) cautions that a dark discolouration of the scrotum, with or without swelling, is abnormal and may be indicative of testicular torsion. This should not be mistaken for the generalised darker pigmentation seen with highly pigmented skin. For girls, the vulva should be examined by parting the labia gently to ensure the presence of the clitoris, and urethral and vaginal orifices. A mucoid discharge may be present, which is normal.

Legs

The legs and feet should be observed for their symmetry, size, shape and posture. To confirm the legs are the same length, straighten them together to compare the two, then flex the hips and knees and place the feet on the surface touching their buttocks. The knees should be at the same height (Galeazzi test/Allis sign); if they are not, it could be indicative of DDH (see p. 490). Both legs should be moving freely; lack of movement may be associated with underlying trauma (e.g. fractures, nerve damage) or poor motor control associated with neurological impairment. The position of the feet in relation to the legs should be noted, as both positional and anatomical deformities may cause the feet to be turned inwards or outwards, upwards or downwards. Some of these deformities require corrective treatment. The shape of the feet should be noted, including oedema or a 'rocker bottom' appearance and the number of toes counted and examined for webbing between them by separating them; polydactyly or syndactyly should be noted.

Spine

The spine is examined by turning the baby over, looking for any obvious abnormality, such as spina bifida, swelling, dimpling or hairy patches; these could indicate an abnormality of the spinal cord or vertebral column. Assess the curvature of the vertebral column by running the fingers lightly over the spine; the spine should feel straight with no scoliosis, lordosis or kyphosis. This may be easier to do by straddling the baby over one hand, while using the other hand to feel the spine (ensure the head is supported). Gently part the cleft of the buttocks, look for dimples or sinuses and confirm the presence of the external anal sphincter. Wilson and colleagues

(2010) caution the buttocks must be parted, as a cursory examination without doing this may result in an anorectal malformation being missed.

Skin

The condition of the skin can be observed throughout the examination, particularly the colour and the presence of any rashes or marks (e.g. birthmarks, bruising). Acrocyanosis is seen when the baby's body is pink but the extremities, in particular the hands and feet, are blue or purple. It is normal during the first few hours of life, often disappearing within 24 hours and is usually physiological, due to the large arteriovenous oxygen difference resulting during the slow blood flow throughout the peripheral capillary beds (Steinhorn 2008). Any obvious swelling or spots should be examined and recorded. A Mongolian blue spot may be evident in some babies, particularly those with an Asian or African ancestry. This appears like bruising, usually over the sacral area, and should be observed over the next few days to enable the midwife to differentiate between the possibility of the discolouration being a bruise or a Mongolian blue spot. 'Birth marks' should be noted, as an infantile haemangioma may present at birth (Leonardi-Bee et al 2011).

Elimination

If urine or meconium is passed it should be recorded, as it indicates patency of the renal and lower gastrointestinal tracts, respectively.

Weight

The weight of the baby is recorded in kilograms; this can be undertaken at the beginning or end of the examination, provided the baby is warm. Many parents may want to know the weight in pounds and ounces and it is useful to have a conversion chart with the scales.

Length

While the crown–heel length of the baby may be recorded, as parents are interested in 'how long' their baby is, it is difficult to measure accurately. The length is measured in two stages using a non-stretchable, disposable tape measure and the baby on his or her side: from the crown (top part of the head) to the base of the spine, and from the base of the spine to the heel. A second person may be required to straighten the legs. Length can also be measured by placing the baby on a disposable sheet and marking the paper where the top of the baby's head is. The baby's legs are then straightened without moving the paper from under the baby and a mark placed where his feet are positioned. The baby can then be lifted from the sheet and the distance between the two marks measured.

Reflexes

A number of reflexes may be seen or looked for during the examination, which reflect the intactness of the neurological system. These need to be undertaken when the baby is relaxed for maximum effect. These reflexes are described below.

Rooting

When the baby's cheek is stroked the baby will turn his or her head in the direction of the stroke to search for the source of the stimulation. The baby's head will move in gradually decreasing arcs until the object is found and he or she may make sucking motions. This is less evident if the baby is sleepy or not hungry.

Sucking

This is seen in response to tactile stimulation around the mouth or when an object (e.g. nipple, finger, teat) is inserted into the baby's mouth.

Snout (also known as 'pout')

If gentle pressure is applied over the philtrum, the baby will pucker his or her lips.

Moro/startle

This response occurs if the baby's head suddenly changes position, particularly downwards or if startled by an unexpected sound. The legs and head will extend while the arms move up and out with palms up and thumbs flexed. The baby will then bring the arms together and clench the fists. It may be accompanied by crying.

Babinski/plantar

When the sole of the baby's foot is stroked firmly, the baby's big toe moves upwards and the other toes fan out.

Palmar grasp

By placing a finger on the infant's open palm, the hand will be seen to close around the finger. As an attempt is made to remove the finger, the baby will tighten the grip. The palmar grasp can be strong, almost allowing the baby to be lifted up if both the baby's hands are grasping fingers.

Asymmetrical tonic neck

This is seen when a baby is lying on his or her back and with the head turned to the side. The arm on the side where the head is facing reaches away from the body with the hand partly open while the opposite arm will flex with a tightly clenched fist. If the baby's head is moved to the opposite side, the reverse happens. This position has been referred as the 'fencer's position' because of its similarity to a fencer's stance.

Stepping/walking

When the baby is held upright and the soles of the feet touch a flat surface, he or she will attempt to walk by placing one foot in front of the other.

DAILY EXAMINATION OF THE NEWBORN

During the postnatal period the midwife will undertake an examination of the baby each day while the baby is in hospital and/or when visited at home to monitor early changes and ensure optimal progress is occurring. Normality is identified and deviations from normal are recognised. NICE (2014b) recommend the use of a postnatal care plan to guide individualised care for the mother and baby; this is updated each visit. Furthermore, parents should be given information and advice that will enable them to assess their baby's general condition so they can recognise signs and symptoms of common health problems for babies and seek appropriate help (NICE 2014b). Although it is referred to as a daily examination, it is not essential to see the baby every day during the postnatal period, but according to clinical need.

Principles of the daily examination

Parental care

The facilitation of optimal infant health and development relies significantly on the skills, education and care given by the parents. This process begins during pregnancy with the midwife working with families in the beginnings of infant health and wellbeing and the development of the postnatal care plan. The midwife teaches by example (e.g. handwashing), as well as with verbal (wherever possible, evidence-based) suggestions. During the daily examination of the baby, the midwife relies on communication with the parents to appreciate the complete picture of how the baby is progressing. Equally, it is a time for guiding, educating and advising parents, as well as supporting and encouraging them in their new role.

Consent

The procedure should be discussed with the parents and informed consent gained, as the baby cannot give consent for the examination. There will be times when the parents may not give consent; for example, the baby is now asleep, having been awake all night. The midwife undertakes a risk assessment, based on detailed conversation, to appreciate whether a physical examination must be undertaken or whether it can be postponed until later. The examination should ideally be undertaken when one or both parents are present, as this provides a good opportunity for discussion as issues from the examination arise.

Reducing infection risks

The baby is considered a 'compromised host' at birth, at risk from infection that can affect morbidity and mortality. Standard precautions should be utilised (see Chapter 1) and it is important to avoid cross-infection from other sources; hand hygiene should be scrupulous (see Chapter 1). If contact with body fluids is anticipated, then personal protective equipment is used (e.g. gloves, apron).

Examination of the newborn

The daily examination is not a copy of the birth examination, but an assessment of progress thereafter. It therefore relies on the fact that all body systems have been screened and deviations from normal are known about, with progress assessed accordingly. It should be undertaken methodically, in a good light and a warm environment.

INITIAL OBSERVATIONS

Observations on entering a woman's personal environment (hospital or home) can give immediate indicators as to the situation and provide the midwife with prompts when giving care advice. The midwife should observe:

- how the parents are feeling by looking at them: peaceful, tired, tearful, happy, etc.
- whether the parents immediately begin to express problems or anxieties
- how the baby is positioned and dressed within the sleeping area
- how the parent(s) handle and react to their baby
- environmental factors such as heat/cold; the presence of smoke, pets, other relatives/siblings/ visitors and their reactions or concerns; and general level of hygiene.

The following observations are likely to lead into more detailed discussion and provide an opportunity for reassurance, education and support.

- The baby's behaviour: Is the baby active, sleepy, contented or unsettled? Does the baby cry a lot? What is the cry like? Can the baby be pacified easily?
- Feeding patterns: Is the baby waking for feeds and how often? What is the approximate feeding pattern? (This will vary according to feeding method.) If breastfeeding, is the mother happy that the baby latches correctly and is achieving an effective feed? (See Chapter 49.) If formula feeding, are amounts taken appropriate for the age of the baby? Is the mother fully conversant with sterilising and preparing feeds? (See Chapter 50.) Is the baby settled after a feed? Is there any vomiting or posseting? In the event of vomiting green bile, or any projectile vomiting, a direct referral is made to a paediatrician.
- Elimination: Do the number and nature of wet and soiled nappies suggest that feeding is progressing and body systems are functioning normally?
- Are the parents feeling confident about other aspects of baby care (e.g. skin care, managing unsettled periods)?
- Do the parents have any other concerns or questions at this time?

GENERAL OBSERVATION OF THE BABY

Observing the baby before undressing it can reveal several potential problems.

- Under-/over-clothed: Advice may be needed as to correct temperature management when indoors to avoid problems associated with hypo- and hyperthermia.
- Position of the baby: The baby should be positioned on his or her back to sleep, but 'tummy time' should be encouraged when awake and someone is with the baby.
- Respirations: The respiratory pattern is noted (often irregular in newborn babies; see Chapter 6), with a normal respiratory rate of 30–40 breaths per minute expected when the baby is at rest with no signs of respiratory distress. The respiratory rate can increase to 60 breaths per minute with crying. Chest movement should be symmetrical (this is often better assessed when the baby is undressed); nasal flaring should not be seen.
- Obvious signs of vomiting or posseting (see above).
- Skin colour: The baby should appear pink all over, reflecting good peripheral perfusion. With skin that is highly pigmented, signs of peripheral perfusion can be assessed by observing the mucous membranes, the palms and the soles. Cyanosis with or without signs of respiratory distress should be reported to a paediatrician immediately. If the baby appears pale, this should be reported, as it could be indicative of underlying illness. Physiological jaundice, seen as a yellow discolouration of the skin (and sometimes the sclera and mucous membranes) is not unusual in babies. Physiological jaundice usually appears from the third day and may deepen over the next couple of days before beginning to subside by the seventh day. If the jaundice appears severe and widespread, particularly if the baby is very sleepy or not feeding, the serum bilirubin level should be estimated. Clinical estimation of the degree of jaundice can be inaccurate and is influenced by the type of lighting, the reflective ability of objects around the baby and the peripheral blood flow (Johnston et al 2003). Arkley (2007) advises that prolonged jaundice (lasting longer than the first 2 weeks) should be considered abnormal and a split bilirubin blood test undertaken. The majority of prolonged jaundice cases will be breast milk jaundice and the parents can be reassured. However, liver disease is sometimes the underlying cause.
- Limb movement: When the baby is active, all four limbs should be moving without any signs of discomfort. If the baby was in an extended breech presentation antenatally, it is likely the legs will continue to maintain an extended position for a few days.
- Head shape: Signs of birth trauma may be noted. The head is examined in greater detail as the examination progresses (see next section).

Following the initial observations, discussions with the parents and general observations, the midwife then undertakes a 'top-to-toe' examination of the baby. Care is taken to only expose the parts that are being assessed, so that the baby does not cool. On picking up the baby, the midwife will appreciate the baby's body temperature and whether the baby is irritable on handling.

PHYSICAL EXAMINATION

Head

With the fingertips, the midwife will feel along the suture lines and fontanelles; moulding should have resolved within the first 24 hours of birth. The anterior fontanelle is palpated and should be level. If raised, it could be indicative of raised intracranial pressure, particularly if the baby is irritable, whereas a depressed fontanelle is suggestive of dehydration. While feeling around the head, note any new swellings. A cephalhaematoma first appears between 12 and 36 hours and is likely to increase in size, taking up to 6 weeks to disappear. It is a firm swelling that does not pit on pressure and does not cross suture lines. A large cephalhaematoma may cause a deepening of physiological jaundice. Any bruised or traumatised areas noted at or since birth should be examined to ascertain that healing is occurring and there are no signs of infection.

Eyes

The eyes are inspected to ensure they are clear, with no signs of discharge. If a discharge is present, the eyes should be cleaned, a swab taken if indicated (see Chapter 12) and the parents shown how to clean the eye. The majority of discharges are not due to infection, but if concerned, referral to a paediatrician or general practitioner is warranted. Jaundice may be noted in the sclera, as discussed earlier.

Mouth

Using a good light source, inspect the mouth, which should be clean and moist. The presence of white plaques on the tongue or inner cheek could be indicative of a monilial infection (if breastfeeding, the mother's nipples should also be assessed), and so warrants further investigation. Oral candidiasis occurs in approximately 4% of babies (Dinsmoor et al 2005) and is common when the mother is taking antibiotics. If the baby has fed recently, sucking blisters may be apparent on the lips. Although this gives the appearance that the skin is peeling from the lips, no treatment is needed and the parents should be reassured this is normal.

Skin

Skin colour should be assessed as discussed earlier. The skin is also examined for the presence of rashes, spots, bruising, signs of infection or trauma. Erythema toxicum appears as a blotchy red rash and is of little significance, as are milia. However, septic spots should be identified early and treatment instigated if required. Areas of excoriation should be looked for, as these may occur due to friction with bedding or clothes, or in cases of excoriation of the buttocks, may be due to an irritant contact dermatitis or fungal infection. The nails should be examined for paronychia. If the baby was postmature, the skin may be dry; parents should be reassured that no treatment is necessary. On exposure of the baby's trunk (non-infective), engorged breasts may be noted in both boys and girls. Parents need reassuring that this is a physiological response to maternal hormones and that no treatment is necessary; as hormone levels fall, the problem will resolve. It is very important that the breasts are not squeezed in an attempt to reduce their size and appearance. This will not only cause discomfort and pain, but may result in mastitis. In the event of redness or signs of infection, the baby should be referred to the paediatrician.

Umbilicus

The umbilical cord and umbilicus should be examined for signs of separation and to exclude infection. The cord usually separates within 5–15 days, often leaving a small stump of cord in the umbilicus, which will fall out over the next few days. Some midwives prefer to remove the cord clamp at 48–72 hours, although there is no clinical indication to do so, and at the time of writing there is no published evidence on the topic to guide clinicians. Early signs of infection may be detected by redness around the umbilicus; the cord may also smell offensive and become sticky. This should not be mistaken for the normal process of cord separation.

Nappies

Elimination acts as a guide for neonatal health, particularly for effective feeding. In the first few days of life, term babies micturate 15–60 mL/kg/day, have a bladder capacity of 40 mL and void 2–6 times per hour (Blackburn 2013). Urine output increases over the first 4 weeks to 250–400 mL/day with one or more episodes of voiding per feed (Blackburn 2013). The midwife should ask the parents how many wet and dirty nappies the baby is having, to gauge if normal output is occurring. It can be difficult to tell if the baby has passed urine with some of the superabsorbent disposable nappies, although the nappy will feel heavier. If there is any concern about whether the baby is passing urine, a folded tissue pressed in the nappy may reveal the presence of urine; alternatively the nappy can be torn open at the back to reveal urine within the absorption crystals. Urine is colourless in the newborn baby.

If the nappy is stained yellow or darker, this could be from conjugated bilirubin due to liver disease (Arkley 2007) and should be investigated, regardless of whether or not jaundice is present. Alternatively, because newborn babies have higher levels of uric acid as a byproduct of nucleotide breakdown (Blackburn 2013), these may sometimes be seen in the nappy as orange or red urate crystals and may be mistaken for blood. Parents need reassurance that this is not a major complication, but care should be taken to ensure that feeding is giving the baby sufficient fluid and nutrition. Parents may notice a tiny mucousy red bleed in the nappy of a female baby, which can be worrisome for them. However, this is likely to be a small pseudo-menstruation caused by the effects of maternal hormones within the baby's system and is harmless.

Meconium is seen for the first 2 days, then a changing stool (greenish-brown) is present for the next couple of days, indicating patency of the upper intestinal tract, followed by a yellow stool thereafter. UNICEF UK (2014) advise the changes to a yellow stool should have occurred by day 5. During the first couple of days, babies pass one or more stools per day; on days 3–4 there are at least two stools passed each day (UNICEF UK 2014). By the end of the first week the UNICEF UK (2014) suggest the baby should be producing six or more wet nappies in a 24-hour period with at least two stools. When feeding is established, a breastfed baby may pass an inoffensive, soft, bright yellow stool every 2–3 days. The baby receiving formula tends to pass a firmer, mustard yellow and mildly offensive stool more often, but will also have a tendency towards constipation. Pale stools should always be investigated, as this could be indicative of liver disease (Arkley 2007).

Weight

A healthy term baby normally loses weight in the first week of life, but this is usually transient and of no significance (NICE 2014b). Birth weight is generally regained by 2 weeks of age. Routine weighing of babies before this time has both benefits and harm associated with it (NICE 2014b) and there is no high-quality evidence to base a recommendation of when to weigh babies. Crossland and colleagues (2008) acknowledge there is little accurate knowledge about weight changes in healthy term babies up to 2 weeks of age. In their small study, babies were weighed each day for 2 weeks. They concluded that 'feeding problems should be considered if weight is not increasing by 6 days, but some healthy babies took 17 days to regain their birth weight' (p. 425). Grossman and colleagues (2012) found that breastfed babies initially lost more weight than formula-fed babies, with over half the babies losing the most weight by day 2. They suggest more research is needed to determine if the smaller weight loss with non-breastfed babies is significant for future adverse health outcomes (e.g. predisposition to obesity in later life [Grossman et al 2012]). Tawia and McGuire (2014) agree that breastfed babies lose a higher percentage of weight initially compared with the formula-fed baby; however, this is physiological and not abnormal. They found babies usually begin to gain weight from around day 4, but the median time for regaining the birth weight was 8.3 days for breastfed babies and 6.5 days for formula-fed babies (Tawia & McGuire 2014). The midwife should be guided by local protocol; however, it is of vital importance that correctly calibrated electronic scales are used each time the baby is weighed. A weight loss > 10% of birth weight would give cause for concern and, if accompanied by suboptimal urine and stooling, feeding would need careful investigation as the mother may require additional support with it.

Identity

If the daily assessment is being undertaken in hospital it is important to ensure that the baby is wearing identity bands according to local protocol.

Screening

Undertaking the examination as a whole is a form of screening for normality. Specific haematological screening (e.g. newborn blood spot screening or serum bilirubin) may also be undertaken with parental consent at the time the examination is carried out.

After the examination

When the examination is complete, the baby should be dressed, the findings recorded in the appropriate documentation and adjustments made to the postnatal care plan if indicated. The findings should form the basis of advice given to the parents regarding the progress and subsequent care of the baby. Any deviations from normal should be acted on accordingly and appropriate care instigated.

SKILL 48.3 Daily examination of the newborn

1. Make a mental note of anything significant on entering the woman's personal environment (see earlier).
2. Discuss the progress of the baby with the parents, allaying their anxieties if necessary.
3. Explain the procedure and gain informed consent.
4. Wash and dry hands (apply non-sterile gloves if contact with body fluids is anticipated).
5. Undertake a general observation of the baby.
6. Ensure there is good light and a warm environment, undress the baby, and undertake the 'top-to-toe' examination described earlier.
7. Weigh the baby if indicated.
8. Redress the baby and give back to the parents.
9. If the timing is optimal, newborn blood spot screening may be taken with consent at the same time as the daily examination is performed. The baby would be re-dressed but with a foot exposed and the baby held by a parent or the midwife, depending on parental preference. The midwife should also suggest or use an appropriate measure to relieve the baby's pain during blood collection: breastfeeding, skin-to-skin contact, and a small volume of a sweet solution (glucose or sucrose) given to the baby orally have each been found to be effective in reducing pain and distress (Harrison et al 2017)
10. Discuss the findings with the parents and made a date for the next visit.
11. Wash and dry hands.
12. Document the findings and act accordingly.

DEVELOPMENTAL DYSPLASIA OF THE HIPS

Developmental dysplasia of the hips (DDH) is used to describe a wide range of conditions related to the development of the hips in babies through to young children. It includes abnormal development of the acetabulum and proximal femur (the femoral head and neck, and the greater and lesser trochanter) through to mechanical instability of the hip joint (Rosenfeld et al 2014). If undiagnosed or left untreated, there is associated long-term morbidity of gait abnormalities, chronic pain, degenerative osteoarthritis and avascular necrosis due to impairment of the blood supply, leading to hip replacement often before the age of 40 years, widening of the perineum and hyperlordosis (Rosenfeld et al 2014, Shorter et al 2013, Wang et al 2013). DDH has also been called congenital dislocation of the hip, hip dysplasia, developmental dislocation of the hip, and acetabular dislocation. In New Zealand the assessment is undertaken by midwives at birth as part of the first examination, while in Australia midwives must have undertaken additional competency-based education to be able to perform it.

What is DDH?

DDH occurs when the femoral head is not sitting centrally in the acetabulum. This can occur during late pregnancy or during the neonatal period. There may be dislocation (total loss of contact between the acetabulum and the femoral head) or subluxation (the femoral head is partially within the acetabulum in a non-centric position). The hip may:

- have instability where the femoral head is reduced (meaning 'within the acetabulum') at rest but not with movement, and there is laxity within the acetabulum
- be subluxable if the femoral head is reduced at rest but can be partially dislocated with examination manoeuvres (also referred to as mild instability)

- be reducible if the hip is dislocated at rest but, with manipulation, the femoral head can be positioned into the acetabulum (Rosenfeld et al 2014).

During the neonatal period the femoral head and acetabular cartilage continue to grow, which is critical for normal hip development, as is reduction and stability of the femoral head (Hart et al 2006). It is normal for babies to have physiological laxity of the hip during the first few weeks of life; however, this usually resolves spontaneously as the acetabulum and femoral head grow and development continues normally (Rosenfeld et al 2014). Rosenfeld and colleagues (2014) suggest that of the 60% of babies who have hip instability in the first week of life, 90% will have stabilised by 2 months. Continued dislocation of the femoral head causes the tendons, muscles and bony structures to develop secondary adaptive changes, which include stretching of the acetabular capsule, leading to the development of abnormal attachments, shortening and contracture of muscles, flattening of the femoral head and acetabular dysplasia, which will eventually result in osteoarthritis in childhood (Hart et al 2006). The degree of dislocation can be classified according to the Graf hip classification type, of which there are five (Rosenfeld et al 2014).

- Type I refers to a fully mature, normal hip that has a deep acetabular cup and an angular acetabular rim with the cartilaginous roof of the acetabulum covering the femoral head.
- Type IIa is seen in infants less than 3 months of age, reflecting the physiological immaturity of the baby's hip joint. The femoral head is situated within the acetabulum, but the acetabulum is shallow and the rim is round, with the cartilaginous acetabular roof covering the femoral head. Ninety per cent will resolve spontaneously (Paton et al 2014).
- Type IIb are abnormal hips seen in babies over 3 months of age and will worsen without treatment. The acetabulum is slightly shallow with a round rim and the cartilaginous acetabular roof covers the femoral head.
- Type III are dislocated hips that have a shallow acetabulum while the acetabular roof is deficient.
- Type IV are dislocated hips where the acetabulum is almost flat and the acetabular roof is significantly displaced.

Hips that 'click' do not signify DDH and the term 'clicky hips' should not be used, as it is misleading. Rosenfeld and colleagues (2014) advise a 'clunk' (or a 'jerk', suggestive of DDH) is a different sensation to a 'click', being one of a high-pitch joint popping movement rather than the clicking or snapping sensation caused by the snapping of tendons or ligaments around the hip and knee.

Risk factors

The hip is thought to develop normally during pregnancy but gradually becomes abnormal for a number of reasons (Hart et al 2006). Towards the end of pregnancy there is pressure on the hip joint, forcing the femur head into an abnormal position within or outside of the acetabulum; thus many of the risk factors within the literature are related to this. However, Choudry and colleagues (2013) suggest there is a lack of known factors in 69–73% of cases.

- Family history: Stevenson and colleagues (2009) propose the risk of DDH increases 12-fold if a first-degree relative has DDH, while the International Hip Dysplasia Institute (IHDI 2018) suggest it is a 1:8 chance, and if a sibling has DDH it is 1:7, but if both a parent and a sibling have DDH the risk increases to 1:3.
- Female gender: Schwend and colleagues (2014) state that 78% of DDH cases occur in females. Hart and colleagues (2006) wonder if this is because female fetuses are more susceptible to the effects of maternal relaxin. However, Bracken and colleagues (2012) point out that cord studies have shown no correlation between relaxin concentration and DDH.
- Breech (extended) presentation ≥ 34 weeks' gestation (Rosenfeld et al 2014, Shorter et al 2013), although if an external cephalic version is undertaken (Chapter 27), the risk reduces from 9.3% to 2.8% (Lambeek et al 2013), and if the baby is born by elective caesarean section, the risk reduces further (Fox & Paton 2010). Schwend and colleagues (2014) propose the highest risk is a female fetus in an extended breech presentation.
- Improper swaddling, whereby the legs are straightened to a standing position, which can loosen the joints and result in damage to the soft cartilage of the acetabulum (IHDI 2018).
- Multiple pregnancy (IHDI 2018).
- Oligohydramnios (Paton et al 2014, Rosenfeld et al 2014).
- First-born babies (Rosenfeld et al 2014).
- Ethnicity: increased in Caucasian babies (McCarthy et al 2005).
- High birthweight babies (Dezateux & Rosenthal 2007).
- Babies with fixed idiopathic congenital talipes equinovarus are not at increased risk of DDH (Paton et al 2014), although those with congenital talipes calcaneovalgus (CTCV) are 5.2 times more likely to have DDH than babies without CTCV (Paton & Choudry 2009).
- DDH may also occur when certain syndromes are present (e.g. trisomy 21, Ehlers Danlos) (Rosenfeld et al 2014).

Incidence

The incidence of DDH varies according to the definition used and whether or not it is a screened population. In recent years the average weighted incidence of the condition in Caucasian Australian and New Zealander babies has been recorded as 6.8 per

1000, while the incidence of neonatal hip instability in Māori infants is just under half that found in Caucasian New Zealander babies; the incidence in Indigenous Australian infants is also half that of their Caucasian Australian counterparts (Loder & Skopelja 2011). Bracken and colleagues (2012) suggest the left hip is four times more likely to be affected than the right; however, Hart and colleagues (2006) suggest the left hip is affected in 60% of cases, the right hip in 20% and both hips in 20% of cases. It is thought the left hip is affected more because the fetus is more likely to lie on the left side of the uterus, pushing the left hip against the maternal sacrum and preventing movement of the hip joint. Late presentation can occur despite the previous tests being normal (Jaiswal et al 2010) and Schwend and colleagues (2014) propose the incidence of this is 1:5000, suggesting the condition may be occult.

When to assess for DDH

It is recommended that all babies have an examination that includes screening for DDH within 72 hours of birth (NICE 2014b). It is also suggested that the assessment is repeated in between 1–2 weeks of age because hips may appear to be more dislocatable than they are during the first 72 hours of life, which could lead to over-referral for suspected DDH and possibly overtreatment (Shorter et al 2013): the majority of cases of DDH detected at birth reportedly resolve spontaneously in the first week of life (Mahan & Kassler 2008). Isolated hip clicks are not pathological, but are a frequent cause of referral and will stabilise as the baby gets older (Mahan & Kassler 2008). However, early detection and treatment is necessary to prevent serious damage to the acetabulum; thus it would seem prudent to screen early, ensuring practitioners are competent in assessing the hips. Midwives who are competent to do this and who do so regularly are in a better position to perform the assessment than are junior medical practitioners on rotation, who may have received little or no training in screening for DDH (Cescutti-Butler 2013, Talbot & Paton 2013). Schwend and colleagues (2014) agree, referring to a study where the most significant DDH cases were identified by a competent practitioner regardless of their profession.

Screening for DDH

DDH screening involves assessing the length and appearance of the legs and skin folds, manipulating the legs using the Barlow's test and/or Ortolani's test, while assessing the range of abduction and **Klisic's sign**. Screening is ideally discussed during the antenatal period and revisited prior to testing to ensure the parents can provide informed consent.

Length of the legs

In the presence of unilateral DDH, one leg will be shorter than the other. This is assessed by lying the baby on his or her back without a nappy on, flexing his or her hips and knees with the knees together, feet flat on the surface and with the heels touching the buttocks. The height of the knees should be the same if there is no DDH, but this may also occur with bilateral DDH. If one knee is lower than the other, it is suggestive of unilateral DDH in the shorter leg. This is known as the **Galeazzi test** or Allis sign. The baby needs to be relaxed to do this, which may be easier to achieve after the baby has fed.

Appearance of skin folds

When both femur heads are in the acetabulum the skin folds should be symmetrical. Bracken and colleagues (2012) advise that isolated asymmetrical thigh and gluteal (buttock) skin folds are common during the neonatal period; nevertheless, asymmetrical skin folds may be indicative of DDH. These can be seen when the baby is on his or her back or front. While Rosenfeld and colleagues (2014) advise asymmetrical thigh skin folds are suggestive of DDH, the IHDI (2018) disagree, cautioning they are rarely indicative of DDH unless the gluteal folds are asymmetrical. These are assessed with the baby on his or her front. Rosenfeld and colleagues (2014) recommend assessing whether the inguinal folds reach beyond the anus, as they do not in the absence of DDH. If one inguinal fold extends beyond the anal opening it is suggestive of unilateral DDH, whereas bilateral DDH is suspected if both extend beyond the anal opening.

Barlow's test

Barlow's test is a manoeuvre that attempts to push the femoral head out of the acetabulum to assess if it is dislocatable. It involves adducting the hip by bringing the thigh towards the midline and applying light pressure in a downward (posterior) direction (Fig 48.1). A positive test occurs if the femoral head dislocates, often felt as a 'clunk'; the normal hip should not dislocate. The test should only be performed by a midwife deemed competent to do so.

SKILL 48.4 Performing Barlow's test

1. Discuss the procedure and gain informed consent from the parents, undertaking the examination in the presence of one or both parents.
2. Wash and dry hands; apply non-sterile gloves if necessary.
3. Lie the baby on his or her back on a flat, firm surface.

SKILL 48.4 Performing Barlow's test—cont'd

4. Ensure the baby is warm and relaxed, then undress the baby from the waist down, removing the nappy.
5. Bring the baby's legs together with the hips and knees flexed.
6. Examining the hips one at a time, hold the knee and hip in a flexed position; then abduct the hip, placing a thumb on the inner aspect of the thigh (over the inner trochanter) and the index and middle fingers over the outer part of the thigh (over the greater trochanter of the femur at the hip).
7. Gently adduct the leg towards the midline while pushing down on the hip laterally towards the supporting surface then gently pulling the leg upwards to try to dislocate the hip laterally.
8. Repeat with other leg.
9. Redress the baby and return to parents.
10. Wash and dry hands.
11. Discuss the findings with the parents.
12. Document the findings and act accordingly.

Source: Johnson R, Taylor W: Skills for midwifery practice, 4th ed., Elsevier, London, 2016.

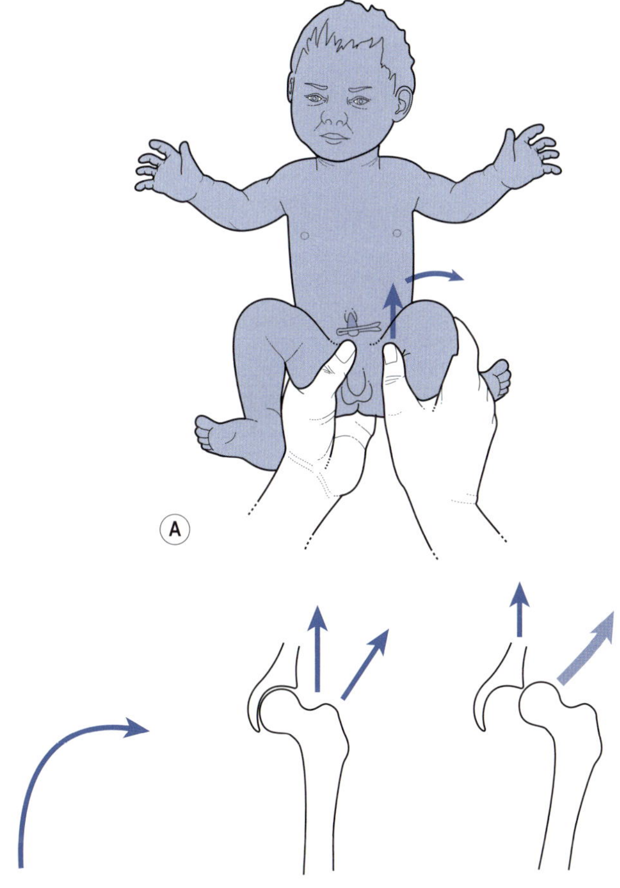

FIGURE 48.1 **Barlow's test.**
Source: Adapted from Farrell P, Sittlington N: The normal baby. In Fraser DM, Cooper MA, eds: Myles textbook for midwives, 5th ed., Churchill Livingstone, Edinburgh, 2009.

Ortolani's test

This manoeuvre is undertaken to relocate a dislocated or unstable femoral head back into the acetabulum by applying pressure on the back of the greater trochanter. If the femoral head relocates (reduces), a clunk may be felt (Fig 48.2). A normal hip will not produce a clunk, as the femoral head is not dislocatable.

SKILL 48.5 Performing Ortolani's test

1. Discuss the procedure and gain informed consent from the parents, undertaking the examination in the presence of one or both parents.
2. Wash and dry hands; apply non-sterile gloves if necessary.
3. Lie the baby on his or her back on a flat, firm surface.
4. Ensure the baby is warm and relaxed, then undress the baby from the waist down, removing the nappy.
5. Bring the baby's legs together with the hips and knees flexed.
6. Examining the hips one at a time, take hold of each leg, placing the thumb on the inner aspect of the thigh (over the inner trochanter) and the index and middle fingers over the outer aspect of the thigh (greater trochanter of the femur at the hip).
7. Flex the knees and the hips 90° and gently abduct the leg (a 'clunk' is felt as the dislocated head of the femur is moved back into the acetabulum; if no clunk is felt, but the leg cannot be abducted fully, DDH is also indicated).
8. Redress the baby and return to parents.
9. Wash and dry hands.
10. Discuss the findings with the parents.
11. Document the findings and act accordingly.

Source: Johnson R, Taylor W: Skills for midwifery practice, 4th ed., Elsevier, London, 2016.

Klisic's sign

With the baby positioned on his or her back, place the index finger on the anterior superior iliac spine and the middle finger on the greater trochanter. An imaginary line is drawn between these two points and should point towards or above the umbilicus if the hip is not dislocated and will be below the umbilicus if DDH is present (Rosenfeld et al 2014). Bilateral DDH may be suspected from this sign if both imaginary lines are below the umbilicus.

Diagnosis

If there is a positive Barlow's or **Ortolani's test**, the baby should be referred for an ultrasound assessment of the hips. This will review the acetabulum and femoral head and measure different angles to determine if DDH is present. The ultrasound should be reviewed by an experienced orthopaedic paediatric surgeon.

Treatment

Depending on when DDH is diagnosed, different treatment options are available. These include using a Pavlik harness, which is designed to gently reposition the baby's hips in a well-aligned and secure position so that the femoral head and acetabulum can grow and develop normally. Other splints include the Von Rosen splint and a variety of hip abduction braces. For late diagnosis, surgery may be required, which is either closed or open reduction, and may also include use of a spica body cast.

Prevention

Swaddling is a major cause of DDH, as noted in cultures where the legs are tightly wrapped so they are positioned together and straight (as if standing). This position does not encourage the femoral head to remain in the acetabulum. This is still a common practice within areas of the Middle East and other countries and DDH rates are high (Clarke 2014). Swaddling tightly with blankets has the same effect, as babies are not able to flex their hips and knees and this is gaining in popularity as an attempt to encourage the baby to settle and sleep for longer and reduce crying. In cultures where babies and children are carried in the straddle/jockey position, DDH is rarely encountered (Graham et al 2015); this style of carrying the baby is similar to the baby in a Pavlik harness. Clarke (2014) suggests that approximately 90% of babies in North America are swaddled in the first few months of life. To counteract the negative effects of placing the hips into forced sustained passive hip extension and adduction while the hips are developing during the first few months of life, the IHDI (2018) suggest the baby should be positioned so the hips are slightly flexed and abducted, with knees flexed, as they would be during late fetal life. The reader is encouraged to watch the video on how to swaddle properly to avoid DDH, available at the IHDI website (see Resources at the end of the chapter). The IHDI also provide advice on how to choose baby carriers, such as slings, car seats and bouncers to encourage the correct positioning of the baby's hips and knees. The midwife can play a vital role in reducing the rates of DDH by advising parents on how to swaddle their baby if this is what they want to do and advise them on how to choose a baby carrier to encourage good positioning of the hips and knees.

Role and responsibilities of the midwife

These can be summarised as:

- being able to competently assess the baby at birth using the Apgar score, and understanding

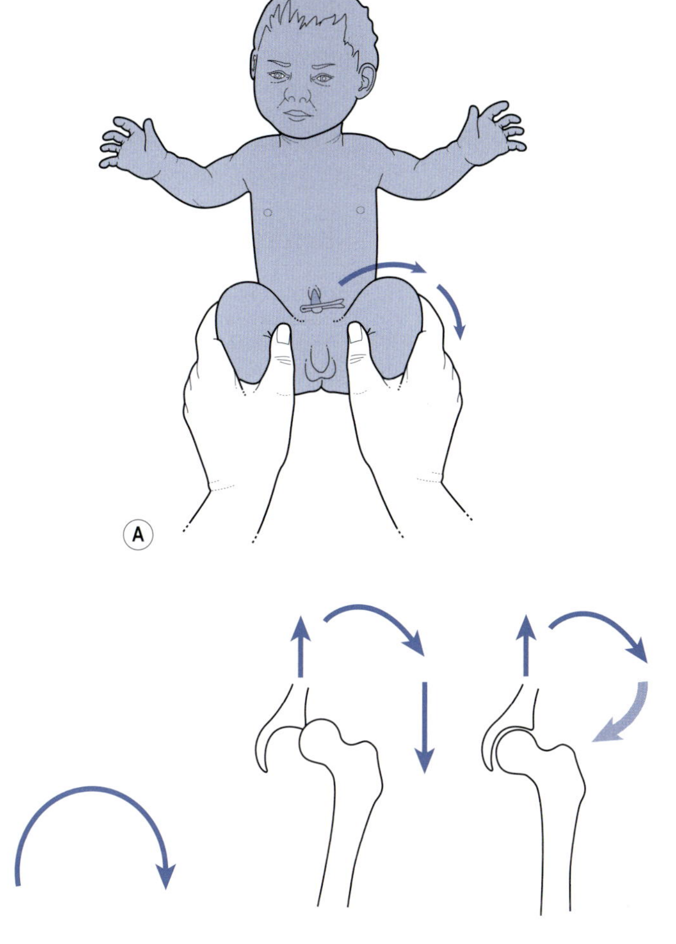

FIGURE 48.2 **Ortolani's test.**
Source: Adapted from Farrell P, Sittlington N: The normal baby. In Fraser DM, Cooper MA, eds: Myles textbook for midwives, 5th ed., Churchill Livingstone, Edinburgh, 2009.

the significance of the score and factors that may influence it
- recognising all the components that encompass the initial gross birth examination and what is normal
- undertaking the birth examination thoroughly and competently, referring on as necessary
- involving parents with the birth examination and informing them gently of any concerns found and of what will happen next (e.g. referral, diagnostic tests, treatment)
- reviewing and adjusting the postnatal care plan
- undertaking all aspects of the daily examination thoroughly and competently, referring on as necessary
- educating and supporting the parents
- discussing the DDH screening test with parents and providing suitable information for them to make an informed decision with regard to DDH screening
- being aware of the risk factors that may increase the incidence of DDH and advising parents on the care of their baby to reduce this
- being able to undertake the assessment procedures for DDH correctly and safely, when appropriately educated
- seeking appropriate referral on if DDH screening test is positive
- undertaking contemporaneous record keeping.

SUMMARY

- Assessment of the baby at birth is an important skill undertaken by the midwife.
- Apgar scoring is quick and easy to undertake, but is subjective and influenced by factors such as lighting and skin pigmentation.

- Birth examination is a thorough physical examination that detects obvious abnormalities; some abnormalities may not be apparent until the baby is older, therefore subsequent examinations should be undertaken as required.
- Examination of the baby during each postnatal visit (whether in hospital or at home) by the midwife is an essential component of the care provided to the mother and baby during the postnatal period.
- The midwife uses skills of communication and observation to ensure that optimal newborn health is achieved.
- The daily examination provides an opportunity to discuss detailed care and advice with the parents.
- An appropriately trained and competent midwife or paediatrician should undertake the assessment for developmental dysplasia within 72 hours of birth, whether in hospital, a birthing centre or at home.
- There are two tests that can be used to assess the ability of the femur head to dislocate: Barlow's and Ortolani's along with assessing leg length, skinfold creases (Galeazzi sign) and Klisic's sign.
- If swaddling the baby, it should be done in such a way that the hips are slightly flexed and abducted and the knees flexed.

Self-assessment exercises

The answers to the following questions may be found in the text.

1. How would a baby who scores one for each category of the Apgar score be recognised?
2. What factors influence the Apgar score awarded at birth?
3. Describe the top-to-toe examination of the baby undertaken by the midwife at birth.
4. Identify six reflexes that a newborn baby has and discuss how these are elicited.
5. What are the roles and responsibilities of the midwife in relation to the assessment of the baby at birth?
6. Describe the different aspects of the daily examination of the baby.
7. What would the midwife do if the baby's mouth had visible white plaques?
8. How should the midwife advise a mother who has seen urates in the baby's nappy?
9. What are the roles and responsibilities of the midwife in relation to the daily examination of the baby?
10. When would the midwife undertake the test for DDH?
11. Describe the two methods of assessment.
12. What would you notice from Klisic's sign and inguinal folds that would lead you to suspect bilateral DDH?
13. What is the significance of the 'clunk' heard during a DDH assessment?
14. What are the roles and responsibilities of the midwife in relation to the assessment for DDH?

Resources

International Hip Dysplasia Institute (IHDI): Hip-healthy swaddling. Online 27 August 2021. Available: https://hipdysplasia.org/wp-content/uploads/2020/05/HipHealthySwaddlingBrochure.pdf.

References

Arkley C: Yellow alert: identification of liver disease in neonates and their appropriate referral—the role of the midwife, MIDIRS Midwifery Digest 14(4):571–573, 2007.

Bailey J: The fetus. In Marshall J, Raynor M, eds: Myles textbook for midwives, 16th ed., Elsevier, Edinburgh, 2014.

Blackburn ST: Maternal, fetal and neonatal physiology: a clinical perspective, 4th ed., Saunders, St. Louis, 2013.

Bracken J, Tron T, Ditchfield M: Developmental dysplasia of the hip: controversies and current concepts, Journal of Paediatrics and Child Health 48:963–973, 2012.

Cescutti-Butler L: Examination of a newborn: whose job—midwife or doctor? You decide ..., MIDIRS Midwifery Digest 23(4):512–515, 2013.

Choudry Q, Goyal R, Paton RW: Is limitation of hip abduction a useful clinical sign in the diagnosis of developmental dysplasia of the hip? Archives of Disease in Childhood 98:862–866, 2013.

Clarke NMP: Swaddling and hip dysplasia: an orthopaedic perspective, Archives of Disease in Childhood 99(1):5–6, 2014.

Crossland DS, Richmond S, Hudson M, et al: Weight change in the term baby in the first 2 weeks of life, Acta Paediatrica 97:425–429, 2008.

Dezateux C, Rosenthal K: Developmental dysplasia of the hip, Lancet 369:1541–1552, 2007.

Dijxhoorn MJ, Visse GHA, Fidler VJ, et al: Apgar score, meconium and acidaemia at birth in relation to neonatal neurological morbidity in term infants, British Journal of Obstetrics and Gynaecology 893:217–222, 1986.

Dinsmoor MJ, Viloria R, Lief L, et al: Use of intrapartum antibiotics and the incidence of postnatal maternal and neonatal yeast infections, Obstetrics and Gynecology 106(1):19–22, 2005.

England C: Recognizing the healthy baby at term through examination of the newborn screening. In Marshall J, Raynor M, eds: Myles textbook for midwives, 16th ed., Elsevier, Edinburgh, 2014.

Fox AE, Paton RW: The relationship between mode of delivery and developmental dysplasia of the hip in breech infants, Journal of Bone and Joint Surgery British Volume 92(12):1695–1699, 2010.

Gardner SL, Hernandez JA: Initial nursery care. In Gardner SL, Carter BS, Enzman-Hines M, et al, eds: Merenstein & Gardner's handbook of neonatal intensive care, 7th ed., Elsevier, St. Louis, 2011.

Graham SM, Manara J, Chokotho L, et al: Back-carrying infants to prevent developmental dysplasia and its sequelae: is a new public health initiative needed? Journal of Pediatric Orthopedics 35(1):57–61, 2015.

Grossman X, Chaudhuri JH, Feldman-Winter L, Merewood A: Neonatal weight loss at a US baby-friendly hospital, Journal of the Academy of Nutrition and Dietetics 112:410–413, 2012.

Habel A, Elhadi N, Sommerlad B, et al: Delayed detection of cleft palate: an audit of newborn examination, Archives of Disease in Childhood 91:238–240, 2006.

Harrison D, Reszel J, Dagg B, et al: Pain management during newborn screening: using YouTube to disseminate effective pain management strategies, Journal of Perinatal and Neonatal Nursing 31(2):172–177, 2017.

Hart ES, Albright MB, Rebello GN, et al: Developmental dysplasia of the hip. Nursing implications and anticipatory guidance for parents, Orthopaedic Nursing 25(2):100–109, 2006.

Iliodromiti S, Mackay DF, Smith GCS, et al: Apgar score and the risk of cause-specific infant mortality: a population-based cohort study, Lancet 384(9956):1749–1755, 2014.

International Hip Dysplasia Institute (IHDI): Home page, 2018. Online 27 August 2021. Available: www.hipdysplasia.org.

Jaiswal A, Starks I, Kiely NT: Late dislocation of the hip following normal neonatal clinical and ultrasound examination, Journal of Bone and Joint Surgery British Volume 92(10):1449–1451, 2010.

Johnston PGB, Flood K, Spinks K: The newborn child, 9th ed., Churchill Livingstone, Edinburgh, 2003, p. 48.

Lambeek AF, De Hundt M, Vlemmix F, et al: Risk of developmental dysplasia of the hip in breech presentation: the effect of successful external cephalic version, BJOG: an International Journal of Obstetrics and Gynaecology 120:607–612, 2013.

Lee HC, Subeh M, Gould JB: Low Apgar score and mortality in extremely preterm neonates born in the United States, Acta Paediatrica 99(12):1785–1789, 2010.

Leonardi-Bee J, Batta K, O'Brien C, Bath-Hextall FJ: Interventions for infantile haemangiomas (strawberry birthmarks) of the skin, The Cochrane Database of Systematic Reviews (5):Art. No.:CD006545, 2011.

Loder RT, Skopelja EN: The epidemiology and demographics of hip dysplasia. International scholarly research network, Orthopedics Article ID:238607, 2011. Online 26 March 2018. Available: www.ncbi.nlm.nih.gov/pmc/articles/PMC4063216/pdf/ISRN.ORTHOPEDICS2011-238607.pdf.

Mahan ST, Kassler JR: Does swaddling influence developmental dysplasia of the hip? Pediatrics 121(1):177–178, 2008.

McCarthy J, Scoles P, MacEwen G: Developmental dysplasia of the hip (DDH), Current Orthopaedics 19(3):223–230, 2005.

McCarthy LK, Morley CJ, Davis PG, et al: Timing of interventions in the delivery room: does reality compare with neonatal resuscitation guidelines? Journal of Pediatrics 163(6):1553–1557, 2013.

Michaelides S: Physiology, assessment and care. In Macdonald S, Magill-Cuerden J, eds: Mayes' midwifery, 14th ed., Elsevier, Edinburgh, 2011.

Ministry of Health: Primary Maternity Services Notice 2021 (DA53), 2021. Online 27 August 2021. Available: https://gazette.govt.nz/assets/pdf-cache/2021/2021-go2473.pdf?2021-07-02_07%3A23%3A24=.

National Institute for Health and Care Excellence (NICE): Intrapartum guidelines: care of healthy women and their babies during childbirth, London, 2014a. Online 23 March 2018. Available: www.nice.org.uk/guidance/cg190.

National Institute for Health and Care Excellence (NICE): Postnatal care clinical guideline 37, London, 2014b. Online 27 August 2021. Available: www.nice.org.uk/guidance/cg190/resources/intrapartum-care-for-healthy-women-and-babies-pdf-35109866447557.

O'Donnell CPF, Kamlin OF, Davis PG, et al: Interobserver variability of the 5-minute Apgar score, Journal of Pediatrics 149(4):486–489, 2006.

Pairman S, Tracy S, Dahlen HG, Dixon, L: Midwifery, 4th ed., Elsevier, Sydney, 2018.

Paton RW, Choudry Q: Neonatal foot deformities and their relationship to developmental dysplasia of the hip, Journal of Bone and Joint Surgery, British Volume 91(5):655–658, 2009.

Paton RW, Choudry QA, Jugday R, et al: Is congenital talipes equinovarus a risk factor for pathological dysplasia of the hip? Bone & Joint Journal 96-B:1553–1555, 2014.

Pinheiro JMB: The Apgar cycle: a new view of a familiar scoring system, Archives of Disease in Childhood. Fetal and Neonatal Edition 94:F70–F72, 2009.

Rosenfeld SB, Phillips W, Torchia MM: Developmental dysplasia of the hip, UpToDate, 2014. Online 23 March 2018. Available: www.uptodate.com/contents/developmental-dysplasia-of-the-hip-epidemiology-and-pathogenesis.

Roth DA, Hildesheimer M, Bardenstein S, et al: Preauricular skin tags and ear pits are associated with permanent hearing impairment in newborns, Pediatrics 122(4):e884–e890, 2008.

Salustiano EMA, Campos JADB, Ibidi S-M, et al: Low Apgar scores at 5 minutes in a low risk population: maternal and obstetrical factors and postnatal outcome, Revista da Associação Médica Brasileira 58(5):587–593, 2012.

Schwend RM, Shaw BA, Segal LS: Evaluation and treatment of developmental hip dysplasia in the newborn and infant, Pediatric Clinics of North America 61:1095–1107, 2014.

Shorter D, Hong T, Osborn DA: Screening programmes for developmental dysplasia of the hip in newborn infants, Cochrane Database of Systematic Reviews (9):Art. No.: CD004595, 2013.

Silverton L: The art and science of midwifery, Prentice Hall, New York, 1993.

Steinhorn RH: Evaluation and management of the cyanotic neonate, Clinical Pediatric Emergency Medicine 9(3):169–175, 2008.

Stellwagen L, Hubbard E, Chamber C, et al: Torticollis, facial symmetry and plagiocephaly in normal newborns, Archives of Disease in Childhood 93(10):827–831, 2008.

Stevenson DA, Mineau G, Kerber RA, et al: Familial disposition to developmental dysplasia of the hip, Journal of Pediatric Orthopedics 29(5):463–466, 2009.

Swanson AE, Veldman A, Wallace EM, et al: Subgaleal haemorrhage: risk factors and outcomes, Acta Obstetricia et Gynecologica Scandinavia 91:260–263, 2011.

Talbot CL, Paton RW: Screening of selected risk factors in developmental dysplasia of the hip: an observational study, Archives of Disease in Childhood 98:692–696, 2013.

Tawia S, McGuire L: Early weight loss and weight gain in healthy, full-term, exclusively-breastfed infants, Breastfeeding Review 22(1):31–41, 2014.

UNICEF UK: Breastfeeding assessment tool, 2014. Online 23 March 2018. Available: www.unicef.org.uk/babyfriendly/baby-friendly-resources/guidance-for-health-professionals/tools-and-forms-for-health-professionals/breastfeeding-assessment-tools/.

Wang TM, Wu KW, Shih SF, et al: Outcomes of open reduction for developmental dysplasia of the hips: does bilateral dysplasia have a poorer outcome? Journal of Bone and Joint Surgery American Volume 95(12):1081–1086, 2013.

Wilson BE, Etheridge CE, Soundappen VS, et al: Delayed diagnosis of anorectal malformation: are current guidelines sufficient? Journal of Paediatrics and Child Health 46(5):268–272, 2010.

SECTION 13

SKILLS FOR SUPPORTING THE WOMAN TO FEED HER BABY

CHAPTER 49

SUPPORTING THE WOMAN TO INITIATE BREASTFEEDING

Learning outcomes

Having read this chapter, the reader should be able to:

- briefly describe the anatomy of the breast and the physiology of lactation
- describe how to facilitate correct attachment at the breast using (1) the traditional approach and (2) the concept of biological nurturing
- discuss the recognition and significance of effective attachment at the breast, feeding cues, feeding patterns and signs of effective feeding
- discuss correct expressing and storage of breast milk
- discuss the advantages, disadvantages and indications for cup feeding
- describe the correct cup-feeding technique
- highlight the potential risks of nasogastric/orogastric feeding tubes
- detail the steps that are taken to ensure that the nasogastric/orogastric tube is correctly placed
- describe how a nasogastric/orogastric tube is inserted and removed safely
- describe how a baby is fed using a nasogastric tube
- provide advice to women about breastfeeding with SARS-CoV-2 (COVID-19)
- summarise the role and responsibilities of the midwife.

There is no doubt as to the suitability of human milk for human infants. It is an internationally recognised recommendation that babies should be breastfed exclusively for the first 6 months of life, and then preferably (with a weaning diet) until 2 years old and onwards (WHO 2011a). The World Health Organization (WHO) and UNICEF assert that every facility that provides maternity services and care for newborn infants should adhere to 'ten steps for successful breastfeeding' in order to support this recommendation (see Resources at end of chapter). Occasionally breastfeeding is delayed, interrupted or not possible for a range of reasons, and in such situations it is vital that the baby still receives breast milk if the woman wishes. Cup feeding is considered to be a viable alternative to using a teat for a breastfed baby, and a nasogastric tube may be necessary where the neonate's gestation or clinical condition requires it. In both cases, it is important that correct techniques for use are followed. A full discussion of breastfeeding, the midwife's role in it, as well as personal, social, political and global perspectives, and an evidence-based framework for understanding, educating, supporting and assisting women and their families with breastfeeding initiation, establishment and maintenance is found in Pairman and colleagues' *Midwifery: Preparation for practice* (2019, Chapter 30).

This chapter is concerned with basic breast anatomy, feeding cues and patterns, assessing for effective feeding, problem-solving and the safe expressing and storage of breast milk. We also provide a brief summary of the evidence at the time of writing (May 2021) related to breastfeeding with SARS-CoV-2 (COVID-19). Indications for cup feeding, the potential dangers and the correct technique are also included, as are safe insertion and removal of nasogastric tubes in neonates, and neonatal nasogastric tube feeding.

BREASTFEEDING

Understanding lactation

Each breast functions independently; it has a rich blood, nerve and lymphatic supply and comprises glandular tissue and fat. Support is provided from ligaments. The proportions of fat and glandular tissue vary for each woman; glandular tissue increases in pregnancy under hormonal influences in preparation for lactation. In some women the proportion of glandular tissue to fat is 2:1. The glandular tissue is an extensive convoluted ductal network separated into lobes. These are subdivided into lobules; within each lobule are alveoli, each of which is a cavity lined with lactocytes surrounded by myoepithelial cells. Under the influence of prolactin, milk is produced in the lactocytes. When the infant suckles (under the influence of oxytocin), the milk is propelled into the network of ducts by the muscular contraction of the myoepithelial cells. The lactiferous ducts branch to join other larger ducts, eventually opening out onto the surface of the nipple. Geddes (2009) suggests that there are 4–18 ducts opening onto the nipple, the average being nine. The network of ducts has been identified much nearer to the surface of the breast than originally thought, and the milk-collecting areas (lactiferous sinuses) are not visible, suggesting that milk is transported directly through the ducts on demand, rather than being stored.

Colostrum is present from about the 16th week of pregnancy, but it is the loss of placental hormones, particularly progesterone, that initiates the rise in oxytocin and prolactin and therefore the availability of increasing volumes of milk for the newborn infant. Colson (2007, 2008) suggests that practice should protect and encourage the mechanisms that stimulate breastfeeding hormones in order to ensure effective transfer of nutrition from mother to child. These include prolonged cuddling and baby holding, skin-to-skin contact, privacy, feeding in biological nurturing positions (below), and maintaining the physical environment in a calm, warm, safe manner (minimal neocortical stimulation).

Early priming of the **lactocytes** is essential for the long-term production of breast milk. This occurs with an early first feed after birth, under the influence of rising prolactin levels. Milk is supplied according to demand; consequently, it is the effective removal of milk from the breast, according to the baby's appetite and feeding action, that stimulates the milk supply. Milk composition changes during the feed (and over time as the infant grows), so that both the hunger and thirst are satisfied. Consequently, babies require nothing other than breast milk for the first 6 months of life. As the baby comes off the breast, the second breast is always offered; the baby will only take from the second one if he/she is still hungry or thirsty.

Feeding cues

Baby-led parenting (Rapley & Murkett 2014) encourages all parents to understand the ways in which babies communicate their needs. **Feeding cues** are one such way; understanding these cues allows parents to respond before their baby becomes distressed, which allows for appropriate prompt care. This applies to whichever method of infant feeding is chosen. As the baby's sleep begins to lighten, rapid eye movements can be seen beneath the eyelids. This is often one of the first feeding cues. The baby may make sucking sounds, begin to 'fidget', begins to 'root' (look for the breast with their mouth), or suck his or her fingers. Movement of the arms and legs becomes more obvious; if there is no response to these cues, the baby begins to cry. Crying is a late feeding cue; a crying baby releases cortisol (stress hormone) and needs to be calmed before feeding can take place. If cortisol is repeatedly stimulated, brain development is affected. Entwistle (2013) discusses the evidence for this in detail.

SKILL 49.1 Supporting the woman and baby to begin breastfeeding—traditional approach

There is no doubt in any of the literature on the topic that an incorrect attachment at the breast potentially damages the nipples and prevents effective transfer of milk. These are the steps for achieving successful attachment at the breast.

- Encourage the mother is comfortable.
- Ensure that the baby's body is turned in, close to the mother's body.
- Keep the baby's head and body in a line.
- The baby should be supported across the shoulders and back so that the baby's head can extend as he or she attaches (to facilitate a deep attachment), and allow the baby to swallow.
- The mother may find it helpful to shape the breast slightly using a 'C' hold. This helps her to direct the nipple towards the roof of the baby's mouth (this is known as an exaggerated latch). Once attached, the mother can release her hold on the breast.
- The baby's nose should be level with the nipple. As the baby's top lip brushes against the nipple, the mouth will open widely.

SKILL 49.1 Supporting the woman and baby to begin breastfeeding—traditional approach—cont'd

- With a wide mouth, the baby is brought swiftly to the breast, chin leading, aiming the nipple to the back of the baby's mouth (Fig 49.1).
- Once attached, the baby's nose should be close but clear and if any areola is visible, there should be more above the top lip than the bottom lip.

Inch (2013) states that breastfeeding is a learnt skill. This means that the midwife's role is both in educating parents (generally using a 'hands-off' approach) and enabling the mother to gain the skills and confidence for herself. Appreciating that the baby is appropriately positioned and attached at the breast allows for feeding to be relaxed and effective. These are some of the signs that the woman can look for.

- The baby has a large mouthful of breast tissue, with his lips curled out.
- The baby's cheeks should be rounded and stay rounded as he feeds.
- Feeding is quiet, no sucks or clicks are heard, but audible swallowing may be heard.
- The initial drawing out of the nipple may feel momentarily uncomfortable for the mother, but thereafter feeding should be a painless experience. If continued pain is felt, the mother should be advised to break the seal from the baby's mouth using her little finger and to attach the baby again.
- Rapid sucks are seen initially; after milk has been 'let down' the sucks become deeper and slower. The baby swallows after every one or two sucks, towards the end of the feed 'flutter' sucking can be seen.
- The baby stays on the breast, pauses from sucking are seen periodically, sucking begins again spontaneously. The baby leaves the breast spontaneously and may fall asleep promptly. (The other breast is offered.)
- At the beginning of a feed the baby's arm is often held tensely upwards, as the baby feeds it relaxes and falls to the baby's side.
- The parents should see adequate urine and stool output (see below).
- From about 2 weeks of age, regular weight gain is seen.
- The breast is lighter and softer after the baby has fed with no visible change to the shape or colour of the nipple.

Source: Johnson R, Taylor W: Skills for midwifery practice, 4th ed., Elsevier, London, 2016.

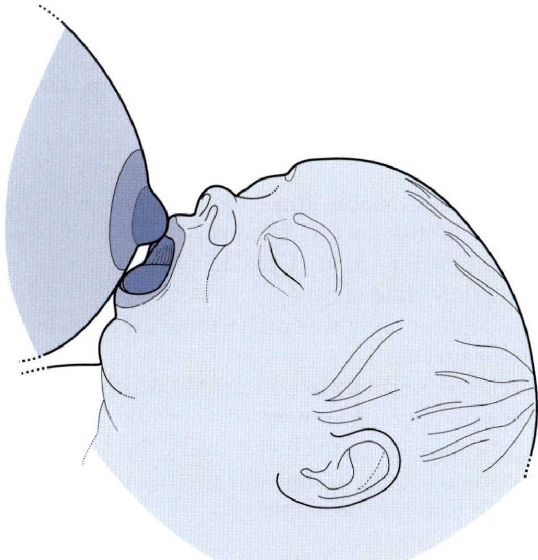

FIGURE 49.1 **The wide gape. Note also the slightly extended head, proximity of top lip/nose to nipple, position of bottom lip and direction at which the nipple enters the mouth.**
Source: Johnson R, Taylor W: Skills for midwifery practice, 4th ed., Elsevier, London, 2016.

Supporting the woman and baby to begin breastfeeding through a biological nurturing approach

Biological nurturing aims to achieve the environment in which babies and mothers exhibit innate reflexes that facilitate infant feeding. The mother is encouraged to adopt a comfortable, sustainable and well-supported, semi-recumbent position. Mother and baby are in skin-to-skin contact (or lightly dressed); the baby lies prone on the mother's abdomen with the head in the area of her breast. In this way the baby is fully supported by her body contours or (depending on position) the feet may be supported by the bed or pillows. It is noted that in this position gravity holds the baby in a naturally chosen position (Batacan 2010); the more traditional approach to breastfeeding practice requires the mother to hold the baby. This difference is noted to be significant, but is yet to be fully explored. The atmosphere should be relaxed and unhurried with plenty of time for cuddling. These positional interactions release the innate reflexes which the baby is born with (Colson et al 2008) (including moderately preterm and small for gestational age infants (Colson et al 2003)). These reflexes encourage the baby, in his or her own time, to find the breast, self-attach and effectively feed. The baby often manoeuvres into the optimal position. Colson (2005) notes that if a baby has not self-attached successfully at the breast, a modification in body lie (the direction of position) may facilitate this. In Colson's studies, babies adopted a similar lie for feeding to their in-utero position: longitudinal, transverse or oblique. Between feeds the baby may sleep in this position or in arms, but Colson and colleagues (2003) proposed that unrestricted access to the breast, including feeding while asleep, for at least the first 3 days of life may increase breastfeeding duration.

Breastfeeding with SARS-CoV-2 (CoViD19)

Emerging evidence at the time of writing (May 2021) about the safety for the newborn of being breastfed by a mother with SARS-COV-2 (CoViD19) strongly suggests that that transmission of the virus via breast milk or breastfeeding is highly unlikely, and the WHO position is that the benefits of breastfeeding outweigh the risk of COVID-19 transmission. If a COVID-19-positive mother chooses to room-in with her newborn, the latest best guidance at the time of writing is that they have a physical barrier (such as a curtain) and a 2 m space between them (DiLorenzo et al 2021).

Case reports started to appear in the literature from late 2020 to indicate that the risk of coronavirus transmission via breastmilk appeared extremely unlikely (e.g. see Perrone et al 2020). More recently, a systematic review that included 73 sources of guidance around breastfeeding and COVID-19 (DiLorenzo et al 2021) confirmed that *vertical* virus transmission from mother to child via breastfeeding appears unlikely, and that COVID-19-positive women or those suspected to have the disease could likely directly breastfeed but that to minimise the risk of *horizontal* transmission of the disease to the neonate, they are advised to practise 'enhanced precautions'. These precautions are detailed as: mask usage, strict hand hygiene, breast cleaning, breast milk expression via a dedicated pump with thorough pump cleaning, and feeding of pumped milk to the newborn by a healthy caretaker (p. 375).

Expressing breast milk

There may be occasions when it is necessary to express breast milk, but this is not a routine part of care when the baby is attaching and feeding well. If there is separation from the baby, problems attaching the baby at the breast, a sleepy reluctant feeder, the baby is preterm with a suboptimal suck reflex, or there is a clinical need to increase the milk supply, then expressing may be undertaken manually by hand or by using a hand or electric pump. Hand expression is more effective and should be the method taught. It allows for the expression of colostrum, something that pumps struggle to do, due to the limited quantity of liquid. It is a part of the midwife's role to guide and support mothers to express breast milk, and to assist where necessary.

SKILL 49.2 Collecting breast milk for the baby who is unable to breastfeed

- To express the milk, the breast is cupped in the hand with the thumb above the nipple and fingers below ('C' hold), approximately 2–4 cm back from the nipple.
- Generally a change in texture can be easily felt by the mother; this change corresponds with the ideal place to position the fingers as it is where the glandular tissue is situated.
- The mother is encouraged to gently compress rhythmically, hold and then release the fingers as the milk begins to flow.
- When flowing well, the position of the hand should be moved around the breast to ensure all lactiferous ducts are emptied.
- A sterilised and wide-necked receptacle is needed to collect the milk in.
- As the flow slows (after a few minutes), expressing should be switched to the other breast (unless purposely expressing one only), as that one slows, the first breast is then recommenced. This pattern encourages a repeated 'let down' of the milk and should be continued until both breasts feel soft and the flow is noticeably slower.
- Expressed breast milk can be kept in the back of the fridge (4°C or lower) for 5 days or frozen (−19°C) for up to 6 months (Department of Health 2013).
- In the event that hand expression is not possible, a hand pump or electric pump may be used.

Source: Johnson R, Taylor W: Skills for midwifery practice, 4th ed., Elsevier, London, 2016.

A link is available from the UNICEF UK (Baby Friendly) website to a demonstration video: search 'hand expression video' (UNICEF 2014).

Milk flow is aided by:

- the application of warmth (flannels, shower, bath) to the breasts
- a relaxed peaceful environment in which the baby (or a photograph) is near
- gentle massage of the breasts using the fingers or clenched fist in a 'rolling downwards' of the breast tissue, towards the nipple
- nipple rolling.

CUP FEEDING

The undisputed ideal way for a newborn baby to feed is to be effectively breastfed. However, when this is not possible, for whatever reason, cup feeding provides a method of feeding that:

- promotes tongue action consistent with breastfeeding

- removes the possibility of nipple/teat confusion
- allows the baby to pace the feed and therefore avoid overexertion
- encourages initial digestion of the milk in the mouth that would not occur if fed via a nasogastric tube.

Samuel (1998) notes that less is taken from a cup than a bottle; the newborn baby's stomach is therefore not overdistended and the feeding pattern is likely to be similar to a baby-led breastfeeding pattern. The randomised controlled study by Yilmaz and colleagues (2014) (522 participants) added to the literature that advocates cup feeding for preterm infants (32–35 weeks gestation in this study). Those who were cup fed were more likely to be exclusively breastfeeding on discharge and at 3 and 6 months of age than those who were fed with a bottle.

Disadvantages

It is recognised that term babies can become addicted to cup feeding if not put regularly to the breast and that they can also lose the skills needed to breastfeed if the cup-feeding technique is incorrect. Aspiration may also occur with an incorrect technique (Thorley 1997) and while milk wastage may be higher, the length of feed can also be longer.

Indications

Cup feeding is recognised as having three valuable uses.

1. As an interim measure for full-term babies when breastfeeding is not yet established (e.g. birth trauma, use of opiates in labour, maternal infant separation, mild palate deformities), or if supplementation is medically indicated. Samuel (1998) describes the way in which babies mature their sucking action and cites examples of the ways in which cup feeding aided term babies that initially lacked the skill. Equally, the breastfeeding mother may prefer her baby to use a cup during periods of absence (e.g. on return to work) rather than a bottle and teat.
2. For the preterm infant without sufficient suck/swallow coordination, who can easily tire if breastfed or bottle fed. Lang and colleagues (1994) suggest that cup feeding is appropriate for babies from 30 weeks gestation. However, Freer (1999) demonstrated that preterm infants underwent greater physiological instability when cup feeding than breastfeeding and so encourages caution. Yilmaz and colleagues (2014) recognised the value of cup feeding for preterm infants as a transition method prior to breastfeeding.
3. Cups are easier to sterilise than bottles and teats and can provide a safe feeding method in an emergency (Australian Breastfeeding Association [ABA] 2012).

The baby should be supported in an upright position and should lap or sip, rather than having the milk poured into their mouth. The experience should not be hurried. Parents can be taught to cup feed easily and may gain greater confidence in relation to their subsequent feeding method, having had the opportunity to learn (Samuel 1998). Parents may choose to feed in skin-to-skin contact and should be supported to do so as a precursor to effective breastfeeding. Term babies often dribble, calculations of the amount taken should consider this, and parents need to be aware that this is normal.

Cup-feeding babies need regular review. Continual observation should be made as to whether there are signs that the baby is ready to breastfeed. Slow pacing will avoid aspiration and enables the baby to rest between swallows (Lauwers & Swisher 2016, p. 515). It should also be established that sufficient nutrition is being achieved with cup feeding and that the baby is not being physiologically compromised or excessively tired by the process.

The cups used should be made of food-grade plastic and should be cleaned and decontaminated as for any other feeding equipment used for a baby, but as noted above, they are easier to clean. Staff training should also be undertaken, as for any skill, both when personnel are new to cup feeding it and for regular revision of technique.

SKILL 49.3 Cup feeding

1. Ensure that the baby is alert and interested. In many circumstances the baby will have been put to the breast first.
2. Gather equipment:
   - expressed breast milk (ideally)
   - sterilised cup (often small, open, slightly shaped and made from polyethylene or similar)
   - bib/napkin
   - baby's records.
3. Wash and dry hands.
4. Sit comfortably with the baby in an upright sitting position, cuddled in close to the parent's body. Consider swaddling the top half of the baby (to prevent hands knocking the cup) and using a suitably placed bib. Parents may choose to feed using skin-to-skin contact.
5. Place the cup (about half-full, if possible) lightly on the baby's bottom lip, reaching the corners

Continued

aspiration is still not possible re-passing the tube may be considered. *Under no circumstances is anything flushed down an NG tube before placement in the stomach is confirmed* (NPSA 2011).

- X-ray is the only other method used to confirm NG tube placement, but it is only to be used if the aspirate cannot be obtained (or cannot confirm pH 5.5 or lower). Equally, an X-ray would not be undertaken unless the baby is being X-rayed for some other reason.
- If an X-ray is performed, it should be read by a competent practitioner prior to permission to use the tube being given. It should also be noted that if deemed to be correct, it is only correct at the time of the X-ray and so pH aspirate screening would still be undertaken.

Despite careful checking, Wilkes-Holmes (2006) is clear that there is no completely reliable bedside method to confirm tube position, and midwives should always be alert to this. Documentation indicating every action and decision taken should be contemporaneous, dated and signed. In many places an NG tube placement record is used detailing issues such as clinical indication, the tube (size, make, batch no., etc.), ease and confirmation of placement, length inserted, length visible externally and date/time/reason for removal. A testing chart may also be used that keeps an ongoing record of each pH at each aspiration.

SKILL 49.5 Nasogastric tube placement and management

1. This should be undertaken in an environment that has working resuscitation equipment (oxygen and suction as a minimum) readily accessible.
2. Gain informed consent from the parents and gather equipment:
   - sterile radiopaque NG tube size FR 6 (for a baby weighing > 1.7 kg) with line markings (straightened if curved in the packaging)
   - sterile water and 2 mL syringe
   - sterile 20 mL syringe
   - tape
   - pH indicator paper with comparison chart
   - non-sterile gloves and apron
   - indelible marker pen.
3. Position the baby in a good light and a safe place (e.g. in the cot or held by an assistant); swaddle tightly so that hands are kept from the face.
4. Wash and dry hands and apply apron and non-sterile gloves.
5. Without touching the skin, hold the tip of the tube near to the nose, measure the distance from the nose to the ear and then from the ear to the xiphisternum (Fig 49.3), noting the distance markers on the tube, and marking the spot with the pen.
6. Pass the tube through the smaller nostril, gently but smoothly; if resistance is felt, stop and try the other nostril, observing the condition of the baby throughout. Stop and remove the tube if there is any gasping, coughing, pallor or cyanosis.
7. Once the tube has been passed through the appropriate length (pen mark at the nose) hold the tube in place, attach the 20 mL syringe, and withdraw approximately 0.5 mL of gastric aspirate.
8. Test the aspirate with the pH indicator paper; the result should be pH 5.5 or below. If the aspirate is hard to withdraw, the tube may have been occluded by mucous on insertion; 1–2 mL air may be injected first (using a 2 mL syringe) and then the aspirate withdrawn.
9. Once the position is confirmed, tape the tube in place across the baby's cheek, flush the tube using an appropriate amount of sterile water for the tube size (1–2 mL), followed by the same amount of air.
10. Dispose of equipment correctly.
11. Remove gloves and apron, wash and dry hands.
12. Document and act accordingly.

Administering a tube feed

Ideally the mother's expressed breast milk is used, alternatively donor milk should be accessed (Entwistle 2013). The amount may be specifically prescribed or calculated based on the baby's daily requirements according to weight, gestation and age. In its review of the evidence for very low birth-weight babies, the WHO recommended bolus feeds rather than continuous feeds, and suggested that if less than 3 hours has passed, the baby could be fed according to his or her hunger cues (WHO 2011b). The tube is flushed with sterile water after each administration, followed by a small amount of air to clear the tube of water. Some guidelines will also suggest that once placement is confirmed the tube is flushed with water before feeding and medicine administration as well as afterwards, this may depend upon the baby's fluid balance.

Parents are supported to undertake the feed themselves if this is appropriate, if not, a good feeding technique is modelled, taught and encouraged.

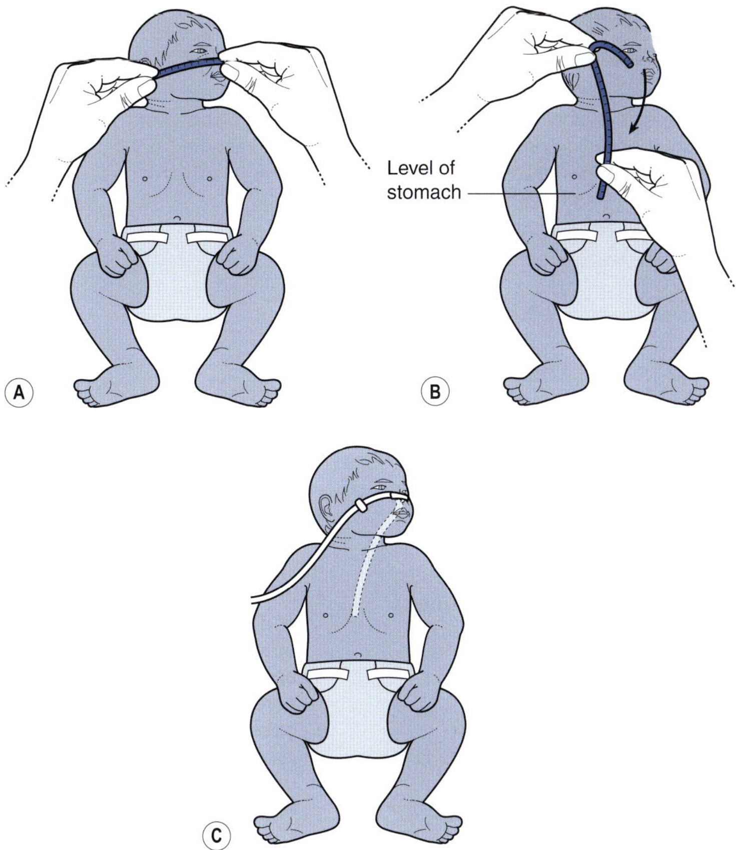

FIGURE 49.3 **A,** **Measuring the length of the nasogastric (NG) tube prior to insertion: measure from nose to ear, then from ear to xiphisternum (NEX measuring), B, noting the distance markers on the tubing. C, Nose to ear to midpoint between xiphisternum and umbilicus (NEMU) measuring would extend to the midway point between the xiphisternum and the umbilicus.**
Source: Johnson R, Taylor W: Skills for midwifery practice, 4th ed., Elsevier, London, 2016.

SKILL 49.6 Nasogastric tube feeding

1. Gain informed consent from the parents, wash hands and gather equipment:
   - 1 × 30 mL sterile syringe and 2 × 5 mL syringes
   - pH indicator paper (with comparison chart)
   - milk, at room temperature
   - non-sterile gloves
   - sterile water for oral use.
2. Position the baby in a good light and a safe place; the baby should be cuddled by one parent and interaction should take place as for any other kind of feed.
3. Wash and dry hands and apply non-sterile gloves.
4. Establish that there are no obvious signs of the tube having moved.
5. Attach a 5 mL syringe and withdraw 0.5–1 mL of gastric aspirate, place it onto the paper, and await the result. If pH 5.5 or less, continue. If pH is greater than 5.5, follow the guidelines discussed above; do not flush or feed.
6. If confident the tube is correctly placed, remove the plunger from the 30 mL syringe, attach the syringe to the tube, but occlude the tube by compressing it gently. (Some protocols will flush the tube using 1–3 mL of water before feeding.)
7. Pour the required amount of milk into the syringe, holding it in an upright position.
8. Release the occlusion on the tube so that the milk begins to flow into the stomach.
9. Regulate the flow by occluding and pausing if it is too fast, or by raising or lowering the syringe height. The feed should be leisurely and enjoyable, as for any other feed.
10. Observe the baby's condition throughout and stop the procedure if necessary (e.g. coughing, vomiting, hypoxic or bradycardic episodes).

Continued

SKILL 49.6 Nasogastric tube feeding—cont'd

11. Follow the feed with approximately 1–3 mL of sterile water drawn up using the other 5 mL syringe to cleanse the tube once the feed is completed (Naysmith & Nicholson 1998), followed by sufficient air (1–2 mL) to clear the tube of water. Water in the tube can affect the pH of the next aspirate tested.
12. Close off the tube, ensure the baby is in a safe place, dispose of the equipment. Remove gloves and wash and dry hands.
13. Complete the records.

Source: Johnson R, Taylor W: Skills for midwifery practice, 4th ed., Elsevier, London, 2016.

Removal of a nasogastric tube

This takes place when clinically indicated, or if the tube needs a routine change, repositioning or replacing because of blockage. To avoid the trauma of unnecessary re-insertion, ensure that removal is definitely indicated before removing it. Unfortunately, babies frequently remove their own NG tubes unless the tube is well secured.

SKILL 49.7 Removal of a nasogastric tube

1. Obtain informed consent; position the baby in a good light and a safe place.
2. Wash and dry hands and apply non-sterile gloves.
3. Remove the tape from the baby's face.
4. Pull out the tube smoothly and quickly, place into a bag for disposal (the baby may sneeze), wipe the baby's nose with soft tissue.
5. Check the tube is complete, dispose of equipment correctly and wash hands.
6. Complete documentation and act accordingly. Ensure that the baby feeds normally following the procedure.

Source: Johnson R, Taylor W: Skills for midwifery practice, 4th ed., Elsevier, London, 2016.

Role and responsibilities of the midwife

These can be summarised as:

- using evidence-based practice with good communication to provide information, support, and encouragement to facilitate the woman's ability to successfully breastfeed, whichever approach is used
- generally using a 'hands-off' approach that contributes towards confidence building for the mother
- monitoring the ongoing health and wellbeing of the mother and child, employing problem-solving strategies should the need arise
- recognising the value of cup and tube feeding as a significant interim measure to support breastfeeding, in babies of various gestations from 30 weeks onwards
- learning and teaching a safe and correct technique
- supporting and encouraging the parents
- undertaking all the techniques safely and competently in line with current best practice
- appropriately supporting and educating the parents
- observing the baby during and following all the procedures; making a referral if indicated
- undertaking contemporaneous record keeping.

SUMMARY

- Whichever method of infant feeding is chosen, uninterrupted skin-to-skin care at birth and during the early postnatal period is the foundation to successful feeding.
- Traditional practice utilising an upright maternal sitting position and the teaching of positioning and attachment skills has been challenged by the concept of biological nurturing. However, while there are differences, both approaches have value and both should be considered.
- Biological nurturing (Colson 2005) encourages the mother to adopt a comfortable semi-recumbent position in which the baby lies prone on the mother and manoeuvres himself or herself to self-attach at the breast. This action utilises innate reflexes.
- Correct attachment at the breast is vital, both to facilitate nutrition and to prevent breastfeeding problems. Midwives need to be able to facilitate this (by whichever approach the woman uses) and to utilise problem-solving strategies accordingly.
- Understanding the feeding cues facilitate baby-led feeding. Midwives should be familiar with the ways to assess that effective feeding is taking place.
- Cup and tube feeding are valuable interim measures; it is important that the baby and the cup are both positioned correctly and that the baby laps or sucks at his or her own pace.

- Nasogastric tubes have a role in feeding babies when oral feeding is limited or not possible.
- The tube must be confirmed to be in the stomach on every occasion. The currently advocated method is the use of pH indicator paper, the aspirate should have a pH of 5.5 or less. The tube is not used unless this is confirmed.
- The condition of the baby must be observed throughout. Efforts should be made to make feed times pleasurable.

Self-assessment exercises

The answers to the following questions may be found in the text.

1. Describe the basic anatomy and physiology of the lactating breast.
2. Discuss how this knowledge is used to promote successful breastfeeding.
3. How can the mother recognise when the baby is ready to feed?
4. Describe to a woman how to successfully attach her baby at the breast using the traditional approach.
5. Describe the features of biological nurturing.
6. Describe the markers used to assess effective breastfeeding.
7. What advice would you give to a woman who needs to hand express?
8. Discuss the advantages and disadvantages of cup and tube feeding.
9. List the circumstances when cup and tube feeding is indicated.
10. Describe how to correctly cup and tube feed a baby.
11. Summarise the role and responsibilities of the midwife when cup and tube feeding.
12. Discuss the possible risks of feeding via an NG tube.
13. Describe how to safely insert an NG tube and confirm its position.
14. Describe how to undertake a milk feed using an NG tube.
15. Describe how to remove an NG tube.
16. Summarise the role and responsibilities of the midwife in relation to each of these aspects of care.

Resources

Ministry of Health NSW: Infants and children: insertion and confirmation of placement of nasogastric and orogastric tubes, 2016. Available: www1.health.nsw.gov.au/pds/ActivePDSDocuments/GL2016_006.pdf.

UNICEF Ten steps to successful breastfeeding: www.who.int/teams/nutrition-and-food-safety/food-and-nutrition-actions-in-health-systems/ten-steps-to-successful-breastfeeding.

References

Australian Breastfeeding Association (ABA): Cup feeding in emergencies, 2012. Online 23 March 2018. Available: www.breastfeeding.asn.au/bf-info/cupfeedemerg.

Batacan J: A new approach: biological nurturing and laid-back breastfeeding, International Journal of Childbirth Education 25(2):7–9, 2010.

Cirgin Ellett M, Cohen M, Perkins S, et al: Predicting the insertion length for gastric tube placement in neonates, Journal of Obstetrics and Gynecology. Neonatal Nursing 40(4):412–421, 2011.

Colson S: Biological nurturing (2): the physiology of lactation revisited, The Practising Midwife 10(10):14–19, 2007.

Colson S: Bringing nature to the fore, The Practising Midwife 11(10):14–19, 2008.

Colson S: Maternal breastfeeding positions: have we got it right? (2), The Practising Midwife 8(11):29–32, 2005.

Colson S, de Rooy L, Hawdon J: Biological nurturing increases duration of breastfeeding for a vulnerable cohort, MIDIRS Midwifery Digest 13(1):92–97, 2003.

Colson S, Meek J, Hawdon J: Optimal positions for the release of primitive neonatal reflexes stimulating breastfeeding, Early Human Development 84(7): 441–449, 2008.

Department of Health: Off to the best start, London, 2013.

DiLorenzo MA, O'Connor SK, Ezekwesili C, et al: COVID-19 guidelines for pregnant women and new mothers: a systematic evidence review. International Journal of Gynecology & Obstetrics 153(3):373–382, 2021.

Entwistle F: Chapter 4. The evidence and rationale for the UNICEF UK Baby Friendly Initiative standards, UNICEF UK, London, 2013. Online 23 March 2018. Available: www.unicef.org.uk/BabyFriendly/Resources/Guidance-for-Health-Professionals/Writing-policies-and-guidelines/The-evidence-and-rationale-for-the-UNICEF-UK-Baby-Friendly-Initiative-standards/.

Freer Y: A comparison of breast and cup feeding preterm infants, Journal of Neonatal Nursing 5(1):16–20, 1999.

Geddes D: Ultrasound imaging of the lactating breast: methodology and application, International Breastfeeding Journal 4(4):1746–1758, 2009.

Inch S: Feeding the newborn baby: breast milk and breast milk substitutes. In Hall Moran V, eds: Maternal and infant nutrition and nurture: controversies and challenges, 2nd ed., Quay Books, London, 2013.

International Breastfeeding Centre: Finger and cup feeding, July 2009. Online 23 May 2021. Available: https://ibconline.ca/information-sheets/finger-and-cup-feeding/.

Jones E, Spencer A: Successful preterm breastfeeding, The Practising Midwife 2(1):54–57, 1999.

Lang S, Lawrence C, Orme R: Cup feeding: an alternative method of infant feeding, Archives of Disease in Childhood 71:365–369, 1994.

Lauwers J, Swisher A: Counseling the nursing mother: a lactation consultant's guide, 6th ed., Jones & Bartlett Learning, Burlington, 2016.

National Patient Safety Agency (NPSA): Patient safety alert: reducing the harm caused by misplaced naso and orogastric feeding tubes in babies under the care of neonatal units, NPSA, London, 2011. Online 23 March 2018. Available: www.cas.mhra.gov.uk/ViewandAcknowledgment/ViewAlert.aspx?AlertID=101559.

National Patient Safety Agency (NPSA): Rapid response report: harm from flushing of nasogastric tubes before confirmation of placement, NPSA, London, 2012. Online 23 March 2018. Available: www.cas.mhra.gov.uk/ViewandAcknowledgment/ViewAlert.aspx?AlertID=101753.

Naysmith MR, Nicholson J: Nasogastric drug administration, Professional Nurse 13(7):424–427, 1998.

Pairman S, Tracy S, Dahlen HG, Dixon, L: Midwifery preparation for practice, 4th ed., Elsevier, Sydney, 2018.

Perrone S, Giordano M, Meoli A, et al: Lack of viral transmission to preterm newborn from a COVID-19 positive breastfeeding mother at 11 days postpartum, Journal of Medical Virology 92(11):2346–2347, 2020.

Rapley G, Murkett T: Baby-led parenting, Vermillion, London, 2014.

Samuel P: Cup feeding, The Practising Midwife 1(12):33–35, 1998.

Thorley V: Cup feeding: problems created by incorrect use, Journal of Human Lactation 13(1):54–55, 1997.

United Nations Children's Fund (UNICEF) UK: Hand expression, 2014. Online 23 March 2018. Available: www.unicef.org.uk/BabyFriendly/Resources/AudioVideo/Hand-expression/.

Wilkes-Holmes C: Safe placement of nasogastric tubes in children, Paediatric Nursing 18(9):14–17, 2006.

World Health Organization (WHO): Exclusive breastfeeding for six months best for babies everywhere, 2011a. Online 23 March 2018. Available: www.who.int/mediacentre/news/statements/2011/breastfeeding_20110115/en/.

World Health Organization (WHO): Optimal feeding of low birth-weight infants in low and middle-income countries, Geneva, 2011b, WHO. Online 23 March 2018. Available: www.who.int/maternal_child_adolescent/documents/9789241548366.pdf.

Yilmaz G, Caylan N, Karacan CD, et al: Effect of cup feeding and bottle feeding on breastfeeding in late preterm infants: a randomized controlled study, Journal of Human Lactation 30(2):174–179, 2014.

CHAPTER 50

SUPPORTING THE WOMAN WHO CHOOSES TO FORMULA FEED

Learning outcomes

Having read this chapter, the reader should be able to:

- discuss in detail the advice and education that new parents need when choosing to formula feed
- describe all the ways in which effective sterilisation of infant feeding equipment can be undertaken
- discuss the principles of correct powdered formula milk preparation and the dangers of incorrect preparation
- explain how to effectively feed a baby with a bottle and teat
- explain the midwife's role and responsibilities in relation to each of these aspects of care.

When a baby is not being breastfed, the midwife has an important role in facilitating safe and effective infant nutrition using formula milk. This chapter considers the significance of effective decontamination of feeding equipment and correct powdered infant formula reconstitution, both within and outside the home, appropriate feeding technique and the midwife's role and responsibilities in this situation.

FORMULA FEEDING

In its *Infant Feeding Guidelines: Information for Health Workers* publication, the Australian National Health and Medical Research Council (NHMRC) (2012) cautions that infant formula 'requires accurate reconstitution and hygienic preparation to ensure its safety, so it is important that health workers know how to demonstrate the preparation of infant formula and how to feed an infant with a bottle'. (p. 73). Similarly, the New Zealand Government has published its own resource for health workers to use with new parents (Ministry of Health 2021) to facilitate safe formula feeding. Women who are using formula milk should be shown how to correctly prepare a feed postnatally before transfer home. All parents of new babies also need to understand effective sterilisation/decontamination of feeding equipment. Redmond and Griffith (2009b) state that for various reasons, the domestic kitchen is not a good place for safe food preparation and therefore healthcare practitioners should take their role seriously in educating parents in these matters. Time has passed since the World Health Organization (WHO 2007) gave new guidance regarding the safe preparation of powdered infant formula at home. Nevertheless, many parents and carers have been found in recent years to still not prepare it correctly (NHMRC 2012), hence the need to educate new mothers and fathers on this topic. In accordance with the *WHO International Code of Marketing of Breast-milk Substitutes* (1981) ('the Code'), which is still current advice despite being 40 years old (WHO 2020), feeding with infant formula should only be demonstrated by health workers (or other community workers if necessary), and only to mothers and other family members who need to use it; further, the Code states that information given should include a clear explanation of the hazards of improper use of formula.

WHAT ARE THE RISKS OF FORMULA FEEDING?

The digestive tract of newborn infants varies in its pH according to feeding method. The formula-fed infant has a more alkaline intestine and so has less protection against harmful microorganisms. Formula milk powder may contain microorganisms; therefore, care should be taken in its reconstitution because of formula-fed babies being at a greater infection risk than their breastfed counterparts to begin with. Minchin (2000) and Inch (2013) both suggest that the production and manufacture of artificial milk has many unanswered questions—its composition, the role of genetically modified ingredients, the potential hazards in manufacture (and to the environment (Inch 2013), to name but a few. Marchant and Rundall (2008) have also stated concerns over misleading advertising claims. The health benefits to mothers and babies of breastfeeding are well documented; however, the long-term consequences of formula feeding are not yet fully realised. There is emerging evidence that it is related to comparatively poorer health outcomes. Parents may also not appreciate the dangers of choking, overfeeding or poor feeding technique alongside those of feed preparation inside and outside their home environment.

FORMULA MILKS

Powdered infant formula milks suitable for newborn babies are predominantly made from modified cow's milk with the amounts of carbohydrate, fat and protein modified to resemble those of breast milk. There is a wide range of regular and diet-specific formula brands available, and each has slightly different constituents; further information about the composition and choice of formula is available from the NHMRC (2012) publication *Infant Feeding Guidelines* (p. 74); however, it is clear that, for whichever milk is chosen, it must be an age-suitable formula (Crawley & Westland 2013). Powdered infant formula milk should be prepared with water at 70°C (or higher, but not boiling). Each container of formula milk powder is supplied with a plastic measuring scoop that is suitable for use with that container's contents only.

Equipment required

The following equipment is suggested.

- Handwashing and drying facilities; clean towel where possible.
- Infant feeding bottles with tops, covers and teats. Wide-necked bottles are often easier to clean. The scale on the side should be clearly visible. Standard flow teats are acceptable (drip rate of 1 drop per second). The woman may make different choices later, according to her baby's needs.
- Sterilising equipment.
- Bottle and teat brushes (non-metallic), hot water and washing-up liquid.
- Plastic spatula or leveller, if not included in milk powder container.
- A safe water supply with kettle or means of boiling water, 1 L of water at least (Crawley & Westland 2013).
- Age-appropriate powdered infant formula, within 'use-by' guidance.
- Equipment for use out of the home (e.g. flask and container for milk powder; possibly a cool bag, depending on the situation).

FEEDING PREPARATION

Potential hazards

The dangers of reconstituting formula feed include the following.

- Use of unclean equipment that has not been properly cleaned and sterilised and is (potentially) recontaminated.
- An incorrectly reconstituted feed. This is a breeding ground for microorganisms and so each feed needs to be prepared as follows.
  - Ideally, prepared freshly at the time of need, although several feeds can be made up in advance for convenience (see below).
  - Prepared with fresh tap water that has been boiled only once, then left to cool for a maximum of 30 minutes. Cooling the water is necessary, as feeds made with boiling water may be nutritionally compromised due to the clumping of some of the ingredients. Crawley and Westland (2013) advocate boiling at least 1 L of water; the temperature of the water after 30 minutes can vary according to the amount of water boiled. Ideally, the water temperature will still be about 70°C; this is considered appropriate to kill the maximum amount of bacteria. Bottled (but not sparkling mineral water or soda water) water may be used (NHMRC 2012). Crawley and Westland (2013) suggest that this should contain less than 200 mg sodium and less than 250 mg sulfate.
  - Carefully reconstituted, by placing the water into the bottle first and adding the correct number of loosely packed level scoops of powder (often one scoop to 30 mL water, but encourage parents to read the packet and use only the scoop that came with that packet). Too much powder may result in hypernatraemia, constipation and obesity, while too little can cause malnutrition.
  - Cooled under cold running water to the required temperature quickly to restrict bacterial growth.

The utmost care should be taken to protect babies against any potential sources of infection because of the immaturity of their immune system: being formula fed is associated with an increased incidence of infectious morbidity, including otitis media, gastroenteritis and pneumonia (Ip et al 2007). All feeding equipment should be carefully cleaned and 'sterilised'; traces of milk can harbour and multiply bacteria quickly (Redmond & Griffith 2009a). The following section outlines the correct use of the different decontamination techniques and the role of the midwife in relation to this.

Sterilisation advice

Most women are now advised to clean feeding equipment in hot, soapy water, rinse with clear hot water and leave to air dry before storing; however, several other methods are also in use. Therefore, it is essential that health workers show parents of new babies correct methods of safe formula feeding, including those related to the range of ways to sterilise and store equipment (NHMRC 2012). Mainstone (2004) has argued that this advice should be a part of general home infection control measures and so should be taught in the parent's usual domestic residence. In hospital, advice is often given as part of antenatal education and prior to postnatal discharge. Particular care should be taken if the woman's first language is not the same as the midwife's; a professional interpreter should be used in that case.

All the equipment used should be compatible with the chosen sterilising method and should also be examined on a regular basis. Bacteria can be harboured in cracks or grooves in older bottles or teats, and bottles with a pattern can make it harder to see if the bottle is clean (Redmond & Griffith 2009a). The chemical bisphenol A (BPA A) is used in the production of some plastic products—including some infant feeding bottles—to prevent cracking and shattering; however, several countries (including Australia and New Zealand) have adopted a voluntary phase-out in response to consumer preference (Food Standards Australia New Zealand 2021).

Cleaning feeding equipment

All equipment needs to be thoroughly cleaned with hot soapy water and using a bottle/teat brush before being sterilised, regardless of sterilisation method (NHMRC 2012). If this step is missed or performed badly, then retained milk may harbour bacteria that survive the sterilisation process. Redmond and Griffith (2009a) indicate that hypochlorite disinfectants are inactivated by food debris, among other things.

Methods of sterilisation (decontamination)

It should be noted that Redmond and Griffith (2009a) suggest that using the term 'sterilisation' is incorrect. Surgical instruments and suchlike may be sterilised; that is, undergo a process that removes all viable microorganisms and spores, but the methods in this chapter used in the home are more akin to disinfection or decontamination. Midwives have a responsibility to help parents understand that items will not be completely sterile and that, therefore, greater care should be taken to carry out these procedures correctly. The method chosen may vary according to ease, convenience and costs, both of the initial outlay and of ongoing use. As well as simply washing in hot soapy water, rinsing and leaving to air dry, there are four additional methods of decontamination (Redmond & Griffith 2009a):

1. boiling
2. chemical (sodium hypochlorite)
3. steam: microwave
4. steam: electrical.

Boiling

Boiling in the home can be a hazardous activity and therefore should be done with great care. Prolonged use of boiling may destroy the teats; they should be examined regularly. A large saucepan with a lid is required and a trivet in the base of the pan prevents the bottles from burning. A good volume of water is required so that the bottles stay below the surface, but care should be taken to ensure that the pan does not boil over or boil dry. According to the NHMRC (2012), boiling is the preferred option and gives consistent and reliable results if the following steps are taken after washing bottles, teats and caps in hot soapy water with a bottle/teat brush.

SKILL 50.1 Decontamination of feeding equipment by boiling

1. Place utensils, including bottles, teats and caps, in a large saucepan on the back burner of the stove.
2. Cover utensils with water, making sure to eliminate all air bubbles from the bottles.
3. Bring the water to the boil and boil for 5 minutes. Turn off—do not allow to boil dry.
4. Allow the equipment to cool in the saucepan until it is hand hot and then remove it—be very careful if children are present.
5. Store equipment that is not being used straight away in a clean container in the fridge.
6. Boil all equipment within 24 hours of use.

Source: National Health and Medical Research Council (NHMRC): Infant feeding guidelines, 2012. Canberra: NHMRC. Online 11 October 2021. Available: https://www.nhmrc.gov.au/sites/default/files/images/literature-review-infant-feeding-guidelines.pdf.

Chemical

Various antibacterial preparations in either tablet or liquid form are available for chemical decontamination. Complete elimination of bacterial contamination will only be achieved if the solution is prepared and used correctly (i.e. it must be 50 ppm hypochlorite and equipment must be completely submersed in it for 30 minutes). Bottles and other equipment must be washed with soapy water prior to submersion in the antibacterial solution (NHMRC 2012).

SKILL 50.2 Chemical decontamination

1. A large enough container with a well-fitting lid and floating cover should be used.
2. Thoroughly wash and dry hands and work on a clean working surface.
3. Prepare the sterilising solution using the correct amounts of water and chemical to produce fluid of the correct dilution.
4. Make sure all equipment to be sterilised in this is made of plastic or glass: the solution will corrode metal.
5. Fully submerge the clean utensils, ensuring there are no trapped air bubbles; place the floating cover and lid on the container, ensuring that all items stay fully immersed.
6. Leave the container undisturbed for at least the required number of minutes; if anything needs to be added to or removed from the solution during this time the timing starts again from the time of addition/removal. Equipment can be left in the solution for longer until needed.
7. When the equipment is required, wash and dry hands, remove the items carefully, handling them by the aspects that will not come into contact with the baby or milk.
8. Shake the excess fluid off the equipment (Redmond & Griffith 2009a): do not rinse or there will be a risk of recontamination.
9. Use removed items immediately.
10. Discard the solution after 24 hours, scrub the container and lid in warm soapy water, and prepare a new solution.

Microwave

Non-metallic equipment can also be sterilised in a microwave using a specific microwave steriliser, prescribed amount of tap water and suitable feeding equipment. Models vary, so the manufacturer's instructions should be followed carefully. It should be noted that the length of time needed depends on the wattage of the microwave, and it should be remembered that the timings often include standing time. The length of time that the undisturbed items remain sterile varies according to steriliser model. Decontaminating in a microwave without the recommended equipment is inappropriate. All items should be placed in the steriliser with the openings facing downwards so that there is maximum exposure to the steam for the inside of the items.

Electric steam sterilisers

Feeding equipment can be decontaminated by steam using an electric steriliser, for which the manufacturer's instructions should be followed carefully. The equipment does need to have complete contact with the steam and so, as above, should be loaded with open ends facing downwards. The cycle length varies (3–15 minutes); the items should be used immediately unless the manufacturer's guidance suggests otherwise. Electric steamers often need descaling on a monthly basis to maintain their efficiency.

Recontamination

There are many ways in which feeding equipment can be recontaminated after decontamination. Clean hands are essential, especially after changing nappies and toileting, food preparation and nose blowing. Redmond and Griffith (2009b) recognise that drying hands thoroughly also contributes to reducing the transfer of microorganisms. Equally, care should be taken at home to use clean hand towels; otherwise, bacteria can be transferred from towel to hand to equipment. The work surface should be clean and uncluttered and, as the feeds are prepared, it is essential that no part of the equipment that will have contact with the milk or baby should be touched.

FORMULA FEEDING AWAY FROM HOME

If feeding outside the home, ready-to-drink formula is commercially available, or parents may wish to prepare their own. Preparation of bottles of infant formula is recommended to occur at the destination to reduce the risk of harmful bacteria developing in warm pre-prepared formula. Parents should therefore ideally carry a freshly sterilised bottle of refrigerated boiled water and the powder in a sterilised container. The bottle of water should first be warmed by standing it in a container of warm water, then the formula added.

STORAGE AND USE OF PREPARED FEEDS

If formula needs to be prepared in advance (e.g. for a babysitter to use), it is recommended that only one bottle of formula be prepared at a time, refrigerated below 5°C until use, and used within 24 hours (NHMRC 2012). Each bottle of formula should be:

- prepared and put in the refrigerator
- cold before transporting
- not removed from the fridge until immediately before transporting
- transported in a cool bag with ice packs
- used within 2 hours of removal from fridge (or replaced in a fridge for up to 24 hours)
- re-warmed at the destination for no longer than 15 minutes.

SKILL 50.3 Preparing powdered formula milk

1. Wash hands and ensure the preparation area is clean.
2. Ensure all equipment has been carefully washed and thoroughly sterilised (decontaminated).
3. Boil fresh water and allow it to cool for at least 30 minutes until lukewarm.
4. Ideally, only prepare one bottle at a time, just before feeding; however, several feeds can be safely prepared in advance if required for convenience (see earlier).
5. Always read the formula packet instructions to check the correct amount of water and powder to use.
6. Add the correct amount of cooled boiled water to the bottle first, then the correct amount of powder: the scoop provided in the packet being used must always be chosen to measure the powder.
7. The correct amount of powder must be added to the correct amount of water. Less or more of either must not be used.
8. Keep the scoop in the packet between uses. Do not wash the scoop as this may introduce moisture into the powder.
9. Place the teat over the bottle, handling it only at the bottom edge. Place the screw ring over and tighten (if this is difficult, sterilised tongs or tweezers can be used), put on a sterilised bottle cover. Shake the milk gently to ensure appropriate mixing of the contents; the powder should be fully dissolved and not show any signs of clumping together.
10. Hold the bottle under cold running water until the feed is cooled to an appropriate temperature. Check it by testing a few drops on the inside of the parent's wrist. The milk should be warm, but not hot.
11. Use immediately. Discard unfinished feeds straight away and thoroughly wash all equipment used in hot soapy water prior to sterilising (decontaminating).

FEEDING TECHNIQUE

The principles of baby-led feeding should be upheld: the baby will feed when hungry, taking as much or as little as desired. All parents should be taught to recognise and understand the baby's feeding cues and feed their baby when the early cues are seen. The recommendation to prepare each formula feed when it is needed will mean a short delay between the baby 'asking' to be fed and the feed being ready; however, this is inevitable. Entwistle (2013) suggests ways in which the feeding experience can be enhanced. These include feeding times that are enjoyable and relaxed, in which the baby feels loved. The baby should be held securely, close to his or her parent in a reasonably upright sitting position (head supported) so that breathing and swallowing are easy. Eye contact should be maintained. UNICEF (n.d.) suggests that babies will feel more secure if most feeds are given by their parents. A baby should never be left unattended to feed, as the milk may flow too quickly and cause the baby to splutter or choke (NHMRC 2012).

As the teat brushes against the baby's lips the baby will open his or her mouth wide and take in the teat. The teat needs to be over the baby's tongue and the bottle just tipped sufficiently for air to be excluded from the teat. The teat should administer regular drops, rather than a stream of milk (Ellis & Kanneh 2000). The baby will suck and pause, retaining the teat in his or her mouth. The pace of the feed should allow for small interruptions that can break the suction that sometimes builds in the teat (move it to the side of the baby's mouth briefly), to wind the baby (gentle back rubbing or patting) or to allow the baby to appreciate whether he or she needs to continue or stop feeding at that time.

The baby will cease feeding when he or she has had sufficient milk.

Role and responsibilities of the midwife

These can be summarised as:

- careful education of the parents; demonstration or observation may be included. Written approved guidance in an appropriate language should be given
- appropriate documentation and ongoing review
- practising with research-based evidence
- using evidenced-based knowledge and application of best practice advice with regard to equipment sterilisation (decontamination), and formula milks, their reconstitution and storage
- educating and supporting parents to ensure safe infant nutrition and feeding technique
- recognition of a healthy formula-fed infant
- contemporaneous record keeping.

SUMMARY

- There are four effective methods of sterilisation/decontamination: boiling, chemical, microwave steam and electrical steam. Items must be compatible for the chosen method of sterilisation and must be thoroughly cleaned before sterilising.
- It is important that the technique is undertaken correctly, whichever method is chosen; babies need to be protected from potential infection.

- It is important that powdered formula milk is reconstituted correctly for each individual feed.
- As well as this, care should be taken to use sterilised feeding equipment, a safe water supply, and, if needed, appropriate storage and transport of a reconstituted feed.
- The midwife has an important role in facilitating parents to develop a loving and safe feeding technique.

Self-assessment exercises

The answers to the following questions may be found in the text.

1. Discuss why decontamination of feeding equipment is necessary, and identify the most common form of feeding equipment decontamination.
2. Describe how to decontaminate feeding equipment when boiling.
3. Demonstrate how to decontaminate feeding equipment using chemical sterilisation.
4. Discuss the different methods of steam decontamination.
5. Summarise the role and responsibilities of the midwife in relation to effective equipment preparation.
6. Describe how to correctly reconstitute powdered infant formula at home.
7. List the times/ways in which bacterial growth could occur while reconstituting a feed or during the feeding process.
8. Demonstrate how to hold the baby and bottle when formula feeding.
9. Summarise the midwife's role and responsibilities when caring for a woman and her baby when the baby is being fed with formula milk.

References

Crawley H, Westland S, Infant milks in the UK: a practical guide for health professionals. London: Nutrition Trust, 2013, First Steps.

Ellis M, Kanneh A: Infant nutrition: part two, Paediatric Nursing 12(1):38–43, 2000.

Entwistle F: Chapter 4. The evidence and rationale for the UNICEF UK baby friendly initiative standards, London, 2013, UNICEF UK. Online 11 October 2021. Available: www.unicef.org.uk/BabyFriendly/Resources/Guidance-for-Health-Professionals/Writing-policies-and-guidelines/The-evidence-and-rationale-for-the-UNICEF-UK-Baby-Friendly-Initiative-standards/.

Food Standards Australia New Zealand: Regulation and monitoring of BPA, n.d. Online 11 October 2021. Available: www.foodstandards.gov.au/consumer/chemicals/bpa/pages/regulationandmonitor5377.aspx.

Inch S: Feeding the newborn baby. In Moran V Hall, Dykes, F, eds: maternal and infant nutrition and nurture: controversies and challenges, 2nd ed., Quay Books, London, 2013.

Ip S, Chung M, Raman G, et al: Breastfeeding and maternal and infant health outcomes in developed countries, Evidence Report/Technology Assessment (153):1–186, 2007. Online 23 March 2018. Available: www.ncbi.nlm.nih.gov/books/NBK38337/.

Mainstone A: Domestic hazard analysis of infant feeding utensils, British Journal of Midwifery 12(6):368–372, 2004.

Marchant S, Rundall P: Safe and appropriate infant nutrition: why does it matter? MIDIRS Midwifery Digest 18(4):566–570, 2008.

Minchin M: Artificial feeding and risk, Practical Midwife 3(3):18–20, 2000.

Ministry of Health: Feeding your baby infant formula, 2021. New Zealand Government. Online 11 October 2021. Available: www.healthed.govt.nz/resource/feeding-your-baby-infant-formula.

National Health and Medical Research Council (NHMRC): Infant feeding guidelines, 2012. Canberra: NHMRC. Online 11 October 2021. Available: www.nhmrc.gov.au/sites/default/files/images/literature-review-infant-feeding-guidelines.pdf.

Redmond E, Griffith CJ: Disinfection methods used in decontamination of bottles used for feeding powdered infant formula, Journal of Family Health Care 19(1): 26–31, 2009a.

Redmond E, Griffith CJ: The importance of hygiene in the domestic kitchen: implications for preparation and storage of food and infant formula, Perspectives in Public Health 129(2):69–76, 2009b.

UNICEF UK: Responsive bottle feeding, London, n.d., UNICEF UK. Online 11 October 2021. Available: www.unicef.org.uk/babyfriendly/wp-content/uploads/sites/2/2019/04/Infant-formula-and-responsive-bottle-feeding.pdf.

World Health Organization (WHO): WHO international code of marketing of breast-milk substitutes, Geneva, 1981, WHO. Online 11 October 2021. Available: www.who.int/publications/i/item/9241541601.

World Health Organization (WHO). Safe preparation, storage and handling of powdered infant formula: guidelines, Geneva, 2007, WHO. Online: 11 October 2021. Available: www.who.int/foodsafety/publications/micro/pif_guidelines.pdf.

World Health Organization (WHO): The international code of marketing of breast-milk substitutes: frequently asked questions on the roles and responsibilities of health workers, Geneva 2020, WHO. Online 11 October 2021. Available: www.who.int/publications/i/item/9789240005990.

PART 4

CARE OF SELF AND OTHERS

Section 14: Skills for working safely

SECTION 14

SKILLS FOR WORKING SAFELY

CHAPTER 51
SELF-CARE

Learning outcomes

Having read this chapter, the reader should be able to:

- understand the importance of self-care
- identify ways to ensure a balance between work and home life
- describe the factors contributing to stress, anxiety and burnout
- identify self-care and stress-reduction strategies
- understand the importance of adequate sleep and the consequences of sleep deprivation.

SELF-CARE FOR MIDWIVES

Self-care is essential for midwives because if they do not look after themselves physically, emotionally and psychologically, they will be unable to provide the best possible care to women and their families. Midwives must make self-care a deliberate priority in order to lead a balanced life that will help avoid burnout, compassion fatigue, stress (Likis 2016), anxiety and depression (Coldridge & Davies 2017). Self-care refers to nourishing activities that sustain and improve health (Reading 2017). Self-care helps individuals cope with stress, aids recovery, provides a buffer against future stress and encourages individuals to be the best they can and to flourish (Reading 2017).

Being healthy and resilient enables midwives to provide high-quality and safe care, minimise errors, provide physical care and remain psychologically receptive over long periods of time (Coldridge & Davies 2017). Emotionally exhausted midwives are less able to perform well (Creedy et al 2017). Burnout decreases the wellbeing of midwives, reduces their ability to provide quality care and increases attrition (Fenwick et al 2017). The symptoms of burnout include fatigue, lack of motivation, decreased productivity, detachment, cynicism and decreased self-esteem (Fedele 2017). Ninety-five per cent of midwives have witnessed traumatic events and around one-third display symptoms of posttraumatic stress (Creedy & Gamble 2016). A United Kingdom (UK) study on the mental health and wellbeing of nurses and midwives found high levels of stress and burnout resulting from escalating workplace demands and declining resources (Teoh et al 2020). Midwives often work in a system with low levels of leeway, high psychological demands and poor support; this places midwives at high risk of reaction disorders such as burnout, anxiety and mood disorders (Pougnet et al 2020).

Organisations employing midwives have a responsibility to address systemic issues increasing workplace stress and impacting on the wellness and self-care ability of midwives (Wright 2020).

To maintain a healthy midwifery workforce requires leadership, suitable support, education, reflective clinical supervision and the opportunity to work in women-centred models of care (Callendar et al 2021). Midwives need a workplace culture designed to mediate the deleterious effect of workplace environments by promoting positive mental health, wellbeing and a healthy work–life balance (Teoh et al 2020). Supporting midwives has the potential to improve outcomes for women and infants through safe midwifery-led continuity of care (Callander et al 2021).

THE TOLL OF MIDWIFERY WORK

Midwifery work can be highly emotional, involving complex, distressing and sensitive issues (Cummins et al 2018), substantial demands and a stressful environment (Coldridge & Davies 2017). Midwives establish close and empathetic relationships with women, which may increase their vulnerability (Coldridge & Davies 2017). Midwives experience high levels of stress, depression, anxiety and burnout (Dixon et al 2017). The COVID-19 pandemic has rapidly changed the way midwives work, including moving to telehealth appointments, reducing the ability to be 'with woman', discontinuation of face-to-face antenatal education, limits on labour support people and use of personal protective equipment (PPE) (Bradfield et al 2021). Midwives have found the changes stressful, difficult, challenging and anxiety provoking (Bradfield et al 2021). Midwives have also noted that visitors and families have become more aggressive, angry and abusive as they deal with their own fears and the restrictions on access to women (Bradfield et al 2021).

Midwives frequently feel psychologically, emotionally and physically stretched, missing meal breaks and working long hours (Coldridge & Davies 2017). A study of Australian nurses and midwives found over one-quarter reported mental health and wellbeing disorders (Smyth et al 2016). A survey in the UK found approximately 50% of midwives suffered from stress related to their work (Howell 2016). Burnout and workload have an impact on the retention of midwives (Australian Nursing and Midwifery Federation [ANMF] 2018). In Australia, almost one-third of midwives have considered leaving the profession (Holland et al 2018).

Australia has an ageing midwifery workforce with an average age of 48 years and 52.2% over 50 years of age (Callendar et al 2021). In New Zealand the average age of midwives is 46.65 years with 44.8% over 50 years of age (Midwifery Council Te Tatau o te Whare Kahu 2020). The potential loss of experienced midwives who will retire over coming years highlights the importance of supporting midwifery retention (Callendar et al 2021).

UNDERGRADUATE AND STUDENT MIDWIVES

Undergraduate and student midwives face the difficulties of combining study, work and the realities of midwifery, which may differ from their original idealised image of the profession (Cummins et al 2018). Incorporating workshops to help students manage feelings, deal with clinical issues (such as domestic violence, sexual abuse, forceps, stillbirth) and explore self-care strategies, including mindfulness and meditation, are beneficial (Cummins et al 2018). Student midwives find mentoring, debriefing and non-judgmental support helpful in their transition to the role of midwife (Coldridge & Davies 2017).

The COVID-19 pandemic has impacted the experience of midwifery students, who have found their clinical situation changed frequently, making it difficult for them to obtain current accurate information and guidance (Kuliukas et al 2021). Midwifery students are also disturbed by the distress they have observed in women, they feel isolated and 'expendable' in the clinical situation and have been more isolated from their peers due to the change from face-to-face classes to online classes (Kuliukas et al 2021).

Compassionate mind training (CMT) can help student midwives cope with the emotional demands and pressures of their work (Beaumont & Hollins Martin 2016). A UK study found student midwives who subject themselves to harsh judgment report high levels of burnout, compassion fatigue and decreased wellbeing, whereas those who practise self-kindness have lower levels of burnout and increased wellbeing (Beaumont & Hollins Martin 2016). Students and recently graduated midwives benefit from working to their full scope of practice and having role models in the workplace (Callendar et al 2021).

IMPACT OF MODEL OF CARE

Midwives working in a caseload model feel more positive about their work and have lower levels of burnout (Dawson et al 2018, Fenwick et al 2017). Although midwives providing continuity of care experience more autonomy, this can result in them being on call with unpredictable work hours (Dixon et al 2017). Self-employed midwives demonstrate improved emotional health and levels of empowerment (Dixon et al 2017). Midwives wish to work to their full scope of practice in a model supporting continuity of care rather than fragmented care (Callendar et al 2021). Continuity of care is considered the gold standard of care for women and is beneficial to midwives. However, in Australia only 8–20% of women receive continuity of care through a caseload model (Styles et al 2020). Therefore, most Australian midwives are working within a fragmented system. In New Zealand 38.15% of midwives work in a caseload model with an average caseload of 37 women per year (Midwifery Council Te Tatau o te Whare Kahu 2020). Midwives working on an employed basis in New Zealand worked fewer hours, but had higher levels of burnout and anxiety (Dixon et al 2017).

BURNOUT

In the UK, the Royal College of Midwives launched a campaign titled 'Caring for You' in recognition of the significant level of stress and burnout reported by midwives (Leversidge 2016). An online survey found Australian midwives reported high levels of personal and work-related burnout, with 64.9% reporting personal burnout (Creedy et al 2017). Approximately 20% of midwives indicated they had symptoms of anxiety, stress and depression. Burnout is implicated in the development of mental health conditions and, in this study, burnout was correlated with depression, anxiety and stress symptoms (Creedy et al 2017).

A UK review of midwives and nurses found concerning levels of burnout with 30–50% reporting poor mental wellbeing (Teoh et al 2020). The review also found midwives and emergency care nurses had the greatest risk for development of posttraumatic-stress

(Teoh et al 2020). Many midwives are unable to take the breaks to which they are entitled, become dehydrated and delay bathroom breaks due to lack of time (Leversidge 2016). Midwives need time to debrief and seek support from midwifery colleagues, friends and family, to retain their passion for midwifery and their resilience during difficult circumstances (Facius 2017).

STRESS

Stress negatively affects the health and wellbeing of midwives and has a negative impact on the women they care for (Warriner et al 2016). In times of stress, fear, anger and confrontation, the body is flooded with stress hormones which increase blood pressure, the heart rate, the release of glucose for energy and respiration, dilate the airways and pupils, halt digestion and send blood to the heart and muscles in preparation for action (Uvnäs Moberg 2011). Stress can lead to burnout. The signs of stress are difficulty sleeping, difficulty switching off, a sense of overstimulation, suppression of the immune system, minor ailments such as headaches, the common cold, muscle aches, physical tension, low mood, decreased concentration and diminished enjoyment of life accompanied by a feeling of being overwhelmed (Reading 2017). Stress also increases anxiety, irritability and reactivity, leading to a tendency to catastrophise and lose perspective (Reading 2017). Compassion fatigue may result from workplace stress and secondary traumatic stress; symptoms include lack of empathy, irritability and anger, hyperarousal, intrusive thoughts, anxiety and an increase in alcohol consumption (Beaumont & Hollins Martin 2016). Over time, stress results in both physical and psychological problems and it is important for the fight- or flight-driven system to be balanced by the calm and connect system to maintain good health (Uvnäs Moberg 2011).

THE BENEFITS OF SELF-CARE

Self-care helps restore balance and reduce stress (Reading 2017). Self-care and relaxation techniques induce the oxytocin-driven calm and connection system, which is associated with trust, friendliness, peace, calm, sensitivity, openness, interest in others, growth and healing (Uvnäs Moberg 2011). The calm and connected state results in lower blood pressure and heart rate, lower stress hormones and more effective digestion. This system is at work when the body is relaxed and provides increased access to problem-solving and creativity. The calm and connection system is the antithesis to the adrenaline-driven fight-or-flight system and can be activated by social interaction, security, warmth, touch, physical exercise, acupuncture, massage, meditation, yoga and tai chi (Uvnäs Mobert 2011). Oxytocin is believed to positively affect social memory, reduce anxiety and stress and increase learning. Under stress and pressure, it is difficult to focus on learning or to think clearly.

POSITIVE SELF-CARE BEHAVIOURS AND ACTIVITIES

Self-care for midwives involves getting to know themselves, being aware of their current behaviour and its consequences and considering the actions needed to provide self-care (Reading 2017). Self-awareness helps to identify factors that can be under one's personal control and those beyond one's individual control (Reading 2017). It is important to deal with unhelpful thinking, such as overthinking which entails excessively going over past actions, feelings and problems; this can cause a cascade of untoward effects such as feeling sad and pessimistic (Reading 2017). Self-care involves taking time out for nourishing activities that provide enjoyment and stress relief, such as reading, meditation, yoga, sport and exercise.

Another factor in self-care is being kind to yourself, practising gratitude, appreciating positive experiences, celebrating accomplishments and not engaging in harsh self-talk. Cultivate self-compassion by observing that inner voice and speaking to yourself as you would to your best friend (Reading 2017). Harsh self-talk is a form of self-sabotage and does not improve performance, health or wellbeing (Reading 2017). When considering actions and intentions, do so in a way that nurtures and enables personal growth (Reading 2017). Manage time by doing tasks or decide on deferring, delegating or dumping them. Manage energy and work towards being at peace with imperfection. Avoid taking on too much and prioritise important tasks.

Exercise, reflective clinical supervision, coping strategies and workplace strategies can be used to enhance work–life balance (Creedy et al 2017). Family-friendly work environments along with a work model that is empowering for midwives may decrease burnout (Fenwick et al 2017).

Howell (2016) lists the following tips for reducing stress.

- See things as they are; stress can result in increased sensitivity and vulnerability. Seeing things as they are helps with deciding if the issue is really something worth becoming stressed about.
- List the issues that result in stress and think about how to prevent stress from occurring in the first place; remember the event will pass.
- Talk about stress with colleagues rather than keeping it to yourself; sharing feelings helps midwives realise they are not on their own.
- Dial down the worry; if there is something to be done about the worry, then take steps to act, otherwise write it down or recognise its presence rather than wasting energy.
- Be positive with colleagues, listen to them and be pleasant by saying something positive about them and their skills or behaviours.

- Practise being grateful by spending some time focusing on the good parts of life and being thankful for them.
- Create a safe area; for example, by imagining having a protective field that deflects negative experiences.
- Ask for help; let someone know when assistance is required.
- Take time to relax; make a list of effective, personalised relaxation strategies.
- Develop strategies to help cope with difficult colleagues; remember it is impossible to change other individuals, only one's own individual reaction can be altered. This helps a person respond calmly, remain in control and avoid being reactive.
- Nourish the body with healthy food and snacks.
- Make a list of everything that needs to be done and divide them into smaller tasks.
- Create mini-breaks in the day by taking some deep breaths and focusing on the feeling in the body.
- Laugh or smile to relieve tension.
- Plan ahead before stressful situations and imagine coping well, remaining calm and being positive.
- Learn to say 'no' and avoid taking on other tasks when already feeling overwhelmed.
- Identify triggers by taking time to notice what causes stressed feelings and consider different ways to react.
- Be kind to yourself and take time to schedule in activities that are enjoyable.
- Learn stress-reduction techniques.

Mindfulness

Mindfulness includes meditation practices, being aware of the breath and observing thoughts, bodily sensations and daily activities (Warriner et al 2016). Research on mindfulness has found it effective in managing 'depression, anxiety, stress, psychosis, body image problems, abuse, trauma, eating disorders, ADHD, nicotine addiction, attention and memory problems, low self-esteem, work-related stress, psoriasis, acute and chronic pain', as well as relationship issues (Sinclair et al 2018, p. 5). Practising mindfulness reduces stress-related symptoms, improves the ability to respond to stress and effectively use coping strategies when under stress (Sinclair et al 2018).

Mindfulness facilitates midwives to consider how they think and feel about stressful experiences (Warriner et al 2016). Mindfulness meditation has been linked to neurological benefits, such as increased emotional intelligence and self-regulation (Warriner et al 2016). Midwives participating in mindfulness training found improvements at home and work, with mindfulness having a beneficial effect on stress and anxiety (Warriner et al 2016).

Mindfulness helps midwives reduce rumination, stress and burnout (Hunter 2016). Mindfulness is a way of being fully aware of the present moment with non-judgmental acceptance which helps avoid worrying about the past and being anxious about the future (Hunter 2016).

Mindfulness facilitates gaining perspective and being attentive and present in the moment, in an open, curious and non-judgmental manner (Hunter 2016).

Regularly practising mindfulness can improve motivation and energy, increase productivity and effectiveness, improve immune system function and general health, reduce stress and other mental health problems, improve communication skills and increase understanding and kindness (Sinclair et al 2018). A midwife who is calm and connected can work with greater focus and clarity (de-Vitry Smith 2016).

SKILL 51.1 Mindful breathing

1. Close your eyes.
2. Start noticing your breath.
3. Notice the natural rhythm and feeling of your breath.
4. Notice the sensation of air entering your nostrils as you inhale and the sensation of air leaving your nostrils as you exhale.
5. Notice the rise of your abdomen as you breathe in and the fall as you breathe out.
6. Remain aware of the natural rhythms of your breath.
7. Notice if there is a pause after you exhale.
8. Focus your attention on your breath.
9. If your attention wanders from your breath, notice the distraction and gently take your attention back to awareness of your breath, and the sensations and rhythm.
10. After a few more breaths, slowly open your eyes and notice your surroundings with the same awareness of the present moment.

Source: Adapted from Sinclair M, Seydel J, Shaw E: Mindfulness for busy people: turning from frantic and frazzled into calm and composed, 2nd ed., Pearson, London, 2018.

SKILL 51.2 The mindful STOP

The mindful stop provides an opportunity for self-connection and to develop wisdom. The purpose of mindfulness is to be aware of whatever is present.

S—stop
T—take three mindful breaths, feeling the breath flowing
O—observe the body, pay attention to any tension and let it go
P—continue your day

Source: Adapted from Bialylew E: The happiness plan, Affirm Press, South Melbourne, 2018.

Sleep

Midwifery often involves shiftwork, overtime and being on call; births may cluster together, resulting in long hours which can disrupt sleeping patterns and adversely impact sleep (Gruenberg 2016). Adequate sleep is essential to good health and fundamental for wellbeing. Sleep is important for cognitive function, including concentration, alertness, decision-making and memory (Lederle 2018). Sleep deprivation impairs emotional and cognitive processing, decreases impulse control and positive emotions, while increasing the intensity of negative emotions (Lederle 2018, p. 78). Due to the nature of their work, many midwives suffer from prolonged wakefulness, which can lead to injuries, errors and accidents (Gruenberg 2016). Midwives who are sleep deprived should sleep before driving home or organise alternative transport to avoid the risk of falling asleep behind the wheel (Gruenberg 2016). Inadequate sleep reduces positive mood, and is linked to cardiovascular and metabolic diseases, hypertension, diabetes, obesity, immune system suppression and hormonal irregularities (Lederle 2018).

Behaviours during the day affect night-time sleep. Behaviours that promote sleep include eating well, staying hydrated and using caffeine in moderation. Having regular mini-breaks during the day helps to minimise stress; this may be as simple as stopping for 30 seconds to notice the environment, how the body feels and focus on the breath (Lederle 2018). Try to do something that encourages a pleasant happy feeling each day and be active. If possible, avoid exercise in the last 3 hours before bedtime, otherwise it may be difficult to fall asleep due to an increased body temperature (Lederle 2018).

To promote sleep, avoid caffeine late in the day and create a bedtime ritual to aid relaxation and help wind down. A comfortable, cosy, dark, quiet and cool bedroom with a temperature of 16–18°C is ideal (Lederle 2018). Have a light, early dinner and avoid blue light from LED devices such as smartphones, laptops and tablets, because these screens increase alertness and suppress melatonin release.

Avoid or moderate alcohol consumption, because although alcohol can help with falling asleep quickly, it often results in a disturbance during the second half of the night (Lederle 2018). Taking time to relax in the evening is helpful. If waking occurs during the night and getting back to sleep is difficult, avoid using a phone or tablet, have an accepting attitude and avoid becoming frustrated. If the mind is racing, cognitive behaviour therapy (CBT) can assist, as well as relaxation and breathing techniques. Multiple websites and books are available to assist in these techniques.

Role and responsibilities of the midwife

These can be summarised as:

- recognising the need for self-care
- undertaking strategies to reduce stress, anxiety and burnout
- engaging in reflective practice
- remaining in good physical, psychological and emotional health
- having adequate sleep and rest to ensure safe care is provided

SUMMARY

- Self-care is essential for midwives and ensures they remain healthy physically, emotionally and psychologically.
- In order to provide high-quality, safe care, midwives need to avoid the negative consequences of stress, anxiety and burnout.
- The midwife should be aware of strategies to reduce or mitigate factors leading to stress, anxiety and burnout.
- Self-care improves the health of midwives.

Self-assessment exercises

The answers to the following questions may be found in the text.

1. List five strategies used to reduce stress.
2. Define self-care.
3. Describe the effects of burnout.
4. Discuss how to avoid sleep deprivation.
5. List the ill-effects of sleep deprivation.
6. Provide a definition of mindfulness.

References

Australian Nursing and Midwifery Federation (ANMF): Stress and bullying among chief concerns for nurses and midwives, Australian Nursing & Midwifery Journal 25(9):5, 2018.

Beaumont E, Hollins Martin C: Heightening levels of compassion towards self and others through use of compassionate mind training, British Journal of Midwifery 24(11):777–786, 2016.

Bradfield Z, Hauck Y, Homer C, et al: Midwives' experiences of providing maternity care during the COVID-19 pandemic in Australia, Women and Birth: Journal of the Australian College of Midwives, 2021.

Callander E, Sidebotham M, Lindsay D, Gamble J: The future of the Australian midwifery workforce—impacts of ageing and workforce exit on the number of registered midwives, Women and Birth: Journal of the Australian College of Midwives 34(1):56–60, 2021.

Coldridge L, Davies S: Am I too emotional for this job? An exploration of student midwives' experiences of coping with traumatic events in the labour ward, Midwifery 45:1–6, 2017.

Creedy DK, Gamble J: A third of midwives who have experienced traumatic perinatal events have symptoms of post-traumatic stress disorder, Evidence-Based Nursing 19(2):44, 2016.

Creedy DK, Sidebotham M, Gamble J, et al: Prevalence of burnout, depression, anxiety and stress in Australian midwives: a cross-sectional survey, BMC Pregnancy and Childbirth 17:1–8, 2017.

Cummins AM, Wight R, Watts N, et al: Introducing sensitive issues and self-care strategies to first year midwifery students, Midwifery 61:8–14, 2018.

Dawson K, Newton M, Forster D, et al: Comparing caseload and non-caseload midwives' burnout levels and professional attitudes: a national, cross-sectional survey of Australian midwives working in the public maternity system, Midwifery 63:60–67, 2018.

de-Vitry Smith S: Mindfulness for midwives, Australian Midwifery News 16(4):36–37, 2016.

Dixon L, Guilliland K, Pallant J, et al: The emotional wellbeing of New Zealand midwives: comparing responses for midwives in caseloading and shift work settings, New Zealand College Of Midwives Journal 53:5–14, 2017.

Facius C: 'Deepening the journey': learning how to midwife yourself, Australian Midwifery News 17(4):44–45, 2017.

Fedele R: The rise of burnout: an emerging challenge facing nurses and midwives, Australian Nursing & Midwifery Journal 25(5):18–23, 2017.

Fenwick J, Lubomski A, Creedy DK, et al: Personal, professional and workplace factors that contribute to burnout in Australian midwives, Journal of Advanced Nursing 74(4):852–863, 2017.

Gruenberg BU: A hard day's night, Midwifery Today 119:36–38, 2016.

Holland PJ, Tham TL, Gill FJ: What nurses and midwives want: findings from the national survey on workplace climate and well-being, International Journal of Nursing Practice 24(3):1, 2018.

Howell M: Resilience and stress management, MIDIRS Midwifery Digest 26(3):277–282, 2016.

Hunter L: Making time and space: the impact of mindfulness training on nursing and midwifery practice. A critical interpretative synthesis, Journal of Clinical Nursing 25(7/8):918–929, 2016.

Kuliukas L, Hauck Y, Sweet L, et al: A cross-sectional study of midwifery students' experiences of COVID-19: uncertainty and expendability, Nurse Education in Practice 51:102988–102988, 2021.

Lederle K: Sleep sense, Exisle Publishing, Dunedin, 2018.

Leversidge A: Caring for midwifery staff will ensure better care for women, British Journal of Midwifery 24(7):463, 2016.

Likis FE: Self-care: taking care of ourselves to optimize the care we provide, Journal of Midwifery & Women's Health 61(1):9–10, 2016.

Midwifery Council Te Tatau o te Whare Kahu: 2020 Midwifery Workforce Survey, 2020. Online: 12 April 2021. Available: www.midwiferycouncil.health.nz/common/Uploaded%20files/Workforce%20surveys/Midwifery%20Workforce%20Survey%202020.pdf.

Pougnet, R., Pougnet, L., Eniafe-Eveillard, M., & Loddé, B. Occupational health of midwives. Medycyna Pracy, 71(4), 473–481, 2020.

Reading S: The self-care revolution, Octopus Publishing Group, London, 2017.

Sinclair M, Seydel J, Shaw E: Mindfulness for busy people: turning from frantic and frazzled into calm and composed, 2nd ed., Pearson, London, 2018.

Smyth W, Lindsay D, Holmes C, et al: Self-reported long-term conditions of nurses and midwives across a northern Australian health service: a survey, International Journal of Nursing Studies 62:22–35, 2016.

Styles C, Kearney L, George K: Implementation and upscaling of midwifery continuity of care: the experience of midwives and obstetricians, Women and Birth: Journal of the Australian College of Midwives 33(4):343–351, 2020.

Teoh K, Kinman G, & Harriss A. Supporting nurses and their mental health in a world after Covid-19. Occupational Health, 72(8), 26–29, 2020.

Uvnäs Moberg K: The oxytocin factor: trapping the hormone of calm, love and healing, Pinter & Martin Ltd, London, 2011.

Warriner S, Hunter L, Dymond M: Mindfulness in maternity: evaluation of a course for midwives, British Journal of Midwifery 24(3):188–195, 2016.

Wright E: The ethical imperative of self-care: a call to action, Journal of Midwifery & Women's Health 65(6):733–736, 2020.

CHAPTER 52
MANUAL HANDLING

Learning outcomes

Having read this chapter, the reader should be able to:

- understand the principles of manual handling
- describe the anatomy of the spine and related structures, relating this to the mechanics of moving and handling
- discuss the responsibilities of both the employer and employee in reducing the risk of injury occurring when undertaking moving or handling
- identify situations that may put the midwife at increased risk of injury
- plan for and minimise, as able, the situations that may increase the chance of injury
- describe and understand strategies for self-care, including good posture.

This chapter provides an overview of manual handling in relation to the role of the midwife. Principles of moving and handling, minimising injury risk, and employers' and employees' responsibilities in relation to injury are discussed. The anatomy and physiology of the spine and its relation to moving, posture and injury are outlined. The risk of musculoskeletal injury in relation to the scope and practice of the midwife is covered and self-care suggestions are included.

WORK SAFETY

Due to the vast amount of changing legislation relating to manual handling in Australia and New Zealand, this chapter does not have the capacity to cover individual state and federal government policies. Midwives are advised to access their local and national legislation and guidelines as appropriate.

In Australia the *Work Health and Safety Act 2011* (Cwth) (Workplace OHS 2011) and in New Zealand the *Health and Safety Act 2015* (Parliamentary Counsel Office 2016) provide a consistent approach to the health and safety of all workers in every workplace. Government policies increase the emphasis on personal responsibility and managerial accountability. All employers should have systems in place to ensure the safety of their staff and must do 'all that is reasonably practicable' to safeguard workers and clients. Similarly, it is expected that all workers will ensure they are aware of policies and procedures in their workplace, including updating training when required (Workplace OHS 2011). Further reading on government policy relating to manual handling can be accessed at the websites of Safe Work Australia and WorkSafe New Zealand (see Resources at the end of the chapter).

Manual handling is defined as 'a hazardous manual task ... that requires a person to lift, lower, push, pull, carry or otherwise move, hold or restrain any person, animal or thing involving factors that stress the body' (Workplace OHS 2018). The Australian Nursing and Midwifery Federation (ANMF) (2018) Occupational Health and Safety Policy has a section on manual handling (Box 52.1).

Midwives are expected to maintain their knowledge of workplace safety in order to provide care for their clients, colleagues and themselves. Midwives are at risk of acute and chronic injuries from manual handling.

As previously defined, manual handling is the moving of items and/or people by lifting, lowering, carrying, pushing or pulling. Injuries can be caused by the impact of the weight of the item being handled, the frequency with which a movement is repeated, the distance an item is carried or moved and the height at which an object is picked up or put down. Manual handling injuries occur not only through incorrect moving and handling techniques and inappropriate moving and lifting, but can also be caused by poor posture, prolonged standing, twisting, bending and stretching (Kay & Glass 2011).

Injury to midwives may occur during non-clinical activities, such as doing computer work, writing

Box 52.1 ANMF's manual handling policy

The ANMF's manual handling policy states that all employees have the right to work within a workplace where:

- manual handling is eliminated wherever possible, or if not possible, reduced as far as possible
- the layout and design of the facility, furniture, fixtures and fittings are conducive to safe manual handling work practices
- appropriate manual handling equipment, aids and furniture are available and maintained in good order
- adequate staffing resources are in place to facilitate safe manual handling work practices
- training in the identification of manual handling hazards, risk assessment and safe work practices is provided
- nurses [and midwives] have input into the design and purchase of suitable equipment for manual handling purposes
- nurses [and midwives] have input into any changes to the workplace, work environment, equipment, furniture, work practices or training relevant to manual handling practices.

(Please note that although this policy only refers to nurses in its original wording; the policy also applies to midwives.)

Source: Australian Nursing and Midwifery Federation (ANMF): Safe patient handling policy, 2018. Online 15 October 2021. Available: www.anmf.org.au/documents/policies/P_Safe_Patient_Handling.pdf.

clinical notes, moving furniture such as beds, pushing wheelchairs, or moving meal trays and linen (Carta et al 2010). Midwives are particularly vulnerable to injuries when supporting women during labour and birth and assisting with breastfeeding.

Historically, health professionals were expected to put their clients' needs before their own, which included the expectation that pain or injury was just a part of the work of a midwife. It is unlikely that incidents or injury will ever be completely eradicated; however, through commitment to risk management and safe manual handling principles it is hoped the most severe cases can be eliminated and the frequency of incidents can be significantly reduced. To achieve this it is expected that midwives and their employers will adopt an evidence-based approach and maintain their knowledge, skills and attitudes towards safety during movement and manual handling.

Most developed countries are now adopting a 'no lift' policy for health professionals. In line with this, the ANMF (2018) has a 'no lift' policy which states that the lifting of people should only occur in *exceptional or life-threatening situations.*

Musculoskeletal disorders (MSDs) are the most common occupational disease in the European Union, accounting for 42–58% of all work-related illnesses with a high occurrence among hospital workers (Magnavita et al 2011). In Australia 17% of serious claims for injury occurred in the healthcare and social assistance industry in 2018–19 (Safe Work Australia 2021). In 2018 the Australian Institute of Health and Welfare (AIHW) compiled a report on the burden of disease in Australia. It included musculoskeletal conditions including back pain among the top five causes of burden of disease.

WorkSafe New Zealand's document *WorkSafe's Strategic Plan for Work-Related Health 2016 to 2026* identifies manual handling and psychosocial work factors as national workplace priorities (WorkSafe New Zealand 2016). MSDs such as back, neck and knee pain have previously been reported to account for the highest incidence of occupational disease in New Zealand, with over 50% of nurses reporting back and neck pain and over one-third reporting shoulder and knee pain (Harcombe et al 2014).

Injuries associated with manual handling can range from acute to chronic, with both having an impact on the workforce and society as a whole. Absence from work due to injuries or pain can affect the entire health system, with reduced staff, staff replacement costs and loss of clinical expertise. This in turn adds increased stress for the remaining work colleagues (Kane 2015, Warren 2016). The literature suggests that workplace injuries are underreported because many health professionals tend to consider pain an inevitable part of their work (Babiolakis et al 2015).

ANATOMY OF THE SPINE

The spine, or vertebral column, supports and is responsible for maintaining the upright posture of the body. The spinal column provides flexibility of movement and protects the spinal cord. The spine consists of 33 separate bones or vertebrae: 24 moveable and 9 fused vertebrae (Fig 52.1):

- seven cervical vertebrae: C1–C7 (the neck)
- twelve thoracic vertebrae: T1–T12 (the upper trunk)
- five lumbar vertebrae: L1–L5 (the lower trunk)
- five fused sacral vertebrae: S1–S5 (the sacrum)
- four fused coccygeal vertebrae (the coccyx).

The vertebrae articulate with their immediate neighbours, with muscles attached, and the thoracic vertebrae meet with the ribs. The coccyx articulates with the sacrum at the sacrococcygeal joint. Each vertebra has a main body, situated anteriorly, which acts as a shock absorber as the person's posture changes. The size of the vertebral body varies throughout the vertebral column, beginning with the small cervical

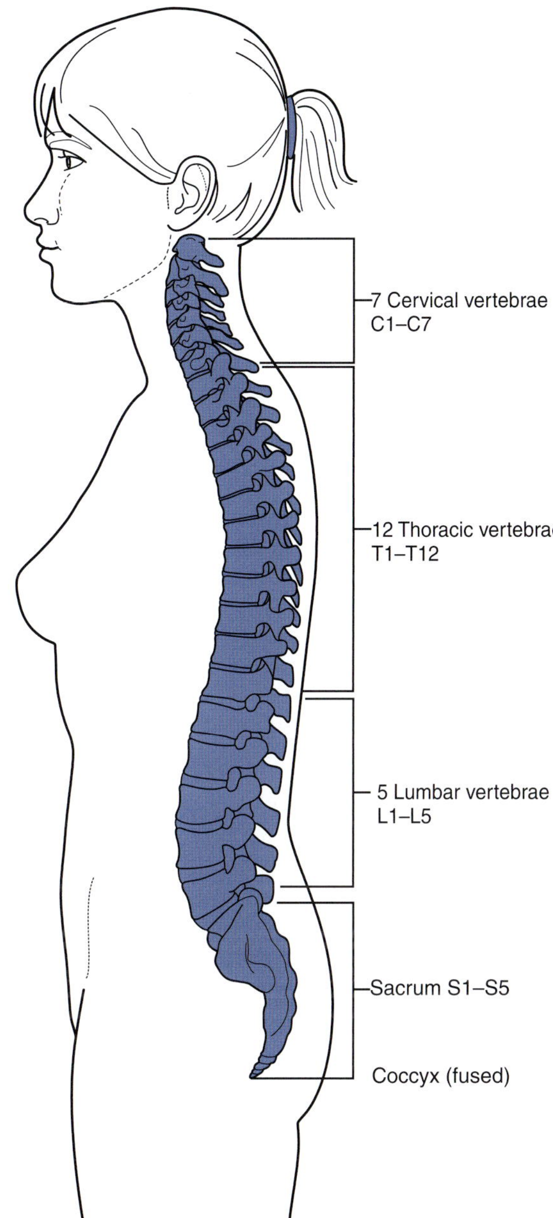

FIGURE 52.1 **Vertebral column: bones and curves.**
Source: Adapted with kind permission from Wilson KJW, Waugh A: Ross and Wilson anatomy and physiology in health and illness, 8th ed., Churchill Livingstone, Edinburgh, 1996.

vertebrae, and increasing in size to the lumbar vertebrae. Behind the body is the vertebral foramen, a large central cavity that contains the spinal cord, with nerves and blood vessels passing out through spaces between the vertebrae.

A flexible intervertebral disc connects the vertebral bodies to each other. These discs, which have a fibrocartilage outer layer surrounding an inner semisolid centre, assist with absorbing shock from movement and affect the flexibility of the spine. The vertebrae and discs are supported by ligaments that help to maintain the vertebrae in position and limit the amount of stress transmitted to the spine by restricting excessive movement. The ligaments do not produce as much support for the lumbar vertebrae, creating an inherent weakness in this area.

The spine supports the whole mass of the upper body. Weights carried in the arms or on the shoulders or excess body fat in an obese person cause increased strain on the spine.

The vertebral column is not straight, but has four curves (see Fig 52.1):

- cervical curve (convex curve anteriorly)
- thoracic curve (concave curve anteriorly)
- lumbar curve (convex curve anteriorly)
- sacral curve (concave curve anteriorly).

The first three spinal curves are important in relation to posture; when they meet in the midline centre of balance, weight distribution is balanced and a healthy posture ensues, protecting the supporting structures from injury. The female spine has an increased lumbar curve spanning three vertebrae (in males this mainly involves two vertebrae). This feature of the female spine is to counteract the effects of pregnancy when the centre of balance tends to shift forwards due to the increase in abdominal size to accommodate the growing fetus. This curves the spine more, which also increases the risk of back pain and injury. The facet joints are also larger and orientated at a slightly different angle in women (Kroemer 2017).

CONSIDERATIONS FOR MANUAL HANDLING

Prior to performing any manual handling, the midwife needs to adopt a risk management strategy that involves considering the hazard and the risk and applying risk controls.

A **hazard** is defined as something that can cause harm. Some examples of hazards with the potential to affect the midwife are trip hazards (e.g. items on the floor), slip hazards (e.g. wet floors) and infection control hazards (e.g. bodily fluids and equipment hazards, including badly stored equipment and clinical supplies). The *risk* is the possibility of harm to the midwife if exposed to the hazard (e.g. the risk of the midwife slipping on the wet floor). **Risk control** relates to the midwife taking actions in an attempt to eliminate health and safety risks. If it is not practical or the midwife is unable to completely remove the hazard, the midwife must attempt to reduce the risk. Totally removing a hazard will eliminate any risks associated with that hazard (Safe Work Australia 2018).

To attempt to control the risk, three levels of controls can be adapted to midwifery practice.

- Level 1 controls: Eliminate the hazard (e.g. remove the clutter to minimise the risk of tripping).

- Level 2 controls: Substitute the hazard with something safer (e.g. rather than lifting and carrying equipment, use a trolley).
- Level 3 controls: Do not control the hazard but rely on human action to reduce the risk, (e.g. wearing nonslip shoes to reduce the risk of slipping; education and training).

Four important categories need to be considered in relation to manual handling as they can affect the likelihood of an injury occurring: the task; the load; the working environment and the individual. These four areas can be made into an acronym to assist with recall: TILE (task, individual, load, environment) (Anderson, Carlisle, Thomson et al 2014, Warren 2016). The four areas will now be discussed in detail.

The task

The task can be divided into two parts: the process and the equipment available to complete the task if relevant.

The midwife should ask the following questions.

- Does the task involve a repetitive movement?
- Does it involve lifting?
- Does it involve pushing or pulling?
- Does it involve twisting or bending?
- What is the distance involved?
- What is the duration of the task?
- Can the task be completed by an individual or team?
- Is any equipment needed to complete the task?
- Does the task require holding an object or load away from the trunk?
- Does it involve reaching upwards or stretching?
- Does the task involve stooping?

Stress on the lower back increases as the load is moved away from the trunk; for example, if a load is held at arms-length, the stress can be approximately five times higher than if it were held close to the trunk. This stress increases significantly if the back is twisted or compressed or when bending over, as can occur when leaning over a bed or birth pool.

The spine has the ability to transit large forces. The larger movements of the trunk, such as bending and twisting, mostly occur in the lower part of the spine; overloading the spinal discs can make the lower back particularly vulnerable to pain and injury (Kroemer 2017). The lumbar vertebrae experience higher levels of stress when the back is bent and the knees are straight when attempting to lift a weight/load (Kroemer 2017). Prolonged stooping may contribute substantially to MSD symptoms (Warren 2016). Manual handling aids are available and should be used to move women who are unable to move themselves; for example, women post-caesarean section or with a high epidural block.

The load

The load should be assessed by asking simple questions. First, is the load an animate or an inanimate object? The answer to this question will obviously result in different assessment outcomes (Warren 2016). The midwife should ask the following questions.

- Is the load heavy? How heavy?
- How manageable is it? Is it bulky, unwieldy or difficult to hold?
- Is the load unstable (e.g. fluid)?
- Is the load harmful (e.g. sharp or hot)?

If the load is deemed to be heavy, consideration should be given to using lifting equipment or getting someone to assist with the task. A load that measures > 75 cm carries an increased risk of injury as it can be difficult to maintain a suitable grip and it can obscure the view in front of and beneath the person carrying it. Bulky objects can put extra strain on the body as holding them can be awkward and unstable loads result in having to continually adjust the body to the shifting weight (Anderson et al 2014, Warren 2016).

When a person needs to be moved, many factors can affect their ability to assist during movement. These can include physical, cognitive and behavioural factors. For example, if trying to assist a woman during labour, pain, fear and anxiety and the effects of medications may need to be considered. The client's safety must always remain a priority, but the midwife must not put themself at risk.

The working environment

Questions should be asked in relation to the environment including the presence of:

- constraints on posture
- wet or slippery floors
- obstructions including objects, doors or people; changes in floor levels; steps to negotiate; carpets or rugs
- adequate lighting.

The environment midwives work in can vary enormously. For example, the midwife attending a homebirth may have to consider household items, low lighting, small children and pets; in contrast the midwife working in the operating theatre may have medical equipment and automatic doors to contend with.

The individual

The individual should consider:

- their level of fatigue
- underlying health problems, injuries or pain
- whether the task is within their usual capabilities
- personal strength
- pregnancy, or recent birth
- if special training is required to complete the task.

The ability to carry out manual handling and physical activities varies between individuals. Considerations include age, gender, height and weight, and level of physical fitness. The individual may also have an underlying illness, be fatigued or have an existing injury. Preexisting medical problems, such as back or limb problems and pregnancy, can limit an individual's capabilities and increase their risk of injury (Govindu & Babski-Reeves 2014, Harcombe et al 2014, Warren 2016). As pregnancy progresses, it becomes more difficult for a woman to hold an object close to her body, and a longer arm reach is required to hold the load in place as gestation increases, placing more strain onto her arms and back (MacDonald et al 2013). Other physiological changes, such as increased joint laxity, may predispose the pregnant midwife to MSDs.

The maximum weight a person should lift is affected by position. Standing enables a person to lift significantly more weight than when they are sitting. The amount of weight lifted is also influenced by whether the elbows are bent or straight and the position of the object to be lifted—higher weights are easier to lift at waist height than at head or feet height. It is therefore important to take these factors into account when undertaking a risk assessment. It is also important to consider that the ability of the individual to carry out manual handling safely can also vary from day to day and hour to hour; just because the midwife was able to perform a manual handling activity at the beginning of the shift does not mean they will be able to do so at the end of the shift.

Applying risk management strategies and taking into consideration the four categories outlined, the midwife may be able to reduce the risk of injury.

ARE MIDWIVES AT RISK?

The majority of women and neonates are healthy; however, midwives may care for women with high-risk conditions or significant illness. Increasing medicalisation has resulted in more women giving birth with epidurals and by caesarean section. In these circumstances women require more assistance with movement and general care. Midwives may also be expected to move beds and other equipment.

Work-related upper quadrant MSD in midwives is not well researched. Long, Johnston and Bogossian (2013) conducted the first English-language investigation into the prevalence and risk factors for neck and upper back musculoskeletal symptoms in midwives as a distinct occupational group. Their study of Australian midwives found that neck and upper back musculoskeletal symptoms were prevalent in Australian midwives. Individual and work-related factors were significantly associated with the symptoms and injuries. Long, Johnston and Bogossian (2013) concluded that many workplace factors are not modifiable; however, the psychological demands of midwifery and the requirement to work in challenging postures when supporting women during birth and breastfeeding require attention from those involved in midwifery care.

The study by Long, Johnston and Bogossian (2013) reported a 'striking finding' which indicated that midwives who worked in awkward positions increased their risk of neck injuries by 35% and upper back injuries by nearly 50%. In all settings, supporting labouring women can be physically demanding. Midwives may be required to sit or stand for extended periods and to physically support the labouring or birthing woman. The woman should be able to birth in any position she finds comfortable; therefore, the midwife may often find themself in awkward positions during the birth, particularly if the woman is birthing: in water; in a standing, squatting or kneeling position; on the floor; or in a confined space. Providing sustained pressure or strong massage to the back and/or sacrum of a labouring woman can increase the chance of injury to the midwife. Psychological demands and stressors can also affect midwives' health and wellbeing. Psychosocial stresses are associated with organisational work practices and have been associated with increased MSD (Govindu & Babski-Reeves 2014, Long, Bogossian & Johnston 2013, Long, Johnston & Bogossian 2013).

Images showing the midwife in challenging positions, with their necks twisted, bent trunks, kneeling, squatting and leaning over birth pools are everywhere, and anecdotal reports still exist of women being told to put their feet against the midwife's hips to aid pushing efforts.

Midwives seem to be aware of the physical risks to themselves when supporting women to birth as they wish. Meyer, Weible and Woeber (2010) found that 75% of midwives worried about physical stressors in relation to supporting women to birth in water. In industrialised countries, the midwifery workforce is ageing; in Australia and New Zealand more than 50% of midwives are over 45 years old.

PRINCIPLES OF MOVING AND HANDLING

A person's centre of gravity changes depending on their body's position. The lower the centre of gravity (the pelvis area when standing), the more stable the person is. The closer a load is held to the body, the less stress there is on the body. The body is most stable when the feet are hip-width apart (Warren 2016). Whether midwives are assisting a client or lifting an object, the basic manual handling principles apply.

The risk of injury occurring when lifting a load can be reduced by straightening the spine and ensuring it is in alignment with the head (which should be raised and facing forwards), relaxing the knees, tightening the core muscles around the abdomen and back, and ensuring feet are shoulder-width apart (Fig 52.2). The compression forces increase with both the weight of the object and the further away from the body it is held, and directly affects the amount of stress placed on the lumbar spine (Kroemer 2017).

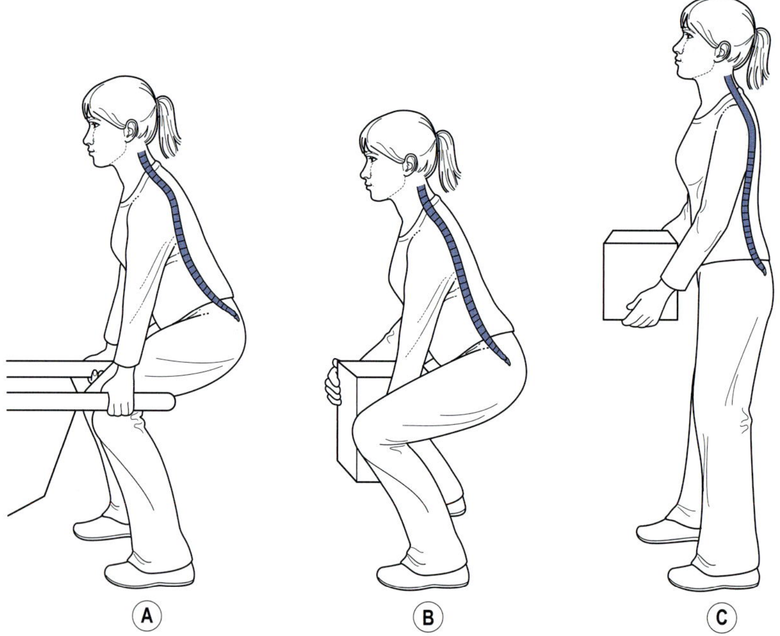

FIGURE 52.2 **The position of the spine when lifting a load.**
Source: Johnson R, Taylor W: Skills for midwifery practice, 4th ed., Elsevier, London, 2016.

SKILL 52.1 Lifting a load

When lifting a load, use the following principles.

1. Place feet shoulder-width apart to provide a wide, firm base.
2. Brace the lower back by tilting the pelvis forwards.
3. Bend from the knees, ensuring the knees do not go over the feet.
4. Lift using the thigh muscles.
5. Keep elbows and load close to the body.
6. Maintain a straight back when lifting or carrying.
7. Lift or carry an object with both hands.
8. Remain forward-facing.
9. Push rather than pull the object.
10. Avoid lifting the object above shoulder height.
11. Avoid repetitive movements where possible.
12. Avoid holding the same position for long periods of time.

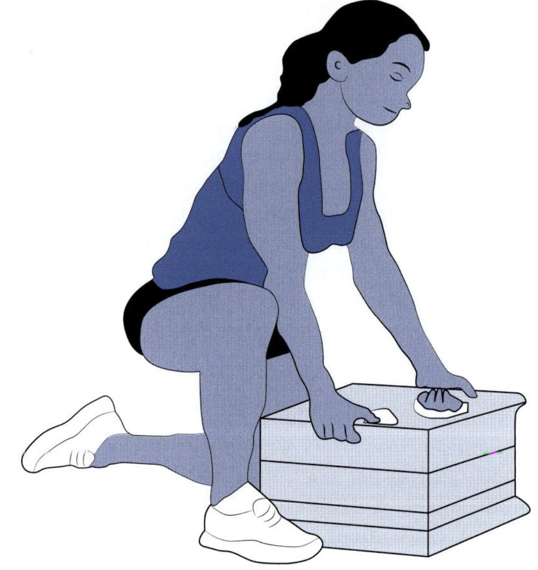

FIGURE 52.3 **The knight's position.**

When lifting a load from the floor, two positions can be used: the squat and the **knight's position**. The knight's position is a half-kneel; it is a very stable position but it may be difficult for some midwives to return to standing (Fig 52.3). The midwife should apply the principles outlined in the skill above and lower into a kneeling position with one knee on the floor beside the load. Lower into a kneeling position with one knee on the floor alongside the object. For the **squat position**, crouch down, apply the same principles as listed above and lower into a crouch position while keeping the spine straight (Fig 52.4).

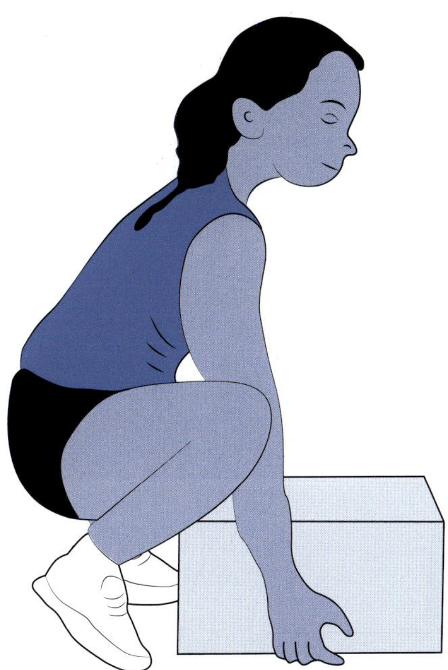

FIGURE 52.4 **The squat position.**

> **SKILL 52.2 Lifting a load using the squat or knight's position**
>
> To lift a load from the floor, use either a squat or knight's position, then the following principles.
>
> 1. Tip the object towards the body.
> 2. Hold the object from underneath.
> 3. Lift the load, applying safe manual handling principles.
> 4. Ensure the spine is straight and the core muscles are activated.
> 5. Use the thigh muscles to bear the weight when standing up.
> 6. Always use a trolley to move an object rather than carrying it.
> 7. Keep the load close to the body.

ASSISTING WOMEN TO MOVE

Ensuring women's independence with mobility is paramount; they must always be actively encouraged to participate in their own care. Manual assistance sometimes has to be offered, but must not involve lifting most or all of a women's weight unless, as previously discussed, it is a life-threatening situation. Always assess the woman's ability and encourage moving within their range of ability. Electric beds allow for variable positioning by having sections under the mattress that raise and lower by pressing a button, thus allowing the woman to raise the head of her bed to bring her to a sitting position or provide a knee break to stop her sliding down the bed. They also require less assistance from the midwife when repositioning.

If women are immobile or not able to move themselves, use appropriate moving and handling equipment. Manual handling aids such as slide sheets are readily available and easy to use. They work by two surfaces sliding over each other. For a semi-independent client, fold the slide sheet in half, placing the open ends in the direction you want to slide the client. When a woman needs to be moved from one bed to another (e.g. following a caesarean section), sliding devices and sheets should be used. Sliding the device underneath the woman, allow her to slide between the two surfaces with minimal effort from the midwives (Fig 52.5). When getting out of bed, the woman should be advised to turn onto her side and push herself upright with her hands, using the elbow nearest the bed as a prop. Once sitting upright, it will be easier for the woman to get up from the bed unaided, particularly if the bed is lowered so she can place her feet on the floor.

> **SKILL 52.3 Assisting a woman to move**
>
> The midwife should always explain the proposed moving procedure and gain consent prior to assisting the woman. Ensure she feels safe and that her dignity is maintained at all times. Explain what to expect and describe her role.
>
> 1. To assist a woman to turn in bed, ask her to move her head in the direction she will be turning.
> 2. The arm on the side she is turning towards should be moved from the side of her body or folded across her chest so she does not roll onto it.
> 3. The outside knee should be flexed and the arm brought across her chest in the direction of the roll. (The woman may need assistance flexing her knee if she cannot do this herself [e.g. with regional anaesthesia such as spinal or epidurals].)
> 4. The woman should then roll onto her side by pushing with her outside foot and reaching across her body or holding onto the bed rail with her outside hand.
> 5. If necessary, the midwife can help direct the roll by placing their hands on the woman's outside shoulder and hip while in a lunge position.
> 6. Using the verbal prompts 'ready', 'steady', 'roll', the woman is rolled onto her side as the midwife transfers their weight to their back foot, keeping their arms straight.

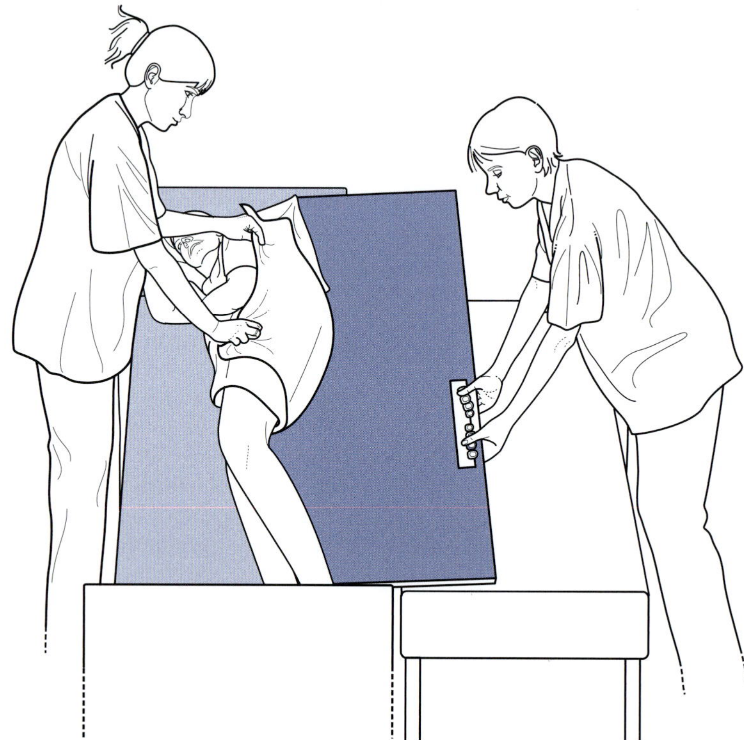

FIGURE 52.5 **Slide sheet placed underneath a woman.**
Source: Johnson R, Taylor W: Skills for midwifery practice, 4th ed., Elsevier, London, 2016.

POSTURES

Chronic low back pain is defined as pain lasting more than 12 weeks. It has a number of causes, including psychosocial factors such as work-related stress; however, the most frequent cause is muscle strain from bad posture. Research shows that when people receive education on improving body posture and ergonomic skills to decrease the load on the spine, their body posture improves and their pain is reduced (Govindu & Babski-Reeves 2014, Jaromi et al 2012).

Situations where bad posture can occur include:

- sitting for long periods (including driving)
- supporting a labouring woman
- assisting a woman during birth
- supporting a woman during labour and birth in water
- perineal suturing
- assisting with breastfeeding
- work involving prolonged bending (e.g. making beds).

Research shows that prolonged bouts of sitting, standing and awkward postures are clearly associated with injuries and pain (Babiolakis et al 2015, Govindu & Babski-Reeves 2014, Harcombe et al 2014, Long, Johnston & Bogossian 2012, Long, Bogossian & Johnston 2013, Long, Johnston & Bogossian 2013, Silva et al 2016). The human body is not designed to stay in the same position for long periods. Regular movement is essential. When kneeling, the midwife should use aids such as knee pads to support the joints. Kneeling for extended periods without moving should be avoided.

Sitting up with a straight back can cause the pelvis to tilt forwards, causing the posture to be maintained by the muscles, which tire quickly. The pressure on the intervertebral discs is increased when sitting compared with a standing position (Kroemer 2017). To reduce the need for muscle effort, slouching and bad posture can occur; rather than using the muscles to support the trunk, the ligaments are used, which places more load on the intervertebral discs and increases the chance of injury. This allows the pelvis to rotate backwards, so the posture and weight of the trunk are maintained more by the ligaments than the muscles. While this is effective in reducing the workload on the muscles, it doubles the force placed on the intervertebral discs, compared with the upright position (Kroemer 2017, Pheasant & Hargreaves 2005). Using a chair with a good back rest can reduce this pressure; the pelvis rotates backwards, as for the slouched position, but the spine flexes again when it comes into contact with the back of the chair. This results in less pressure being placed on the intervertebral discs, which can be reduced further by the use of a pad in the lumbar region, possibly to a pressure that is 30–40% lower than when in a standing position (Pheasant & Hargreaves 2005).

Stooped posture

During situations such as labour, birth and breastfeeding, the midwife may adapt a stooped posture, where the trunk is inclined forwards. In this situation the weight of the upper body is supported by postvertebral muscles. Contraction of these muscles can result in compression of the intervertebral discs.

Asymmetric posture

An asymmetrical posture, involving side bending, is sometimes adopted by the midwife during birth, particularly if the woman is squatting, standing or on all-fours and the midwife is on the floor. This increases pressure on the spine, predisposing the midwife to injury. Whenever the midwife is required to adopt an unusual position, they should carefully consider maintaining a symmetrical posture and avoid maintaining the position for long periods of time to prevent placing undue pressure on the muscles and ligaments.

Employers' responsibilities

Specifically, employers should:

- avoid hazardous manual handling operations as far as reasonably practicable
- assess any hazardous manual handling operations that cannot be avoided
- reduce the risk of injury as far as is reasonably practicable.

Furthermore, if an employee is complaining of discomfort, any changes employed to avoid or reduce manual handling should be monitored to determine if they are having a positive effect. If this is not the case, alternatives must be considered.

A risk assessment should be undertaken for any situation requiring manual handling, ideally before the situation arises to allow sufficient time for measures to reduce the risk of injury (e.g. use of appropriate equipment).

Role and responsibilities of the midwife

These can be summarised as:

- being familiar with the manual handling policy and attending regular training sessions
- informing the employer of any situations in which a risk assessment should be undertaken
- using moving and handling equipment correctly
- knowing how to lift a load correctly
- being able to achieve a good posture in the position adopted
- recognising situations where there is potential for injury and taking steps to reduce the risk
- ensuring that undertaking an activity does not put midwives or others at risk.

SUMMARY

- Be aware of legislation and policies applying to the workplace.
- Always use a risk assessment approach and TILE (task, individual, load, environment) when performing manual handling.
- Encourage support and promote a 'no lift' approach in the workplace.
- Assess manual handling tasks to reduce the risk of injury occurring.
- Incorrect moving and handling techniques can cause serious damage to the health of the midwife and may cause physical and psychological harm to the person being moved.
- The midwife should not be involved in lifting another person without appropriate manual handling equipment unless it is a life-threatening situation.
- Poor posture increases the risk of physical injury.
- Maintaining psychological and physical health helps reduce the risk of MSD.

Self-assessment exercises

The answers to the following questions may be found in the text.

1. What are the responsibilities of the midwife and the employer in relation to moving and handling?
2. Describe the anatomy of the spine and associated structures that are involved in the mechanics of moving and handling.
3. Identify five clinical situations that may place the midwife at increased risk from a manual handling injury and discuss how the midwife can reduce the risk.
4. When lifting a load, how can the risk of injury be reduced?
5. How can the midwife achieve a good posture and what is the significance of a poor posture?

Resources

Safe Work Australia: Model code of practice: Hazardous manual tasks. www.safeworkaustralia.gov.au/doc/model-code-practice-hazardous-manual-tasks.

WorkSafe New Zealand: Manual handling. https://worksafe.govt.nz/topic-and-industry/manual-handling/.

References

Anderson MP, Carlisle S, Thomson C, et al: Safe moving and handling of patients: an interprofessional approach, Nursing Standard 28(46):37–41, 2014.

Australian Institute of Health and Welfare (AIHW): Burden of disease, 2018. Online 15 October 2021. Available: www.aihw.gov.au/reports-data/health-conditions-disability-deaths/burden-of-disease/overview.

Australian Nursing and Midwifery Federation (ANMF): Safe patient handling policy, 2018. Online 15 October 2021. Available: www.anmf.org.au/documents/policies/P_Safe_Patient_Handling.pdf.

Babiolakis CS, Kuk J, Drake DM: Differences in lumbopelvic control and occupational behaviours in female nurses with and without a recent history of low back pain due to back injury, Ergonomics 58(2):235–245, 2015.

Carta A, Parmigiani F, Roversi A, et al: Training in safer and healthier patient handling techniques, British Journal of Nursing 19(9):576–582, 2010.

Govindu NK, Babski-Reeves K: Effects of personal, psychosocial and occupational factors on low back pain severity in workers, International Journal of Industrial Ergonomics 44:335–341, 2014.

Harcombe H, Herbison GP, McBride D, et al: Musculoskeletal disorders among nurses compared with two other occupational groups, Occupational Medicine 64:601–607, 2014.

Jaromi M, Nemeth A, Kranciz J, et al: Treatment and ergonomic training of work-related lower back pain and body posture problems for nurses, Journal of Clinical Nursing 21:1776–1784, 2012.

Kane J: Intervention needed for manual handling safety, Kai Tiaki Nursing New Zealand 21(10):18–21s, 2015.

Kay K, Glass N: Debunking the manual handling myth: an investigation of manual handling knowledge and practices in the Australian private health sector, International Journal of Nursing Practice 17:231–237, 2011.

Kroemer K: Fitting the human: introduction to ergonomics, 7th ed., Routledge, Abingdon, Oxon, 2017.

Long MH, Bogossian FE, Johnston V: Functional consequences of work-related spinal musculoskeletal symptoms in a cohort of Australian midwives, Women and Birth e50–e58, 2013.

Long MH, Johnston V, Bogossian FE: Helping women but hurting ourselves? Neck and upper back musculoskeletal symptoms in a cohort of Australian Midwives, Midwifery 29:359–367, 2013.

Long MH, Johnston V, Bogossian FE: Work-related upper quadrant musculoskeletal disorders in midwives, nurses and physicians: a systematic review of risk factors and functional consequences, Applied Ergonomics 43: 455–467, 2012.

MacDonald LA, Waters TR, Napolitano PG, et al: Clinical guidelines for occupational lifting in pregnancy: evidence summary and provisional recommendations, American Journal Obstetrics Gynaecology 209(2):80–88, 2013.

Magnavita N, Elovainio M, De Nardis I, et al: Environmental discomfort and musculoskeletal disorders, Occupational Medicine 61(3):196–201, 2011.

Meyer SL, Weible CM, Woeber K: Perceptions and practice of waterbirth: a survey of Georgia midwives, Journal of Midwifery and Women's Health 55(1):55–59, 2010.

Parliamentary Counsel Office: Health and Safety at Work Act 2015. New Zealand Legislation, 2016. Online 18 October 2021. Available: www.legislation.govt.nz/act/public/2015/0070/latest/DLM5976660.html.

Pheasant S, Hargreaves C: Bodyspace: anthropometry, ergonomics and the design of work, 3rd ed., Taylor and Francis, London, 2005.

Safe Work Australia: Australian Workers' Compensation statistics 2018–19, 2021. Online 15 October 2021. Available: www.safeworkaustralia.gov.au/collection/australian-workers-compensation-statistics.

Safe Work Australia: Model code of practice: hazardous manual tasks, 2018. Online 18 October 2020. Available: www.safeworkaustralia.gov.au/doc/model-code-practice-hazardous-manual-tasks.

Silva C, Barros C, Cunha L, et al: Prevalence of back pain problems in relation to occupational group, International Journal of Industrial Ergonomics 52:52–58, 2016.

Warren G: Moving and handling reducing risk through assessment, Nursing Standard 30(40):49–58, 2016.

WorkSafe New Zealand: WorkSafe's Strategic Plan for Work-Related Health 2016 to 2026, 2016. Online 18 October 2021. Available: www.worksafe.govt.nz/dmsdocument/1448-worksafes-strategic-plan-for-work-related-health-2016-2026.

Workplace OHS: Work Health and Safety Act 2011. Commonwealth legislation. Online 18 October 2021. 2011. Available: http://workplaceohs.com.au/legislation/commonwealth-legislation.

Workplace OHS: Manual handling, 2018. Online 18 October 2021. Available: http://workplaceohs.com.au/hazards/manual-handling.

CHAPTER 53
WORKPLACE HEALTH AND SAFETY

Learning outcomes

Having read this chapter, the reader should be able to:

- understand workplace health and safety management
- apply workplace health and safety management methods, techniques, processes and practices
- identify workplace stress and burnout and optimise one's own emotional health and wellbeing.

The provision of healthcare occurs in professions and workplaces that pose a range of risks to their employees. Workplace health and safety (WHS) legislation (previously and sometimes still occasionally referred to as occupational health and safety or OHS) has existed to minimise the risk to employees of workplace risk-related illness and injury in some form in both New Zealand and Australia since the late 1800s (Australian Council of Trade Unions n.d., Peace et al 2019), and it is updated regularly. Midwives should be aware of the legislative requirements affecting safety within their workplace and demonstrate a commitment to addressing the health, safety and welfare of all who visit and work in the workplace.

BACKGROUND

Issues affecting midwives

Like other healthcare professionals, midwives are exposed to an ever-changing array of occupational and workplace risks. In New Zealand, WHS is regulated by WorkSafe, which is a Crown agency with a governance board; its members are appointed by the New Zealand Minister for Workplace Relations and Safety. In Australia, the government statutory body Safe Work Australia fulfils the role of developing national policy relating to WHS.

According to SafeWork Australia (2020), 17% of serious claims in 2018–19 were from the healthcare and social assistance industry. Workplace risks and hazards for midwives include body stress derived from muscular stress as a result of manual handling (e.g. pushing, pulling, lifting, carrying, stress from physical movements or repetitive movements). Other work-related injuries comprise of: falls, trips and slipping; hitting objects; being hit by objects; heat, radiation and electricity; and chemical and other substances. Pressures, sound (noise), mental stress and biological factors can also lead to injuries. These come at a high cost to workers and employers. In particular, fatigue, workplace stress and pathogens are the most likely risk factors for midwives, ahead of other factors such as bullying and violence (De Cieri et al 2015).

The need for careful monitoring continues in the workplace (Fig 53.1). Staff have a right to feel safe in their work environment and employers have a responsibility towards ensuring risks are minimised. When midwives experience workplace injuries, it can have a significant impact on their life, career and financial commitments. Workplace injuries also have an effect on the workplace (NSW Nurses and Midwives' Association, 2013). The midwife has a particular skill set based on where they work. When the midwife is injured and unable to work effectively and efficiently, the skill set is compromised. This, in turn, often increases the workload on other midwives. The cost of workplace injuries also adds to the financial burden for the employer. These costs are associated with replacement and re-training of staff, injury investigation and workers compensation premium. Therefore, preventing injuries is of great importance. Midwives work in a variety of positions

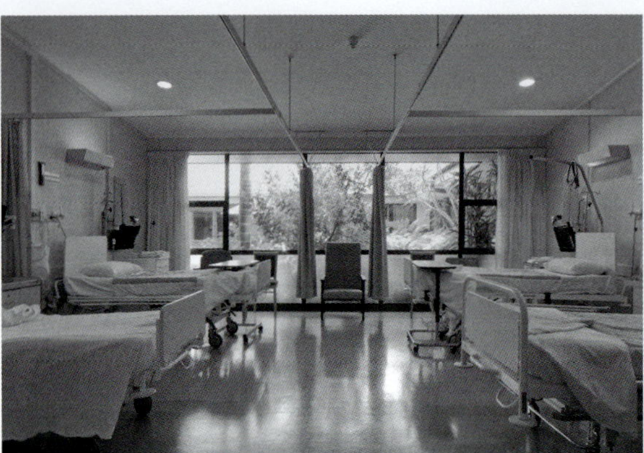

FIGURE 53.1 **Workplace injuries have declined for midwives, but it is still an area of great importance. iStockphoto/ep_stock**

within an organisation – as clinicians, managers and educators – and need to be committed to ensuring a safe workplace.

WORKPLACE HEALTH AND SAFETY AND PATIENT SAFETY

Workplace health and safety also extends to patient safety. When receiving care, patients are also at risk of injury from incidents such as burns, falls or poor manual handling. Therefore, the safety of patients and workers supplement each other. Safety for everyone should be the cornerstone of practice. As identified in Australia's *Work Health and Safety Act 2011* (Cth) and New Zealand's *Health and Safety at Work Act 2015*, the primary duty of care is for the person providing the care to ensure the health and safety of others, including patients, and no one should be at risk of harm. Similarly, patients have obligations to take reasonable care for their own safety and avoid putting others at risk, while at the same time complying with safety regulations.

Workers' compensation

In New Zealand, a no-fault accidents (and injury) compensation scheme exists for all who live there or who sustain an injury while visiting. In Australia, workplace accident and injury compensation is delivered through 11 main workers compensation systems. Each of the eight Australian states and territories have developed their own workers compensation scheme and there are three Commonwealth schemes: the first is for Australian Government employees, the employees of licensed self-insurers and Australian Defence Force personnel with service prior to 1 July 2004; the second is for certain seafarers; and the third is for Australian Defence Force personnel for service on or after 1 July 2004 (Safe Work Australia 2019). The schemes manage work health and safety, workers compensation and laws on injury management. This is achieved by giving advice to the employer and workers that focuses on specific issues, such as returning to work after injury and investigating complaints and incidents. Enforcement and compliance of workplace health and safety is monitored by inspectors through regular assessments of the workplace, as well as evaluating the incidence of harmful incidents and near misses, and the steps taken by the employer to prevent incidents (Lyons 2017). Best practice approach for compliance is through cooperation and persuasion, leading to sanctions when there is inadequate or non-cooperation by the duty holder (Lyons 2017). Various factors are also considered when determining enforcement action, such as the seriousness of the potential breach, the culpability of the duty holder, the extent of the potential risk, non-compliance history, whether the duty holder was registered to practice, whether there was an attempt to minimise the risk, and whether attempts or plans have been made to address the issue for safety.

Midwives form part of the healthcare industry. According to the Queensland Nurses and Midwives Union (cited in Lyons, p. 32), healthcare accounts for the highest employment rate in the state. As reported by Lyons (2017), healthcare is a priority industry for injuries. A survey in Queensland which included nurses and midwives, identified a high incidence of musculoskeletal disorders, followed by mental health conditions requiring sick days off work (Lyons 2017). Hence, midwives need to be committed to compliance for a safe workplace for all.

Further measures to improve compliance are recommended to encourage safe work practices. These include:

- increasing the capability of health and safety representatives (work-elected)
- greater emphasis on the role of the workplace health and safety officer (management-appointed)
- the right to information in order to be proactive in minimising risks
- the health and safety representative's right to access employer information to determine risks
- a timely response to notification of serious incidents.

Role of agencies and organisations

The employer and various organisations play an important role in promoting workplace health and safety. Strategies used include providing a position statement or policy, a policy manual, induction and re-training programs, an annual review of competency skills, and maintaining a database of workers and their completion of annual mandatory educational modules.

An example of a policy statement is one by the Australian Nursing and Midwifery Federation (2021), within which responsibilities for the employer and employee are clearly specified.

LEGISLATION

Legislation on workplace health and safety is designed to support industry and workers so they understand what is needed to comply with the Act for that particular country or state. In New Zealand the legislation is covered by the *Health and Safety at Work Act 2015*, while Australia has the *Work Health and Safety Act 2011*. These each provide a framework within which standards and strategies are derived. Employees need to be given protection in relation to health and safety from their workplace. Employers also need to provide means of protection such as resources, policies and procedures, and strategies to minimise risk (Fig 53.2). Further, service users need to feel safe and experience 'no harm'. Essentially, the legislation is about looking after one another and doing the right thing. Everyone is accountable to ensure a safe workplace and a safe place to receive care.

For the midwives, it is about duty of care for mothers and babies, their families and looking after oneself and colleagues in the workplace. To achieve this, midwives need to focus on several areas, some of which are included below.

- Maintain standards of practice as a midwife as per the relevant registration body.
- If working as an independent midwife, have indemnity insurance.
- Maintain annual registration.
- Ensure professional practice support.
- Establish a work–life balance with regular recreational leave.
- Ensure equipment is serviced regularly (e.g. equipment loaned to clients, handheld Dopplers).
- Maintain optimal means of communication (e.g. mobile phone, paging system, particularly in rural settings).
- Know how to contact emergency services.
- Ensure safe storage of documents and records.

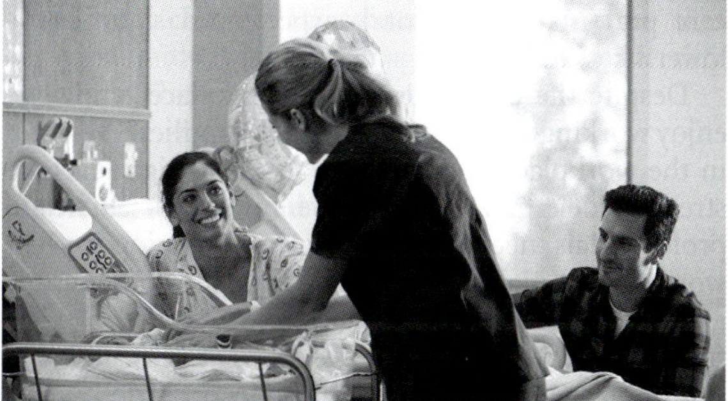

FIGURE 53.2 **Midwives must help ensure the safety of clinical environments. iStockphoto/monkeybusinessimages**

- Consider the possibility of cross-contamination (e.g. use gloves).
- Use barrier consumables where necessary (e.g. disposable gloves) (New Zealand College of Midwives 2017).

Standards for National Safety and Quality Health Service

In Australia, there are eight National Safety and Quality Health Service (NSQHS) standards, provided by the Australian Commission on Safety and Quality in Health Care (ACSQHC), that require strategies implemented in healthcare organisation-wide systems to meet quality and safety outcomes. They are clinical governance, comprehensive care, developing partnerships with consumers of care, safety in medication administration, healthcare-associated infections, therapeutic and effective communication, blood and blood products management, and monitoring for and responding to acute deterioration of illness or condition (ACSQHC 2021). With new and better practices since the first edition of these standards, improvements have been seen in several areas, including a reduction in *Staphylococcus aureus* bacteraemia infection rate from 1.1 to 0.87 cases per 10,000 patient days; a drop in central line associated bloodstream infections; and improved documentation of adverse drug reactions and medication history.

The equivalent body to the ACSQHC in New Zealand is the Health Quality and Safety Commission. The focus for the Commission is to compare healthcare services across the country and to the rest of the world. The measurement and evaluation provides a guide on stimulating improvement in quality care (Health Quality and Safety Commission New Zealand 2017).

Policy and code for practice

Aligned with legislation and standards, policies are developed. Policies on workplace health and safety are promoted by registering and professional bodies, healthcare employers and other organisations, such as unions. The New Zealand College of Midwives provides for a Health and Safety at Work Policy, while the Australian Nursing and Midwifery Federation has a specific policy titled Occupational Health and Safety. Some common features are listed below.

Manual handling

- Avoid manual handling where possible.
- Ensure the layout of the workplace, furniture, fixtures and equipment are beneficial to safe manual handling practices.
- Ensure manual handling equipment is available and maintain it in good order.
- Ensure appropriate staffing and skill-mix to allow for safe manual handling practices.
- Undertake training in manual handling, risk assessment and safe practice.

Role and responsibilities of the midwife

These can be summarised as:

- having an understanding of the hazards and risks involved in the nature of one's work (e.g. violence, contamination, infection, needle-stick injuries)
- adhering to policies and procedures set by the employer
- being familiar with the location and content of policy and procedure manuals
- being familiar with the reporting of incidents that may occur (e.g. falls)
- being familiar with use of resources and processes to ensure safety (e.g. have fire safety knowledge, know evacuation drill)
- reporting hazards or incidents immediately after it is known (e.g. medication error)
- taking reasonable precautions in ensuring the safety of oneself and that of others at all times
- participating in the information session and complying with annual mandatory WHS skills
- developing practical steps to create a fair and productive workplace
- being familiar with the workplace discrimination and harassment policy
- understanding the meaning of bullying, harassment and discrimination
- being informed about the discriminating factors that exist
- knowing how discriminating factors apply to one's own behaviour.

SUMMARY

- Midwives and those they care for are at risk of injury from a range of sources in the clinical environment.
- The primary duty of care providers is to ensure the health and safety of others.
- Workplace health and safety legislation in both Australia and New Zealand provides employing organisations with information to develop a WHS operational policy framework, standards and strategies.
- There are many ways in which midwives can help to protect themselves, their colleagues and those in their care from physical, psychological and emotional harm.
- Safe midwifery practice environments rely on the presence of six key factors.
- Midwives in leadership and management positions have a pivotal role to play in WHS.

Self-assessment exercises

The answers to the following questions may be found in the text.

1. What do you understand by workplace health and safety? What is the other term frequently used?
2. What are some of the issues affecting midwives in the workplace?
3. Identify some of the injuries that can occur in the workplace. Who is responsible for these?
4. What roles do the following people play in ensuring workplace health and safety?
   a. Midwives
   b. Senior management
   c. Other healthcare professionals
   d. Patients
5. In what way is workplace health and safety enforced?
6. Are other agencies and professional organisations involved in ensuring safety for all? In what way?
7. Summarise the responsibilities of the midwife in relation to workplace health and safety.
8. Identify the related legislation in force in your country. How is this translated and sifted down into the workplace?
9. Explain what you understand by the Standards for National Safety and Quality Health Service.
10. What do you understand the term 'manual handling' to mean?
11. What is the impact of high or chronic stress in the workplace? List some of the contributing factors.
12. List some of the protective factors that can help the midwife cope with stress in the workplace.
13. How can good leadership help in promoting a safe and healthy workplace?

References

Australian Commission on Safety and Quality in Health Care (ACSQHC): National safety and quality health service standards. 2nd ed.—version 2. ACSQHC, Sydney, 2021. Available: www.safetyandquality.gov.au/sites/default/files/2021-05/national_safety_and_quality_health_service_nsqhs_standards_second_edition_-_updated_may_2021.pdf.

Australian Council of Trade Unions: Workplace Health and Safety in Australia, n.d. Online 5 October 2021. Available: www.actu.org.au/ohs/about-us/workplace-health-and-safety-in-australia.

Australian Nursing and Midwifery Federation (ANMF): Work health and safety: ANMF Policy. Australian Nursing and Midwifery Federation, 2021. Online 5 October 2021. Available: https://anmf.org.au/documents/policies/P_Work_health_and_safety.pdf.

Australian Public Service Commission: State of the service report 2014–15. Canberra, Commonwealth of Australia, Canberra, 2015.

Banovcinova L, Baskova M: Sources of work-related stress and their effect on burnout in midwifery, Procedia, Social and Behavioral Sciences 132(SupplC):248–254, 2014.

Creedy DK, Sidebotham M, Gamble J, et al: Prevalence of burnout, depression, anxiety and stress in Australian midwives: a cross-sectional survey, BMC Pregnancy and Childbirth 17:13, 2017.

Dabrowski R: Midwives under high levels of stress, The Royal College of Midwives. 7 March 2017. Online 11 July 2018. Available: www.rcm.org.uk/news-views-and-analysis/news/'midwives-under-high-levels-of-stress'.

De Cieri H, Shea T, Sheehan C, et al: Leading indicators of occupational health and safety: a report on a survey of Australian Nursing and Midwifery Federation (Victorian Branch) members, 2015. Online 5 October 2021. Available: https://research.iscrr.com.au/__data/assets/pdf_file/0010/297262/Measuring-the-leading-indicators-of-OHS-Report-for-survey-of-Australian-Education-Union-AEU-Members.pdf.

Fenwick J, Toohill J, Gamble J, et al: Effects of a midwife psycho-education intervention to reduce childbirth fear on women's birth outcomes and postpartum psychological wellbeing, BMC Pregnancy and Childbirth 15(1):284, 2015.

Fidele R: The rise of burnout: an emerging challenge facing nurses and midwives, Australian Nursing & Midwifery Journal 25(5):19–21, 2017.

Health Quality and Safety Commission New Zealand: Health Quality and Safety Commission New Zealand, 2017. Online 15 May 2018. Available: www.hqsc.govt.nz/our-programmes/health-quality-evaluation/about-us/.

Hogan R, Orr F, Cummins A: Sustaining 'super' midwives: building resilience in midwifery students, Women and Birth 28:S18, 2015.

Jepsen I, Juul S, Foureur M, et al: Is caseload midwifery a healthy work-form? A survey of burnout among midwives in Denmark, Sexual & Reproductive Healthcare 11(SupplC):102–106, 2017.

Lyons T: Best practice review of workplace health and safety Queensland: final report. July 2017.

McAllister M, McKinnon J: The importance of teaching and learning resilience in the health disciplines: a critical review of the literature, Nurse Education Today 29(4):371–379, 2009.

Midwifery Council of New Zealand: 2020. Code of Conduct Midwifery. Council of New Zealand. Online 5 October 2021. Available: www.midwiferycouncil.health.nz/Public/Midwifery-in-Aotearoa—New-Zealand/I-am-a-registered-midwife/Standards-of-Clinical—-Cultural-Competence—-Conduct/Public/06.-I-am-a-registered-midwife/1.-Standards-of-Clinical—-Cultural%20 Competence—-Conduct.aspx?hkey=b3251793-36c1-46b8-821f-afb858c8b04a.

Mollart L, Skinner VM, Newing C, Foureur, M: Factors that may influence midwives work-related stress and burnout, Women and Birth: Journal of the Australian College of Midwives 26(1):26–32, 2013.

New Zealand College of Midwives: Health and Safety at Work Policy, New Zealand College of Midwives, 2017. Online 5 October 2021. Available: https://www.midwife.org.nz/wp-content/uploads/2019/06/Health-and-Safety-Policy-2017.pdf.

NSW Nurses and Midwives' Association: Work health and safety essentials for nurses and midwives. New South Wales Nurses and Midwives' Association, 2013.

Nursing and Midwifery Board of Australia: Code of Conduct for midwives, NMBA, 2018. Online 5 October 2021. Available: www.nursingmidwiferyboard.gov.au/codes-guidelines-statements/professional-standards.aspx. Accessed 5 October 2021

Peace C, Lamm F, Dearsly G, Parkes H: The evolution of the OHS profession in New Zealand. Safety Science. 120, 2019, pp. 254–262.

Safe Work Australia: 2020. Key WHS statistics Australia 2020. Online 5 October 2021. Available: www.safeworkaustralia.gov.au/sites/default/files/2020-11/Key%20Work%20 Health%20and%20Safety%20Stats%202020.pdf.

Safe Work Australia: Comparison of workers' compensation arrangements in Australia and New Zealand, 27th ed., 2019. Online 5 November 2021. Available: www.safeworkaustralia.gov.au/system/files/documents/2001/comparison-report-2019.pdf.

Southwick S, Bonanno G, Masten A, et al: Resilience definitions, theory, and challenges: interdisciplinary perspectives, European Journal of Psychotraumatology 5(10):3402, 2014.

Williams A, McDonald C: Five tell-tale signs of burnout, The Australian Journal of Advanced Nursing 25(5): 22–23, 2017.

GLOSSARY

5 moments for hand hygiene: An evidence-based approach to hand hygiene which defines the key moments when hand hygiene should be undertaken by healthcare workers.

abdominal palpation: Palpation of the abdomen to determine fundal height, fetal position and any deviations from normal during pregnancy and labour.

abnormally adherent placentation: The placenta is deeply attached to the uterine wall and does not easily separate during the third stage of labour to allow delivery of the placenta. Incudes placenta accreta, increta and percreta.

active management of third-stage labour (AMTSL): Process whereby the expulsion of the placenta after birth is assisted by a set of medical interventions rather than being left to occur naturally.

active phase (first stage of labour): The period between the cervix being fully effaced and 4 cm dilated and the birth of the baby. **(second stage):** The phase at the end of labour when the woman is actively pushing her baby/ies out.

airborne precautions: In addition to standard precautions, a correctly fitted N95 or P2 respirator mask is worn when entering or leaving a room.

amnicot: Small, disposable, rubber latex fingertip cot with a hook attached, used for artificially rupturing membranes.

amnihook: Long, plastic, disposable instrument with a sharp hooked end, used for artificially rupturing membranes.

amplitude: The sound made by the pulse; a reflection of pulse strength and the elasticity of the arterial wall.

anaemia: A lower than normal concentration of haemoglobin in the blood due to a decrease in red blood cells. Anaemia results in decreased oxygen levels in peripheral tissue.

anaphylaxis: An extreme sensitivity to an antigen, leading to the secretion of histamine and adverse reactions that can sometimes be fatal.

Apgar score: Systematic five-step assessment of the physical condition of a newborn baby. The baby is assessed at 1, 5 and 10 minutes after birth; the score measures breathing, heart rate, colour, tone and reflex irritability.

apnoea: An absence of respiration for a period of 20 seconds or longer.

arrhythmia: A condition in which the heart beats with an irregular or abnormal rhythm.

arterial blood pressure: The pressure exerted on the arterial walls to facilitate blood flow around the body to ensure adequate oxygenation of the tissues and vital organs.

arterial sample: Sample of blood taken from an umbilical cord artery.

artificial rupture of membranes (ARM): Rupture of the amniotic sac using either an amnihook or an amnicot for the purpose of expediting labour.

asepsis: Being free of pathological organisms and the process of destroying or removing organisms to prevent transmission of infection.

aseptic non-touch technique (ANTT): The framework for aseptic practice. ANTT provides a sequential, logical standardised and auditable approach to asepsis management.

assessing uterine activity: Assessment of the length, strength and frequency of uterine contractions.

assisted birth: Birth assisted by medical instruments, either forceps or vacuum extraction equipment.

auscultation: The action of listening to sounds inside the body. In midwifery, auscultation of the fetal heart refers to listening to the fetal heart rate and rhythm.

automated external defibrillator (AED): Portable electronic device that diagnoses common life-threatening cardiac arrhythmias, and is able to treat them through the application of electrical charges that may correct the arrhythmia.

bacteraemia: The presence of bacteria in the blood.

Barlow's test: One aspect of the physical examination performed on infants to screen for developmental dysplasia of the hips (DDH).

baseline rate: Abbreviated term for baseline fetal heart rate (FHR), which is the mean level of the FHR when this is stable, excluding accelerations and decelerations. It is determined over a time period of 5–10 minutes and expressed as beats per minute (bpm).

baseline variability: Minor fluctuations in baseline rate. It is assessed by estimating the difference in fetal heart rate beats per minute between the highest peak and lowest trough of fluctuation in 1-minute segments of cardiotocograph trace.

bilirubinuria: The presence of bilirubin in the urine.

Bishop's score: A score used to determine how favourable the cervix is for birth. Five cervical features are rated: dilation, length of cervix, station, consistency and position.

blood transfusion: The administration of blood products intravenously into the circulation.

body temperature: The temperature of the body which reflects the balance between heat gain and heat loss.

brachial pulse: The pulse in the brachial artery at the anterior (inner) aspect of the elbow.

bradycardia: Heart rate below normal.

bradypnoea: A decreased respiratory rate of less than 10 breaths per minute; may be a sign of impending respiratory arrest.

Braxton Hicks: Uterine tightenings that occur without dilation and effacement of the cervix.

buccal: A potential space or cavity in each cheek, adjacent to the gum beneath the molars, into which oral medication may be administered.

caesarean section (CS): Abdominal surgical procedure used to retrieve a baby that is unable to be born vaginally.

caput succedaneum: A serosanguinous, subcutaneous, extraperiosteal swelling that occurs to a baby's head as a result of sustained pressure on it from the maternal cervix, maternal vaginal walls or the application of instruments applied to the fetal head to assist birth.

cardiopulmonary resuscitation (CPR): Technique combining chest compressions and breathing support performed to try and save a life where the heart is not beating and/or breathing is ineffective.

cardiotocograph (CTC): A machine using ultrasound technology for continuous monitoring of the fetal heart rate over a specific period of time, which can be recorded.

carotid pulse: The pulse in the carotid artery at the side of the trachea.

cell salvage: The intraoperative or postoperative collection of a person's own red blood cells, which can be reinfused into the person in order to avoid exposure to blood components from another person.

central venous access device (CVAD): A device with a single or multiple lumen that allows for long-term venous access for multiple infusions of fluids, blood products, medications and/or parenteral nutrition. The CVAD catheter generally terminates near the heart or one of the great vessels.

chorioamnionitis: Inflammation of the fetal membranes (chorion and amnion), generally the result of a bacterial or viral infection of the amniotic fluid.

closed system of infusion: A system of fluid infusion that does not require external venting. Fluid remains in a closed infusion system and is protected from airborne contamination.

closed vacuum system: Enables blood to be collected via a double needle, attached to a plastic holder, so the blood can go directly into a vacuumed specimen tube.

combined spinal–epidural (CSE) analgesia: The combination of a single spinal bolus injection with an epidural catheter, which can be used for ongoing pain relief.

complementary and alternative medicine (CAM): Therapies that complement conventional medical treatment, but are often considered outside conventional medical treatment.

contact precautions: Procedures to reduce the risk of spread of infection through direct or indirect contact. In addition to standard precautions, a gown and gloves are applied to enter or leave the room.

continuous non-locked suture: Wound closure technique in which continuous suturing begins at the apex of a perineal tear or episiotomy and a knot is not tied until the wound is completely closed.

continuous positive airway pressure (CPAP): Delivery of air through a pump (CPAP machine) via a mask over the airways at pressures high enough to assist or stimulate normal breathing.

controlled cord traction (CTT): Maintenance of manual traction on the umbilical cord to encourage the placenta to separate from the uterine wall after birth.

cord blood gases: Measurements of key gases present in cord blood taken immediately after the birth of a baby.

cotyledons: The discrete small sections of the placenta that make up its whole.

cup feeding: Provision of milk feeds to a baby by a small cup.

Cusco speculum: A self-retaining vaginal speculum with two short, hinged blades which are curved across the width of the blades. Used for examination and procedures within the vagina. The blades are adjusted using a lateral screw.

delayed cord clamping (DCC): Clamping of the umbilical cord after a period of time following birth, during which the cord is allowed to stop pulsing spontaneously and its contents allowed to drain into the baby.

developmental dysplasia of the hips (DDH): A problem with the way a baby's hip joint forms before, during or after birth and which causes instability in that joint.

diarrhoea: Frequent defecation of liquid faeces caused by increased motility of the intestines. Can be due to infection or stress.

diastolic blood pressure (DBP): The pressure exerted on the blood vessel walls during ventricular diastole when the arteries contain the least amount of blood, resulting in the least pressure being exerted on the blood vessel walls.

droplet precautions: In addition to standard precautions, a surgical mask is worn when entering or leaving a room. This is to prevent the spread of droplets during coughing, sneezing and talking.

dyspnoea: Denotes difficulty with breathing; use of accessory muscles of respiration may be observed.

dysuria: Difficult or painful micturition.

electronic medication management (EMM): A system enabling electronic prescribing, supply and administration of medicines. EMM covers the entire medication cycle with the aim of reducing medication errors and improving efficiency.

engagement: When the widest part of the baby's presenting part (usually the head) enters the pelvic brim or inlet.

epidural analgesia/anaesthesia: Administration of medications (generally a local anaesthetic combined with an opioid) through a small catheter into the epidural space to provide pain relief during labour.

episiotomy: A deliberate incision made in the perineum. In labour it is performed most often to facilitate birth where fetal descent is arrested at the perineum, or instrumental assistance is used.

eupnoea: Normal breathing at rest.

extravasation: Escape of fluid from the vessels into the surrounding tissues.

faecal incontinence: The inability to control the passage of flatus or faeces from the anus. The most common cause is childbirth injury to the anal sphincter nerves or muscles.

feeding cues: Signs made by a baby to indicate they are hungry.

femoral pulse: The pulse in the femoral artery in the groin.

Ferguson reflex: Also known as the fetal ejection reflex. The neuroendocrine reflex that occurs when the pressure of the presenting part on the cervix or vaginal walls triggers uterine contractions that assist fetal expulsion.

fetal blood sampling (FBS): The collection of blood for analysis from the fetal scalp during labour.

fetal compromise: When the fetus is compromised by insufficient oxygenation or nutrition.

fetal scalp electrode (FSE): Fetal heart rate sensor which is attached to the fetal scalp using a spiral self-retaining needle.

finger feeding: Provision of siphoned milk feeds to a baby via a fine tube placed along one of the caregiver's fingers.

four Ts: Tone (uterine atony), trauma (Lacerations), tissue (retained placenta or clots) and thrombin (preexisting or acquired coagulopathy): four words that identify the main underlying causes of postpartum haemorrhage.

fundal height: The result of symphysis–fundal height measurement.

fundal palpation: Examination by touch of the top of the uterus to assess whether fetal size is consistent with gestational age.

Galeazzi test: Used to test for developmental dysplasia of the hip. It is performed by flexing an infant's knees when they are lying down so that the feet touch the surface and the ankles touch the buttocks. If the knees are not level then the test is positive, indicating a potential congenital hip malformation. Also known as the Allis sign.

Glasgow Coma Scale (GCS): A tool for assessing the level of consciousness and a measure of brain function. The GCS is divided into three categories: eye opening (4 points), best verbal response (5 points) and best motor response (6 points). The three scores are totalled to score between 15 (fully conscious) and 3 (no response). The score should be recorded as a fraction using 15 as the denominator (e.g. 10/15).

glomerular filtration rate (GFR): The amount of blood passing through the glomeruli of the kidney (measured in millilitres per minute). The GFR is used to determine how well the kidneys are functioning.

glycosuria: The presence of glucose in the urine.

Graves speculum: A bivalve vaginal speculum with wide, curved, arched blades and a shorter anterior blade. Generally used for women who have been sexually active.

haematuria: The presence of blood in the urine.

haemoconcentration: An increase in the proportion of red blood cells relative to plasma. This occurs because of a decrease in the volume of plasma or an increase in the concentration of circulating red blood cells.

haemorrhoids: Varicosities of the rectal vein resulting from enlargement of the venous plexuses. They can occur from chronic repetitive straining to defaecate or the weight of the gravid uterus.

handheld Doppler device: A small, handheld, battery-operated device that uses ultrasound technology to provide audible fetal heart sounds.

hands on: The accoucheur places one hand on the presenting part once it is on view to maintain its flexion and control its emergence, and one hand on the maternal perineum to try and prevent tearing.

hands poised: The accoucheur has their hands closely adjacent to the emerging fetus once the presenting part is on view, ready to assist the birth if necessary.

hazard: Something that can cause harm.

healthcare-associated infections (HAIs): Infections occurring as a result of healthcare provision.

high vaginal swab (HVS): A swab collected high in the vagina, generally from the posterior fornix.

hyperglycaemia: An abnormally high concentration of glucose in the blood.

hypertonic: A fluid with a higher concentration of electrolytes than plasma. IV administration of a hypertonic solution will result in fluid moving from the extravascular spaces into the intravascular space.

hypotonic: A lower concentration of electrolytes than plasma, which will result in fluid moving from the intravascular to the extravascular space.

hypoxic ischaemic encephalopathy (HIE): A type of brain damage that occurs when an infant's brain doesn't receive enough oxygen and blood.

infiltration: The movement of a cannula from inside a vessel into the surrounding tissue. Usually involving inadvertent administration of parenteral fluid into the tissue surrounding a vein.

initial birth examination: The initial post-birth assessment to exclude obvious abnormalities.

intermittent positive airway pressure (IPPV): The process of manually or mechanically ventilating a person, usually via a mask over the airways, who is unable to breathe effectively on their own.

interprofessional care: Care provided by a team comprising members of different healthcare professions.

intradermal (ID) injection/ intradermally: An injection into the dermis, the area just below the epidermis.

intramuscular (IM) injection: An injection into a muscle.

intravascular access: Access into a blood vessel or the blood vascular system.

iron infusion: The administration of an iron-containing solution intravenously into the circulation.

isotonic: A solution with equal concentration of electrolytes and with the same composition as plasma, so the solution will be equally distributed between intracellular and extracellular fluid.

ketonuria: The presence of ketone bodies in the urine, occurring as a result of increased metabolism of fats.

key parts: The sterile parts of equipment used for procedures that, if contaminated, are likely to cause infection (e.g. bungs, needle hubs, syringe tips, dressing packs).

key sites: Any portal of entry on the body that could be infected, including where medical devices access the body (e.g. insertion or puncture sites) and open wounds.

Klisic's sign: One aspect of the physical examination performed on infants to screen for developmental dysplasia of the hips (DDH).

knight's position: A half-kneeling position used for lifting items, where one knee is on the floor beside the object to be lifted.

This position assists with stability when working at a low height.

lactocytes: Milk-producing cells in the breast.

latent phase (of first-stage labour): The period between the onset of regular painful uterine contractions and the cervix being fully effaced and 4 cm dilated.

lateral palpation: Examination by touch of the pregnant abdomen to determine fetal position/lie using two hands.

lithotomy: Position wherein a person is lain recumbent and their legs are placed up in stirrups. In labour, it is used most commonly for instrument-assisted births and for suturing the maternal perineum.

low vaginal swab (LVS): A swab connected low in the vagina, usually 2–3 cm within the vagina.

Luer lock: A fitting, usually part of or attached to intravenous devices, that enables a needleless connection to another piece of medical apparatus.

massive postpartum haemorrhage: Puerperal blood loss greater than or equal to 2000 mL or blood loss that is life-threatening. See also **postpartum haemorrhage** and **severe postpartum haemorrhage**.

massive transfusion: Transfusion of five or more units of blood within a 4-hour period.

mean arterial pressure (MAP): The average pressure required to push the blood through the circulatory system. MAP remains relatively constant during normal pregnancy.

membrane sweeping: The use of a circular movement of the finger to separate the chorioamniotic membranes from the lower uterine segment during a vaginal examination. The fingers gently dilate (stretch) the cervical os, and then separate the membranes from the lower segment (sweep).

methicillin-resistant *Staphylococcus aureus* (MRSA): Strains of *Staphylococcus aureus* that are resistant to methicillin and other closely related antibiotics.

micturition: Urine is discharged from the bladder in the act of passing urine.

Modified Early Obstetric Warning System (MEOWS): A specialised early warning system modified for use with pregnant or postpartum women that aims to improve the recognition, response and management of clinical deterioration. If vital signs are outside the normal parameters, an escalation pathway is triggered which includes repeating/increasing observations, consultation with charge midwife, clinical review or activation of a rapid emergency response.

multidrug-resistant organisms (MROs): Also known as **multiple antibiotic-resistant organisms** and **multi-resistant organisms**. These organisms are resistant to one or more antimicrobial drugs, to which they are normally susceptible.

nasal swab: Sample of secretions collected from the back of the nose that is then analysed for the presence of pathogens. Instructions for collection are detailed in hospital or health service clinical guidelines.

national inpatient medication chart (NIMC): A national standard medication chart available on paper and electronically. The chart utilises best available evidence to communicate medication information consistently.

neurological assessment: May be undertaken when there are concerns about actual or possible alterations in a woman's level of consciousness (e.g. post-seizure, magnesium sulfate toxicity, meningitis, head injury).

newborn bloodspot screening (NBS)/newborn screening test (NST): A blood test offered to all newborns between 48 to 72 hours of life, usually taken from a heel capillary sample, to detect increased risk of a treatable genetic condition. Conditions screened for include congenital hypothyroidism, cystic fibrosis and amino acid disorders such as phenylketonuria, organic acidemias and fatty acid oxidation defects.

nitrous oxide (N_2O): A colourless gas with a slightly sweet odour; also known as laughing gas. Inhaled nitrous oxide has analgesic properties and is a weak anaesthetic agent.

nocturia: Excessive urination at night.

nuchal cord: The umbilical cord is around the emerging fetal neck.

obstetric haemorrhage: Bleeding from the uterus, usually the placental site. Allows haemorrhage-related morbidity and mortality to be identified as obstetric or non-obstetric.

occipitoposterior: A cephalic presentation with the fetal occiput turned towards the sacrum.

operculum: The mucous plug that seals the cervix during pregnancy to protect the fetus and its environment from ascending infection. Loss of the operculum at the onset of labour is colloquially called 'having a show'.

oral/enteral syringe: Syringe used to administer food and medications via the human gastrointestinal tract. In Australia and New Zealand they are generally orange or purple in colour.

Ortolani's test: One aspect of the physical examination performed on infants to screen for developmental dysplasia of the hips (DDH).

Pap smear: Papanicolaou smear, a sample of vaginal or cervical cells obtained for cytological study. In Australia this has been replaced by the cervical screening test, which screens for human papilloma virus infection. The new test can identify women who may be at risk of cancer of the cervix at an earlier stage.

parenteral route: Medications not administered by the enteral route are considered parenteral and include intramuscular, subcutaneous and intravenous medication administration.

passive phase (of second-stage labour): The period during which, after the cervix is fully effaced and dilated, the fetus descends through the maternal pelvis by the force of uterine contractions.

patient-controlled analgesia (PCA)/patient-controlled epidural anaesthesia (PCEA): Self-administered analgesia delivered using a programmable pump directly connected to a person's intravenous line. The pump delivers a pre-set, titrated dose of analgesic when a button is pressed.

Pederson speculum: A flat, narrow vaginal speculum, similar to the Graves speculum but with narrower blades, used for women with narrow vaginal canals.

pelvic palpation: Examination by touch, using either one or two hands, of the abdomen over the lower pole of the uterus to determine fetal presentation, whether the presenting part is engaged and the degree of flexion.

per vaginam (PV): Medicines administered via the vaginal route.

perineal tears, measured in degrees: Tears to the perineal area that are defined by degrees: **first-degree** involves the perineal skin and/or vaginal mucous membrane; **second-degree** involves the perineal skin, posterior vaginal wall and perineal muscles; **third-degree** involves the perineal skin, posterior vaginal wall, perineal muscles and the anal sphincter. Third-degree is further classified as **3a**—less than 50% of external anal sphincter thickness torn, **3b**—more than 50% of external anal sphincter thickness torn, **3c**—both the external and internal anal sphincter are torn; **fourth-degree** is the same as a third-degree with the addition of damage to the structures of the anal sphincter complex and the anal epithelium or rectal mucosa.

perineal trauma: Injury sustained to the perineum during the process of giving birth.

peripherally inserted intravenous cannula (PIVC)/peripheral intravenous catheter (PIVC)/ peripheral cannulae: A thin, flexible tube inserted into a peripheral vein (does not include a peripherally inserted central line).

personal protective equipment (PPE): Clothing or equipment designed to protect a person from injury, illness and the spread of infection.

pharmacodynamics: The action and effects of medicines in the body, their distribution in bodily tissues over time, and their breakdown and excretion.

pharmacogenetics: How the actions of drugs and reactions to drugs differ due to a person's genetic make-up. Pharmacogenetics considers why people respond to drug therapy in different ways.

pharmacokinetics: The way the body affects the drug (e.g. absorption, distribution, metabolism and excretion).

phlebitis: Inflammation of a vein.

Pinard stethoscope: A hollow, wooden, plastic or metal cone-shaped device used to amplify the fetal heart sounds so they can be heard by the listener.

placenta accreta: When the placenta is abnormally adherent to the uterine myometrium (uterine muscle layer) with partial or complete absence of the decidua basalis.

placenta percreta: Placenta accreta with the addition of invasion of the myometrium (uterine muscle layer) through to the peritoneal covering.

placenta praevia: Low implantation of the placenta, so that it partially or completely covers the cervical os.

positive end expiratory pressure (PEEP): The pressure in the lungs (alveolar pressure) above atmospheric pressure that exists at the end of expiration.

postdural puncture headache (PDPH): Inadvertent puncture of the dura mater during placement of an epidural, which results in an occipito-frontal headache. The proposed causes is cerebral spinal fluid (CSF) loss which decreases CSF pressure and/or distension of the cerebral blood vessels.

postpartum haemorrhage (PPH): Puerperal loss of 500 mL or more after vaginal birth and loss of 1000 mL or more after caesarean birth. See also **massive postpartum haemorrhage** and **severe postpartum haemorrhage**.

presenting part: The part of the fetus that is lowermost in the pelvis.

pressure injury: Localised damage to skin and/or underlying tissue that usually occurs as a result of pressure, sometimes in combination with shear and/or friction.

prostaglandins: Lipid hormones with a variety of effects; commonly used for cervical ripening and induction of labour.

proteinuria: The presence of protein in the urine.

pulse deficit: The difference between the heart rate and the palpable pulse (as often seen in atrial fibrillation).

pulse oximetry: A non-invasive method of monitoring arterial oxygen saturation (SpO_2), used in conjunction with respiration assessment.

pulse pressure: The difference between systolic and diastolic blood pressure (SBP and DBP); a normal SBP is around 40 mmHg higher than DBP.

pupillary assessment: The size and shape of each pupil and reaction to light are assessed by shining a bright light from a pen torch into each eye.

Quality Use of Medicines (QUM): One of the central objectives of Australia's National Medicines Policy which refers to: 1. selecting management options wisely; 2. choosing suitable medicines if a medicine is considered necessary; and 3. using medicines safely and effectively.

radial pulse: The pulse in the radial artery at the inner wrist.

rapid immunoassay tests: Fast chemical tests used to detect or quantify a substance or analyte in blood or body fluids using an immunological reaction (e.g. pregnancy test).

rectal route: Medications and fluids administered by insertion into the rectum which are absorbed by the rectal blood vessels and distributed via the circulatory system.

risk control: Actions taken in an attempt to eliminate health and safety risks.

second stage of labour: The period between the cervix being fully effaced and fully dilated and the birth of the baby.

self-care: The ability to maintain one's own health, minimise the development and impact of disease and cope with illness and disability.

severe postpartum haemorrhage: Puerperal blood loss of greater than or equal to 1000 mL. See also **massive postpartum haemorrhage** and **postpartum haemorrhage**.

skin integrity: The degree to which the skin is complete and healthy (undamaged).

skin swab: sample of flora or fluid collected from the skin's surface or a superficial wound that is then analysed for the presence of pathogens. Instructions for collection are detailed in hospital or health service clinical guidelines.

small for gestational age (SGA): The fetus weighs less and has smaller key measurements (e.g. skull, femur length and/or abdominal circumference) than is normal for their gestational age.

somersault manoeuvre: Manoeuvre employed to facilitate birth without clamping and cutting the cord when the nuchal cord is tight around the emerging fetus's neck.

sphygmomanometer: A device used to measure blood pressure that works by exerting a measured pressure on an artery.

spinal anaesthesia/analgesia: A single bolus of medication administered into the subarachnoid space.

squat position: Both knees are bent and the body is in a crouching position.

standard aseptic non-touch technique (ANTT): Used for short and technically simple procedures involving few and relatively small key parts and key sites. Generally uses a small general aseptic field and relies more heavily on a non-touch technique, and can involve non-sterile gloves; clean but not necessarily sterile equipment may be placed onto it.

standard precautions: Healthcare practices applied to everyone, regardless of their diagnosis or infection status; used to prevent or reduce the likelihood of the transmission of infection from one person or place to another and to keep the environment free from possible infectious agents.

stress incontinence: As a result of reduced control of the internal and external sphincter, involuntary voiding of small amounts of urine occurs when the intra-abdominal pressure increases (e.g. during bouts of coughing, laughing or sneezing).

subamniotic swab: A swab taken between the amnion and chorion on the fetal surface of the placenta.

subchorionic swab: A swab taken from underneath the chorion on the fetal surface of the placenta.

subcutaneous (SC) injection: An injection administered into the connective tissue and fat beneath the skin.

subcuticular suture: Stitches made just below the skin surface to secure apposition of the edges of a surgical or traumatic wound.

sublingual artery: A branch of the carotid artery which runs below the sublingual pocket of the mouth.

sublingual pockets: Under the tongue; an area under the tongue where medication is placed to dissolve slowly.

surgical aseptic non-touch technique (ANTT): Used in operating theatres and consists of a surgical hand scrub, full protective gown and sterile gloves; it uses a critical aseptic field managed as a key part, so only sterilised equipment and items can come into contact with it.

symphysis–fundal height (SFH): The distance between the symphysis pubis and the top of the fundus.

systolic blood pressure (SBP): The pressure exerted on the blood vessel walls following ventricular systole when the arteries contain the most blood and is the time of maximal pressure.

tachycardia: Heart rate above normal.

tachypnoea: An increased respiratory rate above 20 breaths per minute.

temporal artery: An artery that is approximately 1 mm beneath the skin of the forehead.

third stage of labour: The time period following birth of the neonate until completed birth of the placenta, which involves separation and expulsion of the placenta and membranes.

throat swab: sample of secretions collected from the back of the throat that is then analysed for the presence of pathogens. Instructions for collection are detailed in hospital or health service clinical guidelines.

thrombus: A fibrinous blood clot formed in a blood vessel, which may cause vascular obstruction.

top-to-toe physical examination (of the newborn): Systematic examination of the newborn from head to toe to assess for obvious physiological abnormalities.

tourniquet: A device used to compress an artery or a vein, applied when obtaining a blood sample or to insert an IV cannula.

transcutaneous electrical nerve stimulation (TENS): A device used to transmit biphasic pulsed electrical impulses in a repetitive manner to relieve pain during labour by stimulating the sensory nerve pathways to reduce pain-related activities within the nervous system.

transmission-based precautions: A strategy used to minimise the transmission of healthcare-associated infections; used in addition to standard precautions when the presence of infectious agents is suspected or confirmed and the risk of transmission is increased and standard precautions may not prevent transmission of infection.

urinalysis: The diagnostic, physical, chemical and microscopic examination of a urine sample.

urinary frequency: Increased need to micturate, often voiding small amounts of urine.

urinary retention: The inability of the bladder to empty, resulting in an accumulation of urine in the bladder.

urinary tract infection (UTI): Invasion and multiplication of microorganisms within the urinary tract, resulting in infection. A UTI is named for the part of the tract infected (e.g. urethritis, cystitis, ureteritis, pyelonephritis and glomerulonephritis).

urobilinogen: A colourless compound formed in the intestines as a byproduct of bilirubin reduction. Urobilinogen in the urine indicates excessive bilirubin in the blood.

uterine atony: The uterus does not contract adequately following birth.

uterotonic drugs: Uterine stimulants which act on the uterus to induce or increase contractions or to increase uterine tone.

vacuum extraction: A method used in the second stage of labour to facilitate the birth of a baby; involves the use of suction via a cup applied to the fetal head.

vaginal examination (VE): Digital examination of the female genital tract. In pregnancy and labour it is used to assess the cervix (e.g. effacement, dilation, oedema) and to: determine what part of the fetus is presenting; to determine the position, lie and attitude of the fetus in relation to the maternal pelvis; and to check the position of the umbilical cord once the membranes have ruptured.

vaginal speculum: A double- or single-bladed vaginal speculum with a groove in the centre, used for examining the vagina and cervix. Does not have opposing blades or an opening mechanism. This was previously known as Sims speculum; a petition to change the name to Lacks speculum is in progress.

Valsalva manoeuvre: Also known as **sustained closed glottis pushing** or directed pushing, this is not recommended in physiological labour. Women in the active phase of the second stage of the labour may be directed to use this manoeuvre to expedite expulsion of the fetus in an emergent situation. The woman is directed to take a deep breath, hold the breath (closed glottis) and push downwards when each uterine contraction starts.

vancomycin-resistant enterococci (VRE): Enterococci (*Enterococcus species*) of bacteria that are resistant to vancomycin, an antibiotic frequently used to treat enterococci infections.

vascular access device: A device inserted into a vein to enable access for diagnostic or therapeutic reasons such as administration of fluids, blood products and medications.

venepuncture: The puncture of a vein with a hollow needle as part of a medical procedure, usually to withdraw a blood sample or for an intravenous injection.

venous blood pressure: The pressure exerted on the walls of the veins, reflecting venous flow to the heart (particularly circulating blood volume) and cardiac function.

workplace health and safety (WHS): Involves the assessment and mitigation of risks that could impact on the health, safety and/or welfare of workers and other people in the workplace including clients.

Z-track technique: A type of intramuscular injection used to prevent leakage of medication into subcutaneous tissue. The skin and subcutaneous tissue are displaced sideways or downwards and held taut prior to the injection and then released to create a zigzag path.

Zika virus: A flavivirus primarily transmitted by Aedes mosquitoes. Zika virus is linked to fetal microcephaly and Guillain-Barré syndrome.

INDEX

Page numbers followed by '*f*' indicate figures those followed by '*t*' indicate tables and '*b*' indicate boxes.

O